Simple
Abundance

ALSO BY SARAH BAN BREATHNACH

Simple Abundance

365 Days to a Balanced and Joyful Life

Sarah Ban Breathnach

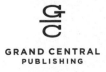

GRAND CENTRAL
PUBLISHING

NEW YORK   BOSTON

Grand Central Publishing
Hachette Book Group
1290 Avenue of the Americas, New York, NY 10104
grandcentralpublishing.com
twitter.com/grandcentralpub

The first edition of this book was published in November 1995.

This Revised Edition: November 2019

Grand Central Publishing is a division of Hachette Book Group, Inc. The Grand Central Publishing name and logo is a trademark of Hachette Book Group, Inc.

The publisher is not responsible for websites (or their content) that are not owned by the publisher.

The Hachette Speakers Bureau provides a wide range of authors for speaking events. To find out more, go to www.hachettespeakersbureau.com or call (866) 376-6591.

LCCN: 2019944327

ISBNs: 978-1-5387-3173-4 (hardcover), 978-1-5387-3502-2 (large print), 978-1-5387-3174-1 (ebook)

Printed in the United States of America

LSC-C

10 9 8 7 6 5 4 3 2 1

Her eye, her ear, were tuning forks, burning glasses, which caught the minutest refraction or echo of a thought or feeling... She heard a deeper vibration, a kind of composite echo, of all that the writer said, and did not say.

—Willa Cather (1873–1947)

For
Chris Tomasino
With dearest love and deepest gratitude
and
Kate
Who is the Deeper Vibration
Always

One moved Heaven for this book,
The other moved Earth.

Gloriana/Alleluia

In a time lacking in truth and certainty and filled with anguish and despair, no woman should be shamefaced in attempting to give back to the world, through her work, a portion of its lost heart.

—Louise Bogan (1897–1970)
America's first woman Poet Laureate

Upon Reading This Book

Preface to the
25th Anniversary Edition of

Simple Abundance

365 Days to a Balanced and
Joyful Life

*For centuries women have been saying many of the things we are
saying today and which we have often thought of as new.*
—Dale Spender
Australian scholar

Dearest Reader,

Welcome. If you're a new acquaintance, I hope that by the end of our
year together you'll think of me as a good friend. And if you're a cherished companion, welcome back. How wonderful to be in your dear
company again! However, no matter the depth of our affinity, I think
that you're in for as much of a treat reading this book as I've had in living and writing it. In fact, this new, updated *Simple Abundance* is the
happiest writing I've ever done.

It's hard to imagine that twenty-five years have passed since *Simple
Abundance* was originally published in 1995. In daily essays, I shared
the revelations that came while trying to reconcile my deepest spiritual
and creative longings with often overwhelming commitments to family
and work. I had long suspected that I wasn't alone in my frustrations and
desires, but nothing could have prepared me for the way women around
the world—millions of you—responded. We began an exciting adventure
together, which is a continuing source of gratitude, grace, and fulfillment
for me. I hope it is for you as well.

First, the Backstory

Story is a sacred visualization. A way of echoing experience.
—Terry Tempest Williams
American author, activist, and conservationist

By far, the most frequent questions I'm asked when I speak or meet with readers pertain to the backstory of *Simple Abundance*. How and why did I write it? How did I manage to express on the page what so many women were thinking? Or the question that everybody wants to know: How did I get on *Oprah*?

Over the years I've learned that the most fascinating part of any book, film, or person is their "backstory," the tale hidden in between the lines. When I glance back at my own, what amazes me the most is how the mystical links in the chain of chance that brought this book into the world, my heart, and your hands came as a result of all my "Unanswered Prayers." This mystery makes me smile in grateful puzzlement, for I have no explanation as to why the tears we shed over our failures prepare our souls for the growth we'll need for our future successes.

Simple Abundance was my third book. I had previously written two books on Victorian family life, and I was about to begin writing the next on Victorian decorative details. However, the thought of ruminating on ruffles and flourishes for a year brought dread to my heart. What I wanted to read was a book that would show me how to reconcile my deepest spiritual, authentic, and creative longings with often overwhelming and conflicting commitments—to my daughter, my marriage, invalid mother, work at home, work in the world, siblings, friends, and community. I knew I wasn't the only woman hurtling through real life as if it were an out-of-body experience. I knew I wasn't the only woman frazzled, depressed, worn to a raveling. But I also knew I certainly wasn't the woman with the answers. I didn't even know the questions.

I could find no such book. The author Toni Morrison, who won the Nobel Prize for Literature in 1993, observed, "If there is a book you really want to read, but it hasn't been written yet, then you must write it." I took her advice to heart.

I wanted so much—money, success, recognition, genuine creative expression—but had absolutely no clue as to what I truly needed. At times my passionate hungers were so voracious I could only deal with them through denial. I was a workaholic, careaholic, and perfectionist. I couldn't remember the last time I'd been kind to myself. Was I ever? More often than it feels comfortable to admit, I was an angry, envious woman, constantly comparing myself to others only to become resentful because of what seemed to be missing from my life, although I couldn't have told you what that was.

Money was an enormous, emotionally charged issue that controlled my ability to be happy because I let it; money was the only way I could measure my success and self-worth. If I couldn't write a check on my accomplishments, they didn't exist. Frustrated and unable to fathom why some women appeared to lead much more fulfilling lives—even though I was conscientiously connecting all the dots—I careened between feeling that I was frittering my life away to feeling that I was sacrificing it on the altar of my own ambition.

I was a woman in desperate need of *Simple Abundance*.

And why did my life need to change? Like fifty million other working mothers, my daily round had become a tug-of-war between other people's demands and expectations and my own genuinely conflicted desires and unrequited needs. I frantically multitasked from one obligation to the next so fast that my spirit felt as if it was constantly sprinting to catch up with me, which it finally did when I collapsed into bed. Mornings were a major source of dread; my first conscious breath was a sigh; my awakening thought was how to make it through the day. Of course, I never complained to anyone else, but I whined to myself and God until, literally, the sound of my own nagging nearly drove me mad.

One morning I woke up physically exhausted and spiritually bankrupt; money was tight, too. I'd lost two lucrative consulting jobs, and the freelance market was shrinking fast because the only story in town was downsizing. I was so sick and tired of concentrating on what was missing from my life, Heaven knows I didn't want to write about it. I felt drained, depleted, discouraged. Worrying about money had squandered my most precious natural resources—time, creative energy, and emotion. So I felt the deep need to sit down at the kitchen table and start writing an inventory of what was *good* in my life, right at that moment. Think Pollyanna on Prozac. When I stopped six hours later, to my great astonishment I'd created a master list of my life's many overlooked blessings. I had more than 150, and none of them had anything to do with money! And then, what I call an everyday epiphany occurred: I realized I didn't need a single thing, except the awareness of how blessed I was. That was the first time that Gratitude beckoned and invited me to use its transformative power, not to revamp my life, but to rejoice in it. The thirteenth-century German mystic Meister Eckhart believed, "If the only prayer you ever say in your life is 'Thank You,' it will be enough." I discovered just how right he was and got so excited that I started writing down five new things to be thankful for every day.

However, before this book could be written, I had to take stock of what was working in my life and what wasn't. Perhaps for the first time, I had to be ruthlessly honest both inwardly and outwardly. During this time of profound introspection, six practical, creative, and spiritual Graces—Gratitude, Simplicity, Order, Harmony, Beauty, and Joy—became the catalysts that helped me define a life of my own. One morning I awoke to the realization that, almost imperceptibly, I'd become a happy woman, experiencing more moments of contentment than distress. Feeling confident again, I proposed writing a downshifting lifestyle book for women who want, as I did then and still do, to live by their own lights.

But the book you're reading bears absolutely no resemblance to the book I began. While I wrote for nearly five years, *Simple Abundance* underwent an extraordinary metamorphosis, as did I. On the page every morning, spirituality, authenticity, and creativity converged into an intimate search for Wholeness. I began writing about eliminating clutter and ended up on a safari of the self and Spirit. No one is more astonished by this than I am.

As *Simple Abundance* evolved from creating a manageable lifestyle into living in a state of grace, I began to barely recognize the woman I once was. *Simple Abundance* has enabled me to encounter everyday epiphanies, find the Sacred in the ordinary, the Mystical in the mundane, and fully enter the sacrament of the present moment. I even laugh more than before, especially at myself.

I've made the unexpected but thrilling discovery that everything in my life is significant enough to be a continuous source of reflection, revelation, reconnection: bad hair, mood swings, car pools, excruciating deadlines, overdrawn bank accounts, dirty floors, grocery shopping, exhaustion, illness, nothing to wear, unexpected company, even losing the final twenty-five pounds. *Simple Abundance* has given me the transcendent awareness that an authentic life is the most personal form of worship. Everyday life has become my prayer.

However, bringing *Simple Abundance* into the world was the biggest challenge of my life. Even though I had been a published journalist for two decades, a nationally syndicated columnist, and the author of two previous books, finding a publisher willing to back me was a demoralizing and difficult battle. Over a two-year period, the proposal was turned down thirty times; eventually, to soften the blow, my agent, Chris Tomasino, would break the news to me a few painful letters at a time. The reasoning behind the rejection? Simplicity wasn't commercial, and a lifestyle book based on gratitude? Forget it.

Twenty-five years, seven million copies, and thirty languages later suggest a different story.

In preparation for this new preface, I went back to my publishing memorabilia files to trace how the miracle came about. Some of the rejection letters are still so difficult to read they make me wince. It's no wonder I cried myself to sleep more nights than anybody can imagine. But the next morning, I'd say, "Let's give it one more shot" and I'd start another meditation. Eventually the thoughts, sentences, paragraphs, and pages began to accumulate, building a creative velocity of their own. Since the beginning I've always felt that *Simple Abundance* was a collaborative project between the Great Creator and me, because the title came to me in flashing neon-colored lights. I pay attention when this happens. My job, as I saw it, was to show up every day and write. The delivery details of finding the right publisher were up to Heaven and Chris.

But I won't kid you, it's very difficult to remain optimistic when the world keeps turning you down, so to keep up my spirits I created a publishing mood board to hang over my desk. One afternoon in 1993, two years before *Simple Abundance* was published, I took a *New York Times* best-seller list, whited out the number one title, and typed in *Simple Abundance* instead and changed the date to June 1996. I pasted it up at the top of my computer screen. I also hung up a beautiful card of a painting by Robert Spear Dunning called a "Harvest of Cherries" painted in 1866, which showed a man's straw hat and a woman's straw bonnet on the grass next to a Shaker basket overflowing with cherries. Here was the perfect depiction of "All you have is all you need." And so there I was, working every day with my future gazing fondly at me. I had to learn to trust that Heaven and the "Book" knew more than I did.

Originally, I conceived *Simple Abundance* as a beautiful full-color lifestyle book, which was quite the trend in the early 1990s; but to no avail. Just as we passed the two-year and thirty-rejection high-water mark, Liv Blumer at Warner Books asked Chris if I would be willing to turn *Simple Abundance* into a daily inspirational book. I thought this was preposterous; how could I give any woman inspiration, when I was so desperately seeking it myself? Chris asked me to sleep on it.

The next morning, I took the existing manuscript and rearranged the text into daily essays. I was stunned by the power of the small and the reassuring nature of having just one story to read and ponder throughout the day. And then I heard that soft and compassionate Voice that I've come to know as Spirit ask, "Can we get to work now?" We did, but it would take another two years to complete. Obviously, I had a lot of things I wanted to talk over with you.

When *Simple Abundance* was finally published in November 1995, my publisher told me it was a "woman's book." That it would be a "slow burn" and depend on women's "word of mouth" recommendations to each other. Actually, "a woman's book," "slow burn," and "word-of-mouth" are publishing euphemisms meaning "no publicity." And sure enough, there was none in those first few months other than through local bookstores.

How heartbreaking and upsetting this was—five years of work, struggle, sweat, and tears and no publicity? *Simple Abundance* was going to just slip through the cracks and disappear? I couldn't let that happen. I had nowhere to go for help except down on my knees. The next day Heaven whispered in my ear: "Send thirty books to *The Oprah Winfrey Show* for every woman on her staff. Let's see if we can't get women talking."

Now this was a very unusual way to publicize books and it was before Oprah began her famous book club, which got women reading and talking about books in a new and exciting way. My publisher's publicity department had already submitted one copy of the book to Oprah's producers, so they were understandably nervous about my suggestion being seen as serious overkill.

In the meantime, it was the holiday season and good friends were generously giving private book parties for me and inviting their friends and friends of their friends. The response was enthusiastic.

I took a booth at the Washington Waldorf School holiday bazaar, which is always packed. People circle the date a year in advance because it is the best holiday bazaar you'll ever go to. I sold a hundred books in a couple of hours, autographing them all. That's when I noticed something unusual. Women were buying multiple copies. They bought it for their sisters, best friends, daughters, daughters-in-law, mothers, mothers-in-law, nieces, cousins, neighbors, bosses, and secretaries. Women who had bought books at the parties later tracked me down to buy some more! It was a wonderful surprise that brought on a very giddy feeling.

But I still couldn't get the idea of Oprah out of my mind. I made my case yet again to the publicity department and offered to pay for the books but asked the publisher to please send them, so I didn't look like the desperate author I really was. I guess they'd heard the passion in my voice because they finally said yes, and graciously sent thirty copies of *Simple Abundance* as holiday gifts to the *Oprah Winfrey* staff. (And I didn't even have to pay for them!)

About a week later, publicity said that while the women all loved the book, the *Oprah* production team claimed it really didn't work as the basis for a show. To save face, I replied: "One day Oprah will pick up *Simple Abundance* and she'll read something that will speak to her, and then it will be a show."

January 1996 arrived, bringing with it blustery weather and, in my house, the heated topic of "When am I going to get a real job?" As I was dropping my daughter off at school after the holiday break, a woman waved at me excitedly and crossed the parking lot. She was breathless, she had so much she wanted to tell me. Putting her hands on my shoulders and looking me straight in the eyes, she began thanking me profusely for writing *Simple Abundance*. She told me that her mother-in-law was a pediatric heart surgeon, but she'd given it up because it was so difficult losing little ones no matter how much she tried.

"We gave her *Simple Abundance* for Christmas and guess what?

She's going back to work because now she recognizes her authentic gift and she's meant to be there." Both our eyes were filled with happy emotions and so much gratitude.

Right then, right there, I completely surrendered to Spirit my attachment to the outcome of *Simple Abundance*. I acknowledged and accepted that it had always been Heaven's book. I had been abundantly blessed to have been the author to write it, and I was very grateful for the opportunity. I just prayed that I might be able to find work using my authentic gifts.

I started receiving letters from readers all over the country thanking me for writing *SA* and saying that they no longer felt so alone.

The first week in February, *The Oprah Winfrey Show* called. Oprah had gone into her hair and makeup room and saw *Simple Abundance* on the counter and wondered, "What's this pink book I keep seeing everywhere?" Oprah opened it and read something that spoke to her, and I was invited to come to Chicago the following week. I asked if I could bring my thirteen-year-old daughter with me. It was the best bring-your-daughter-to-work experience ever!

We arrived in Chicago the afternoon before the taping of the show and took a short walk from our hotel to explore Michigan Avenue and our surroundings. We found the Terra Museum of American Art. It was almost closing time, so we quickly strolled through the museum. On the second floor I turned into an empty gallery. And what do you think I found? Robert Spear Dunning's "Harvest of Cherries." The painting of the postcard that I'd lovingly looked at every day while I wrote *Simple Abundance*. I still get shivers of delight remembering this full-circle moment and the spiritual confirmation that I had never been alone on the journey of unanswered prayers. Neither are you.

The Grace of Gratitude

Nothing is stronger than an idea whose time has come.
—Victor Hugo (1802–1885)
French poet, novelist, and dramatist

I don't know which passage of *Simple Abundance* spoke to Oprah, but I sense it had something to do with Gratitude, and no one spreads the gospel better than Oprah. She generously spoke about the life-changing effect of keeping a gratitude journal and devoted many shows to *Simple Abundance* and the *Simple Abundance Journal of Gratitude*. Before I knew it, "gratitude fever" had swept the country.

Just five years before, in 1991, when I'd begun experimenting with Gratitude as a spiritual catalyst for changing my life, I'd been disappointed at how little I could find written on the subject. The one exception was a slender meditation by the Benedictine brother David Steindl-Rast, titled *Gratefulness, The Heart of Prayer.* Certainly, there was no such thing as the gratitude journal. My answer was to create one, because daily gratitude was such a wonderful new practice for me.

Today when I type the word *gratitude* into search engines there are 154,000,000 books, websites, articles, newsletters, and research project links, and that number increases daily. One of my favorites is the weighty tome *The Psychology of Gratitude,* edited by Robert A. Emmons and Michael E. McCullough, which is the first compilation of the empirical, scientific research on gratitude conducted by prominent scientists documenting the positive effects gratitude has on our mind, body, and spirit.

I'm sharing this with you because if you're new to *Simple Abundance,* then whether you're aware of it or not, you've been hearing about it for years, whenever you encounter conversations about gratitude or gratitude journals. In fact, it's become so ubiquitous within the American conversation that it's almost the pop-cultural, psychobabble equivalent of elevator music.

I wanted to address and acknowledge this directly before you embark on the *Simple Abundance* path to your authenticity. You may think you know about the power of Gratitude, but until you experience the miracle of Gratitude personally, you can't. Throughout this revised version of the book, I have deliberately left the meditation sequence for your own discovery of the power of Gratitude as it was in the original *Simple Abundance.* You will come to these pages just as the women before you did. I want to reassure you that I consider your search for authenticity a sacred undertaking.

Which brings us to the "Authentic Self," another runaway offspring that has been used in so many ways over the last twenty years that it, too, has become its own cliché. But I promise you, if you can just mentally delete anything and everything connected to somebody else's version of the "Authentic Self," you'll have so much fun in discovering Her for yourself.

Truth or Dare

What would happen if one woman told the truth about her life?
The world would split open.
—Muriel Rukeyser (1913–1980)
American poet and political activist

When I was writing *Simple Abundance,* I was writing for only one reader: you. Every day for five years I was creating a private respite for the both of us from the stresses of the world and our own impossible pursuit of perfection. I was telling the truth about my life, and perhaps it mirrored your own. We are kindred spirits.

In many respects, *Simple Abundance* was the original woman's blog because its day-to-day format dealt with everything in our daily round. It also went viral. Women bought *Simple Abundance* to give to others for the holidays, birthdays, anniversaries, and graduations; in turn, they received it from family on Mother's Day, and from their friends when the marriage ended, the job was eliminated, or the diagnosis was devastating. When a phone call sent a woman reeling, dashing her dreams and shattering the life she took for granted, the "pink book" turned up as often as casseroles. Psychotherapists have told me they prescribed it; twelve-step program participants passed it on; abused women found it in a shelter's communal library. Women read it while waiting to receive chemotherapy then left it behind for the nurses who cared for them so tenderly. To celebrate, to commiserate, to comfort, to cheer, but above all, to communicate, women around the world—from Connecticut to Croatia to China—shared *Simple Abundance* with each other and blessed the life they found in between its lines: their own.

Why This Book, Why Now?

People have to learn sometimes not only how much the heart can take, but how much the head can bear.

—Maria Mitchell (1818–1889)
America's first female astronomer
and discoverer of Miss Mitchell's
Comet in 1847

As women, we've been separated into age groups from birth that no longer fit or serve us. What are our descriptive choices right now? Millennial, Generation X, Boomer? *Simple Abundance* readers defy these limiting categories. I wouldn't be writing this updated version today if it hadn't been for some new millennial readers who wrote to tell me how much they loved *SA*, but could I possibly update it for them? Michelle Obama, who in my heart is the poster woman for the Authentic Self, tells us: "If you don't get out there and define yourself, you'll be quickly and inaccurately defined by others."

So let's get to it by meeting in the middle. We are the glorious and stunning Mid-Century Moderns. But no matter what our age or attitude, our hearts and heads need a little homegrown comfort, balance, and joy for what ails us. And I think you'll discover it in between these covers. How about serenity, one sentence at a time? Today's rapidly changing, complex, and mostly alarming 24/7 "Breaking News" culture engulfs us at every turn, depleting our sense of security and diminishing our capacity for happiness, leaving us feeling exhausted and vulnerable. We're fraught, fragile, and frightened.

Most of us on any given day will admit that we hardly know whether we're coming, going, or where we've been; we feel constantly distracted—even in the company of those we love. We're often on the verge of tears "for no reason" and feel that there's no one we can talk to who will understand. More bewildering is that this continuous sensation of being anxious, overwhelmed, and emotionally overwrought has somehow become our culture's accepted "New Normal." Virtually every woman I know admits that she wakes up worn out and weary, on edge, and more likely to imagine difficulties ahead than ever before. But this behavior is *not* normal or healthy. And someone needs to say so.

I'll go first.

This is not normal.

We are living through extraordinary times, but they are not the New Normal, because there is nothing normal about what is unfolding every day. And the only way to safeguard ourselves and those we love is by realizing and acknowledging that technology must have its limits. How do we do this? The way women have always protected their own: by creating emotional and psychological safe havens that shelter what we hold sacred. That's why I'm back.

The last revision of *Simple Abundance* was done for its tenth anniversary in 2005. But fourteen years ago, technology had not expanded to its dominance over our lifestyle as it has today. Where technology once enhanced our lives, now we're often held hostage to it. Stanley Kubrick's 1968 science-fiction film *2001: A Space Odyssey* has become our prophetic living history. But instead of the sentient HAL floating in outer space, we've got Alexa to do our bidding at home and Siri giving us directions in the car. And we wonder why we don't have the patience to hear ourselves complete one thought?

I've approached the total revision with a reader in mind not of twenty-five years ago, but of today. I've freshened some meditations, revamped others, replaced many. The soul of *Simple Abundance* remains intact: All we have is all we need. All we need is the awareness of how much we've been blessed with every day. For those of you who already are treasured friends, there's plenty new to ponder. For our daughters, there are the gentle nudges that we needed at that age, and much encouragement to embark on their own safari of the self. But here's the magic: While I was rewriting this version, I was reunited with the girl I'd left behind, and I'm now on my *own* new safari. I hope that everyone who reads *Simple Abundance* will be so inspired.

At the end of every month, besides updated "Joyful Simplicities," there's a section called "Do Try This at Home." In it you'll find suggestions on how to prepare a "Caution Closet." This emergency closet will hold everything we might need if forced to evacuate our homes quickly. At the very least, you'll have enough supplies to help you make it through the next Snowmageddon, which seems to be occurring with increasing regularity these days.

The Divine Art

The divine art is the story.

—Isak Dinesen (1885–1962)
Pen name of Danish author Karen
Blixen-Finecke

Being an Irish writer, I trust the unseen more than the visible. I agree with the nineteenth-century writer Franz Kafka that writing is the most personal form of prayer. On every page, in between the lines are my thank-you notes to the Great Creator—in whom I move, write, live, love, find my being and my meaning.

Emily Dickinson believed Home was another name for God. Helen Keller described God as the "Light in my darkness, the Voice in my silence." The thirteenth-century mystic Julian of Norwich told her novitiates, "God is our clothing that wraps, clasps, and encloses us." Every time I slip into my beloved comfy robe at the end of a long, harrowing day, I know how right she was.

In the Hebrew tradition, so holy and hidden is the Almighty's identity that the proper name of God cannot be pronounced. But in English it is written as YHWH—four sacred letters representing the past, present, and future tense of the verb *to be*. God told Moses to call on the great "I AM," and when Moses did, the seas parted, and his people were fed daily while wandering in the wilderness for forty years. Many of them probably looked up to the sky calling God *Manna*, the name of the heavenly sustenance that kept them alive.

Every woman who believes in God calls the Holy One by a particular name; just as those who have no faith or experience one different from yours or mine will choose another word to describe God, such as the Cosmos or the One, or Good Orderly Direction. In my books, I often use the word *Spirit* for God because I do not want to impose on my readers my own view of Divinity, which is always expanding, thank Heavens. I feel inspired by my Irish ancestors' Celtic spirituality, which has many exquisite and descriptive names for Divinity, all of which honor the sacred in the ordinary: *Source of All Mystery, Piercer of Doubt, Kindler of Hope, Ever Present Provider, Compassionate Listener, Guardian of the Hearth, Holy Source,* and *Mother Plenty,* who is a constant source of guidance for me.

Here's a hint: If you come across a word beginning with a capital letter, I am trying to describe, however feebly, an aspect of Divinity that has comforted, sustained, and delighted me.

May reading *Simple Abundance* remain a comforting conversation with a good friend who's grateful that our paths have crossed. When I look down our unfolding path of everyday grace, I see delightful days ahead. Blessed are we among women, and how wonderful that, finally, we both know it.

Dearest love, boundless thanks,
blessings on your courage,

Sarah Ban Breathnach
May 2019

JANUARY

And now let us welcome the New Year
Full of things that have never been.

—Rainer Maria Rilke (1875–1926)
Twentieth-century German poet

January, the month of new beginnings and cherished memories, beckons. Come, let winter weave her wondrous spell: cold, crisp, woolen-muffler days, long, dark evenings of savory suppers, lively conversations, or solitary joys. Outside the temperature drops as the snow falls softly. All of nature is at peace. We should be, too. Draw hearthside. This is the month to dream, to look forward to the year ahead and the journey within.

JANUARY 1

A Transformative Year of Delight and Discovery

There are years that ask questions and years that answer.
—Zora Neale Hurston (1891–1960)
African-American writer and anthropologist

New Year's Day. A fresh start. A blank page. A new chapter in life waiting to be written. New questions to be asked, embraced, and loved. New answers to consider and then, new choices to make in this transformative year of delight and self-discovery.

Can you carve out a quiet interlude for yourself in which to dream? What are your hopes for the future? As you reflect on the years that have passed, don't concern yourself too much with what's gone before. Today you've been gifted with another chance. And is there anything more precious than that? Dame Good Fortune has traveled through time and space to sweep us off our feet with lush possibilities—a bounty of grace and favor. Let's make the most of it.

Each year we are presented four glorious seasons, twelve months of mystery, fifty-two weeks of wonder, and three hundred and sixty-five daily rounds, each one of them crowded with twenty-four measures of time—the gifts of dawn, matins, noon, dusk, twilight, and eventide. Hours and minutes. Moments and heartbeats. There will be surprises that trigger smiles as well as deep sighs, wisdom gleaned and eventually appreciated, landscapes larger than the ones we can see right now, beckoning. More blessings than we can count and carry in our saddlebag.

Only dreams give birth to change. Gradually, as you become curator of your own contentment, you will learn to listen to the gentle yearnings of your heart. But this New Year, instead of resolutions, write down your most private aspirations. Those longings you have kept tucked away until the time seems right. Trust that now is the time. Ask the questions. The *Simple Abundance* path brings confidence that the answers will come, and you will discover—day by day—how to live them.

JANUARY 2

Loving the Questions

You only live once—but if you work it right, once is enough.
—Joe E. Lewis (1902–1971)
American entertainer

How often in the past have you turned away from all that is unre-solved in your heart because you feared the questioning? But what if you *knew* that a year from today you could be living the most creative, joyous, and fulfilling life you could imagine? What would it be? What changes would you make? How and where would you begin? Do you see why the *questions* are so important?

"Be patient toward all that is unsolved in your heart and try to love the questions themselves," the twentieth-century Austrian-German poet Rainer Maria Rilke urges us. "Do not now seek the answers which cannot be given you because you would not be able to live them, and the point is to live everything. Live the questions now."

The answers to your questions will come, but only after you know which ones are worth asking. Pause and ponder. Read between the lines of your personal story up until now. Invite your questions. Become open to the changes the answers will inevitably bring. This may take some time, but time is the New Year's bountiful blessing. Believe in yourself. And believe that there is a loving Source—the Sower of Dreams—just waiting to help you make your dreams come true. A simply abundant year to be savored.

JANUARY 3

What Are You Doing for the Rest of Your Life?

May I have the courage today
To live the life that I would love,
To postpone my dream no longer
But do at last what I came here for
And waste my heart no more.

—John O'Donohue (1956–2008)
Irish poet, author, philosopher

Still, we hesitate. Is it because the gift of new beginnings comes wrapped in life's plain brown wrappers? Have we learned to temper our New Year's enthusiasm with steely resolve, and weariness? Or is it because we have learned that every beginning starts with an ending? Perhaps the ending you never expected has already occurred, and you are still grappling with new circumstances and challenging changes. You haven't a clue of how to begin again.

"Beginnings often frighten us because they seem like lonely voyages into the unknown. Yet, in truth no beginning is empty or isolated," the Celtic mystic, philosopher, and poet John O'Donohue reassures us in his profound book on the power of blessing, *To Bless the Space Between Us*. "We seem to think that beginning is setting out from a lonely point along some line of direction into the unknown. This is not the case. Shelter and energy come alive when a beginning is embraced. A beginning is ultimately an invitation to open toward the gifts and growth that are stored up for us. To refuse to begin can be an act of great self-neglect. There is nothing to fear in the act of beginning. More often than not it knows the journey ahead better than we ever could. Perhaps the art of harvesting the secret riches of our lives is best achieved when we place profound trust in the art of beginning."

So there seems to be only one question that needs to be answered. What are you doing for the rest of your life?

JANUARY 4

Things Come Suitable to Their Time

You don't think your way into a new kind of living. You live your way into a new kind of thinking.
—Henri J. M. Nouwen (1932–1996)
Dutch Catholic theologian and writer

When you close your eyes to imagine a different way of life, what does your day look like? Can you pull focus on just one scene? Or do you find your thoughts are scattered in a thousand different directions—a frustrating jumble? Can you conjure up any new happy images? This isn't a trick question, because I've had a bit of difficulty with this exercise recently myself, and if you have, too, there's a good reason. Sometimes just when we think we've gotten through whatever it was that we'll never get over (and we all have something), we find "it" everywhere, staring us down, daring us even to think about leaving the past where it belongs—in the rearview mirror.

Perhaps you were trying to organize a closet, so all the holiday decorations finally are in one place, and there's a battered brown box stuffed all the way in the back. You open it and it's full of memorabilia and photographs of all those happy times before they became ugly. In a split second your good mood is extinguished. Suddenly you're exhausted and disoriented. You feel as if you've been sucked back into an enormous bog of the unfair and the unresolved by a dangerous undertow.

You have. Me, too. Let's meet the two secret agents of self-sabotage, the Regret and Remorse twins. These twisted sisters are up to no good and they're determined not to let you move one inch without them. That's because they feed off our sad and dark emotions. They need for you to be down and out, disillusioned and depressed, so they'll distract you for as long as they can, however they can. For what you are doing this year is not just increasing the amount of light in your own life but increasing the light you bring to the world. And this scheming duo will attempt to quash it with a bushel basket of painful memories at the first glimmer of your happiness, healing, and hope.

So utterly discouraged, we leave all the mismatched holiday decorations strewn across the spare bedroom and perhaps we polish off the eggnog (can't let that go to waste) as well as any leftover holiday treats we can find. Or why not that bottle of wine we were saving for a special occasion? (I hear you: "And *when* is that going to *ever* happen?") And after we finally make it to the couch or bed, why don't you finally unfriend the old boyfriend on Facebook, especially now that he's married. (As I remember, you broke up with him.) So let's flick on the remote control, looking for some old movie or TV show to help our swollen eyes glaze over.

Maybe our distraction of choice is an online fashion flash sale, or home shopping network, never more persuasive than it is just before the sun comes up. If you stare long enough, you start to believe the attractive, energetic hosts who promise luxury, style, wrinkle-free skin, or a figure without a dimple of cellulite, which all can be yours for six easy-pay installments. Dream fixes for all the items you apparently need, right at this moment, to help you cope, look, live, and feel better—now that you've remembered your world has completely crashed and burned and, yes, you must start all over again.

"Aren't you, like me, hoping that some person, thing, or event will come along to give you that final feeling of inner well-being you desire? Don't you often hope: 'May this book, idea, course, trip, job, country or relationship fulfill my deepest desire,'" the brilliant Dutch Catholic theologian Henri J. M. Nouwen confides in his reassuring *Life of the Beloved: Spiritual Living in a Secular World*, explaining why finding the Sacred in the ordinary is such an unexpected and comforting revelation, sure to nourish souls and heal broken hearts.

"But as long as you are waiting for that mysterious moment you will go on running helter-skelter, always anxious and restless…never fully satisfied. You know that this is the compulsiveness that keeps us going and busy, but at the same time makes us wonder whether we are getting anywhere in the long run. This is the way to spiritual exhaustion and burn-out."

Discombobulated days and long dark nights come to all of us. However, when we can learn to be kind to ourselves in small, nurturing ways, believe it or not, we'll find unexpected rewards. Just save some peppermint bark for me.

JANUARY 5

Simple Abundance: The Inner Journey

simple, adj. 1: without embellishment; 2: clarity of form and thought; 3: fundamental

abundance, n. 1: an ample quantity, profusion; 2: wealth; 3: plentifulness

simple abundance, 1: an inner journey; 2: a spiritual and practical course in creative living; 3: a tapestry of contentment

Today I want you to become *aware* that you already possess all the inner wisdom, strength, and creativity needed to make your dreams come true. This is hard for most of us to realize because the source of this unlimited personal power is buried so deeply beneath the bills, the car pool, the deadlines, the business trip, and the dirty laundry that we have difficulty accessing it in our daily lives. When we can't access our inner resources, we come to the flawed conclusion that happiness and fulfillment come only from external events. That's because external events usually bring with them some sort of change. And so we've learned to rely on circumstances outside ourselves for forward or backward momentum as we hurtle through life. But we don't have to do that any longer. We can learn to be the catalysts for our own change.

At the heart of *Simple Abundance* is an authentic awakening, one that resonates within your soul; you already possess all you need to be genuinely happy. The way you reach that awareness is through an inner journey that brings about an emotional, psychological, and spiritual transformation. A seismic shift in your reality occurs, aligning you with the creative energy of the Universe. Such change is possible, when you invite Spirit to open the eyes of your awareness to the abundance that is already yours.

Simple Abundance is restoring passion, finding comfort, and discovering the Sacred in our ordinary. *Simple Abundance* is re-imagining the spirit, style, and substance of your daily round. *Simple Abundance* is considering what you need now to experience contentment; embracing what you want to do, want to have, want to be, or what you want to experience in your life, regardless of anyone else's opinion about what your choices are, because they are *your* choices.

Simple Abundance is recovering the part of yourself you might have abandoned long ago to be practical. Perhaps you've put other people's wants before your needs. We all have. Taking care of others before ourselves is a woman's default response.

Think of *Simple Abundance* as daily, strictly confidential personal prompts to encourage you to reclaim your lost dreams or create entirely new ones. You will build from the ground up the lifestyle for which you have been yearning for years.

There are six Graces that will act as guides as we make our journey over the next year. These are the six threads of abundant living that, when woven together, produce a tapestry of contentment that will wrap us in well-being, happiness, and a reassuring sense of serenity. First there is *Gratitude*. When we do a mental and spiritual inventory of all that we have, we realize that we are very rich indeed. Gratitude gives way to *Simplicity*—the desire to clear out, pare down, and realize the essentials of what we need to live truly well. Simplicity brings with it *Order*, both internally and externally. A sense of order in our life reveals our longing for *Harmony*. *Harmony* provides us with the inner quietude we need to appreciate the beauty that surrounds us each day, and seeking *Beauty* opens us to *Joy*. But just as with any exquisite needlepoint tapestry, it's difficult to see where one stitch ends and another begins. So it is with *Simple Abundance*.

Pick up the needle with me and make the first stitch on the canvas of your life. Invite Spirit to open the eyes of your inner awareness. Be still and wait expectantly, knowing that in the warp and weft of your daily round as it exists today are the golden threads of a simply abundant tomorrow.

JANUARY 6

This Isn't a Dress Rehearsal

When you perform...you are out of yourself—larger and more potent, more beautiful. You are for minutes heroic. This is power. This is glory on earth. And it is yours, nightly.
—Agnes de Mille (1905–1993)
American dancer and choreographer

You've probably heard the expression "Life's not a dress rehearsal." Unfortunately, many of us unconsciously act as if it were. Like an actress just going through the motions to conserve her creative energy and focus for opening night, we hold back. Are you still eating off mismatched china? Do you sleep well on a comfortable mattress? Have a decent reading light on your nightstand? Dry yourself off with threadbare towels and then relax in a faded and frayed T-shirt? Perhaps you're like me and rarely dress up when you're home alone. If we're not playing to an audience, does it really matter?

Now that's a question to ask as the New Year begins and we examine the quality of our real-life journey. It does take more effort to set an inviting table, but it enhances our enjoyment of eating. Single or married, eighteen to eighty, we all feel brighter and more energetic when we walk into a clean kitchen in the morning. And those few extra minutes to fix our hair and put on makeup are an investment in our repose during the day, because when we aren't thinking about what we look like (good or bad) we can focus on other people, which is the essence of charm. Every actress knows the magic power of props and costumes to create special moods both onstage and off.

None of us can be expected to perform every minute of our lives. But a lot more of us might tap into the power, excitement, and glory of real life more frequently if, for once, we cast ourselves as the leading ladies in our own lives.

JANUARY 7

The Woman You Were Meant to Be

Many women today feel a sadness we cannot name. Though we accomplish much of what we set out to do, we sense that something is missing in our lives and—fruitlessly—search "out there" for the answers. What's often wrong is that we are disconnected from an authentic sense of self.

—Dr. Emily Hancock
American psychologist and author

Has this ever happened to you? You're washing your face and suddenly you don't recognize the woman staring back at you. "Who's this?" you ask the mirror on the wall. No reply.

The woman looks vaguely familiar but bears little resemblance to the one you were expecting to see there. Psychologists call this phenomenon a "displacement of self," and it usually occurs during times of great stress (which for many of us is an everyday occurrence).

But what's wrong? What is this sadness we cannot name? Can we give this question the loving meditation it deserves today? Perhaps the heart of our melancholy is that we miss the woman we were meant to be. We miss our Authentic Selves. But the good news is that even if you have ignored her overtures for decades ("Wear red...Cut your hair... Study art in Paris...Learn the tango..."), your Authentic Self has not abandoned you. Instead she has been waiting patiently for you to recognize her and reconnect. Turn away from the world this year and begin to listen. Listen to the whispers of your heart. Look within. Your silent companion has lit lanterns of love to illuminate the path to Wholeness. At long last, the journey you were born to take has begun.

JANUARY 8

Standing Knee-Deep in a River
and Dying of Thirst

When I'm hungry, I eat. When I'm thirsty, I drink. When I feel like saying something, I say it.

—Madonna
American singer, songwriter, actress

The first time I heard Kathy Mattea's beautiful rendition of the country song "Standing Knee-Deep in a River (Dying of Thirst)," I was driving to my daughter's school to pick up the afternoon carpool. Suddenly I had to pull over because I was crying so much, I couldn't see the road in front of me. Until then, it had been a busy but good day. I was not consciously aware of being sad or depressed. So why was I crying?

As Kathy sang of friends who had been taken for granted, sweethearts she had known, and a wonderful world full of strangers just waiting to make a connection with us (while we turn our eyes away), something deep within me stirred. There was so much I was taking for granted. I didn't want to continue to live unconsciously.

The revelation that we have everything we need in life to make us happy but simply lack the conscious awareness to appreciate it can be as refreshing as lemonade on a hot afternoon. Or it can be as startling as cold water being thrown in our face. How many of us go through our days parched and empty, thirsting after happiness, when we're really standing knee-deep in the river of abundance?

Yet make no mistake about it. The Universe will get our attention one way or another—with a sip or a splash. Let's choose today to quench our thirst for "the good life" we think others lead by acknowledging the good that already exists in our own lives. We can then offer the Universe the gift of our grateful hearts.

JANUARY 9

How Happy Are You Right Now?

Perhaps if one really knew when one was happy one would know the things that were necessary for one's life.

—Joanna Field (1900–1998)
British psychoanalyst and writer

How happy are you right now? Do you even know? Most women know what makes their parents, partners, or children happy. But when it comes to an awareness about the little, specific things in life that bring a smile to our faces and contentment to our own hearts, we often come up short.

In 1926 a young Englishwoman, Marion Milner (writing as Joanna Field), began to feel that she was not living a truly authentic life because she didn't know what made her genuinely happy. To remedy this, she embarked upon a seven-year experiment by keeping a journal devoted to what specifically triggered the feeling of delight in her daily life. The journal, *A Life of One's Own*, was published in 1934. It was written, she confided, in the spirit of a detective who searches through the minutiae of the mundane in hopes of finding clues for what was missing in her life.

What's missing from many of our days is a true sense that we are enjoying the lives we're living. It's difficult to experience moments of happiness if we are not aware of what it is we genuinely love. We must learn to savor small, authentic moments that bring us contentment. Take the time to slowly arrange a bouquet of flowers to appreciate their colors, fragrance, and beauty. Find a bakery near your work and allow yourself the indulgence of two cookies in different flavors; you're strictly a chocolate chip gal, so why not try butterscotch shortbread? Put the ingredients on your grocery list for a personal bake-off over the weekend. Enjoy a few while they are warm from the oven and freeze the rest so that there's always a treat available for you "just because." If you're a tea drinker, did you know there are 1,500 varieties of tea in the world? Experiment with a different tea blend for a week, and you just may find a new favorite. Pause for five minutes to pet a purring cat or play with the dog. There are countless simple pleasures waiting to be enjoyed every day. Let's make room for the ones so often overlooked or dismissed.

Joanna Field discovered that she delighted in red shoes, good food, sudden bursts of laughter, reading in French, answering letters, loitering in a crowd at a fair, and "a new idea when first it is grasped."

Let us each grasp a new idea this year. Let us grasp the awareness of what it is that makes us truly happy. Let's consider our personal preferences (provocative though they may be), and compassionately give ourselves permission to recognize, indulge, and enjoy moments of genuine happiness that are uniquely our own.

The Underrated Duty

There is no duty we so much underrate as the duty of being happy.
By being happy we sow anonymous benefits upon the world.
—Robert Louis Stevenson (1850–1894)
Scottish novelist, poet, and travel writer

Perhaps you think you'll be happy when you get a bigger kitchen, or a new job, or the perfect someone with whom to share your life. But don't you want to start making happiness a habit right now? Every morning when we wake up we've been given a wonderful gift—another day of life—so let's make the most of it. No one can do it for us. "Happiness is not a possession to be prized," the British author and playwright Daphne du Maurier wrote in her most famous novel *Rebecca*, published in 1938. "It is a quality of thought, a state of mind."

Let's adopt a new state of mind about happiness. Let's stop thinking that things outside our control will bring us happiness.

Admittedly, remodeling the kitchen, landing the job we've been dreaming of, or finding that special someone can make us feel—at least momentarily—happier. But the magic seeds of contentment are planted deep within us. Happiness that the world cannot take away only flourishes in the secret garden of our souls. By tending to our inner garden and uprooting the weeds of external expectations, we can nurture our authentic happiness the way we would nurture something that's fragile, beautiful, and alive. Happiness is a *living* emotion.

But more than that, *your happiness is not a frivolous, expendable luxury.* Read that sentence again. Now say it aloud slowly as if you were speaking a foreign language: *My happiness is not a frivolous, expendable luxury.* It feels like a radical idea, doesn't it? But that doesn't make it any less true.

Indeed, the *pursuit* of happiness was considered so important by America's Founding Fathers that it was deemed an inalienable right *guaranteed* in the United States. Now, they didn't guarantee what would make us happy, but they certainly did guarantee our right to pursue it. To find out. They also pledged their lives, their fortunes, and their sacred honors to make our *pursuit* of happiness not just words on a dusty old parchment but a Divine blessing here on earth. Two centuries later, this legacy of love, protection, and care deserves to be cherished.

Ultimately, genuine happiness can only be realized once we commit to making it a personal priority in our lives. This may be new behavior for most of us and a bit intimidating. Be gentle with yourself. It will all unfold in time. Today you may not be familiar with the happiness habit. But like any new behavior, the *pursuit* of happiness can be learned.

JANUARY 11

What Is It You Truly Need?

In my life's chain of events nothing was accidental. Everything happened according to an inner need.
—Hannah Szenes (1921–1944)
Hungarian poet and spy for Great Britain

Do you have everything you need right now? What about your wants? Few of us have everything we want, and at times our wants can seem positively all-consuming. Our sensibilities become confused and over-stimulated by a mass media that glorifies beautiful people and expensive objects. It's easy to lose clarity about what we need to live authentically. Most of us *are* hungering for something more in our lives. But do you really think the answer can be found in a glossy magazine, on a stunning website, or a television reality program?

If we are to live happy, creative, and fulfilled lives, it's crucial for us to distinguish between our wants and our needs. Unfortunately, many women, including me, blur the distinction and then wonder why we feel so diminished.

Making peace with the knowledge that you can't have everything you want exactly when you want it teaches us many creative and spiritual lessons: the mysteries of cycles; the immense fulfillment of delayed gratification; and blessings of unanswered prayers which, in my own life, seem to be messengers of miracles. Why should this be so? Because in order to love our lives truly, madly, and deeply, we must separate our wants and our needs: until we learn to notice how they often overlap, seem to merge, or act as an unseen ally in our search for happiness. That's because, like infants, we feel contentment when our essential needs are met.

Be courageous. Ask yourself: What is it I truly need to make me happy? These deeply personal answers will be different for each of us. But trust the loving wisdom of your heart. It is only after we acknowledge our inner needs that we can harness the creative energy necessary to manifest them in our lives. "It is inevitable when one has a great need of something, one finds it," Gertrude Stein, the early twentieth-century American poet and Parisian avant-garde art collector, reassures us. "What you need you attract like a lover."

JANUARY 12

Until It Is Carved in Stone

It's only when we truly know and understand that we have a limited time on earth—and that we have no way of knowing when our time is up—that we will begin to live each day to the fullest, as if it was the only one we had.

—Elisabeth Kübler-Ross (1926–2004)
Swiss-American psychiatrist

Visiting old cemeteries can be very illuminating in unexpected ways. In fact, during the late nineteenth century, visiting graveyards with a picnic became a Victorian pastime that grew from the collective grief brought on by the Civil War. Whether they wore blue or gray, no family was left untouched. And so landscape architects, such as Frederick Law Olmstead, who designed Central Park and the US Capitol, re-imagined cemeteries as "landscapes of remembrance" and a source of solace, beauty, art, and history.

I love old cemeteries. When I was growing up in Massachusetts there was a small graveyard behind our house that had been built in 1789. When I moved to London, I learned the art of brass stone rubbing at ancient gravesites, and when I was living in Paris writing my play about Sarah Bernhardt, I tended her grave in Père Lachaise Cemetery every week. It seems to me that old cemeteries whisper that until it is carved in stone, pursuing our heart's desire is our soul's prime directive if we are to recognize what makes us truly happy.

In the 1938 Pulitzer Prize–winning play *Our Town* by Thornton Wilder, a deeply poignant scene takes place in a graveyard. The play is set in the fictional American small town of Grover's Corners, New Hampshire, between 1901 and 1913, and the audience is given an opportunity to glimpse the daily life of two neighboring families—the Webbs and the Gibbs—as their children grow up, fall in love, marry, and have children of their own. In Act Three, we are observers at a funeral. Ghosts comfort the young heroine, Emily, who has recently died in childbirth. Still longing for the life she has just left so abruptly,

Emily wishes to revisit one ordinary, "unimportant" day in her life. The ghosts warn her that she will be able to watch but not speak to her loved ones, nor change her choices. When she gets her wish, she realizes how much the living take for granted.

Eventually her visit is too much for her to bear. "I didn't realize," she confesses mournfully, "all that was going on and we never noticed... Good-bye, world. Good-bye, Grover's Corners... Mama and Papa. Good-bye to clocks ticking... and Mama's sunflowers. And food and coffee. And new-ironed dresses and hot baths... and sleeping and waking up. Oh, earth, you're too wonderful for anybody to realize you."

On our new path we will become seekers of what I call Everyday Epiphanies: those fleeting moments when, like Emily, we recognize the Sacred in our ordinary. Hopefully we'll realize in our own sunflowers, in the aroma of fresh coffee brewing, and in hot baths that none of us can afford to throw away even one "unimportant" day by not noticing the wonder of it all. We must be willing to discover and then appreciate the authentic moments of happiness available to each of us every day.

JANUARY 13

Gratitude: Awakening the Heart

The eyes of my eyes are opened.
—e e cummings
Edward Estlin Cummings (1894–1962)
American poet

Has this ever happened to you? You're reading a book and suddenly a sentence leaps off the page as if it had been written just for you. Or you hear a revelation in the lyrics of a song. Sometimes a stranger casually makes a comment in a checkout line, and it seems as if an angel has whispered in your ear. We call these moments "synchronicity," which was explained by the Swiss psychiatrist Carl Gustav Jung (1875–1961) as surprising coincidences that have deep personal meaning or connection with us.

One ordinary morning I woke up feeling drained and discouraged. Money was tight, too. I'd lost two lucrative consulting jobs and the freelance market was shrinking fast because businesses were downshifting left and right. I was sick and tired of concentrating on what was missing in my life and all the things I wanted but couldn't afford. Goodness knows, the last thing I wanted to do was write about it. Worrying about money had squandered my most precious natural resources—time, creative energy, and emotion. I had no reserves left. What I hungered for was an inner peace that was impervious to the world's unpredictability. I asked Spirit for help and committed to following wheresoever She would lead me. For the first time in my life I discarded my carefully plotted five-year goals and became a seeker, a pilgrim, a sojourner.

After I sent my daughter off to school, I heard a Voice I knew was not my own, which instructed me to "Sit down at the dining room table and write down every blessing in your life and give thanks for each one of them. And none of them can be about money."

Well, until that moment, the only Inner Voice I've ever heard in my head and heart had been my own, so I did what I was told. Six hours and several pots of tea later, to my great astonishment, I had more than 150 overlooked blessings on my list. And then, my first Everyday Epiphany occurred: I realized I didn't need a single thing, except the awareness of how blessed I was. This was the first time Gratitude beckoned and invited me to use her transformative power—not to revamp my life, but to rejoice in it. The thirteenth-century German mystic Meister Eckhart believed, "If the only prayer you ever say in your life is 'Thank You,' it will be enough." I discovered how right he was and got so excited that I started writing down five new things to be thankful for every day.

And what was included in the inventory of my life's assets? My health, a wonderful husband, a beautiful and happy daughter, their health, our home (small but comfortable), and three precious pets who daily lavished me with love, faithful companionship, and great joy. There was always plenty of good food on the table and wine in the pantry. We were also blessed with many wonderful friends who cared deeply about us and who share in our lives.

Once I started, my list grew. I loved my work; it was being sent out into the world and had been well received. Many women had let me know that my first book on Victorian family celebrations had enriched their lives. I truly believe that what you give to the world will be returned to you—maybe not all at once or in the way you expect it—but if you give your very best, the very best will come back to you. Now was the moment to live my beliefs.

When I looked at my life's ledger, I realized I was a very rich woman. What I was experiencing was merely a temporary cash-flow problem. Finally, I came to an inner awareness that my personal net worth couldn't possibly be determined by the size of my checking account balance. Neither can yours.

It doesn't matter how awareness arrives. What matters is that it comes. My heart began to overflow with gratefulness. I started giving thanks for everything: daisies in a jelly jar on my kitchen windowsill, the sweet fragrance of my daughter's hair, the first sip of tea in the morning, the pork roast with apples and golden potatoes for Sunday supper, the woman at our farmer's market who made the best sour cherry pie ever, hearing the words "I love you" before I went to sleep. Each day began to offer me authentic moments of pleasure and contentment. But hadn't they before? The difference was that I was now noticing and appreciating each day's gifts. The power of gratefulness caught me by surprise.

All I ask you to do today is to open "the eyes of your eyes" and give your life another glance. Are your basic needs met? Do you have a home? Food on the table? Clothes to wear? Do you have dreams? Do you have your health? Can you walk, talk, see the beauty that surrounds you, listen to music that stirs your soul or makes your feet want to boogie? Do you have family and friends whom you love and who love you?

Then pause for a moment and give thanks. Let your heart awaken to the transforming power of gratefulness. "No trumpets sound when the important decisions of our life are made," Agnes de Mille reminds us. "Destiny is made known silently."

JANUARY 14

The Gratitude Journal

Gratitude unlocks the fullness of life. It turns what we have into enough, and more. It turns denial into acceptance, chaos to order, confusion to clarity. It can turn a meal into a feast, a house into a home, a stranger into a friend. Gratitude makes sense of our past, brings peace for today, and creates a vision for tomorrow.

—Melody Beattie
American author

There are several tools that I'm going to suggest you use as you begin your inner exploration of *Simple Abundance*. While all of them will help you become happier and more content and will nurture your creativity, this first tool could change the quality of your life beyond belief: It's what I call a daily Gratitude Journal. I have a beautiful blank book and each night before I go to bed, I write down five things that I can be grateful about that day. Some days my list will be filled with amazing things; most days, though, they're just simple joys.

Mikey got lost outside in a fierce storm, but we found him shivering, wet and scared on a neighbor's roof. They had a ladder and rescued him. I baked some banana bread to thank them. It was delicious!

I listened to Puccini while cleaning and remembered how much I love opera.

There were a couple of batteries in the back of the junk drawer and I didn't have to go out and buy new ones. Finally finished transcribing the interview.

The tech guys in College Park were able fix the computer in a day. Glory be!

Other days—rough ones—when I doubt I have even five things to be grateful for, I'll write down my basics: my health, my husband and daughter, their health, my animals, my home, my friends, and the comfortable bed that I'm about to get into. And even sometimes just the fact that the day's over. That's okay. Real life isn't always going to be perfect or go our way, but the recurring acknowledgment of what *is working* in our lives can help us not only survive but surmount our difficulties.

The Gratitude Journal must be the first step on the *Simple Abundance* path, or it just won't work for you. Simplicity, Order, Harmony, Beauty, and Joy—all the other Graces that can transform your life can't blossom and flourish without Gratitude. If you want to travel this journey with me, *the Gratitude Journal is not an option.*

Why? Because you simply will not be the same person two months from now after consciously giving thanks each day for the abundance that exists in your life. And you'll have set in motion an ancient spiritual law: The more you have and are grateful for, the more will be given to you.

The *Simple Abundance* path is a transformative process. We're going to work on each Grace for two months at a time, weaving their beautiful threads into the fabric of our daily life.

Let's begin today with Gratitude. Select the prettiest, most inviting, or most pleasing blank book you can find for your Gratitude Journal. Note the fabric or design of the cover. The look and feel of the paper. The size. Do you prefer ruled pages or blank? Many women keep their thoughts in bullet journals, which are notebooks of graph paper that you can customize any way you'd like. Perhaps you can find one with a pen loop, ribbon bookmark, or an elastic closure. Having a pen that enables you to write beautifully—such as a calligraphy marker—is a fantastic nudge to write, as are colored inks. One of my most valuable *Simple Abundance* lessons is that it's in the smallest details that the flavor of life is savored. If you'd rather have a journal that's already set up for you, I've also created a monthly diary, *The Simple Abundance Journal of Gratitude*, that you might enjoy.

Now, of course, being a woman with her wits about her, you're not going to let finding the "perfect" journal delay you from experiencing serenity. Perfectionism isn't the point here. When I began caring for my soul with the Grace of Gratitude daily, I noticed that the more I used it, the more fragments of thankfulness floated across my mind. However, if I didn't write them down immediately, they were lost from my appreciative grasp. So in the beginning, I started using Post-it notes and index cards, carrying some in my purse as well as stashing them in different places around the house. You may be used to taking notes on your phone, so if this works for you, by all means grasp your gratitudes this way. You'll be amazed how so many pleasant, comfortable, or often overlooked moments of pleasure occur in an hour. We need to acknowledge them before they evaporate into the ether of every day.

As the months pass and you fill your journal with blessings, the tectonic plates of your daily round will start shifting. Soon you'll be delighted to discover how content and hopeful you're feeling, especially when "nothing" seems to have changed with your outer circumstances. This is because you are growing in subtle but profound ways. As you focus on the abundance rather than on the lack in your life, you'll be designing a wonderful new blueprint for the future. This sense of fulfillment is Gratitude at work, transforming your dreams into reality.

A French proverb reminds us that "Gratitude is the heart's memory." Begin this day to explore and integrate this beautiful, life-affirming Grace into your life, and the miracle you have been seeking will unfold to your wonder and amazement.

JANUARY 15

Simple Gifts: Embracing Simplicity

'Tis a gift to be simple,
'Tis a gift to be free,
'Tis a gift to come down
Where we ought to be
And when we find ourselves
In the place that's right
T'will be in the valley
Of love and delight.

—Nineteenth-century Shaker hymn

Is there a woman alive who does not yearn for a simpler life? Or, to be completely honest, any life other than the one now running us ragged? But for what do we yearn? To chuck it all in and become a caretaker of fifty-five cats on a Greek island? Sorry, the last time I checked 35,000 other women had applied for that job before us. How about scaling the

Inca trail to Machu Picchu? Organizing African safaris to save endangered species? Or making spiritual pilgrimages from Chartres to Angkor Wat, with a little antiquing on the side to find inventory for that fabulous shop you're going to open in Big Sur? Mind you, none of these enterprises sound simple, but their fantasies trigger simply exquisite dreams, surely better than whatever we're dealing with today, which, of course, is too, too much.

Or could we really be seeking a fundamental simple pleasure, such as concentrating on one task at a time? When was the last time you were able to concentrate on only one task until it was finished? That's what I thought. Looking for simple? Better we head back to the Inca trail.

Here's the good news. Once we take stock of our lives and let Gratitude begin her transformative work, the next step on the path unfolds naturally. When we appreciate how much we have, we feel the urge to pare down, get back to basics, and learn what is essential for our happiness. Don't give up on your dreams. Just rank them in order of importance. Is it more important for you to work overtime to buy that new dining room set or to attend Little League games? Perhaps you could add a colorful runner, some new cushions, and a seasonal centerpiece for a pleasing freshening up. These choices are part of simplifying our lives. These choices are also creative brushstrokes on the blank canvas of our everyday. Welcome them. They *are* the authentic journey.

Many people believe simplicity implies doing without. *Au contraire.* True simplicity as a conscious life choice illuminates our lives from within. True simplicity is both buoyant and bountiful, able to liberate depressed spirits from the bondage and burden of extravagance and excess. True simplicity can elevate ordinary moments, dreary lives, and even inanimate objects—as anyone who has ever looked at an exquisite piece of Shaker furniture will attest—from the mundane to the transcendent.

Less can mean more for those of us on the *Simple Abundance* path. Today just think about how appealing simplicity can be. Visualize a bouquet of bright yellow daffodils in a white milk jug on a pine mantel, sunlight streaming through sparkling clean windows, the shine of beautifully varnished wooden floors, the shimmering glow and fragrance of pure beeswax candles. Trust that through the balm of simplicity your frazzled and weary soul can discover the place where you ought to be. Every day offers us simple gifts when we are willing to search our hearts for the place that's right for each of us.

A Sense of Order: Cultivating Contentment

Order is the shape upon which beauty depends.
—Pearl S. Buck (1892–1973)
First American woman to win the Nobel
Prize for Literature (1938)

For years I have suspected that in happy and fulfilled lives domesticity and spirituality are invisibly but inexorably connected—one a golden thread, one a silver filament—which, when woven together, create a tapestry of contentment.

The Shakers, a religious communal sect that flourished in America during the mid-nineteenth century, invoked a prayer each morning for the grace that would enable them to express their love of God through their daily tasks—tasks as simple and mundane as making a bed. And the seventeenth-century Carmelite friar Brother Lawrence wrote in his devotional classic *Practicing the Presence of God* that he frequently felt the spirit of God among the pots, pans, and potatoes in his kitchen as he was preparing a meal for his fellow monks.

Whenever I am feeling overwhelmed by outside circumstances—worries about money, concern over a sick family member, or anxiety over prolonged business negotiations—instinctively I turn to home-grown rituals to restore my equilibrium. There is an immediate emotional and psychological payoff to getting our houses in order. We might not be able to control what's happening externally in our lives, but we can learn to look to our own inner resources for a sense of comfort that nurtures and sustains. I have even noticed that there is a direct correlation between the days when I'm feeling depressed and the days when the house is in disarray. I suspect that I'm not alone. "It's not the tragedies that kill us," the sassy Jazz Age literary wit Dorothy Parker observed, "it's the messes."

If you feel constantly adrift but don't know why, be willing to explore the role that Order—or the lack of it—plays in your life. No woman can think clearly when constantly surrounded by clutter, chaos, and confusion, no matter who is responsible for it. Begin to think of order not as a straitjacket of "shoulds" (make the bed, wash the dishes, take out the garbage) but as a shape—the foundation—for the beautiful new life you are creating. It may be as simple as putting something back that you take out, waking up to a clean kitchen, hanging something up after you take it off, or teaching those who live with you that they must do the same for the common good of all.

There is a Divine Order—a Sublime Order—inherent in the Universe.

We can tap into this powerful source of creative energy when we are willing to gradually cultivate a sense of order as to how we conduct our daily affairs. Invite Divine Order into your life today and a more serene tomorrow will unfold.

JANUARY 17

Harmony: Achieving Balance in Our Lives

The notes I handle no better than many pianists. But the pauses between the notes—ah, that is where the art resides.
—Artur Schnabel (1882–1951)
Austrian classical pianist

A Chopin piano nocturne played by a novice musician will not sound the same as one played by a virtuoso. That's because the Polish composer Frédéric Chopin (1810–1849) spent his lifetime composing and discovering through discipline and devotion when to pause, and when to color the notes with passion and bravado.

So it is with the concerto of our lives. Individual notes must be learned, played, and practiced daily before we achieve harmony. Above all, we must learn how to pause and set boundaries in our personal and professional lives, which is the hardest task every woman faces each day.

Today's rapidly changing, complex, and mostly frightening 24/7 "Breaking News" culture assaults us at every turn with shocks that regularly catapult us into the realm of the unspeakable. Unless we avoid television and the internet altogether, we find ourselves "embedded" with news anchors around the world who are covering every harrowing natural disaster or appalling terrorist atrocity. The three most terrifying words in the English language have become "shelter in place."

Lassoed by our heartstrings, we helplessly watch strangers in danger, as these tragic events unfold in *real* time. Our daily round becomes a hostage, as our sensibilities and sympathies are poked by a virtual cattle prod of terrors that wear us down physically, emotionally, and psychically. What should be the ordinary task of getting through the day with all our loved ones accounted for drains our energy, depletes our sense of security, and diminishes our capacity for happiness, leaving us exhausted and vulnerable. We have forgotten that silence—the pauses—is the most important part of any symphony, especially the ones our souls long to compose. Usually, when the distractions of daily life press for attention the first thing we eliminate is the thing we need the most: quiet, reflective time. Time to think, time to contemplate what's working and what's not, so that we can make changes for the better. Even time to dream.

Harmony is the inner cadence of contentment we feel when the melody of life is in tune. When somehow, we're able to strike the right chord—to balance the expectations of our families and our responsibilities in the world on the one hand with our inner needs for spiritual growth and personal expression on the other.

When *Simple Abundance* was originally published, technology was just beginning. Personal computers were rare new tools used only by the tech-minded, the internet was rudimentary at best, and even the concept of smartphones nonexistent. These were new and very inviting instruments for sharing our lives with our friends and family, and it was incredibly exciting to blend our personal worlds with the bigger one out there.

But the drawbacks to this kind of technological immersion weren't far behind. Did you ever see the movie *Gremlins,* the 1984 American comedy-horror film about Billy Peltzer, a teenager who receives a strangely adorable creature called a *mogwai* as a Christmas gift? There are only three rules of care for the mogwai: (1) keep him in the dark, (2) don't get him wet, and (3) don't feed him after midnight.

Well, of course these safeguards are immediately ignored, and overnight the furry ball of fun multiplies into repugnant reptilian little monsters called "gremlins," hell bent on causing mayhem. I think of technology in the same way—it looked harmless, its tools appealingly clever gizmos. But then artificial intelligence hooked up with multimedia platforms and the internet morphed from a plaything into an enormous badass robot, ready to absorb our very souls, bit by bit, into the collective.

On the *Simple Abundance* path, we begin to learn how to pause. We need to push the pause button so that we can see how much of our lives have become an artificial intelligence hologram. We can't dismantle what we can't see, and unwittingly our internet use is written out using invisible ink by us, formulated by code breakers known as hacks. As we bring the Graces of Gratitude, Simplicity, and Order into our lives, Harmony emerges. We learn to balance demands with pleasures, moments of solitude with a need for companionship, work with play, activity with rest, consciously connecting the wider world through the internet, and withdrawing from it for the sake of our sanity and serenity.

Today, just try slowing down. Approach the day as if it were an adagio—a melody played at an easy, graceful pace. Listen to music that soothes and uplifts your spirit. And while you listen, pause to consider how all the individual notes come together harmoniously to give expression to the entire score.

Beauty: Opening Our Eyes to the Beauty
That Surrounds Us

*There is nothing more powerful or radical or stunningly beautiful
than a woman who chooses to rebuild her life day after day after
day. No matter how many pieces there are to pick up, or how many
mistakes she must spin into gold.*

—Cara Alwill Leyba
Author and motivational coach

While the *Simple Abundance* path is gentle, its lessons are powerful.
First, we learn to be grateful no matter what our circumstances may be.
In offering Gratitude for our real lives, we discover how to change them
for the better. As we embrace Simplicity, we learn that less is truly more.
This freedom encourages us to bring order to our affairs and cultivate
Harmony in our inner world. Going at our own pace, learning to rec-
ognize our limitations, appreciating our progress, we weave the lessons
into the fabric of our daily moments until they become a part of us.

Suddenly one day we feel very much alive and desire more beauty in
our personal quest. We come to a deep awareness that creating a beautiful life is our highest calling. "It was as if I had worked for years on the
wrong side of a tapestry, learning accurately all its lines and figures, yet
always missing its color and sheen," the journalist Anna Louise Strong
confessed in 1935. We understand her sentiments as life's color, sheen,
and beauty call to us. But with piles of work upon our desk that must be
finished immediately, if not sooner, we don't know how to respond to
this inner urge, other than to ignore it and work through lunch, as we
push our inner desire for a beauty reprieve down even further.

What is needed, then, is a plan. Look at your calendar for the next
two weeks. Can you find one lunch hour in the next ten workdays to
call your own? Quick, while no one's looking, block that hour out with
a yellow highlighter. Now if someone asks you to do something on that
yellow-hued hour, you can honestly say, "Sorry, I've got an appointment I can't break." Between now and then, scout your local newspaper
and see if you can find an art exhibition near you. That's where you're
headed. And I'll meet you there.

The rest of today, look for unexpected shapes, form, and color. I
once discovered the most perfect color scheme of blush and green from
an heirloom peach at a farmer's market. Beauty surrounds us. We just
don't notice it. Let your eyes seek and find the beauty that surrounds
you. Look around your office for a compliment to bestow on another.
You'll be so pleasantly surprised (so will she) to find something of

beauty in the everyday of one of your coworkers, it will make you both feel fabulous.

Tonight, gaze into the faces of those you love, set the table with care, and relish the preparations you make for dinner, delighting in the presentation of your meal. Light the candles, pour wine or sparkling water in your prettiest goblets, and celebrate this new awareness. It is in the details of life that beauty is revealed, sustained, and nurtured.

Outside, winter's darkness closes in. Inside, you have found your own Light.

JANUARY 19

Joy: Learning Life's Lessons with a Light Heart

I cannot believe that the inscrutable universe turns on an axis of suffering; surely the strange beauty of the world must somewhere rest on pure joy.

—Louise Bogan (1897–1970)
American Poet Laureate

The *Simple Abundance* journey takes us to undiscovered territory. We learn each day how cultivating Gratitude tills the soil of our soul and then how the seeds of Simplicity and Order send their roots down deep into the earth of our everyday existence.

As we work with each Grace and find unexpected contentment, Harmony inspires us with quiet courage to create an authentic life for ourselves and those we love by setting boundaries with imaginative choices. With patience, Beauty blossoms in unexpected places of our daily round and our hearts experience not only happiness, which is often fleeting, but a wellspring of unexpected Joy that refreshes and renews. We have found our true place in the world. "With an eye made quiet by the power of harmony, and the deep power of joy," the eighteenth-century English poet William Wordsworth (1770–1850) wrote, "we see into the life of things."

Seeing into the life of things is what engages us at this point in the transformative process. From deep within there comes a longing to reject the path of struggle to learn life's lessons. Finally, we are ready to embrace the path of Joy.

Learning to live in the present moment is part of the path of Joy. But this requires a profound inner shift in our reality. Many of us unconsciously create dramas in our minds, expecting the worst from a situation only to have our expectations become a self-fulfilling prophecy. Inadvertently, we become authors of our own misfortune. And so we struggle from day to day, from crisis to crisis, bruised and battered by circumstances without realizing that we always have a choice.

But what if you learned how to stop the dramas and started to trust the flow of life and the goodness of Spirit? What if you began to expect the best from any situation? Isn't it possible that you could write new chapters in your life with happy endings? For many of us this is such a radical departure from the way we have been behaving for years that it seems, well, frankly, unbelievable. Yet it is possible. Suspend your disbelief. Take a leap of faith. After all, what have you got to lose but misery and lack?

Begin today. Try it for an hour. Try it as a lark. Try it as a dare and discover your truth. Declare out loud to the Universe that you are willing to let go of struggle and eager to learn through Joy. It just may take you at your word. What's more, you'll discover, much to your amazement and delight, that such blessings have been waiting patiently for you to claim them all along.

JANUARY 20

Simple Abundance: The Basic Tools

There are no wrong turnings. Only paths we had not known we were meant to walk.

—Guy Gavriel Kay
Canadian author of fantasy fiction

There is no companion so companionable as Solitude," the nineteenth-century American poet and philosopher Henry David Thoreau reminds me as I carry a hot cup of tea back to bed. The house is hushed now after the hustle and bustle of a weekday morning. The cats follow me up the stairs, scurrying for nests in the rumpled bedcovers. Even they know that a reassuring ritual is about to take place, a civilized ceremonial for a common day.

Although it is still too early to receive business calls, to avoid interruptions I turn off my phone. My next hour is spent going within: in prayer and reading one chapter in the inspirational book I'm currently enjoying, and then reflecting on my Gratitude Journal. Usually there's something I've forgotten to acknowledge and give thanks for. Also, when you glance back at the blessings that have gone before, you get an understanding of how yesterday's worries worked themselves out with unexpected grace. And so will today's.

What I do *not* do is turn on the radio, television, or my computer, because if I do, and I'm not grounded, then the day is usually lost to some urgent "Breaking News" just waiting to suck the life out of me and my day. People ask, "What if something important is happening?" Don't worry, I'll find out about it when I finally turn my computer on. But at least I've allowed myself an hour of solitude to collect my thoughts and set the day's priorities.

See if you can't give yourself the gift of one hour a day to journey within. You need enough breathing space to allow your heart to ponder what is precious. Or perhaps you can let your imagination soar to the twilight where dreams first dwell. If you feel a solid hour is too much of a luxury in the beginning (it isn't, but we'll go gently), break up the time during the day. Start with a half hour in the morning and another half hour before you retire in the evening.

Most days after my inner excursion is over, it appears as if nothing has happened that has dramatically changed my life. I've just spent an hour alone. I'm not aware of any new insights, inspiration, or guidance. But sometimes I can bring the larger picture into sharper focus. You will, too.

This much I know: If you go deep enough, often enough, something good is bound to come back to you. Very often glimmers of the inspiration I desire or the insights I need will come later in the day when I'm driving, walking, preparing supper, or in the shower. But whether or not revelations have been part of my morning ritual, each day offers its own gift.

JANUARY 21

The Illustrated Discovery Journal

Knowledge of what you love somehow comes to you; you don't have to read nor analyze nor study. If you love a thing enough, knowledge of it seeps into you, with particulars more real than any chart can furnish.

—Jessamyn West (1902–1984)
American Quaker author

The key to loving how you live is in knowing what it is you truly love. "To know what you prefer instead of humbly saying Amen to what the world tells you you ought to prefer, is to keep your soul alive," Robert Louis Stevenson reminds us. Keeping our soul alive and nurturing our creativity is what interests us today.

One of the most pleasurable ways to start finding out your personal preferences is by creating an *Illustrated Discovery Journal*. This is your explorer's log as you begin to make your way into the darkest terra incognita: your authentic inner world. We feed our imaginations and get in touch with our authenticity by gathering together beautiful images that speak to our souls. You didn't know that the sun-drenched colors of Santa Fe called to you? Then why do they keep popping up in your pictures? You thought mid-century modern was your style, but rose-covered chintz is what you're collecting on paper? And what's that arts and crafts bungalow doing here? Not very modern, but you love the way the architecture seems grounded in the earth with stone plinths and deep protective covered porches that act as strong branches against the winds of life.

Isn't that interesting?

Now, here is a perfect occasion when one picture speaks a thousand words. And it speaks to you. Meditating on one visual image a day can jump-start your creativity and lead to revealing insights.

Today get a blank, black-bound artist's sketchbook, a pair of sharp scissors, double-sided sticky tape, and your favorite magazines and mail order catalogs. Magazine subscriptions are pricey these days (which is why print is quickly disappearing), so I love to look at specialty magazine lots on eBay (with a ten-dollar limit) such as the southern lifestyle *Garden and Gun* and American Express's member monthly *Departures*. Friends who travel know my favorite treats are foreign home and fashion glossies and bring them back for me. Once you start looking for new sources of images, you'll find them.

But you say you already collect pictures that you love on Pinterest or one of the other image-collecting online sites. And you're not alone. Millions of other people share their delights online that way. You can find recipes, home decorating ideas, style inspiration, and more on their zillions of boards. There are even boards about the *Simple Abundance Illustrated Discovery Journal*! But these weren't started by me. And here's why: I'm ever so gently trying to help you create boundaries of privacy and sanity by reconsidering what you put online for the rest of the world to see, and I'm trying to do the same for myself.

Besides, be honest. Haven't you already forgotten three-quarters of the images you've collected on these photo-collecting online sites? I'd be willing to bet you haven't even looked at most of the things on your own boards in ages. Every time the next inspirational photo comes into view it's easier and easier to fall down the rabbit hole of overstimulation and stress. Seeing other women's perfect images of how they live, dress, decorate, travel, and get married just sets up an impossible, deceptive shell game that diminishes our sense of self-worth and increases our sense of lack.

Instead, the *Illustrated Discovery Journal* puts you on the *Simple Abundance* path of pure intuition and feeling. It's slow and steady, tactile and reassuring. The more you do, the more you'll feel connected to your authenticity. Over this year, I hope to encourage you to learn to trust yourself once again and come to view your intuition or sense of "knowing" as your soul's compass, pointing bravely toward your own creative and spiritual True North.

Gather them all in a basket and keep it by your bed. At night before you go to sleep, when you're in a drowsy, relaxed, and receptive state, flip through the magazines. When you see an image you love, rip or cut it out and paste it in your book. Don't try to arrange the pictures in any specific sort of way. Let the collages you are creating simply evolve. Soon they will give you directions about where your heart wants you to go. I have also added quotes, sketches, greeting cards, and art postcards to my discovery journal, crafting with paper what the English-American poet W. H. Auden called "a map of my planet."

Start collecting ephemera, random images culled from periodicals or catalogs, photographs, or postcards. As you reverently and reflectively assemble collages that reveal just about anything you might ever have wanted to know about yourself, you'll feel a gravitational pull toward your passions. Your preferences. What tickles you. What ticks you off. What makes you happy. From discovering why a certain shade of blue makes you smile to suddenly comprehending the source of a problem in a friendship, to recognizing your deep spiritual beliefs, the *Illustrated Discovery Journal* will lead you to the hidden side of your Authentic Self as no other exercise book can.

JANUARY 22

Your Personal Treasure Map

For *where your treasure is, there will your heart be also.*
—Matthew 6:21
New Testament

No self-respecting, swashbuckling buccaneer would set out in search of buried treasure without a map. Why should you? A personal treasure map is a collage of your ideal life that you create as a visual tool to focus your creative energy in the direction you wish to go.

First, you'll have to visualize your ideal life. And this is not so easy. Take a moment to get quiet and go within. Close your eyes. Now see how you live and who lives with you. What does your dream house look like? What part of the world is it in? Do you have children? How many? What type of garden do you have? Have you started your heirloom vegetable kitchen garden surrounded by a white picket fence? Your arbor of old-fashioned climbing roses?

Do you have any pets? What kind of job do you have? Are you publishing your own blog, directing a feature film, or raising thoroughbred horses? Now see if you can't find pictures in magazines to match your ideal images. Cut them out and create a collage in your *Illustrated Discovery Journal*. If you can't find visuals to match your dreams, tap into the creativity deep within you and draw a picture. When you're finished, find a photograph of yourself that you especially like. Make sure it's a picture of you looking radiant and happy. Cut yourself out and place yourself in the center of your treasure map collage.

When making your personal treasure map, think fun. Think delight. Think seven years old. This is not an intellectual exercise. This is a wish list to the Universe. Our deepest wishes are whispers of our Authentic Selves. We must learn to respect them. We must learn to listen. "Put your ear down next to your soul and listen hard," the Pulitzer Prize–winning poet Anne Sexton (1928–1974) advises.

Above all, remember that no one needs to be privy to your personal treasure map, nor should anyone but you. Our wishes for the future, our hopes, our dreams, and our sacred aspirations are our truest treasures. Guard yours in the sanctuary of your heart. Keep your personal treasure map in the back of your *Illustrated Discovery Journal* and look at it often. When you do, give thanks for the wonderful life you are leading. Even realizing that you want to live another way is the most fabulous blessing. The greatest secret to living a happy and fulfilled life is the realization that everything is created in our minds before it manifests itself in the outer world. And before our minds, it is a spark in our heart. We must believe it before we can see it. You must know what you're digging for, before X can mark the spot.

JANUARY 23

Creative Excursions: The Gift of Time

Cherish your solitude. Take trains by yourself to places you have never been. Sleep out alone under the stars. Learn how to drive a stick shift. Go so far away that you stop being afraid of not coming back. Say no when you don't want to do something. Say yes if your instincts are strong, even if everyone around you disagrees. Decide whether you want to be liked or admired. Decide if fitting in is more important than finding out what you're doing here.
—Eve Ensler
American playwright and performer

Now that you've met your Authentic Self, wouldn't you like to get to know her better? You can when you start going on creative excursions together.

Creative excursions are regular solo rendezvous with your Authentic Self designed for this purpose. In the beginning of any intimate relationship the best gift you can offer another person is the investment of quality time together. So it is with your Authentic Self. You have probably been ignoring her for decades; now it's time to make amends.

What will you do? Celebrate yourself, find pastimes that make your heart light and your spirit sing. Take in a movie (one of those English period dramas you love), have an early breakfast before work at a new French café, cruise the aisles at that incredible Italian market, go for a morning hike or take the evening yoga class, explore a fabulous thrift shop, browse in used-book stores, visit an art supply store and imagine all the wonderful ways in which you can begin expressing yourself. When you embark on creative excursions, your Authentic Self will lovingly reveal to you the beautiful mystery that is *you*. This occurs spontaneously as you make the pursuit of personal growth a sacred endeavor.

Having encouraged you, now let me warn you. This is not as easy as it sounds. In fact, for me the *hardest* part of the *Simple Abundance* path was creative excursions. I was simply not used to seeking *fun* by myself. It seemed too frivolous, too self-indulgent. Be prepared for strong, emotional resistance. Excuses will be plentiful: You're too broke, you're too busy, who will watch the kids, maybe next week when you're not so frazzled or you've made that deadline. Every excuse known to womankind will present itself. I know. For the first few times I took myself out on a date, I felt delinquent. Eventually I realized that the often mischievous, always clandestine aura that hung around a creative excursion was in fact its irresistible come hither. I stopped resisting and became better for it.

Creative excursions require an investment of time, not money. Remember that seemingly random suggestion of yellow-highlighting an hour to call your own in your calendar a few days ago? I suggested you find an art exhibition in which to wander. How did that go? I hope wonderfully. Now let's make creative excursions a self-nurturing habit: I want you to yellow-highlight an hour a week for the next month.

None of us are too busy to find an hour a week. If we are, we seriously need to reconsider our personal priorities. Hire a babysitter, let your spouse watch the kids, carve out time when they are in school, use your lunch hour at work. Once we realize that nurturing our imaginations and developing a relationship with our Authentic Selves is an investment we can no longer afford to put off, we'll find ways to do it. This week commit to a weekly creative excursion with your Authentic Self as you follow the *Simple Abundance* path. Expect nothing less than signs and wonders to follow.

There Is No Scarcity

When money is plenty this is a man's world. When money is scarce it is a woman's world. When all else seems to have failed, the woman's instinct comes in. She gets the job. That is a reason why, in spite of all that happens, we continue to have a world.

—Ladies' Home Journal, October 1932

When you are worried about your health or the health of a loved one, your concentration focuses like a laser. Suddenly there's a clarity about all of life because you realize what is important. Living is important. Every day is a gift. You ask for another chance to get it right. Most of the time you're given it, and you're very grateful.

But worries about money mock you. They steal the joy of living because they follow you around all day like a dark, menacing shadow. At night they hover at the foot of your bed waiting to rob you of sleep. When you're worried about money you dread the days and you agonize at night. Without thinking, you throw away every one of the precious twenty-four hours that come your way. You cease to live and instead merely exist.

If you are worried about money today, take heart. You have the power to change your lifestyle and move from a feeling of lack and deprivation to a feeling of abundance and fulfillment. Money ebbs and flows in our lives. What should remain constant is our realization that abundance is our spiritual birthright. The American gospel singer Mahalia Jackson (1911–1972) once said that "It is easy to be independent when you've got money. But to be independent when you haven't got a thing—that's the Lord's test."

This is what I have learned and share with the seeker in you. The simpler we make our lives, the more abundant they become.

There is no scarcity except in our souls.

Acres of Diamonds

Your diamonds are not in far distant mountains or in yonder seas;
they are in your own backyard, if you but dig for them.
—Russell H. Conwell (1843–1925)
American minister, orator, and philanthropist

Few motivational talks have influenced or inspired as many people as the famous Victorian lecture that was known as "Acres of Diamonds." Russell H. Conwell, a former newspaper correspondent and minister, delivered his speech more than six thousand times between 1877 and 1925. When it was published it became an immediate best-seller and a classic in inspirational literature. Conwell later founded Temple University in Philadelphia, Pennsylvania.

The story Conwell told in his lecture had enormous appeal. It recounted the life of a Persian farmer named Ali Hafed who sold his farm and left his family to travel the world in search of wealth. He looked everywhere but he could not find the diamonds he lusted after. Finally, alone and in despair as a homeless pauper, he ended his own life. His search for riches had consumed him. In the meantime, the man who bought the land from Hafed was grateful for every blade of grass that was now his and lavished love and hard work on his farm. At night, surrounded by his family and eating the fruits of his labor, he was a contented man. Finally, one day he made a remarkable discovery. In the backyard that Ali Hafed had abandoned was a diamond mine—literally an acre of diamonds. The simple farmer became wealthy beyond his wildest dreams.

Conwell used this parable to illustrate an extraordinary and wonderful message: Within each of us lies a wellspring of abundance and the seeds of opportunity. For each of us there is a deeply personal dream waiting to be discovered and fulfilled. When we cherish our dream and then invest love, creative energy, perseverance, and passion in ourselves, we will achieve an authentic success.

Where is your acre of diamonds? If you could do anything in the world, what would it be? Yes, that very thing right now that you believe is impossible! Would you open a store, nurture a family, design a dress, write a screenplay, go back to school to finish your degree in microbiology?

We all have an acre of diamonds waiting to be discovered, cherished, and mined. We all have a place from which to begin. Let your imagination soar, for it is your soul's blueprint for success. On the *Simple Abundance* path, you will discover that your own opportunity for personal success, authentic happiness, and financial serenity is as close as your own backyard.

JANUARY 26

Letting Go of Limiting Illusions

I like living. I have sometimes been wildly, despairingly, acutely miserable, racked with sorrow, but through it all I still know quite certainly that just to be alive is a grand thing.
—Agatha Christie (1890–1976)
British writer and best-selling author
of all time

For some of us the thought of trusting a power outside ourselves to help make our dreams come true is a threatening concept, especially if we're used to being in control—or, rather, used to the illusion of being in control.

Many more of us go through life trapped by another illusion: that an uncaring, capricious fate determines our destiny. Shell-shocked from some of the acutely miserable things that life throws our way, we are deeply afraid to believe that a loving, generous Creative Force supports our endeavors. We're afraid to trust that the same Spirit that created the Universe probably knows how to help us apply for the grant, get the promotion, go back to school, launch a start-up, or move to a new city. Like mirrors in a carnival fun house that distort appearances, what we see with our eyes is not real. We buy in to the illusion that external events possess the ultimate power to deny our dreams.

And we wonder why we're so unhappy?

Can you be willing to let go of limiting illusions that have held you back from knowing that just to be alive is a grand thing? That's all, just be willing. Become your own research and development team. Conduct an experiment with a loving, supportive Universe that embraces even skeptics. I've learned that skeptics make the best seekers. Today, be willing to believe that a companion Spirit is leading you every step of the way and knows the next step.

JANUARY 27

The Prosperity of Living

*Woman must be the pioneer in this turning inward for strength. In
a sense she has always been the pioneer.*

—Anne Morrow Lindbergh (1906–2001)
American pioneering aviatrix and author

These are challenging times in which to live. But we are not the only
generation of women to have known difficult days. It is comforting to
realize that others before us have persevered and prospered.

During the dark days of the Great Depression an editorial in the October 1932 issue of *Ladies' Home Journal* encouraged readers to remember
that "The return of good times is not wholly a matter of money. There
is a prosperity of living which is quite as important as prosperity of the
pocketbook." But the magazine stressed that "It is not enough to be willing to make the best of things as they are. Resignation will get us nowhere.
We must build what amounts to a new country. We must revive the ideals
of the founders. We must learn the new values of money. It is a time for
pioneering—to create a new security for the home and the family...Where
we were specialists in spending, we are becoming specialists in living."

I remember the exact moment when I found that quote. I was mining my acre of diamonds: seated on the floor of an antique shop perusing
women's periodicals from the past for hints on how to live successfully
today. I had been on the *Simple Abundance* path for a year and felt like a
pioneer. In fact, I felt exactly like a woman who had packed up her family
and all her worldly possessions in Boston to start across country in a covered wagon in search of the Promised Land. For two thousand miles I had
kept the dream of a better life alive while enduring epidemics, drought,
blizzards, tornadoes, snakes, and salted beef. By this time, I was in the
Nebraska Territory with a thousand more miles to go, but I had come
too far to turn back. Like that pioneer woman, I was discouraged and
exhausted. When I found that magazine, I immediately embraced it as a
telegraph message to my soul. "Keep going. Don't stop. You're on the right
path and you are not alone." From that moment, I have never looked back,
and my exhaustion was transformed into creative energy. I learned firsthand that the *Simple Abundance* path has the power to transform lives.

Are you ready to become a pioneer? Then it's time to invest your soul
with all the creative energy at your disposal. Think of me as your scout,
your own personal pathfinder. I've gone ahead and cleared brush from
the trail. This much I'll tell you at the outset. The path spirals and takes
time—it will take us a year—but it is comforting and nurturing. It can
also be undertaken only one day at a time. Don't be afraid. We are not

alone. Like pioneers on the trail, we will learn to live by our own lights and the stars of heaven, for that is all we need. There is no obstacle that true grit and Amazing Grace cannot overcome.

JANUARY 28

The Golden Mirror Meditation

Almost always it is the fear of being ourselves that brings us to the mirror.

—Antonia Porchia (1885–1968)
Argentinian poet

For years I have used a special meditation I call the golden mirror meditation. I visualize in my mind an enormous mirror the size of a room, with an elaborately carved, 24-karat gold frame. This is my materializing mirror. Those dreams I wish to materialize in my life are first viewed here.

Now let me share with you an amazing coincidence that a French proverb would suggest is "God's way of remaining anonymous." After I had been doing the golden mirror meditation for about a year, I was invited on an all-expenses-paid business trip to Dublin, one of my favorite cities. I was to stay at one of Dublin's oldest, most beautiful, and expensive hotels, the Shelbourne, where I had never been before. When I arrived at the hotel and walked into the lounge, what should I see but the physical manifestation of my daily meditation: a beautiful mirror with a gold-leaf frame that was so large it took up an entire wall of the lounge. I laughed with delight when I saw my reflection in it, for here was the Universe's way of demonstrating to me that whatever we visualize in our minds can come to pass in the physical world.

Today, find a few minutes to get quiet and journey within. Close your eyes. Visualize a beautiful, large golden mirror surrounded by shimmering white light. This light is Love and it surrounds you, enfolds you, enwraps you, and protects you. Look into the mirror. Do you see the reflection of an extraordinary woman? She is beautiful and radiant. She possesses a strong, healthy, vibrant aura. Her eyes are sparkling, and she is smiling warmly at you. Do you know who this woman is? You feel as if you have known her all your life. And you have. She is your Authentic Self. Spend a few moments with her now. What is she doing? How is she doing it? Visit her as often as you like. She is waiting to help you find your way as you make the journey of self-discovery.

There are days when we all fear the harsh glare of the looking glass, but there is never a time when you should hesitate to encounter the woman in the golden mirror. She is the highest reflection of your soul, the embodiment of the perfect woman who resides within and she sends you Love to light your path.

Accepting Real Life

Everything in life that we really accept undergoes a change.
—Katherine Mansfield (1888–1923)
New Zealand modernist short story writer

Accepting and blessing our circumstances is a powerful tool for transformation. In fact, this potent combination is a spiritual elixir that can work miracles in our lives.

What is acceptance? Acceptance is surrendering to what is: our circumstances, our feelings, our problems, our finances, our work, our health, our relationships with other people, the delay of our dreams. Before we can change anything in our life, we have to recognize that this is the way it's meant to be *right now*. For me, acceptance has become what I call the long sigh of the soul. It's the closed eyes in prayer, perhaps even the quiet tears. It's "all right," as in "All right, You lead, I'll follow." And it's "all right," as in "Everything is going to turn out all right." This is simply part of the journey.

Over the years I have discovered that much of my struggle to be content has arisen when I stubbornly resisted what was happening in my life now. But I have also learned that when I surrender to the reality of a situation—when I don't continue to resist but accept—a softening in my soul occurs. Suddenly I can open to receive all the goodness and abundance available to me because acceptance brings with it so much relief and release. It's as if the steam of struggle has been allowed to escape from life's pressure cooker.

What happens when we accept our circumstances? Well, first, we relax. Next, we change our vibration, our energy pattern, and the rate of our heartbeat. Once again, we're able to tap into the boundless positive energy of the Universe. Acceptance also illuminates reality so that we're better able to see the next step. Whatever situation exists in your life right now, accept it. Natalie Goldberg, the world-renowned writing instructor and author of *Writing Down the Bones*, believes that "Our task is to say a holy yes to the real things of our life as they exist." Cast a glance around and acknowledge what's going on. This is my tiny kitchen with the dirty floor, this is how much I weigh, this is my checking account balance, this is where I work. This is what is really happening in my life now. This is okay. This is real life.

Today, let go of the struggle. Allow the healing process of change to begin.

You're ready to move on. To begin again.

JANUARY 30

Blessing Our Circumstances

Bless a thing and it will bless you. Curse it and it will curse you...
If you bless a situation, it has no power to hurt you, and even if it
is troublesome for a time, it will gradually fade out, if you sincerely
bless it.

—Emmet Fox (1886–1951)
Early twentieth-century New Thought
spiritual leader

All faiths have shared one type of invocation for Heaven's intercession, and it's known as a "blessing." Very often, the thanksgiving spoken before a meal is also called a "blessing." However, most of us are under the impression that it is only clergy who can offer blessings, but that is not the case.

Since ancient times, a blessing has been considered an invisible cloak of Divine protection, good fortune, health, and wealth. "Traditionally in Ireland, the act of blessing was not separate from daily life," the Celtic poet and mystic John O'Donohue tells us in *To Bless the Space Between Us,* his book on retrieving the lost art of blessings for solace in today's hectic and chaotic world. "What is a blessing? A blessing is a circle of light drawn around a person to protect, heal, and strengthen. Life is a constant flow of emergence. The beauty of blessing is our belief that it can affect what unfolds... When we bless, we are enabled somehow to go beyond our present frontiers and reach into the source. A blessing awakens future Wholeness. We use the word *foreshadow* for the imperfect representation of something that is yet to come. We could say that a blessing 'forebrightens' the way. When a blessing is invoked, a window opens in eternal time."

In my own spiritual journey, I have discovered how the power of blessings—my spoken word—over a perplexing situation or disheartening undertaking has often changed the outcome of circumstances. However, the first step is any blessing is always first accepting my circumstances, no matter how difficult or unfair the situation seems. Then I must bless the misery facing me.

That's right.

Through gritted teeth if necessary. Usually we don't know why something has occurred and we won't know until there's enough distance to take a backward glance. Maybe never. However, blessing whatever vexes us is the spiritual surrender that can change even troublesome situations for the better. Blessing the circumstances in our lives also teaches us to trust. Over the years my easiest and most joyous lessons have been learned through blessing. If you're sick and tired of learning life's lessons through pain and struggle, blessing your difficulties will show you there's a better way. I'm so convinced about the enormous power of our words that when I hear something I don't want to, I've been known to shout out loud: "I'm calling you a blessing! I'm calling you a blessing" as many times as I need to in order to calm down.

A powerful set of blessings that I learned from the teachings of Stella Terrill Mann, a Unity minister who wrote during the 1940s, encourages us to greet the morning with the affirmation "Blessed be the morn for me and mine." At noon declare, "Blessed be the day for me and mine," and in the evening, invoke this prayer: "Blessed be the night for me and mine." As you go about your work at home or in the office, affirm, "My work is a prayer for good for me and mine." These affirmations of good will bring many blessings into your daily life, as they have in mine.

Start to count your blessings. Start today. Literally. Make a spiritual inventory of all your blessings. See if you can't get to one hundred. So much good happens to us, but in the rush of daily life we fail even to notice or acknowledge it. Writing it down focuses our attention on the abundance already within our grasp and makes it real.

JANUARY 31

Working with What You've Got

If your everyday life seems poor, don't blame it; *blame yourself; admit to yourself that you are not enough of a poet to call forth its riches; because for the creator there is no poverty and no poor indifferent place.*

—Rainer Maria Rilke (1875–1926)
Twentieth-century German poet

Up until now many of us have secretly believed that we had to wait until things calmed down a bit before we started to get our acts together.

Tomorrow we'll begin discovering authentic pleasures. Tomorrow we'll treat ourselves better. Tomorrow we'll take the time to enjoy ourselves. Tomorrow, when everything calms down. Well, this I can report from the trenches of the front lines: Life *never* calms down long enough for us to wait until tomorrow to start living the lives we deserve.

Life is always movement, always change, always unforeseen circumstances. There will always be something trying to grab your attention: the phone, the child, the email or text alert, the deadline, the car breaking down, the check that never arrives in the mail. Let's just acknowledge that as far as real life is concerned, we are only one step away from dealing with dysfunction.

So what are we going to do about it? We can stop waiting for life to become perfect and start working with what we've got to make it as satisfying as we can. We can accept, bless, give thanks, and get going.

Today, we can begin to call forth the riches from our everyday life. Today we can move from lack to abundance. Procrastination has robbed us of too many precious opportunities. Call a friend for lunch, begin to read or even write that novel, organize your papers, try a new recipe for dinner, smile at everyone you meet, sit and dream before a blazing fire, pick up your needlepoint again, act as if you're grateful to be alive, scatter joy.

Think of one thing that would give you a genuine moment of pleasure today and do it. Great! The first steps in the journey are always the most difficult to take. "Life begets life. Energy creates energy," the legendary Victorian French actress Sarah Bernhardt reminds us. "It is by spending oneself that we become rich."

EMBRACING JOYFUL SIMPLICITIES

Year by year the complexities of this spinning world grow more bewildering and so each year we need all the more to seek peace and comfort in the joyful simplicities.
—Woman's Home Companion, December 1935

As we become curators of our own contentment on the *Simple Abundance* path, one of the great payoffs is that we start to seek peace and comfort in the Joyful Simplicities. Little things begin to mean a lot to us. Joyful Simplicities nourish body and soul by engaging our senses. They teach us how to live in the present moment. Life comes together when we seek out the Sublime in the ordinary.

We all have days in our lives that are marked by great moments of rejoicing and celebration: The baby is born, the promotion comes through, the new apartment rental agreement is signed, the wedding vows are made and cheered. But life is not an endless round of cake and champagne. There's a lot of drudgery to most of our days: sheets to be changed, dry cleaning to pick up, garbage to put out. To keep our daily round from being all drudgery, we've got to savor the art of the small: discovering diminutive delights that bring us peace and pleasure.

In 1949, the British playwright J. B. Priestley gathered together such moments in a book of essays entitled *Delight*. Among his favorites: waking in the morning to the smell of coffee, eggs, and bacon; reading detective stories in bed; suddenly doing nothing in the middle of the day; buying books; and enjoying the company of (instead of just tolerating) small children.

It's a winter's day. Can you make a pot of homemade soup for supper? If not tonight, then this weekend? I relish this Joyful Simplicity once a week during the winter. Chopping, paring, and scraping are very calming activities. Really look at the colors of the vegetables—the orange of the carrots, the bright green celery, the pearly white onion. You have a beautiful still life in front of you. Don't rush through the process but enjoy the *mindfulness*, or the Zen, of cooking. Isn't the fragrance of homemade soup wonderful? It makes you glad to be alive or at least at your own house for dinner.

Can you see how we must seize the essence of life, while we have it? We must embrace every moment. "People need joy quite as much as clothing. Some of them need it far more," Margaret Collier Graham, a California short story writer, observed in 1906. Today, make discovering those Joyful Simplicities that bring you personal comfort and make your well-being one of your highest priorities.

Joyful Simplicities for January

It is winter proper; the cold weather, such as it is, has come to stay. I bloom indoors in the winter like forced forsythia; I come in to come out. All night I read and write, and the things I have never understood become clear; I reap the harvest of the rest of the year's planting.

—Annie Dillard
American Pulitzer Prize–winning author

☞ When you want to make a personal change, try planting some spring bulbs indoors to bloom on the edge of a sunny window. Mix miniature daffodils, paper whites, hyacinths, and tulips—to brighten your spirits and home with color and fragrance. Stake them with the new good habit you desire and watch both the habit and the bulb grow.

👉 Serve a traditional New Year's Day dinner of Hoppin' John: black-eyed peas (for luck), rice (for health), collard greens (for prosperity), baked ham, and cornbread (for delicious eating!). I make a scrumptious winter salad of cooked black-eyed peas, diced green and red peppers, and red onion dressed in a French vinaigrette, which is served at room temperature.

👉 Go through your personal papers at home and organize your desk to get a fresh start on the new year. Discard as much as you can. Hang your new calendars on the wall. Try to make your personal space at home where you do paperwork as inviting as possible.

👉 Visit an art supply shop if there is one nearby and simply look around. Take in all the different ways that you can begin to express yourself: in vivid color, on paper, canvas, in clay. If you can't find my *Simple Abundance Journal of Gratitude* or *The Illustrated Discovery Journal: Creating a Visual Autobiography of Your Authentic Self* pick up a black-bound spiral artist's notebook to use for your collage therapy.

👉 If you're truly devoted to Pinterest, print out images that resonate with you and use them in your collages. Use search words that speak to your design aesthetic, or emotions that you are feeling, or places that bring you peace. Look at other artists' work and see what media they use to express themselves.

👉 Use acrylic magnetic picture frames to create a gratitude collage for your refrigerator. Place in them photographs of those you love and are grateful for, such as family, friends, and pets. Also, reminders of the little things you're thankful for, like the car repair bill that was less than you had anticipated. Or create a bulletin board for your Gratitudes, and as the seasons change take them down and place them in an album. When New Year's Eve rolls around, glance through all your blessings. This is a marvelous ritual, because we lose sight of our blessings so quickly. If there's something you particularly want to have come into your life, place a picture of it here and give thanks for it ahead of time.

👉 Prepare for a winter's idyll. Stock the pantry with real cocoa, tiny marshmallows, and a bar of good chocolate (for a shaved-chocolate topping). Get some whipped cream and keep it in the refrigerator. Prepare your pleasures so you can take time to enjoy them over a quiet weekend or if you're lucky to have an unexpected day off. When snow comes and you're home, lounge about in your pajamas. If you're lucky enough to have a fireplace, keep the fire stoked all day. If you have "littles" living or staying with you, build a snowman together, go sledding, then have tomato soup in mugs and toasted cheese sandwiches for lunch. Afterward, take a nap.

🖎 Yes, you can find the most unbelievable bargains online, but if there's a great local thrift store nearby, go there. Every woman needs a great thrift store in her repertoire.

🖎 Bake a pan of dense, dark, moist gingerbread for after-school tea with the children or for dessert. Read Laurie Colwin's delightful *More Home Cooking: A Writer Returns to the Kitchen*. Laurie's most important tip is not to use ordinary molasses. Instead she "wholeheartedly" recommends C. S. Steen Syrup Mill of Abbeville, Louisiana. The company is over a hundred years old. Visit them on the web (http://www.steensyrup.com/links.html). British cooks can use Lyle's Golden Syrup, available at British food websites.

🖎 Browse through gardening blogs this month. Cut out your favorite flowers and create your ideal garden on paper. If your passion is for an herb garden, indulge in creating a gardening collage and keep it in your *Illustrated Discovery Journal*. Pretend you're creating a secret garden for solitary sojourns. What does it look like? What gardening accessories and furniture appeal to you? Add them to your collage. Let your fantasies come to life on paper first.

🖎 Why not make a wish list to restock the pantry with deliciousness when you next make it to the market? Winter days can be celebrated with seasonal sweet and savory treats: steel-cut oats porridge, waffles with warm blueberry syrup, pancakes with orange-flavored butter, brioche French toast, hot cinnamon buns in the middle of the afternoon, café au lait, spiced cocoa, mugs of consommé, lemon verbena tisanes, stout pots of new-to-you tea and crumpets, glass tumblers of glogg, hot buttered rum or hot whiskey toddies redolent of lemon and cloves and guaranteed to cure whatever ails you. Let us remind ourselves to gracefully receive the flavors of winter and count our blessings.

FEBRUARY

China tea, the scent of hyacinths, wood fires and bowls of violets—
that is my mental picture of an agreeable February afternoon.
　　　　　　　　　—Constance Spry (1886–1960)
　　　　　　　　　　　Legendary British floral designer and author

February arrives cold, wet, and gray, her gifts disguised for only the most discerning spirits to see. Gentle is our path. Gratitude is the thread we weave into the fabric of our daily lives this month, giving thanks for our simply abundant lives and asking for the gift of one thing more: grateful hearts.

The Authentic Self Is the Soul Made Visible

You never find yourself until you face the truth.
— Pearl Bailey (1918–1990)
American actress and singer

When I suddenly begin to weep as I write, I know that I'm getting close to the wondrous truth of my assignment. Inadvertently my subconscious scrawl has hit a deeply hidden psychic sciatic nerve. I've got no choice but to go on and go deep, the way a deep-tissue masseuse will work on a painful knot of stress energy trapped in our backs or shoulders.

"The line of words fingers your own heart" is how the incomparable Pulitzer Prize–winning author Annie Dillard describes the process of releasing truth while writing. "It invades arteries and enters the heart on a flood of breath; it presses the moving rims of thick valves; it palpates the dark muscle...feeling for something, it knows not what."

As I knead my own nerve steadily, I chance upon a gnarled knot from the past—suppressed sorrows, calcified regrets, shards of remorse—entangled and embedded, buried deep in my heart's cavity. I tap the keys, my prose probing close to memory just as the masseuse kneads my shoulder with the palms of her hands. Something I've been resisting is struggling to be heard.

Making the absolute best of ourselves is not an easy task. It is a pleasurable pursuit, it is the reason we were born, but it requires spiritual moxie, the quixotic blending of passion, patience, persistence, and perseverance. For many of us it also requires prayer. That's because we find it far easier to learn to live by our own lights when we access a Higher Source of Power to illuminate our path. The American creativity teacher, author, and artist Julia Cameron calls this switching on "spiritual electricity" that transcends our own limitations.

In my own journey I have found this to be very true. Usually I limited the times I requested that the Power be turned on for the occasions when I was appearing in public: giving workshops, lecturing, holding business meetings. Then it occurred to me this was like living in a house with electricity but turning on the lights only for a couple of hours every few months. And I wondered why I was frequently bumping into obstacles?

So I started to ask for the Power to be switched on in my daily life: as a mother, a writer, an artist, and a friend. When I asked, it was turned on. When I didn't, I stayed in the dark. You don't have to be a master electrician to understand what's going on here: Someone must turn on the switch. Asking is the only way to activate spiritual electricity. When there is Light, we see remarkably well. We see with clarity. And what we can see if we look deep within is that *the Authentic Self is the Soul made visible.*

Your Authentic Self is your Soul made visible to the world.

I remember the day that spiritual truth pushed through my creative resistance. Up until then I was under the impression that *Simple Abundance* was a book about eliminating clutter from our lives.

I'd casually glanced at the page currently coming from the printer and was jolted by a sentence I hadn't remembered writing. I felt a shock, like static electricity, which I now call creative energy. To put it simply, the Great Creator and the work in progress, which became *Simple Abundance,* were having an editorial meeting without me.

The Authentic Self is the Soul made visible.

As I began to ponder this unexpected detour, I realized that the clutter isn't only the objects that no longer serve us, but the clutter of other people's opinions: about our lives, our jobs, our partners, our wardrobes, our weight, our children, our decorating style. All the usual riff-raff we wade through every day just to get to a level playing field, to find space for our own thoughts. And you wonder why you're tired?

Don't try to remake yourself into something you're not. Just try making the best of what the Great Creator made in you. The sacred art of nurturing our soul is the artisanal craft of *Simple Abundance.* Begin today by flipping the switch to turn on the Light.

FEBRUARY 2

Beginning to See the Light

We don't get offered crises, they arrive.
—Elizabeth Janeway (1913–2005)
American author and feminist

Since the Middle Ages, February 2 has been known as Candlemas day, an ancient European feast day when candles were blessed and sent home with parishioners so that Divine Light could guide their earthly steps.

Prudent country women would also do a midwinter inventory of their Caution Closets, which included the pantry and larder where the preserved, pickled, and potted were stored, as well as homemade tinctures, medicinals, and remedies. However, the most important items at this midwinter point were the beeswax candles because it was still dark before dawn and everyone dressed by candlelight. Midwinter's darkness would continue for several more months.

Of course, in America, today is known as Groundhog Day, when the legendary groundhog Punxsutawney Phil crawls out from his den searching for his shadow. If he sees himself, it will be six more weeks of winter; if he doesn't, it will be an early spring. Either way, there's a good chance that another big storm is headed our way, whether it be snow, sleet, or a nor'easter.

And what do you know, we've just lost the power again.

Wouldn't it be fabulous to walk to our own Caution Closet and put our hand on the candles and matches, not to mention the camping lanterns and a fully charged battery for all our personal electronic devices? Wouldn't it just.

"The great crises of life are not, I think, necessarily those which are in themselves the hardest to bear, but those for which we are least prepared," Mary Adams wrote in her 1902 self-help manual *Confessions of a Wife*. It seems astonishing to think that over a century later her very apt observation of being unprepared for a crisis resonates in many women's hearts. At least it does in mine.

Why?

Let's see. It's a typical weekday morning. As the coffee brews we anxiously listen to the news for what's happened overnight, recalibrate our way to work based on weather and traffic reports, while checking email for anything that "just can't wait." Like a mother prairie dog poking her head out of the burrow, instinctively measuring the vibrations of miles to minutes before the buffalo stampede, we simultaneously ignore and respond to this vague but increasing urgency to be prepared.

But our dogged determination to shrug it off wins again, and in our rush to get out the door, we can't hear, never mind decipher, the spiritual dots and dashes of our soul's Morse code: *Get Ready.* So we begin to feel this confusing unease in our body as a "fight or flight" response, even as we're standing alone in our kitchens.

Because the truth is, we are not prepared. We are not ready. For anything. We know this. We aren't prepared for a heart attack (the leading cause of death for women in their forties, fifties, and sixties). We aren't prepared for the raging wildfire, mudslide, sinkhole, tornado, earthquake, tsunami, or flash flood. We aren't ready for two weeks of downed power lines when the entire family is snowed in without heat, electricity, or food during the "storm of the century" which seems to occur awfully frequently these days.

Truth or Dare: If there was a pounding on your door right now and someone in a yellow emergency vest told you to evacuate your entire household in ten minutes because there was a dangerous gas leak nearby, how do you think you'd do?

I didn't do very well. Being the woman in her nightgown rolling one screeching cat in a carrier down the street while desperately looking for the two missing ones is not among my most cherished visions of myself. It was hard to tell who was more relieved when the all-clear was signaled, the gas man or my daughter, on the receiving end of my sobbing cell phone call.

Yes, the world is frightening and seems to become more so each day. Our emotional equilibrium is continually in free fall. But could our lack of emergency preparedness skills also explain why we awaken exhausted, remain on edge, and are more prone to imagine difficulties than before? I think so. And it's because we know we're not prepared.

Consider this: We are the *first* generation of women since Eve left the garden to be *completely* dependent on outside sources for our survival—power grids, communication, food, clean water, first aid, medicine, transportation, shelter.

I'm not trying to panic you. But the unpredictable has shown its face too many times for us not to be wary. I've come to believe deeply that Emergency Preparedness 101 is a sacred imperative for whatever extreme rite of passage each of us may face, either alone or with loved ones expecting us to behave as if we're Mother Courage.

It takes basic skills to become our own First Responders, ready for the next crisis. We need to have a plan and supplies in place so we can evacuate if necessary or completely cope at home for at least several days.

Here's what I've learned and share with the seeker in you. Being scared is a *sacred* warning signal triggered to keep you and yours out of harm's way. Just change the position of the letters "a" and "c" and *scared* becomes *sacred*. Being scared is a primordial instinct meant to keep you alive in dangerous situations until you can get the hell out of them. Think of it as a spiritual shortwave radio frequency processed through a woman's sixth sense—your intuitive sense of Knowing. The more scared I am about any situation or circumstance, the more imperative it is for me to acknowledge it, face it, and learn how to push through to overcome it.

My prime directive now (and here's your invitation to join me) is to become the calmest, most capable woman during any challenge or crisis in which we could find ourselves. The more chaos that surrounds us, the calmer we'll become—anyplace, anytime, anywhere. And then, when we believe in ourselves, when we trust in Spirit and our strength to rise to any occasion and when we *know* what needs to be done, we will be exactly the women that we would want to call upon in an emergency.

That's why this year, we're going to create a Caution Closet, calmly and methodically, with everything we might need "just in case." I feel better already. I hope you do, too. Blessings on our courage.

The World Is Too Much with Us

Change your life today. Don't gamble on the future, act now, without delay.

—Simone de Beauvoir (1908–1986)
French philosopher and feminist

The world is too much with us," the English Romantic poet William Wordsworth complained in 1807. "Getting and spending, we lay waste our powers." Two hundred years later, many women, including me, would agree with him. We're worn to a raveling, chronically exhausted from the "getting"—the amount of time, creative energy, and emotion spent juggling the demands of work and home. And this week, with the arrival of the holiday credit card bills, it seems as if we'll be paying our festive "spending" until summer.

However, despite all the doom and gloom that constantly assaults our senses, there is a way for us to ransom our lives and reclaim our futures: It consists in turning away from the world in order to recognize what in life makes us truly happy. For each of us, this will be different. But once we obtain this crucial inner knowledge, we will possess the ability to transform our outer world.

"You can live a lifetime and, at the end of it, know more about other people than you know about yourself," the pioneering aviatrix, race-horse trainer, adventuress, and author Beryl Markham (1902–1986) confessed in her stunning memoir, *West with the Night*. Even though she was the first person to fly solo nonstop across the Atlantic Ocean from east to west in 1936, Markham didn't give herself much credit for her astonishing achievement.

What about you? Do you rack up savvy accomplishments without acknowledging your wins as you pursue the next triumph? I know a woman like that. You might, too. She gives her personal best to everything and everyone from the moment she rolls out of bed each morning, but her self-confidence never registers any of her remarkable feats, and then she continually wonders why she feels so unfulfilled.

I don't suppose anyone's called you *self-centered* recently. Why would they? Most women, like ourselves, recoil from the thought of personal descriptions that even include the word *self*, which is too bad, because this self-effacing and self-defeating modesty eliminates a lot of flattering adjectives: self-poised, self-assured, self-accomplished. All the traits that we marvel at in other women. So why do we self-consciously shrink from self-admiration?

Probably because ever since our hands were slapped as we reached for the last cookie on the plate all those years ago, we've viewed satisfying our needs, desires, and wanderlust as selfish. But now that you're all grown up and ready to rediscover how amazing you really are, it's time to realize that the cheeks that once burned with embarrassment can now radiate with the vibrant glow of a self-possessed woman.

Today, I am going to ask you to deliberately turn away from the world—deep breath here—but only for a week. Shun the glossy magazines, websites, and media outlets. Wean yourself from the opinions of others—however talented, creative, and celebrated they may be—including your favorite blogs or Instagram influencers. There's a fine line between those becoming corrosive intravenous drips and their being sources of renewal and inspiration.

Here's a provocative thought worth pondering: Why are social media posts called "feeds" when what they often do is starve our souls?

Ask yourself this every time you're tempted to look. And trust me, you will be. Instead, for the next week, be willing to absorb the shock that comes after you realize that many of your preferences and opinions aren't really your own. By osmosis you've unconsciously adopted other people's points of view.

Begin to listen for the whispers of your Authentic Self. What do you *really* want to be doing? The next choice you make, step you take, task or urge you follow may come from something as simple as clearing your desk to find that buried adult extension course brochure. Weren't you interested in botanical drawing or discovering more about French art deco design? Sign me up with you. Learning something new every week is such a glorious gift. Starting in this New Year we're going to play that game. Why, we've already started. For only when the clamor of the outside world is silenced will you be able to hear the Deeper Vibration. Listen carefully. Spirit's playing your song.

FEBRUARY 4

Becoming Mrs. Miniver

*Certain films—like certain lovely people, glorious works of art
or music, and special instances of prayer—seem a grace expressly
given for our edification.*
—Marsha Sinetar
Author, educator, and Christian contemplative

Have you ever lost yourself so completely in a book or a movie that
you became part of it? Something about the story, the writer's voice, the
heroine, or the conversations in the dialogue struck a profound mystical
chord in you.

However, when millions of people around the world have the very
same reaction, it is the work of Spirit, even if it springs from a human
heart, mind, and hands. The 1942 Oscar-winning English wartime
saga *Mrs. Miniver* starring Greer Garson is such a Divine inspiration
for me. It depicts an English middle-class family's heroic efforts to preserve what was precious in their daily life as they learn to cope during
wartime.

Mrs. Miniver is the embodiment of a sacred archetype of a woman
defending her family and home from all danger through her faith, intelligence, strength, courage, determination, unshakeable optimism, and
love. And she's such a powerful heroine because each of us can see ourselves in that role.

I met Kay Miniver after September 11, 2001. At that time, I had an
apartment in New York and my daughter, Kate, had just enrolled in
New York University. As America reverberated from the shock of terror
on our own shores, I was frequently asked to give advice and comfort
to other women. But I felt so inept. Secretly I needed a woman in my
life whom I could emulate, one who possessed "repose of the soul." I
needed a grown-up heroine to help me remember what mattered most:
making a safe haven in a scary and tumultuous world for my daughter
and myself. That's when Mrs. Miniver and I found each other.

I want to share my love of Mrs. Miniver because she has inspired
me to create a Caution Closet for emergency preparedness. Preparing for the unexpected is a task I've known I should tackle, but every
time I'd tried, the plethora of disaster scenario books would scare the
heebie-jeebies out of me. Instead, I'd watch *Mrs. Miniver*. Finally, I
made the connection between my role model and the Caution Closet.
And "Becoming Mrs. Miniver" became my metaphor and mantra. I'll
be invoking her wisdom and calm presence throughout the coming
months, and I know she'll become a great friend of yours, too. At the

end of every month from here on out, you'll find a meditation called "Do Try This at Home," which will focus on one aspect of our Caution Closets' preparation.

Start by watching the movie *Mrs. Miniver,* directed by William Wyler, which is available on many movie streaming sites. However, before Greer Garson so beautifully embodied Mrs. Miniver on the screen, she was the figment of English journalist Jan Struther's domestic reveries, written anonymously and featured in the London *Times* between 1937 and 1939. Known for her stylish prose, witty poems, and modern hymns, Jan had been asked by her editor to write "about an ordinary sort of woman who leads an ordinary sort of life—rather like yourself."

Charm makes everyone feel better, and during this time, threats of war were daily headlines in Britain. English readers adored Mrs. Miniver's musings about the little things in her daily round because it mirrored their own. As one reader said, Mrs. Miniver was the only cheerful and bright bit in the papers.

Nothing in Mrs. Miniver's life was too insignificant that it couldn't become an uplifting source of reflection, revelation, or renewal, and she reminded readers how much they had to be grateful for in the small particulars of their (and our) everyday epiphanies: the familiar route to a holiday home; unread library books to look forward to; the comforting feel of the banister beneath your hands as you climbed the stairs; having another's hand to hold and eye to catch at a dinner party; the small indentation at the nape of your child's neck, so perfect for a quick kiss; the pang of parting from the old family car; finding the perfect calendar to give pleasure throughout the year; the notches on the nursery door as the children grew; a hat with a floppy bow; the mingling scent of roses and a fire in the hearth; crumpets for tea on a rainy afternoon; choosing beer over wine if on a budget.

But even in her readers' darkest hours, Mrs. Miniver's repose of the soul was a comfort in between the lines. By September 1940 at least two million British children and pregnant women had been evacuated from London to escape the nightly German bombing campaign that lasted nine months. Here Mrs. Miniver is preparing to evacuate what's left of her beautiful home so that her children would be out of danger. As Mrs. Miniver thought to herself: "Another thing they had gained was an appreciation of the value of dullness. As a rule, one tended to long for more drama, to feel that the level stretches of life between it, a waste of time. Well, there had been enough drama lately. They had lived through seven years in as many days; and Mrs. Miniver, at any rate, felt as though she had been wrung out... She was tired to the marrow of her mind and heart, let alone her bones and ear-drums; and nothing in the world seemed more desirable than a long wet afternoon at a country vicarage with a rather boring aunt."

Fifty years after Mrs. Miniver comforted the brave and courageous women of the British and American home front, Greer Garson recalled that "Like the whiff of a certain perfume wafted from an earlier period of one's life" Mrs. Miniver brings back a time when the Western world was in turmoil. "It was suddenly a world of quiet heroism, compassion, faith, and all the best in the human character—the world, in other words, of Mrs. Miniver—summoned to combat the worst... Bless Mrs. Miniver with her unpretentious ways, her resolute serenity, her matter-of-fact courage and humor. She shows us a pretty good view of human nature. Welcome back. We need you. And we do enjoy you."

FEBRUARY 5

Discovering Your Authentic Self

To love oneself is the beginning of a life-long romance.
—Oscar Wilde (1854–1900)
Anglo-Irish poet, playwright, and legendary
raconteur

One of the surprises that comes when you catch glimpses of your Authentic Self is the discovery that she's such a positive, upbeat woman. She's always smiling. She's always calm. She's always reassuring. She exudes confidence. Who is this woman, you might ask, and does she bear any resemblance to you?

Yes and no. This is who you are on the inside. The real you. If you don't act this way all the time, and certainly I don't, it's probably because we're continually censoring ourselves unconsciously, anticipating another's disapproving opinion of us before we even make our choices. However, it's really our own censoring that frightens the heck out of us, but we'll handle our shadows another day.

The American spiritual teacher, author, and political activist Marianne Williamson believes this will come when we move past our understudy role to become the leading lady in our own lives. "When a woman falls in love with the magnificent possibilities within herself, the forces that would limit those possibilities hold less and less sway over her," she tells us in *A Woman's Worth*.

But occasionally we get glimmers of what it's like on this higher plane: on a good-hair day; when we've had eight hours of sleep; when we soar through a business meeting because we're thoroughly prepared; when we fit into last year's clothes; when we throw a great party, and everyone—including us—enjoys themselves immensely. When moments like these occur, we tend to think that all's right with the world. Everything just fell into place. What we don't realize is that all's right with ourselves. We're in the flow of life and loving it. *We're in place*: that special alignment when authenticity and reality merge into Wholeness.

But how do we tap into this spiritual energy source more often? How do we access the flow of life more frequently?

Meditation helps. So does separating every activity with a five-minute pause before we jump to the next item on our to-do list. Making a mini ritual for every coffee or tea break, so it really becomes a pause that refreshes. Trying to find new places to take a walk. Long soaks in scented baths using essential oils, washing our hair a day before it needs it, smiling at everyone we meet, being gentler with ourselves, especially in our self-talk monologues. Catching a stunning sunrise or a sublime sunset and allowing ourselves the length it takes to really see it. Petting an animal, playing with a child, discovering a new favorite cologne. Four pieces of chocolate and a new book, a hot water bottle at the bottom of the bed on a wintry night, having some small pleasure to look forward to every day, and being grateful for all of them. You see? There are more ways to tap into this feeling of joy and elevation than you thought.

But above all, be open to change. Welcome it. "Watch. Wait. Time will unfold and fulfill its purpose," Marianne Williamson advises. "While we wait, we must not go unconscious. We must think and grow. Rejoice and dream but kneel and pray. There is holiness in the air today; we are giving birth to goddesses. They are who we are, for they are us: friends, therapists, artists, businesswomen, teachers, healers, mothers. Start laughing, girls. We have a new calling."

FEBRUARY 6

Knowing What You Love

Perhaps loving something is the only starting place there is for making your life your own.
— Alice Koller
American philosopher and author

It should be straightforward, this knowing what we love. But it seldom is. After decades of letting other people influence us—social media, the magazines, our mothers, our sisters, our friends—we're going to have to go cold turkey. The only opinion that counts from now on is your own.

This week try an experiment. Plan to go on a browse in a home furnishings and decorative accessories shop. Go somewhere you've never been before, so that you're looking at everything with fresh eyes. What startles you, calls to you, excites you? Write it down in a small spiral notebook or on your phone, so you can keep it in your purse.

Is it a fragrance in the shop, or the shape of a teapot? Is it the music that you've never heard before, the colors of a hooked rug, the textures in an exquisite flower arrangement? You'll know what you love the moment you see it. It's that familiar "wow" reaction. Trust the impulse, capture the encounter, record the clues. These will be important later.

Then next week on another creative excursion, go window shopping (not to buy) at a new-to-you fashion boutique. You know, that place that always intrigues you, but you stay away from because it's too expensive. The spring collection should be on display now. See what's new. See what's you. Your spirit perks up at the sight of a goldenrod linen blazer. So why are you always dressed in black? A fabulous flowered georgette pleated skirt and tunic top wows you, but you always wear jeans because they're more practical. Maybe, just maybe, feeling gorgeous outweighs practicality. Be open to authentic aspirations.

Remember this is the year for asking questions. The most essential one we can ask is: What is it I truly love? Be patient. We're not going to overhaul our lives, our work, our homes, or our wardrobes in a week. Trust that your authentic life will unfold naturally and with grace.

FEBRUARY 7

Remaking Your Own World

I have made my world and it is a much better world than I ever saw outside.

—Louise Nevelson (1899–1988)
American sculptor

Many creation myths say it took only six days to make the world. It will take us a little longer to remake our own. But we can begin where Spirit did by declaring that there be Light to illuminate our journey of self-discovery.

The Quaker tradition teaches that this Light is within each of us. The Quakers, or members of the Religious Society of Friends, are a perfect example of individuals who manage the delicate balance of living in the world but not belonging to it. This is because they refuse to segment their lives into the Sacred and the secular. Instead, Quakers believe that all of life's daily experiences are spiritual in nature, from preparing a family meal to protesting political policy. The British writer George Gorman has observed that "the essence of Quaker spirituality is the certainty that everything we do has religious significance. It is not cutting ourselves off from life but entering deeply and fully into it."

Simplicity is the common thread that stitches together Quaker lives, homes, and dress. Their weekly worship service, or meeting, is a silent meditation. Rhythm, reverence, and reflection are their hallmarks. These touchstones can help us as well as we attempt to remake our personal world.

Restoring a sense of rhythm to our lives is the first step. How much rhythm do you have in your personal world? Children are not the only ones who need regular bedtimes, mealtimes, and quiet times. Their mothers do, too. Think of the steady, reassuring rhythm of the natural world—the ebb and flow of the tides, the recurring cycle of the four seasons, the monthly phases of the moon, and the daily progression from day into night. Rhythm needs to be the cornerstone in our personal world as well. All of us lead busy lives, some more frantic and frazzled than others. We need to learn where to draw the line and how to say no.

Today be willing to reflect quietly on the role that rhythm plays in your daily round. Your heart will always tell you what's working and what's not. Restoring rhythm to the way you conduct your affairs can bring you contentment and a sense of well-being that will nurture and sustain you when the cares of the world can't be left behind.

FEBRUARY 8

An Artist Is Someone Who Creates

Living is a form of not being sure, not knowing what next or how...
The artist never entirely knows. We guess. We may be wrong, but
we take leap after leap in the dark.
—Agnes de Mille (1905–1993)
American dancer and choreographer

Most of us feel more secure when we play it safe. We wear a string of pearls, for example, instead of the hand-painted glass beads we glimpsed and passed up at the craft fair. Yet it is precisely those red and purple glass beads around the neck of another woman that stop us dead in our tracks. "Wow," we mumble as we pass her on the street, "she looks fantastic." We also wonder how she knew she would.

She probably didn't. She just took a leap in the dark and trusted her instincts. She trusted her own sense of style. The necklace whispered,

"Try me!" and she listened. She played at living—in a small way, to be sure, but relevant all the same—by taking a chance.

Every day we're given chances to embrace the new. It could be serving focaccia at dinner tonight instead of garlic bread. It could be choosing a pair of floral socks instead of your usual black. You could choose a leopard print scarf or a bodacious pair of black fishnet booties that show off your beautiful ankles. I'm just saying you could.

While we're at it, let's prime the pump of your imagination. It could be trading in your messy bun for a chic French chignon. The difference will startle you. Miss Messy Bun may walk into the coffee shop, but when she walks out, they'll all be singing "Mademoiselle from Armentieres." That's because of a feminine interpretation of Sir Isaac Newton's third law of motion: For every action, there's an equal and opposite reaction. If you spend the time to master the French twist, you'll soon be adding lip color and a smoky eye. Maybe statement earrings. See where this is leading? Away from the bed-head and once more with wonder into the world she goes.

Psychologist Susan Jeffers suggests we "take a risk a day—one small or bold stroke that makes you feel great once you have done it." Today, take a real risk that can change your life: Start thinking of yourself as an artist and your life as a work-in-progress.

Works-in-progress are never perfect. But changes can be made to the rough draft during rewrites. Another color can be added to the canvas. The film's flow can be tightened during editing. Art evolves. So does life. Art is never stagnant. Neither is life. The beautiful, authentic life you are creating for yourself is your art. It's the highest art. "Since you are like no other being ever created since the beginning of time," the brilliant 1930s writer Brenda Ueland reminds us, "You are incomparable."

Hold that thought.

FEBRUARY 9

You Are an Artist

It takes courage to not only accept our limitations but embrace our potential.
    —Erwin Raphael McManus
    Author, futurist, and founder of MOSAIC
    church

Most of us feel uncomfortable thinking of ourselves as artists, but we are. We think artists write novels, paint pictures, choreograph ballets, act on Broadway, throw wet clay on a potter's wheel, shoot feature films, dress in black, drink absinthe, and line their eyes with kohl. And it's true, some do. But many more don't.

Each of us is an artist. An artist is merely someone with good listening skills who accesses the creative energy of the Universe.

When I'm in the process of writing a book, after flipping on the spiritual electricity, I pray to get out of my own way. After months of stoking embers, showing up every day at ten a.m., one morning I'll arrive at the computer, expecting nothing, and suddenly something erupts; I can literally sense the book hovering and swirling over my head.

But here's the thrilling part: If I raise my arm above my head it feels as if I can literally pull words down onto the page. It's magical and miraculous, but it's also the only way I know how to write. Remember, though, it can take months of methodical work to get this boiler blazing. Sometimes the entire day is rewriting one paragraph over and over. Or as Oscar Wilde so brilliantly admitted, "I spent all morning putting in a comma and all afternoon taking it out."

I also trust that "the Book" always knows more than I do. The hardest part of creating for any artist is trusting the Work, especially when the rest of the world doesn't.

"True creativity does not come easily," Erwin Raphael McManus tells us in *The Artisan Soul: Crafting Your Life into a Work of Art*. "Creativity is born of risk and refined from failure. If we are at the core both spiritual beings and creative beings, then the artisan soul is where we live when we have the courage to be our truest selves."

So it is with creating your authentic life. With every choice, every day, you are creating a unique work of art. Something that only you can do. Something beautiful and ephemeral. The reason you were born was to leave your own indelible mark on your personal world. This is your authenticity.

Today, accept that you are creating a work of art by making big and little choices between playing it safe and risking. Is there something you'd like to do that's new and different? Why not order an espresso at lunch, if you've never tried one? Savor the simplicity of goat cheese on sourdough olive toast for supper. Create a different music playlist for various moods or tasks. For example, I listen to movie soundtracks when I write, opera when I clean, and the Great American Songbook of Cole Porter, George Gershwin, Jerome Kern, as I putter around the house.

Or for something completely different, try St. Hildegard of Bingen's favorite brew, fennel tea, for an afternoon treat. Abbess, artist, author, composer, mystic, pharmacist, poet, theologian, and saint, St. Hildegard (1098–1179) wowed the Dark Ages. I'll have whatever she's sipping.

Each time you experience the new, you become receptive to inspiration. Each time you try something different, you let the Universe know you are listening. "This is the courage of the artisan—to know ourselves and be true to that knowledge," Erwin McManus explains. "The artisan rejects all that makes us false and takes the huge risk of being true. To embrace our authentic selves and live in that raw expression of being fully human is our greatest risk and our richest reward."

Trust your instincts. Believe your yearnings are blessings. Respect your creative urges. If you are willing to step out in faith and take a leap in the dark, you will discover that your choices are as authentic as you are. What is more, you will discover that your beautiful life *is* your art.

A Fresh Canvas Every Twenty-Four Hours

Another real thing! I am not dead yet! I can still call forth a piece of
soul and set it down in color, fixed forever.
—Keri Hulme
New Zealand poet and novelist

Before a painter begins a new work, she takes preparatory steps to get ready. She's probably made preliminary sketches of the scene she is trying to capture. She mixes her pigments to achieve the right colors. She's also prepared the canvas with a fixative coating called a primer, so that the paint will adhere to it. All of this takes time.

Of course, we don't see the preparations when we look at her completed work. We only see the entire vision. And as American abstract expressionist artist Helen Frankenthaler (1928–2011) once commented, "A picture that is beautiful or that works looks as if it was all made at one stroke. I don't like to see the trail of a brushstroke or a drip of paint."

Preparatory steps are necessary in all the arts. They are also necessary in life if we want to live authentically. Every twenty-four hours we are given a fresh canvas to prime, to make ready for the vision. Quieting our minds, carving out time to dream and express ourselves with our Gratitude and *Illustrated Discovery Journals*, becoming aware of our true preferences, and slowing down to concentrate on completing one task at a time—these are the preparatory steps we need to take if we wish to experience contentment. A trick of mine (as well as of makeup artists) is to use a makeup "primer" in the morning on my face both for psychic as well as physical reasons, as I announce to the mirror, "Okay—we're primed and ready to go."

Whatever preparation an artist takes in front of the mirror, canvas, dance barre, or in her heart is never in vain. For when we are in the flow of life, savoring the moment, the brushstrokes don't show. Today, don't rush through your inner preparations as you get ready to set down a piece of your soul on life's canvas.

FEBRUARY 11

Creating an Authentic and Artisanal Lifestyle

It's a funny thing about life; if you refuse to accept anything but the best, you very often get it.
—W. Somerset Maugham (1874–1965)
British playwright, novelist, and short story writer

It's far easier to live an elegant, beautiful life when you're not on a budget. When cash is readily available, you don't have to learn the lessons that delayed gratification teaches us. But having money does not guarantee that we live authentically. Or that we make artisanal choices. Nor does being surrounded by beautiful objects guarantee a lifetime of happiness. If you receive heartbreaking news, it's not more comforting to sob into a damask and silk-tasseled cushion.

When I was beginning the *Simple Abundance* path and started to wean myself from worldly distractions for several months by choosing not to read magazines and newspapers, or watch and listen to the news, and especially not to go shopping (except for groceries and essentials), the symptoms I experienced were like withdrawal pains. At times, I felt achy, shaky, and even dizzy. When this occurred, my Authentic Self would reassure my conscious self (who didn't think much of the new program) that I was undergoing a deep inner, transformative shift. I needed empty space to adjust.

For the first time in my life I was learning to differentiate between my needs and my wants, and this powerful lesson had to be mastered before I could move forward. I had to learn what I could live without. Whatever I needed I could budget for—in other words, I could have— but self-knowledge had to come first.

When you learn what you can live without, you are able to ask life for the very best because you possess the gift of discernment. You develop patience that enables you to wait gracefully and gratefully until the best arrives, because you know it will. You can create an authentic life for yourself and those you love because you are able to make conscious, well-crafted choices.

"Long afterwards, she was to remember that moment when her life changed its direction," the British author of fifty novels Evelyn Anthony (1926–2018) writes in *The Avenue of the Dead*. "It was not predestined; she had a choice. Or it seemed she had. To accept or refuse. To take one turning down the crossroads to the future or another."

Turning away from the world and toward your own happiness is the path of authenticity and the most important choice you will ever make. Keep going, my brilliant girl. You've got this!

FEBRUARY 12

Divine Discontent: Learning to Live by Your Own Lights

Discontent and disorder [are] signs of energy and hope not despair.
—Dame Cicely Veronica Wedgewood (1910–1997)
British historian

When we practice switching on the "spiritual electricity," what should we expect? More energy and inspiration, amazing and delightful coincidences, and the ability to accomplish goals with grace? Yes, certainly. That has, at least, been my experience.

But one thing you might not expect—the one thing that might throw you—is how dissatisfied you may suddenly feel when the Power is not present; when you are in the dark because you forgot to turn the switch on. Or to use your Gratitude Journal for the last few days. Or maybe you're doing both, but everything still seems to be rubbing you the wrong way.

The dissatisfaction you can feel manifests in various annoyances. Suddenly you don't like any room in your house. Decorating mistakes from past lives haunt you. Your clothes don't fit or look right on you anymore, not to mention all the clothes with tags still on them, untried for ages and stuffed in the back of the closet. Don't fret, we'll deal with that.

You're bored with the meals you're cooking. Or the same local takeout. You're sick of covering your head before opening the front hall closet for fear of what will tumble out. But worse, that expansive, even giddy hopefulness that came from starting to integrate Gratitude into your life gives way now to restless discontent. You didn't just roll out of the wrong side of the bed today, babe, you slept on the floor. You begin to think that the *Simple Abundance* path might work for some women, but it's not right for you.

Hold on.

The transformative process is working. Think of an adorable baby who loves to smile. Suddenly she's crying, cranky, and stuffing as many Cheerios as she can get her hands on into her mouth. Please put this child down for a nap. To your amazement she sleeps most of the afternoon and then again all through the night.

In the morning as you dress your happy little baby/big girl, you realize she's grown an inch overnight! The baby was going through a growth spurt, and those growing pains are real.

You're going through a spiritual and authentic growth spurt as well. I call it Divine Discontent. This is the grit of sand in the oyster that eventually creates the pearl. This creative second chance is when we come into our own. When we finally claim our own lives and wrestle our futures from fate. When we learn how to spin straw into gold. When we realize gratefully that we can live by our own lights if we access the Power.

"Discontent can be a blessing," Barrie Dolnick reassures us in her marvelous guide *Instructions for Your Discontent: How Bad Times Can Make Life Better.* "It is an intensely creative state that nags and pokes you to get yourself going and accomplish what you really want in life."

Ask for it. Claim it. Today.

FEBRUARY 13

Once Upon a Time You Trusted Yourself

Don't look down at your feet to see if you are doing it right. Just dance.

—Anne Lamott
American inspirational writer

Today, try to find a photograph of yourself when you were about ten. Make sure you're smiling. Put it in a pretty frame and place it on your dressing table, desk, or in your *Illustrated Discovery Journal* and look at it every day. Send love to that young girl.

Try to travel back in time and imagination. See yourself at ten: at home, at school, and at play. Where did you live? Can you see your house or apartment, and the street? Walk through the rooms in your childhood home. What did your bedroom look like? Did you share it with your sister? Did you have maple twin beds and white dot chenille bedspreads or Ikea bunk beds?

Who were your friends? Did you have a best pal? Who was she? What was your favorite color in the Crayola pack? Did you play a musical instrument? Put on backyard plays in the summer? What was your most treasured toy that you still love? Even if it sits on a shelf, instead of your bed.

What was your favorite book? *Nancy Drew, National Velvet? The Babysitters Club, Little House on the Prairie,* something by Judy Blume?

What were your favorite foods? What subject did you like best in fifth grade? Can you remember? Try to recall yourself at ten as you get ready to close your eyes at bedtime. See what you remember in the morning.

Have fun with this exercise, because age ten was probably the last time you trusted your instincts. You weren't bound to the opinions of your mother, your sister, or your friends because you had your own.

I remember watching my then ten-year-old daughter in the dressing room of a department store. It was a revelation. "No, that's not me," she'd frequently say as I brought her outfits to try on. With an assurance that I still envy, she reached for a tapestry vest and a black felt slouch hat. "There," she announced with satisfaction, "this looks like me." And she was right, beautifully so.

I remind myself that once upon a time, I trusted my instincts. You did, too. Once upon a time there weren't second and third guesses. It can be that way again. Play with me here, because discovering your authenticity is not a spectator sport.

Try to contact the girl you once were. She's all grown up now. She's your Authentic Self, and she's waiting to remind you how beautiful, accomplished, and extraordinary you really are. What's more, She's missed you as much as you've missed her.

FEBRUARY 14

The Great Romance

What if—what if Life itself were the Sweetheart?
—Willa Cather (1873–1947)
American Pulitzer Prize–winning novelist

Women often confuse love and romance. God knows I did, four decades and three marriages' worth. However, I've learned this crucial lesson now and will never again forget that while romance and love are frequently in each other's company, they're not the same. Think of love as emotion. Romance is its evocative expression.

Romance reveals the depth and breadth of a lover's feelings in a certain, tangible way. Love can be conveyed in an email, but when a woman receives a handwritten letter, she's being courted. The time it took, the glimpse of her name in another's handwriting—these are the things that make her heart beat faster. Or should you reveal the depth of your feelings to your sweetheart, and "Ditto" is the disappointing echo you hear back, you might have love, but you definitely don't have romance.

Women want and need love, but our constant craving is for romance. However, the most delicious midlife secret for a woman is the discovery that while love's tango might require two, living a deeply rewarding romantic life requires only one singular sensation: you.

"When you're living from the heart, every moment brings another chance to fall in love," the life coach and writer Martha Beck reminds us in *Finding Your Own North Star: Claiming the Life You Were Meant to Live*. Years ago, Martha found herself alone in Paris, but instead of feeling isolated, she almost swooned with enchantment. "Walking in the streets of Paris in a thin spring rain, breathing the smell of apple blossoms and coffee, I realized that you don't have to wait around for the perfect companion to have a richly romantic life. There are people who have relationships but no romance and there are those whose lives are full of romance even when they're not paired up."

If you want a romantic life, act as if you're in the throes of a passionate affair in your personal preparations. Every woman has her own secret ritual of beauty pleasures and indulgences when she's in love. Even if you're not sharing your fabulous *très soigné* self with another, surround yourself with the things that you love, so that your home is a sanctuary, not just a dwelling place.

Indulge in beautiful lingerie. Escape into armchair adventures, unusual sleuths, film noir. Reconsider red—lips, nails, shoes, walls. Slip on bangles and treat yourself to brioche. Curl your hair, cinch your waist. Remember that chocolate becomes you, so show off your curves. Find your perfect scent and don't start or end your day without it. Or find one for the daylight hours and one for your nights, and not only for you, but your home. Above all, be willing to learn how to become your own courtesan.

"The only thing you must do to live a deeply romantic life is to base every decision you make on love," Martha Beck tells us. "Self-love, love of others; love of ideas, activities, and places; love of smells, tastes, sights, sounds, and textures. Living this way brings romance into the smallest, most ordinary moments and leads to a lot of large and extraordinary ones."

A Woman with a Past

Women...are born three thousand years old.
—Shelagh Delaney (1938–2011)
British dramatist and screenwriter

During my twenties I lived in England, Ireland, and France. My primer on authenticity began when I had the blessed good fortune to meet one of the most amazing persons in the world, who became my first mentor, a true Renaissance woman who showed me the extraordinary hidden depths beneath my ordinary.

When I first encountered Cassandra, I was painfully trapped in an impenetrable shell of self-consciousness. Whenever I found myself lured by her gracious hospitality to dinner parties or country weekends, I would politely excuse myself after being introduced and seek refuge in an empty room far from the crowd. Eventually she'd come looking, only to discover me happily settled in an ample armchair before a cozy fire, my head buried in a book.

One night, after taking the book from my hand and before leading me back to the dining room, she drew out my social discomfort. I confessed a terror of exposing myself or risking ridicule in even the most casual conversations. Cassandra promised me that I need never worry about being uncomfortable in social situations again, if I could regale strangers with stories of daring, folly, and risks.

"Well, there are some wonderful books about Victorian women explorers in your library," I told her. "I'll see what I can find."

"*Find?*" she teased me with mock horror. "Sarah, you can only *borrow* other people's stories after you've started *living* your own. You must become your own heroine. Most people have lives crowded with incident but without purpose. You must start seeing each day as a blank page waiting to be filled up with amusing anecdotes, profound turning points, provocative choices, and pursuits of passion. The world adores storytellers but deplores those who refuse to live or tell their own stories."

Now some four decades later, I have certainly collected enough of my own stories to fill a dozen books, many of which I never thought I'd live through, never mind be able to tell the tale. I suppose those are really the most riveting in anyone's life. The close calls, great escapes, and the "Oh, you didn't really?"

I've been thinking about stories and storytellers quite a lot lately, especially since most of the storytellers I want to share with you, the Women with a Past whom I cherish, are no longer writing or living and their daring exploits have fallen through the cracks of domestic and literary history.

I don't know how successful you've been with learning to cherish yourself above all others. But that doesn't mean we can't join the Woman with a Past club, because along the way we've all racked up a past whether we wanted to or not; and what's more, we've all paid our dues.

There's nothing more alluring, intriguing, and romantic than being perceived as a Woman with a Past. Except, of course, knowing that you are one, which makes you glorious. Magnificent. Powerful, even if you'd still like to lose ten, twenty, or thirty pounds. A Woman with a Past has loved and been loved passionately. She celebrates her quirks, exults in her extravagances, feels secure in her own skin, faces down her fears, and learns to treasure her foibles. Because of that, she's grounded in the soul knowledge that there is no other woman like her. Never has been. Never will be.

Unlike the rest of us, a Woman with a Past does not secretly mourn a love lost, a love that could have defined her, or a love that she denied. She claims them all and honors even the unbidden gifts. The rest of us turn away from such loves all too often, especially the cringeworthy ones: the love that couldn't be returned, the love that frightened us, the love that challenged us, the love that would cost more than we were willing to pay, the love that bankrupted us, the love that was unconventional. And in discounting what once made our hearts beat faster, our cheeks flush, our knees weak, and tears flow, we rob ourselves of the grandeur of hard-earned, well-deserved wisdom.

This week ponder and ruminate on how full we might feel if we called back to ourselves and were grateful for a female confidante, worldly and wise, soulful and sincere, compassionate and calm, graceful and generous, who finds no fault and only seeks to comfort us. Call back your Woman with a Past, your Authentic Self.

"All the great blessings of my life/Are present in my thoughts today," the Civil War poet Phoebe Cary (1824–1871) reminds us. Let us hold this thought tenderly and let us hold on to each other profoundly, but most of all, let us hold on to our own true selves passionately and fiercely.

Loving Your Authenticity

A sobering thought: what if, right at this very moment, I am living up to my full potential?

—Jane Wagner
American writer, director, and producer

Take a deep breath, relax, and laugh. Jane Wagner is the comedic collaborator and partner of Lily Tomlin and the author (among many works) of *The Search for Signs of Intelligent Life in the Universe*; so her rhetorical question possesses both wisdom and irony, which is another definition for truth. Jane also points out that the "ability to delude yourself may be an important survival tool." She has a very good point.

The reassuring news is that you've not completely lived up to your potential or you wouldn't be drawn to this book. You're still striving, still dreaming, still yearning, still doing. *I'm* in the same boat, or I wouldn't be writing this book—again! We're both on an exhilarating adventure, but sometimes we need to remind ourselves not to look down.

We're both staring at a blank page right now. For all its glorious promise, this blank page is intimidating, especially since we're hoping to fill it with passion and purpose, love and longings, wisdom and, above all, a happy ending. We might not have an inkling as to how to begin or where we're headed, but today let's agree with Audrey Hepburn, who believed that nothing we set our heart, soul, and imagination to is impossible: "Why, the very word says 'I'm possible.' "

Buried Dreams

Who is this woman?
You know her better than yourself.
Except when you don't know her at all.
A wind sweeping through every part of your life.
Re-arranging even the past.

—John Peterman
American entrepreneur

It takes great love and courage to excavate buried dreams. Once we were going to set the world on fire. Remember? Today we all have our share of ashes, along with the memory of a few bright sparks, to show for our efforts. Our precious passions hidden in plain sight behind sighs and shrugs and the inevitable, "It doesn't matter."

Our dreams—how did we love and lose you? Let us count the ways: naïveté, good intentions, relinquishment, bitter failures, detours, disappointments, rejections, wrong choices, bad timing, bungled efforts, stupid mistakes, unforeseen circumstances, whims of fate, and missed opportunities. It's no wonder that we'll need courage to retrace our steps.

But as we find our way back to our Authentic Selves, we'll discover buried dreams waiting patiently for us to start over again.

A wise woman once advised me not to be a "would-be-if-I-could-be or a could-be-if-I-would-be. *Just be.*" And while I have learned that dreams need doing as much as they need being, I have learned that the being always comes first.

Today is a day for being. Be with those you love, be kind to yourself. Be with your own thoughts. Be quiet and call forth the dream you buried long ago. The ember is still glowing in your soul. See it in your mind, warm yourself tenderly in your heart. "The dream was always running ahead of one," the French-American novelist, poet, and diarist Anaïs Nin (1903–1977) confessed. "To catch up, to live for a moment in union with it, that was the miracle."

FEBRUARY 18

A Studio of Your Own

A woman must have money and a room of her own if she is to write fiction.

—Virginia Woolf (1882–1941)
Influential twentieth-century modernist writer

During my flush years, I enjoyed the great delight of being able to collect works of art that I discovered by casting a very wide net ranging from high school art school exhibitions to major auction house events, both in the United States and in Europe. This was an enormous source of pleasure for me; buying a young artist's work always brought great joy to both the artist and to me, and bidding on paintings that hadn't seen the light of day for decades at Christie's and Sotheby's was a thrill, too.

I rarely attended the auctions in person, because I'm a stay-in-the-background kind of gal and novice art collector. I also rarely bought art and collectibles for investment, which was a good thing, because those "sure things" always resulted in costly losses that left me shocked and incredulous. Another story for another day. But the things I bought for love and beauty—the art, antiques, and collectibles—have remained with me long after I needed to sell them, imparting in their fading traces valuable lessons and precious memories.

One of the paintings I rescued from oblivion was "buried" in a Sotheby's 1998 catalog for "Important European Paintings." These sales were usually filled with portraits of ancient Italian cardinals in their Roman Catholic red pomp; exotic looking women with long, dark hair, rounded bellies, translucent harem pants, and gold coin necklaces dripping between their abundant décolleté; and still life paintings of long tables displaying dead animals, fish, furs, and antlers. Just the type of paintings you'd love for the breakfast nook. If you've ever wondered where the art world's cloying clichés come from, look no further than the salons of European painters during the eighteenth and nineteenth centuries.

Ah, but *A Studio of Their Own* was a one of a kind. Painted in 1886 by a mysterious Elizabeth Pillard, it depicted eight Victorian women in a closed-door art studio, painting a black man dressed as an African chieftain. I had never seen anything like it—it was amazing and brought to life a slice of women's history so vibrantly. The camaraderie of the women, the buzz of creating, the feeling of liberation and escape behind a closed door.

It seemed a small picture, maybe a two-inch square in the catalog, so imagine my surprise when it required three strapping men to carry it into my small Maryland townhouse, with the freight charges from London doubling the purchase price. You see, I'd not bothered to check the size of the painting before bidding. So, my two-inch *Studio* in its massive gray wood frame ended up over seven feet long and equally high. It was enormous, and there was only one wall in the house just barely big enough to display it.

I thoroughly enjoyed my hours spent daily with these ladies and relished my feeble attempts to unravel the mystery of exactly who Elizabeth Pillard was. Was she English or French? Where, when, and how did she paint this gigantic, fascinating studio portrait? It had to be in a woman's art school because this wasn't something you dashed off on the back porch after hanging the laundry. Even after searching for several years, I never found out more about her. Then the trajectory of my life changed, and I moved to England. *Studio* was sold again at auction (I always hoped to a museum), and if any of you ever find it, please drop me a line and let me know where she reigns.

Virginia Woolf was only four when Elizabeth Pillard painted *A*

Studio of Their Own, but artist studios were popular subjects during the Victorian decades of Virginia's formative years and she was born into an intellectual family. For many years the influential art magazine *The Studio,* first published in London in 1898 (which championed the arts and crafts movement and art nouveau) carried pages of advertisements for studios for women artists. It always seemed to me that at some point Virginia Woolf might have seen Elizabeth Pillard's painting in an exhibition and the seed of a title for her *A Room of One's Own* essay published in 1929 could have found inspiration in Elizabeth's brushstrokes or women artists like her.

Since time began, the essential ingredients for women to create seem to be private space and money, and you won't get an argument from me, especially since I was blessed with both for a few years when I lived at Newton's Chapel in Britain. But idyllic conditions come and go in our lives in a spontaneous cycle. Granted, once we obtain entry to Paradise, we hardly expect to be evicted, but nothing stays constant except change. And change is disruptive before it can be dynamic. Heaven knows I wish I'd learned that lesson early on, but I'm just making peace with it as I write this.

However, I think this deeply embedded cultural notion that we need *all the perfect conditions* before we can birth a dream, create art, start a new business, or, more importantly, cultivate a lifestyle that we feel passionate about, is a subtle but sophisticated form of self-sabotage.

So is it lack of time, space, creative energy, emotion, difficult relationships, or money that you feel is holding you back today? Bet you that at least two out of those six very real reasons have you rooted in discomfort and discouragement. I know what it's like to feel timid, and unsure, even after, or should I say, *especially* after worldly success.

But in all honesty, if I pull down the yellowed scrim of memory and return to the most creative time of my life when I was first writing *Simple Abundance,* I must admit that my circumstances were hardly ideal. I had a young child, a marriage with trouble brewing, thirty publisher rejections, and no money to spare. The space of my own where I created everything out of nothing was my side of the bed.

Women have always spun straw into gold threads out of desperate need. But what miracles might come if we give thanks first for the desperate need even before we're rewarded with the golden threads?

For truly, the space in which a woman needs to create is safeguarded within her imagination, to be hidden in the crevices of her heart until she's ready to make it come true. I hate to be the one to break it to us both, but sometimes a woman finds her destiny in between sighs or sobs, staring at a blank wall, in the same bed she took to to escape it.

Meeting the Inner Explorer

Tell me, what is it you plan to do with
your one wild and precious life?
—Mary Oliver (1935–2019)
National Book Award and Pulitzer
Prize–winning poet

I craved to go beyond the garden gate, follow the road that passed it by, and set out for the unknown," the French explorer and author Alexandra David-Néel (1868–1969) wrote in 1923, recalling her daring journey to the Himalayas in search of spiritual truth and high-spirited adventure. Her thrilling exploit is heady enough, but we can up the ante of her story: Alexandra was fifty-five years old when she did it.

The Paris-born explorer was also a former actress, so she knew to dress in costume, as a Buddhist pilgrim making her way into the heart of Tibet—the closed and sacred city of Lhasa. Never had a woman from the West seen its face.

As I drove the afternoon car pool, I wondered, how does a woman today satisfy such wanderlust? How do I reconcile the dream of visiting the temple of Egypt's Queen Hatshepsut near ancient Thebes with the reality of transporting a minivan of high-spirited kids from school to soccer practice? Or maybe you're at a cubicle desk in an open plan office. Little privacy and even less conviviality. Glance around. Do you see anyone you'd like to ask to tag along?

If you, too, crave scenes beyond the garden gate, do what I do to keep the spark of adventure alive: Journey within to meet your authentic explorer. Keep a seductive and glamorous "someday" box to hold your secret petitions. My "someday" contains a travel promotion on heavy stock paper about great train journeys I hope to go on someday: the elegantly restored glamorous South African Rovos Rail between Cape Town and Pretoria; the art deco Orient Express from London to Venice with stops in Paris, Innsbruck, and Verona. The seven-night journey on India's shocking pink Golden Chariot from Bangalore to Mysore, and the Nagarhole National Park where I disembark...

You get the idea. If you could go anywhere in the world, all expenses paid, babysitter/pet-sitter at your disposal, where would it be? Why? Who would you be with? How long would you stay? What would you do?

Yes, this is a first-class fantasy, and it's supposed to be fun. To inspire your far-flung creative imagining, you're encouraged to do some online research. There are so many marvelous women's adventure travel sites offering treks to places like Antarctica following the footsteps of Ernest Shackleton, Charles Darwin's Galapagos Islands, and the secret kingdom of Bhutan! Let your fingers do the wandering and your imagination soar. Read about famous women explorers. It astonishes me to think of these plucky Victorian women and where they went—up mountains, sailing mighty rivers, trekking through jungles and across deserts dressed in those long, heavy skirts and petticoats. I've acted in Victorian plays, and in full garb; it's a feat just to make it across the stage.

You can find lots of inexpensive travel magazines (*Travel & Leisure, Conde Nast Traveler, National Geographic Traveler,* American Express's *Departure,* and *Wanderlust*) online. Collect ideas for "someday" into that bedtime basket and tuck your visions into your fertile and fearless subconscious mind before bed. No one needs to know that you're traveling in your armchair (for now), indulging your imagination on a cold winter's night as you consider exploration as a personal metaphor.

And why, you might ask? Because, as the American Pulitzer Prize–winning novelist Alice Walker astutely observes, we're learning day by day that "the most foreign country is within." We are our own dark continent; we are our own savage frontier. Many marvels await discovery as we continue the path to authenticity.

FEBRUARY 20

The Heart Is a Lonely Hunter

All we can do is go around telling the truth.
—Carson McCullers (1917–1967)
Southern Gothic novelist, short-story writer, and playwright

When we begin to make authentic choices, we discover our true place in the world for the first time. But this self-knowledge is not easily acquired. It takes tenacity and daring to travel to the darkest interior of one's self. Who knows what we might find there? "It does not do to leave a live dragon out of your calculations, if you live near him," advises the English fantasy writer J. R. R. Tolkien, author of *The Hobbit* and *The Lord of the Rings*.

Our dragons are our fears: our day stalkers, our night sweats. Fear of the unknown. Fear of failing. Fear of starting something new and not finishing. Again. Or the real fear, the one that sends shivers up our spines: the fear of succeeding, of becoming our Authentic Selves and facing the changes *that* will inevitably bring. We might not be happy with the way we are living now, but at least it's familiar.

"I want—I want—I want—was all she could think about," Carson McCullers wrote in her novel *The Heart Is a Lonely Hunter*. "But just what this real want was she did not know."

We don't know where we are headed, and it's very scary. Old dreams are resurrecting, new desires are wooing. Instead of clarity, we feel confused. At moments like this, it is comforting to consider that there is really nothing to fear from self-awareness, because at the end of all our personal exploration, we will be reunited with our own Authentic Self: the woman who's been missing, not just from the center of our life, but even from its fringes.

Women have always known how to deal with dragons hiding under beds or lurking in closets. We turn on the lights and reassure worried souls with love. We need to slay the dragons in our minds the same way.

Today, if you feel frightened or unsure about the future, pick up the double-edged sword of Light and Love. Always remember, it's simply not an adventure worth telling if there aren't any dragons. But as in the best old tales, at the end of your exploring, you will live your happily ever after and the dragons of discouragement will either be slain or tamed.

FEBRUARY 21

A Safari of Self and Spirit

There is something about safari life that makes you forget all your sorrows and feel as if you had drunk half a bottle of champagne bubbling over with gratitude for being alive.
—Baroness Karen Blixen-Finecke (1885–1962)
Danish writer known as Isak Dinesen

In the summer of 1893, an English woman named Mary Kingsley traveled to the wildest and most dangerous part of the French Congo in search of herself. Both her parents had recently died, and suddenly, at the age of thirty-one, Miss Kingsley found herself "not only desolate with grief but bereft of purpose." Her adventures in West Africa changed all that. Several years later her writings and naturalist discoveries, including the documenting of unknown species of fish and animals, were applauded by the Victorian scientific community.

Mary Kingsley was a hunter of a dream: the knowledge of who she really was and her place in the world. So are you. Yet even without encountering the daily dangers she faced—wild animals and deadly diseases—you have embarked upon a heroic adventure as exciting as that of any explorer. Uncovering the source of the Nile or charting the course of the Amazon are outward parallels to the inner journey you are on today—a safari of the Self and the Spirit.

In Africa, to go on *safari*—the Swahili word for *journey*—is to leave your accustomed comfort and safety to venture into what for you is wilderness. Each time you listen to the woman within—your Authentic Self—you do the same. Remind yourself of this often.

"The grand African forests are like a great library, in which, so far, I can do little more than look at the pictures," Mary Kingsley wrote in her explorer's log, "although I am now busily learning the alphabet of their language, so that I may some day read what these pictures mean."

Remember Someday always comes before Yesterday.

FEBRUARY 22

Safari Life

I have a trunk containing continents.
—Beryl Markham (1902–1986)
Pioneering aviatrix and adventuress

Winter is the dry season in Africa, the time of safaris. We can learn from the dry seasons in life, and from life on safari.

"You could expect many things of God at night when the campfire burned before the tents," the British-born, Kenyan-raised pioneering bush pilot and safari guide Beryl Markham confided about safari life. "You were alone when you sat and talked with the others—and they were alone...What you say has no ready ear but your own, and what you think is nothing except to yourself. The world is there, and you are here—and these are the only poles, the only realities. You talk, but who listens? You listen, but who talks?"

A safari of the self and Spirit is at times lonely. But we know we are never alone. It is a comfort to realize that this sense of isolation is necessary if we are to encounter mystery, which is very much a part of a safari. Each day in the wilderness brings with it the struggle to survive and a heightened awareness of how wonderful it is just to see the sun set and rise again in the morning. Each day on safari is lived to the fullest because it is all that is guaranteed. If only we could learn this lesson as well in our everyday lives.

Today, expect many things as you sit around the campfire of your heart. Someone is listening. Someone is talking to you, encouraging you to take that next step as you embrace the mystery of the wilderness within.

Expect to have hope rekindled. Expect your prayers to be answered in wondrous ways. The dry seasons in life do not last. The spring rains will come again.

FEBRUARY 23

The Story Beneath the Story

I have come to believe that falling obsessively in love is one of life's necessary assignments. It cracks us open. We put everything at risk. In the process we discover the dimensions of our own appetites and desires. And life, to be lived fully, demands desire.
—Rosemary Sullivan
Canadian biographer, academic, and author

A biographer is a clandestine cartographer of the heart, mapping out certain milestones to search for the secret story beneath her subject's surface life. Because all writers know that true lives are lived between the lines.

We will be taking on different roles as we search for our Authentic Self: biographer, explorer, adventuress, and authentic archaeologist. For each specialist possesses skills to unearth remnants of memory buried deep within the fertile soil of our subconscious minds and in the deepest caverns of our hearts. Archaeologists read artifacts much the way a detective reads clues. The reason we want to awaken the authentic archaeologist is to excavate the true you. The you that is the story beneath your story.

Among the most powerful touchstones of our lives is how and what we love. "In literature and art, love is a myth we tell ourselves. By myth I mean not an invention or falsehood but rather a narrative that enfolds our deepest beliefs and longings," Rosemary Sullivan writes in her brilliant *Labyrinth of Desire: Women, Passion, and Romantic Obsession.* "The story of obsessive love is a story about wanting something so badly that we will risk everything to gain it. As we hurtle down the highway at break-neck speed to meet our lover, as we defy all prescriptions for rational behavior, we are living a drama, and nothing else in the world matters."

In this fascinating book, which explores famous romantic couples such as the French philosophers Simone de Beauvoir and Jean-Paul Sartre and the Mexican painters Frida Kahlo and Diego Rivera, Sullivan asks a provocative question: Does a woman fall in love out of a need to release a pent-up passion that she's unable to express artistically in her present situation?

Wow. Whoa. Wisdom—it's a beautiful thing.

As you ponder this question, think about where you were, and who you were with or not, when you last fell obsessively in love and perhaps made some bad choices because of that romance. I certainly have my list, but now to possess an understanding of what lay beneath those loves is a beautiful blessing, a soothing balm that heals toxic memories.

When a woman cannot access or express her own passions, desires, and artistic expression, or when she denies the authentic part of herself to care instead for the needs of others, especially lovers and spouses, eventually she arrives at a three-forked intersection where choice, circumstances, and chance are patiently waiting for a painful head-on collision.

However, when we can understand the prequel of a great passionate love, that the romance we are seeking is with ourselves, we don't have to crash and burn to rearrange the shape and structures of our lives.

"For better or worse, obsessive love awakens the whole range of primitive emotions of the needy self and we find ourselves caught in a world of mirrors, looking in astonishment at the multiple selves that occupy our inner world," Rosemary Sullivan explains. "Obsessive love sends us deep inside the caverns of our own psyches, where, if we have the stamina, we will discover how rich, how resonant, how numinous we are."

FEBRUARY 24

The Authentic Dig

Sometimes a person has to go back, really back—to have a sense, an understanding of all that's gone to make them—before they can go forward.

—Paule Marshall
American novelist

How we remember, and what we remember, and why we remember form the most personal map of our individuality," writer Christina Baldwin reminds us in her wonderful book *Life's Companion: Journal*

Writing as a Spiritual Quest. Today, become willing to remember. Prepare yourself for a gentle but authentic dig that will help you discover the mystery in which your soul abides.

Whether you realize it or not, you have lived many lives, and each one has left an indelible mark on your soul. I'm not referring to reincarnation. I'm referring to the episodic way in which our lives evolve: childhood, adolescence, college years or early career, marriages, motherhood, perhaps life as a single mother, widowhood, and onward. At each stage in our lives, we have both laughter and tears. But more important for our interests, we develop personal preferences. Each life experience leaves a layer of memory like a deposit of sediment: things we've loved and moments of contentment we've cherished that, when recalled, reveal glimmers of our true selves.

Some women are hesitant to recall their past because they're afraid they'll dredge up painful memories. But just as each illness brings us unexpected gifts, so each painful memory comes bearing a peace offering. There is nothing to fear. The past asks only to be remembered.

Unearthing a mosaic is one of the most exciting discoveries on an archaeological dig. Mosaics are pictures or decorative patterns formed by inlaying thousands of small, multicolored chips to create a larger visual representation. Early mosaics tell sacred stories about ancient worlds—how people lived and what was important to them—providing archaeologists with revealing and riveting glimpses into the past.

On the authentic dig we shall also go in search of a mosaic: what brought us moments of happiness and contentment in our past lives. When taking a backward glance, always bear in mind that memory is fickle. She must be wooed and courted if she is to succumb to our charms. Sometimes she surprises us with her generosity, and we recall moments with astonishing clarity. Most of the time, however, our memories are fragmented, like small colored chips. When this happens, we need to be patient as we brush away the sediment of the past.

Today, prepare for your personal dig in a thoughtful way. Let your authentic archaeologist gather artifacts that can coax memory: old photographs, letters, mementos. Carve out time when you can be alone and take a leisurely trip back in time. Enjoy a glass of wine or a cup of tea. Listen to your favorite music from yesterday: the Beatles, Bruce Springsteen, Faith Hill, Whitney Houston, Cowboy Junkies, Joni Mitchell, Phil Collins, Abba, Carole King, Amy Winehouse, Sting, Alanis Morrisette, Beyoncé, Celine Dion.

Peruse the photographs, flip through your high school yearbook, read the old love letters. Trace your life back to when you were ten, sixteen, twenty-one, twenty-five, thirty, thirty-five, forty, and onward. See what memories are triggered as you reacquaint yourself with the girl and woman you once were. Linger only on the happy times. What you are searching for is a pattern of personal, authentic pleasures and preferences. These are the chips in your mosaic.

"The events in our lives happen in a sequence in time, but in their significance to ourselves they find their own order," the acclaimed American Southern writer Eudora Welty (1909–2001) confides. With patience and quiet observation, these events will provide the seeker in you with a "continuous thread of revelation."

Excavating the Real You, Part I

Maybe being oneself is always an acquired taste.
—Patricia Hampl
American memoirist, lecturer, and educator

Excavating is not glamorous work on an archaeological dig. It demands painstaking effort in often harsh conditions. Tons of dirt must be removed carefully from the site if the search to uncover treasures from the past is to be successful. No matter how impatient everyone on the dig is, the excavation process cannot be rushed. The thrill of discovery wouldn't be as great if time weren't invested in slowly digging in the dirt.

We must dig patiently to excavate our real selves. "As long as one keeps searching, the answers come," Joan Baez, the iconic American folk music singer and songwriter, tells us. And for what are we searching? Shards of our authentic style.

For centuries women have displayed their innate sense of style to the world through choice: in their personal appearance, in the way they decorated their homes, in how they entertained, in their work, and in the pursuit of their personal passions. The more we learn about ourselves and our preferences, the easier it is to make these choices. And creative choice is at the heart of authenticity.

Choice confers freedom—the freedom to embrace the new because it speaks to your soul and you are listening. Today be willing to consider the choices you have made in the past as you trace your life. Have they been the right ones for you? Do you make choices with your heart, mind, or gut? Are you comfortable with your style of making choices, or do you wish to try a different approach? Was there something you did not choose in the past that, with hindsight, you now wish you had?

Perhaps a long-buried dream still calls to you from a road you chose not to take. If this is true, then stop telling yourself that it's too late. The delay of our dreams does not mean that they have been denied. Perhaps now you have the wisdom to make alterations in your dream so that it can come true. Perhaps now you have the wisdom to choose differently.

Have a dialogue with your Authentic Self. Ask her about the choices you have made or didn't make. Listen for the wisdom she has to offer.

Excavating the Real You, Part II

My memory is certainly in my hands. I can remember things only if I have a pencil and I write with it and I can play with it. I think your hand concentrates for you. I don't know why it should be so.
—Marjorie Kinnan Rawlings (1896–1953)
American author, 1939 Pulitzer Prize winner

We're back at the site of your soul this morning for some more digging. Perhaps you wonder why we are spending so much time excavating. Maybe you balk at having to search your past for clues as to how to live contentedly in the present. Please be open: The excavation process expands your sense of the possible because it provides you with inner knowledge. Now you'll be using your pen to dig with.

Let's return to the home of your childhood.

How was it decorated? Do you remember? Take a walk through the rooms and see them once again. Did you clean your room? Was the door usually kept closed? What was your favorite spot in the house? Was your mother a good cook? Do you ever prepare any of her special recipes for yourself?

How did your mother comfort you when you were sick? When was the last time you had alphabet soup and saltines for lunch on a tray in bed?

Where did you go on vacation? Did you visit your grandparents? Can you remember the neighborhood where they lived? Is there a sense memory you associate with childhood vacations? The hydrangea bush beside the driveway?

Now fast-forward to your teenage years. Were there any girls in your class that you admired? Envied? Who were they and why? Did you go to a prom? Describe your gown. How did you fix your hair? Who initiated you into the feminine rituals of good grooming? Was there an older girl or woman in your life whose sense of style impressed you? When you were a teenager, who was the most glamorous woman in the world for you?

Let's move ahead to when you set up your first home, either as a young working woman or when you first lived as a couple. Where was it? How was it furnished? Are you still living with some of your early decorating choices? Do they reflect who you are now, or have you outgrown them? Are you living with things that you've inherited from your family? Do they really suit you?

Now slowly let your attention return to the room. You have excavated some more chips to place into your authentic mosaic. "Minor things can become moments of great revelation when encountered for the first time," the great English prima ballerina Dame Margot Fonteyn (1919–1991) observed. We tend to think it is the major events that mark our lives, when really it is the minor moments that resonate in memory. Lovingly pick one pleasant recollection and think about it today. Maybe even write about it in your Gratitude Journal or commemorate it in pictures in your *Illustrated Discovery Journal.*

FEBRUARY 27

Passion: The Authentic Muse

What is passion? It is surely the becoming of a person.
—John Boorman
English filmmaker

Many women long to live passionate lives, to be swept away—but at a safe distance and in small doses. That's why we are drawn to juicy novels, time-travel trysts, all shades of gray, three-hanky movies, soap operas, platonic flirtations, and personality journalism that glorifies lives larger than our own. Passion, after all, means the abandonment of reason in the reckless pursuit of pleasure: rushing off with an Argentine polo-playing paramour instead of driving your daughter to the orthodontist.

Passion is wild, chaotic, unpredictable. Permissive. Excessive. Obsessive. Glenn Close in *Fatal Attraction* as the single working executive who won't be toyed with still registers on our personal Richter scale. Passionate women can't help but exult in their emotions, revel in their desires, howl at the moon, act out their fantasies, lose all control, boil a pet rabbit for revenge.

The rest of us have real-life responsibilities that leave little room (or so we think) for giving in to passionate impulses: runny noses to wipe, dogs to walk, Brownie snacks to prepare, conferences to attend, trains to catch, deadlines to meet, supper to put on the table. There goes the day. There goes a life, and not with a bang, but a whimper and a whine.

What we don't realize is that passion is the muse of authenticity. It's the primordial, pulsating energy that infuses all of life, the numinous presence made known with every beat of our hearts. Passion does not reveal herself only in clandestine, romantic, bodice-ripping clichés. Passion's nature is also cloaked in the deep, subtle, quiet, and committed: nursing a baby, planting a rose garden, preparing a special meal, caring for a loved one who is ill, remembering a friend's birthday, persevering in a dream. Encouraging a child to not give up *her* dream.

Every day offers us another chance to live passionate lives rather than passive ones, if we will bear witness to passion's immutable presence in the prosaic. If we will stop denying ourselves pleasure. If, as James Joyce's heroine Molly Bloom whispered, we can only learn to say "...and yes I said yes I will Yes."

Passion is holy—a profound Mystery that transcends and transforms through rapture. We need to accept that a sacred fire burns within, whether we're comfortable with this truth or not. Passion is part of Real Life's package because we were created by Love, for Love, to Love. If we do not give outward expression to our passions, we will experience self-immolation—the spontaneous combustion of our souls.

Did you know that both the Koran, the sacred book of Islam, and the Jewish Talmud teach that we will be called to account for every permissible pleasure life offered us but which we refused to enjoy while on earth? Dorothy L. Sayers, the deeply spiritual Christian writer, as well as mystery author, believed, "The only sin passion can commit is to be joyless."

Go now. Depart in peace and sin no more.

FEBRUARY 28

Do Try This at Home: Vital Records

Courage can't see around corners, but goes around them anyway.
—Mignon McLaughlin (1913–1983)
American journalist and author

Better to be safe than sorry is an old adage which we may well take to heart in war time," *House and Garden* magazine encouraged their readers in 1942. "Have you an Air Raid closet where all the supplies that pertain to this emergency are kept together? It may be only a cupboard but it should be intelligently planned."

So let's begin. Since just the idea of having to evacuate your home is overwhelming, we're going to keep this low intensity. This is just a great opportunity to get organized. Plan for two hours at a time on a couple of weekends, and you will not believe the relief of knowing where everything is instantly.

We'll be adding things to the Caution Closet as the year goes along, but for now, the first file will be a collection of our vital records. Most likely, all these papers will be in separate files. Gather these originals and keep them all in a storage box while you complete this task. Make photocopies of them, and if you have a scan function on your computer and printer you can also scan your information, which will give you a vital documents file to keep on a backup disc, thumb drive, or in the cloud. The originals can be placed in a personal storage box or briefcase that is both fireproof and waterproof.

I like to keep each category of documents in a clear (nine-by-thirteen-inch) plastic envelope file with a snap. This way I can immediately identify the file.

Birth certificate or adoption decrees

Marriage license; divorce papers, if any

Wills

Banking information

Any powers of attorney, legal and medical

Insurance papers: life, home, and auto

Deeds or leases

Copies of credit cards

Auto registration and car documents

Social Security cards and papers

Passports, visas, green cards

Income tax files for the last three years

Medical records

When you're done with this enormous project, keep the clear folders and disc or thumb drive in a backpack that is used only for this information. Keep the backpack inside a closet that is closest to the door you use to exit from when you leave your home. While previous generations have relied on paper copies, today electronic versions of vital records are the norm and are infinitely easier to transport.

I call this project "You'll Never Need to Know This, But..." Once you have assembled your documents, take photos with your smart phone and email them to yourself with a searchable subject line, which in my case would be something like: Family Docs—SBB—Birth. Save all the photos in one folder on your computer for easy access or upload them directly to the digital storage service of your choice. On an extended trip abroad, a friend uploaded all relevant documents to a shareable Google Drive and sent the link to her family. At any time, her children or siblings had access to her information from the other side of the world. Fortunately, her family never needed to know this information, but knowing they had it reassured everyone.

By the way, preparing digital vital records for someone who isn't a tech wiz is a great gift. It will give someone you love such comfort.

FEBRUARY 29

Now That I've Gotten Your Attention

Sometime in your life you will go on a journey.
It will be the longest journey you have ever taken.
It is the journey to find yourself.

—Kate Sharp
American independent filmmaker

For nearly two months we have contemplated the inner journey to authenticity together. Hopefully you've started to let Gratitude till the soil of your soul, preparing it for the seeds of *Simple Abundance*: finding the sacred in the ordinary, realizing that all you have is all you need, and welcoming choice as a creative energy booster.

Maybe you've set aside time to begin a daily gathering of well-spent moments in your Gratitude Journal; indulged in the pleasure of searching for your Authentic Self in images with the *Illustrated Discovery Journal*. Hopefully you tried to wean yourself away from the outer world, especially the internet, for a week or even a few days, just so we can compare what your daily round is like when you're plugged in and on those days when you are the composer of your own soundtrack.

Then again, maybe you haven't.

I've been where you are now. I know. I know how days, weeks, months, even years can escape your grasp. I know what it's like to put everyone else's needs before your own so that you can't find a half hour a day for yourself. I know how easy it is to find heartfelt excuses for why you can't begin something new even if you yearn to, desperately. I know how easily the word *tomorrow* slips out unconsciously. Tomorrow you'll begin. Tomorrow. All this I know. All this I've lived.

But what I know most of all is that reading about a journey is not the same thing as taking one.

Now that I've gotten your attention, let me tell you about the rest of the year. Each day from now on we're going to use the daily grist of our real lives as a cause for celebration. That's right, celebration. I have learned many lessons on the *Simple Abundance* path. Chief among them is that the details of our days do make a difference in our lives, that no experience is ever just for drill, and that everything can be a springboard for inspiration if we are willing to be open to the goodness of life.

How many times in the past have we chosen not to change our lives for the better simply by *not* choosing? Today, make a choice. Choose to continue the *Simple Abundance* path or close this book now. If you choose to close the book, my blessings accompany you. May peace and plenty be your portion. Pass this book on to a friend or donate it.

If you are still with me, you know what you need to do *today*, not tomorrow. Take another look at your life. Give thanks. Accept your circumstances. Give thanks. Count your blessings. Give thanks. Show up for each day's reflection. Be willing to give the basic tools a fair chance. They can help you find your way. Above all, have faith in your spiritual moxie and Divine Change.

"One does not discover new lands without consenting to lose sight of the shore for a very long time," the French author and 1947 Nobel laureate for literature André Gide reassures us.

Set the sails. Pull anchor. Cast away. Feel the wind at your back. Keep your eyes on the horizon.

Or stay on shore.

But choose.

Joyful Simplicities for February

You are discontented with the world because you just can't get the small things that suit your pleasure.
—George Eliot (1819–1880)
Pen name of celebrated Victorian writer Mary
Ann Evans

⚜ Light candles all over your home on Candlemas day, February 2. Bask in the glow. Relax and see how different the world seems without electricity to blur the distinction between night and day. Consider that you might like to live by candlelight more often. I love a large scented room candle. Decorative flameless candles are popular, but the ambiance is not the same. Invest in beeswax dripless candles. They come in a rainbow of exquisite colors and reflect the light beautifully. (Amazon has a huge variety.) Store them in the freezer and they will burn twice as long without dripping.

⟿ Create a sacred space for yourself to celebrate, concentrate, and consecrate your inner work—on a small table, bookshelf, a window ledge, the top of a bureau. Julia Cameron shares with the seeker in us: "In order to stay easily and happily creative, we need to stay spiritually centered. This is easier to do if we allow ourselves centering rituals. It is important that we devise these ourselves from the elements that feel holy and happy to us." I collect different prayer beads and change their setting seasonally.

⟿ A winter comfort beloved by the preeminent American food writer, the sublime M. F. K. Fisher, is hot chocolate soup for supper. Layer pieces of hot buttered toast (about ten to twelve pieces) in the bottom of a soup bowl. Sprinkle with a heaping handful of fresh mini marshmallows, and slowly ladle real hot cocoa over the toast. Savor with soup spoons. After all the toasty bits are gone, you can continue with animal crackers.

⟿ Have you found a wonderful picture of yourself when you were ten? If you have, find the perfect frame for it and put it on your bureau or dressing table. If you haven't yet, ask your mother or whoever keeps your family photographs to help you.

⟿ A bedtime ritual for blissful mornings is to arrange a pretty tray for your morning tea or coffee and leave it ready on the kitchen counter. Finding it waiting for you begins your day gracefully and if you really want to know what it's like to be pampered, you'll also find a clean kitchen and empty sink to greet you. It doesn't take much to make us happy, and these simple perks are among those things that money can't buy.

⟿ Are you growing any indoor bulbs? Most supermarkets and garden supply stores have discounted holiday bulb kits now. To create splendor in the pot, mix daffodils, tulips, crocus (whatever is on sale) and plant them all in one pot—you'll have a riot of fragrance and color in a month. Or just get supermarket pots of hyacinth, daffodils, and tulips and then gather them together in a round basket or pot.

⟿ A mixed-colors basket of primroses on the kitchen windowsill is a mood lifter. It's amazing how often 3 little pots of primroses make an appearance in many of my Gratitude Journals.

⟿ Wear perfume every day.

⟿ Try a red lipstick.

⟿ Listen to the music of Cole Porter.

⟿ Make a batch of old-fashioned chocolate fudge for Valentine's Day.

⟿ I love to read a group of books about people and places to get as true an interpretation as possible. February is the month safari life begins, so here's a wonderful list of books that have given me enormous pleasure:

❧ For an understanding of British colonial life in the Kenya Colony between 1920 and 1950:

West with the Night by Beryl Markham (her memoir)

Straight Till Morning: The Life of Beryl Markham by Mary Lovell

Isak Dinesen: The Life of a Storyteller by Judith Thurman

Out of Africa by Isak Dinesen

Too Close to the Sun: The Audacious Life and Times of Denys Finch Hatton by Sara Wheeler

❧ For a passionate and compelling glimpse of post-colonial Africa after 1960 there is the marvelous Nigerian author Chimamanda Ngozi Adichie and her two international award-winning novels: *Purple Hibiscus* and *Half of a Yellow Sun*.

❧ *Mrs. Miniver* by Jan Struther is a collection of the original essays, and *The Real Mrs Miniver* by her granddaughter Ysenda Maxtone Graham is a fascinating biography of Jan Struther's backstory, as she attempted to have a private life that unfolded in the imagination of a public audience.

❧ Did you know there is an original soundtrack to our *Simple Abundance* journey, called *Sarah Ban Breathnach's Simple Abundance: Music of Comfort and Joy?* It's available for streaming on Amazon Music, iTunes, and Spotify.

MARCH

This is the month of sudden changes... In March, winter is holding back and spring is pulling forward. Something holds and something pulls inside of us, too. We are caught between two forces and sometimes nearly torn asunder... Some days confidence shrinks to the size of a pea, and the backbone feels like a feather. We want to be somewhere else and don't know where—want to be someone else and don't know who.

—Jean Hersey (1902–1993)
American naturalist and author

March arrives, the last hurrah of winter and the first whisper of spring. Slowly our spirits reawaken, along with the natural world, from a long winter's slumber. Branches that just days ago were bare now blossom with new growth. Deep within we feel stirrings of hope. Turn over the earth in the inner garden. This month we plant the seeds of the second *Simple Abundance* Grace—Simplicity—in the fertile soil of our souls.

MARCH 1

Restoring Serenity to Your Daily Endeavors

*God, give us the grace to accept with serenity the things that cannot
be changed; courage to change the things which should be changed
and the wisdom to distinguish the one from the other.*
—Dr. Reinhold Niebuhr (1892–1971)
American Protestant theologian

When thinking about serenity, many people immediately associate the
famous prayer written by Protestant theologian Dr. Reinhold Niebuhr
for a sermon he delivered in 1934, which was printed in the *New York
Times*. Coming in the middle of the Great Depression, the simplicity
and directness of his words gave comfort to millions of Americans
who felt powerless to change the circumstances of their lives. Among
those millions was Bill W., the founder of the twelve-step community
Alcoholics Anonymous in 1935, who wrote, "With amazing speed the
Serenity Prayer came into general use and took its place alongside our
two other favorites, the Lord's Prayer and the Prayer of St. Francis."

I'm among the millions of people who love the Serenity Prayer. However, I think the time has come for us to stop associating serenity with
things that cannot be changed. For we can dramatically change the
quality of our lives when we consciously seek to restore Simplicity's gift
of serenity to our daily endeavors.

How exactly can this be accomplished in our lifetime? Well, how
about beginning each day by not having to delete over a hundred emails
trying to sell you peace of mind? Of course, this means that we'll need to
invest a half hour consciously unsubscribing to this onslaught of junk,
but you will feel so unburdened after completing what I call the "well-
spent moments" that it takes that it will be worth at least one Gratitude
Journal entry.

However, if you frequently feel as if you're about to spin off this
planet, it's probably because you are. I know a woman who will begin
to brush her teeth only to start making her bed while she is still foaming
at the mouth. And why? Because from the corner of her eye she saw the
rumpled sheets. Before she could rinse, she had flung herself into the
next task. Needless to say, a day that starts off this frenzied can only go
from bad to worse.

Serene women do not become sidetracked. Sidetracked women who
scatter their energies to the four winds never achieve serenity. Nervous
breakdowns, to be sure, but not serenity. It's as simple as that.

This is not how the cool, glamorous, and regal Hollywood icon
Grace Kelly (1929–1982) spent her days after she became Her Serene

Highness the Princess of Monaco. Nor should it be how we should spend ours. And while I'm sure Princess Grace had somebody else making her bed, the point is still valid.

What I do find fascinating is that despite Grace Kelly's beauty and assured public poise, which distinguished her Oscar-winning film career, she had to be tutored on how to perfect the biggest role of her life, as the wife of Prince Rainier. If Grace Kelly could learn how to become a Serene Highness, then so can we. And in doing so, we can recover our sanity.

So here's the plan: Concentrate slowly on completing one task at a time, each hour of the day, until the day is over. Like the members of twelve-step programs, we will act "as if" we are serene (think Grace Kelly), by bringing all our attention and conscious awareness to whatever we are doing—from brushing our teeth to putting the children to bed. What we will gain from this exercise is the inner peace that comes from living fully in the present moment.

I realize, of course, that for most of us, accustomed as we are to performing six tricks simultaneously, what I'm proposing sounds ridiculous. You wonder how you'll get everything done if you don't do everything at once. But I assure you that you will accomplish all you set out to do with much more ease, efficiency, pleasure, and satisfaction when you merge mind, body, and spirit with the task at hand.

And surprise!—you will experience serenity.

MARCH 2

Meditation: Many Paths to the Present Moment

Meditation is simply about being yourself and knowing about who that is. It is about coming to realize that you are on a path whether you like it or not, namely the path that is your life.

—Jon Kabat-Zinn
American Professor Emeritus
of Medicine and author

If you do not already practice meditation, when you hear the word *meditate* you probably conjure up the unpleasant image of sitting uncomfortably in a lotus position, back aching, mind racing ahead to all the things you need to be doing, and hyperventilating because now you are concentrating on whether you are breathing or not.

This unappealing image isn't what meditation is all about. But it goes a long way toward explaining why many people do not meditate.

However, there are compelling physiological, psychological, and spiritual reasons why we should engage in regular meditation—"time off for good behavior," as I like to call it. It is the mortar that holds mind, body, and Spirit together.

There are many ways of meditating. Dr. Joan Borysenko, the gifted and inspired psychologist, scientist, and spiritual teacher, explains that meditation is intentional concentration on one thing, which can be either secular or spiritual.

"Perhaps you have become so absorbed in gardening, reading or even balancing your checkbook that your breathing slowed, and you became as single-pointed as a panther stalking her dinner! In this state creativity flowers, intuition leads to a deeper wisdom, the natural healing system of the body is engaged, our best physical and mental potential manifests itself and we feel psychologically satisfied," she writes. Spiritual meditation, on the other hand, "will help you become aware of the presence of the divine in nature, in yourself and in other people. The love and joy that are inherent in Spirit—that are the very essence of Spirit—will begin to permeate your life."

I have many different ways of meditating, depending on my inner needs: concentrating on a sacred word in a centering prayer, focusing on a poetic phrase to find deeper personal meaning, or setting out on a walking meditation. I also listen to one song on repeat for as long as it takes for my heart to stop racing.

I also love meditating on antiquing jaunts, musing as I meander on how the past still speaks to me, especially in artifacts that were once part of someone else's vibrant life. There are so many paths to the present moment, but it begins with concentrating on and finishing one task at a time. Joan Borysenko's "all-time favorite meditation is a small, moist piece of chocolate cake eaten with exquisite attention and tremendous gratitude. Any time we are fully present in the moment we are meditating."

Today, retreat to a quiet place where you can sit or even lie down in a comfortable position so that you can relax your body. Now close your eyes and let your breathing become slow and steady. Get in touch with the silence within. Consider how you might be able to carve out twenty minutes a day to meditate. That is all, merely consider. Actually doing it will be the next step.

MARCH 3

Setting Aside a Personal Sabbath

Anybody can observe the Sabbath but making it holy surely takes the rest of the week.

—Alice Walker
American Pulitzer Prize–winning novelist

It was all right for the Great Creator to rest on the seventh day, but many contemporary women assume they just can't take the time off. After all, we're not creating the world six days a week, just carrying its weight on our shoulders.

"Some keep the Sabbath going to Church," Emily Dickinson confided. "I keep it, staying at Home." So do I. There are some Sundays, especially in winter or when it rains, that I don't even get out of my pajamas. Long ago, I stopped feeling guilty about this, because I've learned how to honor my Sabbath by keeping it holy and happy. Many people look upon the Sabbath as Sunday; others keep the Sabbath from Friday at sundown through Saturday. It doesn't matter what day of the week you set aside as your own personal Sabbath, it just matters that you keep one.

Here is a short guide to what you should *not* be doing on your Sabbath: strenuous household chores (preparing meals is fine, but they should either be easy or festive, depending on your choice); catching up on work that you didn't complete last week, or getting a head start on work you're supposed to start on Monday.

This is what the Sabbath is for: reverence, rest, renewal, rejuvenation, reassuring rituals, recreation, rejoicing, revelation, remembering how much you have to be grateful for, and saying "thank you!" You can do this in a church, mosque, temple, or synagogue, on a walk, swimming, horseback riding, taking a hike with the dogs, sitting in bed propped up on pillows reading something wonderful with a breakfast tray, working the crossword puzzle before a roaring fire, attending a marvelous art exhibition or movie matinee, or listening to opera in the kitchen as you sip sherry and prepare a fabulous feast.

What matters is that you do something different that speaks to your soul and refreshes your body and mind on whatever day you decide to take a personal Sabbath. I like to think of the Sabbath as a spiritual sanctioned "time out" so that we can just have a few hours of relaxation, regardless of our personal faith. Your activities on the Sabbath should uplift you and provide enough inspiration to sustain you during the week to come. Well, at least that's what we're aiming toward!

"Sunday is sort of like a piece of bright golden brocade lying in a pile of white muslin weekdays," the Japanese-American author Yoshiko Uchida (1921–1992) wrote in *A Jar of Dreams*. If this is not what the Great Creator intended when She created the Sabbath, then I have no idea what is Sacred.

MARCH 4

Priming the Pump for Inspiration

The well of Providence is deep. It's the buckets we bring to it that are small.

—Mary Webb (1881–1927)
English romantic novelist and poet

Whenever I prepare to write, I have a carefully crafted ritual of comfort that eases me into creating. I work from my bed with a fresh pot of tea on my bedside table and music—film soundtracks—that I only listen to when I'm writing. Each writing project has its own soundtrack. Next to me are a new spiral notebook and my favorite pens, along with a revered pile of dog-eared books. You see, I am not alone but in the company of my circle of saints—my beloved women writing mentors—Joan Didion, Annie Dillard, Mary Cantwell, and Merle Shain—each of whom has an authentic voice and a special message for me. I savor the work of their hands, hearts, and minds once again to get my own creative juices flowing.

My writing ritual is what I refer to as "priming the pump for inspiration." When you must pump water from a well the old-fashioned way, by hand, you need to pour a pitcher of water down the pump to get it going. I prime my personal pump in a very particular way because the repetitiveness of the process activates the right side of my brain where creativity dwells: I use the same Belleek porcelain mug for tea, listen to the same music, write with the same type of pens and notebooks, reread the same books. The instantly recognizable ritual informs my brain that we're now working, picking up from where we left off yesterday. Before I realize it, I'm jotting down notes as if I'm taking dictation from Spirit. When I've got a rough draft written in longhand, I head into my office to work on the computer. Now the real writing begins. But once again, I have coaxed inspiration into helping me through the power of ritual. Fledgling writers always love to discover the personal "secrets" of other writers, and mine is harnessing the discipline of rhythm and routine. I'm at my desk by ten a.m., so that the Muse knows where to find me.

You need to create a reassuring ritual for yourself to access your inner reservoir—that place deep within you inhabited by imagination. Why not create an inviting one for when you work with your *Illustrated Discovery Journal*? If you find that you can't work on it during the week, it could be a perfect Sunday pastime to search for the visual images that reveal your authentic preferences. Make the process as appealing as possible. Perhaps you can take a long, leisurely soak in the bathtub. Then, after you are comfortable and relaxed, bring the basket containing your magazines, scissors, and journal over to your bed. Prepare a special mug of cheer to enjoy only at this time. Light a pretty candle on your dresser to invoke inspiration.

This week consider the importance of creating a special way to prime your personal pump. Carry a large bucket to the well of Providence with a ceremony of comfort.

MARCH 5

The Thrill of Thrift

There is satisfaction in seeing one's household prosper
In being both bountiful and provident.
    —Phyllis McGinley (1905–1978)
    Pulitzer Prize–winning poet and essayist

I don't know a woman alive who doesn't get a thrill out of thrifting—finding the perfect item at the perfect price. But thrifting is so much more than a bargain bagged at a garage sale, flea market, or on eBay. For centuries, thrifting has been the heart of the homemaker's honorable estate and a sacred trust that included the right apportionment of her personal and domestic resources: time, creative energy, emotion, industry, strength, skill, craft, and labor; the management of property of all kinds, including money; the exercise of prudence and temperance; and the distribution of charity to those less fortunate.

In other words, all those homespun virtues necessary to keep a family healthy, prosperous, and secure were contained in the Heavenly boon of this one expansive word.

But to truly understand the reassuring and redeeming spiritual qualities of thrift and how it balances our daily round, let's clear away all the old, hackneyed cobwebs that surround this marvelous quality.

Let's begin with what thrift isn't: parsimonious, frugal, mean, scrimping, paltry, shoddy, stingy, or cheap.

What thrift is: bountiful, generous, compassionate, vigorous, growing, abundant, blooming, copious, healthful, efficient. Thrift is practicing the art of elegant economies, such as Gratitude, Simplicity, Order, Harmony, Beauty, and Joy (interestingly, all the six Graces of *Simple Abundance*). Thrift is thriving, increasing, expanding, and plentiful. Through the artisanal craft of thrift, we become balanced in all areas of our lives.

We can trace the role that thrift has played in the English household back to the fourteenth century bard Geoffrey Chaucer's *Canterbury Tales* as well as William Shakespeare's *The Merchant of Venice*. Probably the earliest meaning of the word *thrift* was "the condition of one who thrives" or being endowed with good luck, good fortune, wealth, and health. But what made thrift such an honorable aspiration was that its bounty was not conveyed by celestial benediction or favor of the crown—but rather through the everyday choices made by prudent housewives who were neat, clean, industrious, imaginative, honest, clever, enterprising, and generous. Women who found the mystical in the mundane rituals of their daily round and cherished the bounty of their everyday.

The invocation of thrift was considered as crucial to a bride's happy marriage as tossing rice, releasing doves, or wearing something old, something new, something borrowed, and something blue. Beginning in the sixteenth century, English nuptials introduced the custom of the bride's father or guardian slipping a silver sixpence coin into her left shoe as a harbinger of wealth and protection against want. The symbol of the sixpence represented the "reward" due to those drawn to the honorable estate of matrimony.

Intriguingly, *thrift* is also the name of a charming English flower, a pink perennial that blooms from April through September and flourishes in rocky crevices, requiring little soil for sustenance while acting as a barrier to protect marshes from the ebb-and-flow erosion of the sea. As a metaphor for our own goal of balanced and joyful lives, the metaphysical boundary of thrift protects us from the ebb and flow of emergencies. It enables us to create our own protective barrier to cushion us from want and distress through our savings, or what the Victorians called the "Margin of Happiness." Isn't this a fabulous name? It makes you want to have one immediately.

Without thrift "there can be little solid domestic happiness," the Pulitzer Prize–winning poet and essayist Phyllis McGinley tells us in her *Sixpence in Her Shoe* (1964), written as an answer to Betty Friedan's groundbreaking *The Feminine Mystique*, published the year before. "For thrift is neither selfishness nor cheese-paring, but a large, compassionate attribute, a just regard for God's material gifts. It has nothing in common with meanness and is different even from economy, which may assist thrift."

Phyllis McGinley is a woman after my own heart. She loved being a wife, a mother, a homemaker, an author, and a poet. She reveled in combining all the facets of her daily round in her writing, working on her poems, essays, or books while a pot of stew or soup simmered on the stove. And she saw no contradictions in combining all the aspects of her life into a tapestry of contentment—from meeting her husband's train to being celebrated at a White House reception for her work.

In her inspirational essay "The Pleasures of Thrift," she describes how passionate thrift is the guardian of domestic bliss: "Meanness inherits a set of silverware and keeps it in the bank. Economy uses it only on important occasions for fear of loss. Thrift sets the table with it every night for pure pleasure but counts the butter spreaders before they are put away."

As we learn how to create a sustainable lifestyle protected from life's storms, "Thrift saves for the future because the children must be educated and because one must not be a burden in old age," McGinley tells us. "Thrift keeps the house painted and the roof in repair, puts shoe trees in shoes, but bakes a jar of cookies for neighborhood children. It is never stingy..."

What I adore about McGinley's view of thrift is that "it has to be a personal joy" that every woman must work out for herself. First, what are your authentic extravagances? You know, the purchases that pinch a little, even as you pull out the plastic?

Do you love to cook? Then quality knives, organic chickens, and virgin olive oil might be your affordable luxuries—but through your prudent meal planning, the chicken will stretch to three delicious suppers. That means the fresh baked sourdough bread accompanying your homemade chicken noodle soup doesn't have to come from your own kitchen. The thrill of thrift invites trade-offs, not trade-downs.

"Every woman has to learn to be thrifty in her own idiom. Her economies must be like her luxuries cut to the shape of the family budget or the family dream and they must never descend to indignities. Thrift implies dignity," Phyllis McGinley reminds us. "It might lie for one person as a thing so small as properly balancing her checkbook or for another in something so large as learning to make all the draperies for her windows... And, like laughter or sachets in bureau drawers, it is a pleasant thing to have around the house."

I believe that once we approach thrift not as a straitjacket of "can't haves" but as a homegrown remedy for contentment and creativity, this ancient art can boost our morale, and increase our "Margin of Happiness," and that, after all, is why we seek the sacred in the ordinary.

MARCH 6

The Margin of Happiness

Annual income twenty pounds, annual expenditure
Nineteen, nineteen six, result—happiness.
Annual income twenty pounds, annual expenditure
Twenty pounds and six, result—misery.
— Charles Dickens (1812–1870)
Victorian British novelist who wrote
A Christmas Carol

The Margin of Happiness was the euphemism Victorian literary domestics—women columnists who wrote about achieving domestic bliss—used when referring to the household budget. As Charles Dickens points out in his novel *David Copperfield*—published in 1849 and based on his father's stint in debtor's prison during Dickens's childhood—the difference in life between happiness and misery can be as little as six shillings of overspending. Because overspending rarely stops at six shillings, which was then about seventy-two cents!

I think creating a "happy margin" in our financial affairs is a splendid way for us to reframe the concept of personal budgets. When we create a buffer of relief between necessary expenses and saving accounts, with our own "Margin of Happiness" account, we get to balance our wants and needs.

Before we go further, we need to remember the power of our words, and *budget* is not among my favorites. "The word 'budget' seems to frighten some people. They think of it as of a beast which will devour, or as a tool by which the homemakers arbitrarily, almost automatically cut themselves off from all possibility of ever obtaining the things they want," the home arts magazine *Modern Priscilla* told readers in January 1928. "On the contrary, it does, if well-made and well used, prevent careless experience for things outside the scheme of life. It prevents wandering thoughtlessly into debt. It ensures the purchase of many things which, however desirable, would have been counted among the impossibilities or extravagance, if the careful survey demanded in making the budget had not shown them to be possible."

While budgets sound punitive, a Margin of Happiness account is a promising and wonderful introduction to the joys of delayed gratification. You'll feel differently about personal budgets if you believe you're an artist of the everyday, actively creating tangible happiness by deciding to allot a regular sum—however small in the beginning—to your Margin of Happiness.

MARCH 7

Outfitting a Comfort Drawer

Life begins at the end of your comfort zone.

—Neale Donald Walsch
American inspirational author

Life requires that we prepare ourselves for the inevitable times that try our souls, particularly on those days when we push past our comfort zone in pursuit of our Authentic Self. After tough days, when I want to pull the covers over my head and never come out again, I've discovered that when worn to a raveling my comfort drawer is a lovely prescription for frazzled hearts and minds.

My refuge is the bottom drawer of my dresser, where I stockpile small indulgences throughout the year. But many of my comforts were originally gifts that I simply saved for whenever a homegrown unhappiness remedy might be required.

Let's see what we find: a box of chocolate truffles; miniature (one-serving size) fruit cordials and after-dinner drinks; an aromatherapy bath treatment to promote serenity; assorted new-to-me cozy mystery novels; a small vial of Bach's Rescue Remedy (a homeopathic essence available at health food stores); a velvet herbal sleeping pillow to induce pleasant dreams; a satin eye mask to shut out distractions; rose-scented bubble bath and talc; old love letters tied with a silk ribbon; a scrapbook of personal mementos; a tin of fancy biscuits; and an assorted gift sampler of unusual teas.

Notice the simply abundant pattern of pleasure? Here is all that is required for the spoiling and pampering of a world-weary woman: a fabulous bath, something scrumptious to nibble, something sentimental to conjure up happy memories, something lovely to sip, and something delightful to read. Now change your sheets, fill your hot water bottle, and assemble a half dozen white votive candles on a tray. Place the tray on your dresser in front of a mirror, strike a match, and ceremoniously create your own northern lights. Play some soothing music and put on your favorite pajamas or nightgown. Get into bed and luxuriate. If this doesn't work, take two aspirins and call me in the morning.

When outfitting your comfort drawer, be sure to line it with a patterned shelf paper that makes you happy just to look at it and tuck in some scented sachets so that the drawer will delight your senses. Wrap your comforts in pretty jewel-colored tissue paper and tie them with beautiful ribbons. This way, when you open your drawer, you'll see a dazzling array of wonderful presents—gifts of the heart for the most deserving woman you know.

MARCH 8

Taking the Plunge

Until you make peace with who you are, you'll never be content with what you have.

—Doris Mortman
American novelist

Simplicity gains importance in our lives as we begin to make peace with ourselves. This is because we gradually come to the inner awareness that we don't need to gild the lily. Some of the trappings can be relinquished because the Real Thing is finally ready to be revealed.

I call this point in the *Simple Abundance* process "taking the plunge" because it involves a courageous leap of faith in the most intimate way: exploring the way we express ourselves to the outside world through our personal appearance. But this is much more than just how we dress or style our hair. It's about the many subtle ways we choose either to celebrate or conceal our authenticity. It's about finally acknowledging and accepting the woman within. It's about learning to become comfortable with who we really are.

"We are not born all at once, but by bits. The body first, and the spirit later," Mary Antin, the Slavic-American novelist and immigration activist, wrote in her stunning 1912 novel *The Promised Land*. "Our mothers are racked with the pains of our physical birth; we ourselves suffer the longer pains of our spiritual growth."

The famed French feminist, writer, and philosopher Simone de Beauvoir (1908–1986) put it another way: "One is not born a woman, one becomes one." This becoming takes time. We need time to consider, time to reflect, time to make creative choices, time to emerge from the cocoon, time to clean out our closets, and time to clear away psychic cobwebs so that we might pare down to our essence.

Some of us have remained dormant for years—oblivious to our genuine beauty—drugged senseless by our own numbing disapproval, nagging doubts, and benign neglect. Coping strategies that once brought a sense of relief now only offer regret. To undo the damage and reconnect with our authentic selves we need to take the plunge, confident that Spirit is holding the net. Above all, we need to treat ourselves gently with the kindness we would bestow on amnesiacs who need the patient reassurance as well as a reintroduction to their true identities.

MARCH 9

A Radiant Reflection: Projecting
Your Authentic Self

*So many women just don't know how great they really are. They
come to us all vogue outside and vague on the inside.*
—Mary Kay Ash (1918–2001)
American businesswoman and founder
of Mary Kay Cosmetics, Inc.

Few women know how great they really are. If truth were told, we'd all
probably admit to feeling pretty vague about our personal appearance.
Many of us would like to trade ourselves in for a sleeker version. Some
of us have been wearing our hair the same way for the last decade—
not because it's so flattering but because it feels safe. Still others of us
haven't changed our makeup since our twenties, even though the face
in the mirror no longer wears the color fuchsia as well as she once did.

Even when we don't consciously know how to pull together our outside packaging, there is someone who does. As we become more intimate with this wonderful source of style, personal fashion know-how,
and comfort, we will begin to awaken to our own radiance. This source,
our Authentic Self, is waiting to help us each evolve into the woman we
were meant to be.

An easy way to let her begin is to gather different images of style
influencers—women whom you admire. Whenever you have a quiet
moment to yourself, sit down and spread out the pictures of the women
you think are attractive and the clothing you'd love to wear. Don't even
consider whether you can afford anything you select or whether you can
fit into it today. This is a creative brainstorming session. Always remember that dreams—your creative visualizations—must come before their
physical manifestations. Play with the pictures in your *Illustrated Discovery Journal*. Create a collage mood board of your ideal woman:
Find the perfect hairstyle, put together a fantastic wardrobe for home
and work. Have fun with this. Pretend you're ten years old and playing
with paper dolls. See what you discover. Does anything in your *Illustrated Discovery Journal* collage resemble anything hanging in your
closet? Consider this carefully.

Now make yourself a promise. Since you have embarked on this
adventure to awaken your authenticity and discover your own sense of
style, be willing not to buy another item of clothing unless you absolutely cannot live without it. No more settling for something that's not
you or that's second-rate. On the *Simple Abundance* path, you're going
to discover the joy of surrounding yourself only with things you love,

and the pleasure of wearing only clothes that make you look and feel fabulous and project your authentic sense of style. Let the potent power of simplicity begin to work in your life. If it's not authentically you, live without it.

You Are Not Your Appearance, but Does the Rest of the World Know That?

The tragedy of our time is that we are so eye centered, so appearance besotted.

—Jessamyn West (1902–1984)
American Quaker author

All of us can pull ourselves together some of the time. Some of us can pull ourselves together all of the time. But none of us wants to be "pulled together" every single moment of our lives. Let's consider those days when you just don't give a damn or are too exhausted to remember to pick up a brush. Can we find inspiration in dirty jeans, an unwashed face, stringy hair? Can there be incarnational revelations when the skirt is too tight and the pantyhose pulls at your hips or the zipper doesn't go up all the way?

I hope so. For I know those days and those days know me.

Probably you were taught, as I was, that how we present ourselves to the world is very important. Unfortunately, our outside packaging counts for far more than it really should. Often, when we don't live up to the world's expectations of how we should look or behave, we fall victim to a vicious circle of self-loathing and denial that can be difficult to escape from unscathed. At times like these, it's a comfort to remember that our souls are more dazzling than our selfies.

"Beauty is an internal light, a spiritual radiance that all women have but most women hide, unconsciously, denying its existence. What we do not claim remains invisible," Marianne Williamson, the American spiritual teacher and best-selling author, observes in her beautiful meditation on power and femininity, *A Woman's Worth: Toward a More Enlightened Feminism.*

But as you become more intimate with your Authentic Self—as you recover your true, incandescent identity—there will come a gradual but undeniable physical transformation. It is absolutely impossible to commit to your spiritual growth, awaken to your own radiant Light, and not have it reveal itself on the outside. "It is God's will that we be beautiful, that we love and be loved and prosper in all good things," Marianne Williamson reminds us. "It is God's will that we all become the goddesses we were created to be."

MARCH 11

Sending and Receiving Personal Signals

If you will resolve to work each day for self-realization, your whole world can change... The two women you are, they can make you over.

—Pond's Cold Cream advertisement,
Good Housekeeping, December 1947

I had not seen my friend in months. At first when she approached through the crowd of strangers, I literally did not recognize her. Her hair, always beautifully styled, was disheveled; her unmade-up face was red and puffy with large dark circles under her eyes, and she was wearing a pair of jeans and a lumpy sweater instead of the coordinating outfits she normally favored. I was absolutely stunned. What was wrong with this picture?

When we sat down together to talk over a cup of coffee, she told me about a serious life crisis she was experiencing. But even before she confided in me, I knew only too well that something was seriously wrong.

Each of us transmits personal signals about our self-esteem every day in myriad ways. Most of them are not as dramatic as my friend's but are rather subtle. When we are feeling on top of the world there's a spring in our step, a smile on our face, and a sparkle in our eyes. Then there are those occasions when, through lack of time, energy, or emotion, we become careless about our attire and our personal grooming. We literally begin to care less—until it looks as though we don't care at all. Of course, deep within, we care very much.

But there is an important reason why we *should* give a second thought to our personal appearance, even when we're alone: the inner joy we experience when we look our best. "Many women feel in their hearts that they have missed full self-realization," another advertisement for Pond's Cold Cream in the March 1949 issue of *Good Housekeeping* advised readers. "Yet they need not accept this—help is within themselves. You can feel it within you—an inner drive for happiness. The close interrelation between this Inner You and this Outer You, the almost uncanny power of each to change the other—can change you from drabness to joyous self-fulfillment."

When I first discovered this "New Age" series of beauty advertisements from the late 1940s, I was amused—and then grateful. For one of the most marvelous lessons you learn on a path of personal transformation is that when your heart is open to change, you're able to recognize the personal signals of encouragement your Authentic Self is constantly sending, no matter how unlikely the source.

How Do I Look?

How women look and how their looks change in the course of their lives, is not a frivolous question... "How do I look?" she asks as her eyes meet the eyes in the mirror. She listens carefully for an answer, because it might prove quite illuminating.
                                          —Kennedy Fraser
                                          English essayist and fashion journalist

How do I look?" is a question all of us have spent our lives asking others. But now that you are on the path toward your authenticity you have reached the point when you need to gently ask *yourself* this loaded question. And, once having asked, you need to listen carefully for the answer. Better yet, when you gaze into the mirror you should ask, "How do I feel?" because how you feel about yourself on any particular day will influence how you look more than what you are wearing.

After years of concentrating on the glitz of the outside packaging, we need to change our approach to beauty completely. Personal transformation begins with a strong inner life. We need to let Spirit show us the way, whether it's changing our wardrobe, losing weight, or finding the right hairstyle. Twenty minutes of meditation a day, quiet reflection, or a restorative walk seeking your Authentic Self will do more for your looks than you will believe. But of course, you'll believe it when you see it.

So what are you waiting for? Start today. Choose one inner tool and make it part of your daily beauty ritual. "If we go down into ourselves we find that we possess exactly what we desire," the French philosopher and mystic Simone Weil (1909–1943) believed. Remember this.

MARCH 13

Accepting Yourself as You Are Today

Seek not outside yourself, heaven is within.
—Mary Lou Cook (1908–1944)
American actress

Today, we make peace with the past: with the bodies and faces we were born with and those that have evolved. Today, we embrace the lines that stare back at us, the parts that sag in the middle or stick out where they shouldn't, the hair that never keeps a curl or never loses it. We begin when we invoke the Tibetan poet, teacher, and earliest Buddhist sage Saratha's song of praise. "Here in this body are the sacred rivers: here are the sun and moon as well as all the pilgrimage places...I have not encountered another temple as blissful as my own body."

It will take a bit of doing, learning to love all our personal pilgrimage places. However, before genuine love can flourish, we must finally accept ourselves exactly as we are today. Not tomorrow or next week or when we lose twenty-five pounds. Remember, acceptance is acknowledging the reality of a situation: that we're heavier than we'd like to be, for example, or that our complexion is ruddy or sallow, or that we've got gray streaks, or that leggings just don't work for us.

Most of us think of other women as beauties, never ourselves. But every woman was created by Spirit to be a genuine beauty. We learn how to reveal to the world our unique radiance only after we acknowledge it ourselves. Today, take as your personal mantra: "I am what I am and what I am is wonderful."

MARCH 14

Loving Yourself into Wholeness

I did not lose myself all at once. I rubbed out my face over the years washing away my pain, the same way carvings on stone are worn down by water.
—Amy Tan
Chinese-American novelist

Life batters us whether we are rich or poor, public or private. The wound we suffer may be an open cut or a slow, silent hemorrhage of the soul. On the outside we may look as if we've got our act together, but each of us encounters those dark, stormy days when we feel very small, very fragile, and very frightened, as if we might shatter into a thousand pieces and break into heartrending sobs at something as simple as "How are you?"

When this happens, we have to be kind to ourselves, not beat ourselves up. Leave that to the rest of the world. Our feelings are valid, our fears very real, even though they are probably not based on reality. Always remember that the best description of fear is "false evidence appearing real."

False Evidence Appearing Real.

When these occasions occur in your life, recall that your first duty is to love yourself into Wholeness. How to do this? By pampering yourself with simple pleasures and small indulgences. By treating yourself like the baby you are right now. Could you order something wonderful for dinner tonight from a Chinese or Indian carryout? Grubhub, the online food service, now can deliver from 85,000 different restaurants across America. There's bound to be something you'd like.

Could you treat yourself to some of the potted primroses, daffodils, or tulips that are appearing in the shops about now? Could you take the afternoon off and go home? If not, how about streaming a movie marathon or limited series with a big bowl of popcorn? Yes, it's called a binge. Why not delight in an ice-cream cone for lunch, taking it to a park to bask in the sunshine and hear the birds singing? What about saying no to the next request for you to do something?

Yes, you can. You don't have to do everything and be everything for everyone else all the time. If you think you can't possibly do one more thing without screaming or crying, you're probably right. Start by saying, "No, I'm sorry, I've got a prior commitment."

For, of course, you do. Today you need to be there for yourself. Remember, we did not lose ourselves all at once. But we recover our authentic selves one kind gesture at a time.

MARCH 15

Self-Nurturing: The Hardest Task You'll Ever Do

Any little bit of experimenting in self-nurturance is very frightening for most of us.

—Julia Cameron
American author and artist

Why should self-nurturance be so frightening for most women? Why is it for you? If you don't think this is true, how many creative excursions have you been on in the last month? Have you outfitted a comfort drawer for yourself? Have you been working in your *Illustrated Discovery Journal* or writing in your *Journal of Gratitude?*

Perhaps we are all Scrooges when it comes to self-nurturing because if we were kind to ourselves, our creativity might begin to blossom like a plant moving toward the light. Of course, this would mean we'd want to make some changes in our lives, and we all know how we feel about changes, even positive ones. We may be in a rut, but at least our own familiar grooves are comforting in their own insidious fashion.

The way to take giant leaps and strides toward our authenticity, however, is through small changes. The great nineteenth-century Russian novelist Leo Tolstoy believed that "True life is lived when tiny changes occur." Take an honest look at how good you are to yourself. How much sleep are you getting? Are you walking often or getting enough exercise? Have you given meditation a fair chance? How much time do you have every week just to relax? To dream? To engage in personal pursuits that bring you pleasure? When was the last time you laughed? "There is a connection between self-nurturing and self-respect," Julia Cameron, who wrote *The Artist's Way*, one of the most important books on recovering our creativity, reminds us.

Self-care has been a struggle for me. But believe me, I have slowly learned on the *Simple Abundance* path that if you want your life to come together, you have to start treating yourself better. No one else can do it for you. Today, make a list of ten nice things you could do for yourself. Now select one and do it. You have absolutely nothing to lose from experimenting with self-nurturing and everything to gain.

MARCH 16

What Do You Like about Yourself?

If you want to find the answers to the Big Questions about your soul, you'd best begin with the Little Answers about your body.
—George Sheehan (1918–1993)
American physician, athlete, and author

Like most of us, you see yourself in the mirror every day. But when was the last time you nodded your head in approval at what you saw? Today, I'd like to ask you to try something radically different: Look at yourself lovingly and begin to appreciate what you see.

This exercise is more than just skin deep, because I want you to take an inventory of what you like about yourself. Most of us are very quick to criticize ourselves. We're always finding things wrong with the way we look. Today we're going to discover and give thanks for what pleases us.

Tonight, set aside an hour to celebrate how marvelous you really are. Prepare an inviting bath, using scented oil or bubble bath. Bring a candle into the bathroom and bathe by candlelight. Allow yourself at least twenty minutes to soak in the warm water to renew yourself. Ask your Authentic Self to bring to your conscious mind all the special things you should discover tonight. After you pat yourself dry, gently apply some body crème or lotion to your body. Give yourself a slow massage and as you work your way down from your shoulders to your toes, visualize each body part surrounded by the most beautiful white light imaginable. This light is Love, and you are sending it to every cell in your being. In your most nurturing voice, tell yourself aloud how wonderful you are.

Now go into your bedroom, and before getting dressed for bed, take a compassionate look at yourself in the mirror. Continue to gaze approvingly into the mirror until you find ten things that you absolutely love about your face and your body—maybe a perfect nose, beautiful hands, trim ankles. Start at the top and work your way down. Consider everything. You may not like the way your hair is styled, for instance, but you love its color. Write all ten down in your Gratitude Journal. Now think about aspects of your personality that you like. You're a gifted improviser, an empathetic listener, an inspired cook, a patient and loving mother, a great woman for detail. Write it all down. Do not stop until you have at least ten things about your personality for which to be grateful.

And if you think you can't find twenty things to love about yourself, go back to the mirror. Do this exercise every day until you can. "Nature never repeats herself and the possibilities of one human soul will never be found in another," the American suffragist and abolitionist Elizabeth Cady Stanton wrote in *Solitude of the Self* in 1892. "Self-development is a higher duty than self-sacrifice." Today, be willing to search genuinely for your glorious possibilities and rejoice in your Divine authenticity. And if you're having difficulty, don't just dismiss the suggestion, lower the number of your discoveries to just one a day. And if you can't find one thing to love about yourself today, then come back tomorrow. Seek only to be gentle and loving to yourself in small ways and watch your self-care increase.

Ponder this today: Self-development is a *higher duty* than self-sacrifice. And that's from the mind, heart, and soul of a woman who dedicated her entire life to women's equality.

MARCH 17

Accentuating the Positive

If one is a greyhound, why try to look like a Pekingese?
—Dame Edith Sitwell (1887–1964)
British poet and critic

In an age when a woman's beauty was considered her most prized possession, the famed English poet Dame Edith Sitwell, born in 1887, stood out in a crowd, but not for the reasons you might expect. As a young girl she was so homely, awkward, and thin that her family fretted constantly over the fact that marriage would not be in her future.

Needless to say, "poor little E," as she was known, endured a miserable, lonely, and frustrated childhood until her beloved governess introduced her to the world of literature and music. She fell in love with the poetry of the Victorian lyric poet Algernon Charles Swinburne and the late nineteenth-century art movement known as the symbolists, which rejected realism in art and poetry. In finding her kindred spirits, Dame Edith fell in love with her Authentic Self.

This authenticity found expression in her poetry and in an eccentric personal style rooted in fantasy and drama. She became famous for her long, flowing Pre-Raphaelite dresses fashioned from brocades or upholstery fabrics, for her furs, and for her extraordinary hats that highlighted her strong, bony profile and became her own distinctive trademark. To accentuate her long, slender fingers (of which she was very vain) she grew her nails to Mandarin length, painted them red, and wore massive rings.

Dame Edith's flamboyant sense of style is not for many of us. But her glorious way of celebrating her Authentic Self and of accentuating the positive can speak to every woman. By now you should have discovered wonderful things about your own face and body. Each of us has at least one special feature that can set us apart. Do you accentuate your assets? Are your eyes your most beautiful feature? Then make them up every day, even if you are staying at home with the children or working from home. You're turning gray? Have you thought about letting your head shimmer in silver? You're blessed with a beautiful smile and full, luscious lips? Think about wearing red lipstick to call attention to them.

"I have often wished I had time to cultivate modesty," Dame Edith confessed toward the end of her life, "but I am too busy thinking about myself." Most of us don't spend nearly enough time thinking good things about ourselves. Today, follow Dame Edith's example. Discover, flaunt, and celebrate your authentic assets.

MARCH 18

Awakening Sleeping Beauty

When Sleeping Beauty wakes up
She is almost fifty years old.

—Maxine Kumin (1925–2014)
American Poet Laureate

In every one of us there lies a sleeping beauty waiting to be awakened through love. Because she has slumbered for so long, she must be awakened very gently. But instead of waiting for Prince Charming to storm the palace gates, you must summon the magic powers of your Authentic Self to break any cruel enchantment that has left you unaware of your own glory.

Let me tell you a story about a pretty girl I knew when I was young. Once upon a time there was a garbage strike in our town. For weeks the garbage piled up in front of trim suburban homes. One day a photographer from a newspaper drove up in front of a house and asked if there were any children present. He wanted to photograph children near the garbage pile to emphasize how much had accumulated. The little girl was shyly standing behind her mother when he came to the door, so she was selected and propped up on piles of garbage for the photograph. After the photograph was printed in the newspaper, some children in the schoolyard taunted the little girl by calling her "just a pile of garbage." In order to handle this public humiliation, she became numb to her own beauty for a very long time. Sitting on the pile of garbage was the same thing as pricking her finger on a spindle and falling into a deep sleep.

"It's hard to tell our bad luck from our good luck sometimes. Hard to tell sometimes for many years to come," the late Canadian author Merle Shain (1935–1989) gently reminds us. "And most of us have wept copious tears over someone or something when if we'd understood the situation better we might have celebrated our good fortune instead."

If that young girl had not pricked her finger, would she have retreated to her bed every afternoon after school and sought comfort in the world of books? When she became older would she have studied theater to learn the secrets of make-believe? Would she have traveled to London and Paris to write about fashion in order to learn about style? I think not, and I should know.

What was your spindle? Was there a moment when you pricked yourself and fell into a deep slumber? Or did you just slowly shut down? Perhaps the cruel enchantment was caused by overly critical parents, by sexual or domestic abuse, by a devastating breakup, or by a numbing reliance on food, drugs, or alcohol.

It is time to awaken, sleeping beauty. Your creativity, imagination, and authentic sense of style are far superior to any sorcerer's spell, no matter how strong. "One can never change the past, only the hold it has on you," Merle Shain reassures us, "and while nothing in your life is reversible, you can reverse it nevertheless."

MARCH 19

Repose of the Soul

Repose is a quality too many undervalue...In the clamor one is irresistibly drawn to the woman who sits gracefully relaxed, who keeps her hands still, talks in a low voice and listens with responsive eyes and smiles. She creates a spell around her, charming to the ear, the eye and the mind.
—*Good Housekeeping*, November 1947

We have all met her, that special woman who draws you into her orbit with a radiant smile. Her eyes light up as you tell her how you've been. She attracts men, women, children, and animals, for her complete attention is soothing and hypnotic. When you walk away from her you feel as if you have been bathed in a beautiful, warm light.

You have. It's called Love, and this ancient beauty secret is available to all of us. When we are genuinely interested in others, a graciousness comes over us that is compelling. "She did not talk to people as if they were strange hard shells she had to crack open to get inside. She talked as if she were already in the shell. In their very shell," the African-American playwright associated with the Harlem Renaissance Marita Bonner wrote of a soulful woman in 1926. Would that each of us were such a woman. Would that each of us could become one.

We can.

Most of us have more harried moments in our daily lives than tranquil ones. But by taking the time to step outside our own sphere to embrace others, we open ourselves up to the power of Spirit. We are suddenly lit up from inside, and this illumination can transform our looks more effectively than any fancy salon beauty makeover.

Today, act as if you are a woman with repose of the soul. Greet everyone you meet with a warm smile. No matter how busy you are, don't rush your encounters with coworkers, family, and friends. Speak softly. Listen attentively. Act as if every conversation you have is the most important thing on your mind today. Look your children and your partner in the eyes when they talk to you. Stroke the cat, caress the dog.

Lavish love on every living being you meet. See how different you feel at the end of the day.

MARCH 20

Inner Beauty, Outward Charm

Don't you love it when some incredibly beautiful woman like...
Cindy Crawford tells us that the real beauty secret is finding your
inner light? No shit. But I've done the same things these women
have done to find my inner light and while it's true I'm happier, I
still don't look like them.
                                            —Marianne Williamson
                                            American author and spiritual teacher

We can't all look like Beyoncé, but we *can* each look our best. Simplicity plays a part in striking the right chord of self. This occurs naturally as we begin to rethink how to put together our best look. Our authentic look. Gradually we learn that the "less is more" approach applies to makeup and fashion as well as to decorating and entertaining.

Ironically, this desire to look our best comes *after* we have committed to our inner work. As we go within, searching for spiritual growth, we begin to blossom on the outside. Time well spent in meditation gives us more serenity, and it shows on our faces. Learning to love ourselves exactly as we are gives us the motivation to move forward, whether in searching for a healthier way of eating or finding the right exercise regime. Perhaps we're starting to wear makeup more frequently and caring how we dress even when we're just working from home, doing errands, or driving children to afternoon activities. These are subtle changes that have a profound impact on how we feel about ourselves.

Why does working on our inner beauty produce outward charm? Perhaps it is because the two are inexorably connected. A Gnostic axiom teaches "As is the inner, so is the outer." Women who realize their full potential delight the Great Creator with their brilliance. Marianne Williamson tells us that the process of personal transformation—whether it be in our lifestyle or in our appearance—"is the true work of spiritual growth." I believe her.

Coming into Balance

I dream of an art of balance, purity, tranquility, devoid of disturbing, or disquieting subject matter . . . something akin to a good armchair.

—Henri Matisse (1869–1954)
French Impressionist painter

As I write, I'm recovering from an hour spent falling down and then picking myself up, just to fall down again. I'm bruised, out of breath, still wobbly (even though I am sitting down), and exhausted. Exactly the way I'm supposed to be, according to my fencing instructor, who placed me in the center of a core board and expected me to stay standing as I lunged my way to humiliation.

Hopefully, I'll be returning to fencing and horseback riding as personal sports, but I'm flummoxed to discover that I have to get in better physical condition to do either activity. And I'm thrown off to realize how unequal the right and left sides of my body are with regard to balance and strength. But I'm told, in sports and in life, you can't find your balance until you completely lose it. And then, if you don't use it, you *will* lose it.

"All too often when we think of living in balance, we approach balance in the same frantic, rushing way that we approach the rest of our lives," Anne Wilson Schaef, author of *Meditations for Living in Balance*, reminds us. "We want to balance work and home. We want to balance relationships. We want to work out and exercise and eat good food. We want to stay healthy so we can do more. We want to fill everything up, ourselves, our time, our activities, our relationships and our lives. If we are not careful, we will add balancing our lives as another task on our long lists of doing too much."

This week is the vernal equinox, when light and darkness find equal balance in the natural world. It's also a perfect time for us to consider how we can find more balance in the many aspects of our busy lives.

For most of us, doing too much feels normal. In any twenty-four hour period, we're constantly pulled in a dozen different directions— work, children, personal relationships, chores, errands, friends, family, finances, promises to others, health concerns, deadlines, and our own unfulfilled dreams and desires—which leaves little time for reflection, renewal, and recreation, the holy trinity of balance. Let's start thinking of them as rites of passage to contentment.

So get off the teeter-totter of your to-do list and find an armchair. One of the more delightful ways to find balance is to realize that not everything that needs doing has to be done today. "Many tasks and issues in our lives will take care of themselves if we will but let them," Anne Wilson Schaef recommends. "The impossible task that *had* to be accomplished immediately looks very different tomorrow or next week. Often, I have found that when others are pushing something as *urgent*...my best response is just to slow down."

Or, as the Zen koan reminds us: "Sitting quietly, doing nothing, spring comes, and the grass grows by itself."

MARCH 22

Why Self-Confidence Can't Be Bought but Can Be Borrowed

I was thought to be "stuck up." I wasn't. I was just sure of myself.
This is and always has been an unforgivable quality to the unsure.
—Bette Davis (1908–1989)
American actress and Hollywood legend

It would be wonderful if we could simply waltz up to a cosmetic counter and purchase a bottle of self-confidence the way we can buy "revitalizing" or "performance" creams for our faces. Unfortunately, this spiritual elixir, like an expensive perfume, is different on every woman because of individual chemistry.

When I was younger, my self-confidence potion was heavily scented with attitude, optimism, and faith; experience, knowledge, and wisdom had to come later. But even today, every new opportunity or challenge requires that I prepare a special batch of moxie for myself. I do this by becoming as thoroughly prepared as possible and by looking the part—wearing an outfit, for example, that exudes self-confidence even when it's hanging in the closet. Next, I say my prayers and ask for the Power to be switched on. Then it's "showtime." I *act* as if I'm self-confident and the world takes me as such.

When you're unsure of yourself but life requires you to be otherwise, it is comforting to remember that you can always borrow a self-confident attitude from your Authentic Self. She knows how terrific you are and can give you that little boost, which is all you really need. Our subconscious mind cannot distinguish between what's real and what's imaginary (which is why creative visualization works). If we act as if we're confident, we become so. At least for a little while.

"You must do the thing you think you cannot do," Eleanor Roosevelt (1884–1962), the longest-serving American first lady, once observed, and her life was spent proving the point. When life challenges arise, you can surmount them by calling on Spirit and borrowing the scent of self-confidence from your Authentic Self.

MARCH 23

Always Be a First-Rate Version of Yourself

Always be a first-rate version of yourself, instead of a second-rate version of somebody else.
—Judy Garland (1922–1969)
American actress and legendary entertainer

I make a terrible Judy Garland but I do a pretty good Sarah Ban Breathnach. It's taken me nearly my entire lifetime to come to this awareness, but I've not been the same woman since I did. Neither will you be once this truth awakens in your heart.

You see, whether we are consciously aware of it or not, we're constantly programmed by the world to be other women, not ourselves. Sadly, one doesn't have to look very far or wide to see how starved the modern woman remains for daily inspiration. Despite the fact that there are now thousands of women's lifestyle websites and blogs, every month brings another onslaught of lifestyle coaches offering advice on how to dress, decorate our homes, "handle" our relationships, raise geniuses, halve our weight, and overhaul our personal ambitions. It boggles the mind.

I don't know about you, but as a busy, exhausted, and very often frazzled woman (what can I say, enlightenment ebbs and flows around here), I don't need another exhortation of trends, but I am seeking gentle encouragement, brief dollops of common sense, compassionate reminders, and comforting reassurances. If *Simple Abundance* often reads like a six-hundred-page permission slip nudging you toward self-nurturance, that's because it is.

You must *believe* your happiness and well-being are not indulgent but a spiritual prime directive.

According to *Webster's Dictionary*, to be authentic is to be "not imaginary, false or imitation." To be authentic is to be "genuine, veritable, bona fide, being actually and precisely what is claimed." The only thing that we can genuinely claim to be is ourselves. But our best is good enough, even on a bad day. I know a woman who is a high-powered advertising executive in New York. There is no one I know on the planet who is more creative, articulate, accomplished, and funny, but some days she doesn't see it that way. She grew up in a home where performance was always graded, and as a result she's extremely hard on herself. Her personal grade of C-minus is probably everybody else's A-plus.

We are all so hard on ourselves. We not only want to be other people; we want to be perfect versions of them.

Let me tell you about another woman I know. When her first book was published, close friends will testify, she acted like a raving lunatic. Instead of congratulating herself on producing such a beautiful book after years of effort, she was about to throw herself off a cliff because she had used the wrong verb tense in one sentence. Instead of celebrating her achievement, she robbed herself of joy.

Now she knows better, thank God. Did you know that Amish quilters will deliberately add a mismatched patch to each quilt to remind themselves that only Spirit can create perfectly? We need to remember that. We should only strive to be first-rate versions of ourselves. And our best is always good enough.

MARCH 24

The Secret Saboteur: When You're Feeling Blue

Listening to your heart is not simple. Finding out who you are is not simple. It takes a lot of hard work and courage to get to know who you are and what you want.

—Sue Bender
American author

After self-nurturance, listening to the whispers of our hearts is probably the hardest task we've ever attempted. Some days the *Simple Abundance* path comes naturally. You realize that all you have is all you truly need. Other days, it's impossible to quiet down the wants. It seems as if you have too many unfulfilled desires and delayed dreams. You're sick and tired of waiting for inner changes to manifest themselves on the outside.

When the dark days come, we need to remember that even if a secret saboteur—depression—is at work temporarily derailing our progress (or so it seems), each day offers us a gift if we will only look for it. Sometimes we're sad for a very apparent reason—an overwhelming loss, for example, or worries over money or health. Other times we don't know why we feel so bad, which makes us feel even worse. It could be for a million different reasons—an appalling lack of appreciation (by ourselves and by others), exhaustion, the weather, hormones, the advent of the flu, or simply part of the process of personal transformation.

I wish I could tell you that spiritual and creative growth was smooth, predictable, and without pain. "All the best transformations are accompanied by pain," the acclaimed British author Fay Weldon tells us. "That's the point of them." Personal growth also comes in spasms: three steps forward, two steps back, and then a long plateau when it seems as though nothing is happening. But it's important to realize that this dormant period always seems to precede a growth spurt. Unfortunately, during the dormant period we very often become depressed and decide to give up.

It's on days like these that you can barely get yourself dressed and out the door. You look like hell and couldn't care less. You can't remember if you took a shower yesterday or when the last time was you washed your hair. The children's voices are insistent and yours is shrill. You haven't any patience. Life seems bleak, not bright with promise. It's taking more work than you expected to discover who you really are, and now you're no longer sure you even want to find out.

When dark clouds hover, what should you do besides hold on and ride out the storm? You have two choices. One is simply to give in, stop resisting. You've got the blues, so sing them, baby. But before you do, ask for grace. Then have a good cry. Leave work early. Take a nap and try to sleep it off. Indulge—without guilt—in something purely for medicinal reasons, like a piece of cheesecake or a bowl of Häagen-Dazs, but don't eat it standing in front of the refrigerator. Sit down, eat your treat slowly, and savor it. If you have the energy, fix comfort food for dinner tonight. If you don't, order in or fix something simple, like sandwiches. Stream a three-hanky movie. Put the kids to bed early. Soak in a hot tub. Raid your comfort drawer. Pull up the covers and snuggle down. Find five things for which to be grateful. The day is done. There's one. You'll catch up tomorrow. Turn out the light.

The alternative blues-kicker is to shift gears. Ask for Grace. Call a good friend and talk. Put the kettle on for a fresh pot of tea. Wash your face, comb your hair, put on some lipstick, perfume, and earrings. Smile at yourself in the mirror. Straighten the living room so that you can find a place to sit down. Take a walk around the block and clear your head. If you're working in an office, give yourself permission to put off that new project at work until tomorrow when you can concentrate. Instead, clean your desk and organize your papers. On the way home treat yourself to a bouquet of daffodils and your favorite takeout.

No matter which route you take, within twenty-four hours another day will begin. Tomorrow should be better. But if it's not, nor the next day, or the next, then know that it's okay to ask for help from friends, a support group, a therapist, a doctor, or your Higher Power. Dark days come to all of us. Yet discouraging days bring with them golden opportunities when we can learn to be kind to ourselves. Believe it or not, today offers you a hidden gift, if you're willing to search for it. Or as Fay Weldon reassures us: "Nothing happens, and nothing happens and then, everything happens."

Real Life: Clothes That Fit Your Lifestyle

*"I haven't got a thing to wear" does not, of course, mean that we
must resort to nakedness or seclusion; it means that our wardrobes
contain nothing that might match our mood or offer a just reflection of our current lives.*

—Kennedy Fraser
English essayist and fashion journalist

Most of us have had the experience of looking at a closet full of
clothes and finding nothing wearable that matches our mood. With
a sigh of resignation, we resort to a well-worn and time-tested "uniform," whether it be a black dress and pearls or a denim skirt, sweater,
and boots.

Actually, most of us wear, with few exceptions, the same thing or its
incarnation over and over again. The outfits may vary according to the
season, but not our dependence on a few staples, which, in their own way,
offer a revealing reflection of how we view our current lives. The legendary editor-in-chief of *Vogue*, Diana Vreeland, was famous for favoring the
same style black couture skirts and sweaters every workday for many years.

So what do we do with all the clothes we don't wear? Nothing.
They just hang there abandoned, because of their size or color or lack
of appropriateness, because they itch, or because we had that last terrible fight with our ex-husband in that sorry dress and don't want to
be reminded of the pain. Sometimes clothes hang around season after
season, phantoms waiting for some unforeseen occasion in the future
that never comes.

Spring is the perfect time to take stock of our wardrobes and reconsider our relationship to clothes. The wind of refreshing change is in
the air. We long to shed our heavy coats and sweaters for lighter garb.
Let's shed our outmoded attitudes about what's fashionable and replace
them with new ideas about what works for us in our real lives and truly
reflects our authenticity.

What if everything hanging in your closet was something you
loved—something that made you look beautiful or made you feel wonderful when you put it on? Think of how good you would feel every
day. Embracing the second *Simple Abundance* Grace of Simplicity can
spiritually induce such a miracle.

Later you'll clean out your closets and dresser drawers, but not
today. Today, I only want you to consider your real life and the clothes
you wear every day. Do they really reflect the woman within? What

about the clothes that speak to you from the pages of your *Illustrated Discovery Journal*? What about the clothes that hang abandoned in your closet? Every dress, skirt, pair of slacks or jeans, blouse, sweater, T-shirt, and jacket tells a story. "Clothes have a life that is quite independent of their shape and color," Kennedy Fraser reminds us in *The Fashionable Mind*. Get quiet, go within, and be willing to really listen to the tale that the threads of your life have woven.

MARCH 26

The Unspoken Language of Authenticity

To choose clothes, either in a store or at home, is to define and describe ourselves.
—Alison Lurie
American Pulitzer Prize–winning novelist

Most of us do not think we're carrying on a conversation with our psyches, our families, and the outside world when we get dressed in the morning, but we are. Alison Lurie tells us in her fascinating book *The Language of Clothes* that the vocabulary of our wardrobe conveys much more than we ever dreamed possible. "Long before I am near enough to talk to you on the street, in a meeting, or at a party, you announce your sex, age and class to me through what you are wearing—and very possibly give me important information (or misinformation) as to your occupation, origin, personality, opinions, tastes, sexual desires and current mood. I may not be able to put what I observe into words, but I register the information unconsciously; and you simultaneously do the same for me. By the time we meet and converse we have already spoken to each other in an older and more universal tongue."

After you begin searching for your Authentic Self, one of your more startling insights will occur when you discover that for years another woman has been carrying on conversations for you—at home, at work, in social situations, even on errands. At first this revelation can be disconcerting, even discouraging. But on reflection, it can be an exciting discovery, because now that you're beginning to cherish and channel your authenticity through creative choices, you can learn how to become not only bilingual but fluent in expressing yourself. As the famous French fashion designer Gabrielle "Coco" Chanel confessed, "How many cares one loses when one decides not to be something but to be someone."

Never Fall for Fashion, Always Be in Style

Fashion fades. Only style remains.

—Coco Chanel (1883–1971)

Madame Coco Chanel is continuing our private tutorial today. What is the difference between fashion and style? So glad we asked.

Women frequently want to have a mad passionate fling with fashion, but given a choice, most of us would marry style. That's because style, like a good partner, doesn't let you down. When fashion seduces you, the affair usually burns itself out before the next season.

Fashion is a show-off, concerned with the cutting edge. Style has seen it all before and knows that the classic tenets of simplicity, beauty, and elegance have staying power. Fashion is a cult; style is a philosophy.

Fashion mocks individuality; style celebrates it. Never forget that fashion, while frequently a charmer, is also a self-centered, frivolous bore. Style is high-spirited and generous, given to touting your best features for all the world to see. Fashion is a provocateur; style prefers to soothe. Fashion is self-congratulatory; style waits for the inevitable compliments. "Fashion can be bought," Edna Woolman Chase, the editor of *Vogue* during Madame Chanel's era, observed. "Style must be possessed."

Fashion guesses, so it can only bluff. Style knows. Fashion is impatient and eventually passes away. Style is steadfast and waits for every woman's awakening, because authentic style is born of Spirit.

Clearing: Parting with Fashion Mistakes

It's never too late—in fiction or in life—to revise.

—Nancy Thayer
American novelist

Revising your wardrobe to reflect your authenticity begins when you ruthlessly part with the fashion mistakes and mismatches that crowd your closets and confuse your cluttered mind. But let's be realistic for a moment. Most women I know have to be psyched up before they can tackle a project like this. Clearing out closets and dresser drawers is daunting to contemplate (all that money, all those bad choices) and hard work once you're at it. But few things are as satisfying as bringing order to a closet in which chaos once reigned. A change of seasons provides the perfect opportunity to get to work because it's time to pack away winter clothes and bring out spring and summer ones. With a plan of attack, you can also clear away the past.

Find three hours for this activity; for many women Saturday afternoon is perfect. Make sure you gather enough boxes and large plastic garbage bags ahead of time so that after you begin, your energy won't be scattered by constantly having to leave the room to find more containers. Play some delightful music; I like Broadway show tunes for clearing chores. Take a deep breath. Now start by taking everything out of your closet and putting it on the bed. There, it's too late to turn back now.

Go through your wardrobe, item by item. Try things on if you're not sure and look at yourself in a full-length mirror honestly but with compassion. Edit your fashion accessories as well: jewelry, scarves, purses, hats, shoes. Keep *only* those things you love—things that make you look beautiful or feel fabulous. This is simplicity at work. What if some of the items don't fit you today but you still love them? Save only one size smaller than you're wearing now, because getting back into it is a realistic goal and something to work toward.

Consider the various real lives you lead and the clothes you need for them: work, dress-up, and comfort. If you haven't worn something in a year, why not? Be willing to part with it, even if it was expensive. Don't save it unless it has tremendous sentimental value. For example, I went through a phase where I wore nothing but Laura Ashley. Today the cottage sprig look doesn't suit me. But because I have so many happy memories of dressing alike with my daughter, I can't bear to part with our shared Laura Ashley past, so it's packed away in the attic for my daughter to consider when she's older, although she rolls her eyes and assures me, "That look is never coming back." Who knows? If you have room to pack away sentimental favorites, then do so. If you don't, be willing to pass them on to someone else who will love them as much as you once did.

Now take the plunge and give away the rest to those who will bless your generosity. In return, you'll experience a sense of grateful abundance when you realize how much you can give away. This positive attitude is essential for attracting more prosperity into our lives. A very therapeutic way of dealing with your expensive discards is donating them to organizations like Dress for Success, which helps women entering the job market with clothes in order to go on interviews. This makes it easy to edit your wardrobe because, really, you're helping other women in a wonderfully positive way. A friend is extremely well dressed and regularly finds gorgeous clothing at unbelievable prices. She always donates clothing every year. She thinks she's just lucky. I think it is the Universe's way of rewarding her for keeping a "cycle of good" continuing.

Every woman has fashion mistakes that clutter up her sense of style and tempt her to whine about her wardrobe. Clearing our closets of past incarnations provides the space and freedom for us to choose clothing in the future that authentically reflects the women we are becoming.

MARCH 29

Comfort Clothes and What They Mean

I base my fashion taste on what doesn't itch.
—Gilda Radner (1946–1989)
American comedian

Most women feel passionately about their comfort clothes. I have a beloved pair of paisley cotton knit pajamas that I would wear twenty-four hours a day, seven days a week, if I could only figure out how to get away with it. During the day they wait patiently on a hook in my bedroom closet; at night they whisper my name. Because I wear these pajamas so religiously, I wash them often, which is why they have become as soft as a baby's cheek. Alas, I have searched in vain to find another pair so that I might have more variety in my at-home wear, but either the style or the fabric doesn't quite match the perfection of my paisley, so the holy quest continues.

I used to own a special sweater that was an incredible silk-cotton blend. I wore it and washed it so often that it began to unravel at the sides. I wore it anyway. I called it my lucky literary sweater because the days I wore it were incredibly productive. This synchronicity occurred because I felt such exquisite pleasure and experienced such divine comfort all day long that I was free to be a creative conduit. Finally, when the book I was writing was completed, my daughter's father beseeched me to discard the ratty old thing. Since I was then known to strangers in our town as simply "the mayor's wife," I reluctantly agreed. One of our cats made a nest on my lost love in the basement. Her look of unadulterated bliss at having inherited such a treasure somewhat alleviates the loss. Somewhat, but not quite.

I'm convinced that we are our own best selves in comfort clothes. Somehow, through the alchemy of fiber and fit, we are once again restored to Paradise, this time not naked before the Great Creator, but reveling in the clothes She intended for us to wear.

Unfortunately, comfort clothes exist for most of us only as a footnote to our lives, not center stage as they would if a sensible woman were in charge of the earthly scheme of things. Perhaps we feel good for eight hours out of every twenty-four, but that is not nearly good enough. The rest of the time we're squeezed into uncomfortable things that pull, pinch, tug, choke, itch, hike up or down, and make the days of our lives miserable. We wear these creations of torture, we tell ourselves, in order to be agreeable to the rest of the world. But why shouldn't we find a way of making the world agreeable to us instead?

This week play detective. Examine closely the items in your wardrobe you reach for when in need of comfort. Look for clues to help you bring more comfort into your life. What fabrics feel good against your skin? Make a note of it on your phone or the small spiral notebook you're carrying in your purse. What size are you really comfortable in? Be honest, not vain. It has been my experience that comfort clothes are usually our *true* size, or even a tad loose. You don't squeeze into comfort; you slip into something that's more comfortable. What collar style suits you? Yes, these details make all the difference. Expand the comfort concept to how you care for your wardrobe. In the future look for clothes that are easy to maintain—no labels that say "Dry clean only."

Now see if you can't find clothing that matches your personal preferences and be willing to wait until you do. Consider budgeting and saving for quality comfort clothing you can wear all day long and love for years. The *Simple Abundance* path encourages us to be patient until we find what's perfect for us, rather than continue to waste our money, energy, and emotion settling for second-best or second-rate.

MARCH 30

Developing a Sense of Style

Taste concerns itself with broad, lifetime progress and never makes mistakes; style moves by fits and starts and is occasionally glorious.

—Kennedy Fraser
English essayist and fashion journalist

Celebrating your authentic style through the clothes you wear is an art form. But like any of the arts, a sense of style is one that needs to be nurtured after it is initially divined and devised. Style begins when you seek and discover your strengths, then bank on them for all they're worth. Personal style flourishes when you realize that you really don't need as much clothing, accessories, jewelry, or makeup as you once thought you did because you've got attitude.

Remind yourself today that you are an artist. In searching for your authenticity, you will uncover your own signature look. It may be the great way you wear hats, highlight stunning eyes with smoky gray kohl, showcase a chic short cut with fabulous earrings, show off gorgeous slender legs with sheer stockings and elegant pumps, or have enough pluck to pair a white cotton T-shirt with a tailored wool jacket.

This year, be willing to experiment with a sense of adventure, to find out what works for you and what doesn't. Then stick with what works, no matter what everybody else is wearing.

MARCH 31

Do Try This at Home: First Aid

The only real security is not insurance or money or a job, not a house and furniture paid for, or a retirement fund, and never is it another person. It is the skill and humor and courage within, the ability to build your own fires and find your own peace.
—Audrey Sutherland (1921–2015)
Solo kayak explorer, adventurer, and author

When my daughter was completing eighth grade her class was planning a camping trip. Since I'd begun writing during the blur of her grammar school years, I'd never been a trip chaperone, so when she asked me, of course I agreed. However, my last camping trip had been many years before when I was a Girl Scout, so you would be correct in assessing my camping skills as zilch.

Nonetheless, I must have felt Mrs. Miniver's spirit unconsciously, because I was determined to be prepared for a camping crisis, should one occur. That meant a trip to our local REI, the outdoor and camping purveyors, where I filled up the shopping cart with first aid and camping gear. Every time I put another "must-have" into the cart, Kate would take it out and say: "We won't be needing this."

I was almost done when I added an emergency tick removal kit. Since the kids would all be outfitted in long johns and rain gear, Kate rolled her eyes and sighed when she saw the box; *nobody else's mom brought this stuff when they were chaperones, why was I embarrassing her*…If you've ever had a heated exchange with a thirteen-year-old, you know it's not pleasant to linger. I seem to recall the conversation ending with an exasperated warning from Kate: "Okay, bring it, but don't let anyone see it."

The camping trip to watch the Assateague ponies in Maryland was terrific fun. There were no medical emergencies, thank Heavens, except for one of the boys, who got bitten by a tick. Fortunately, some resourceful parent had included a tick removal kit with the first aid supplies, and so all's well that ends well.

Emergency Medical Information

This month we'll continue mirroring Mrs. Miniver's calm practicality as we start to get our first aid kit and health records in order.

"When an emergency happens, whether it's a heart attack or a hurricane, it's critical that medical service providers have access to health information for anyone who needs assistance," the Mayo Clinic recommends. "While you can't predict when an emergency may happen, you can be prepared."

So let's start.

As you did with your vital papers last month, we'll begin compiling a family health records file. Gather them all together to be kept in one box while you prepare the individual files, including a digital scan so you'll have a thumb drive as well as a printed version. Again, this is a project that can be spread out in two-hour blocks over a couple of weekends. It took me about four hours to do by myself over two weekends. Two hours is enough for one session, however; even just starting with one hour is great. The point is to start.

For every member of your family, you'll create a file. You'll need: name, age, and sex, address, blood type, any medical conditions, such as high blood pressure, diabetes, or epilepsy, allergies.

Our smartphones are also equipped to keep all our medical information in the medical ID available on the home screen. When we update the setting called "show when locked on," emergency medical personnel have access to all our vital information. Do this for your mother, aunt, or grandparent for the gift of a lifetime. Don't forget to set up the in case of emergency data. If an emergency was activated (check your phone's system on the specifics), a phone call is made to everyone on the list to notify them that first responders have been called.

You'll also need a list of each person's prescriptions. Tell your family's physicians that you're preparing an emergency first aid kit and would like to have an extra month's worth of medicine, issued separately.

If you have immunization records, include that with your digital scans as well as your printout. Who can remember the last time anyone had a tetanus shot?

Have any of you traveled recently outside the United States? Make note of that.

Each person should have a medical consent form and any other documentation or special products to deal with individual health concerns, and make sure you have a signed medical proxy authorization.

If you have any x-rays from recent medical conditions (or as part of your mammogram records) bring them in a waterproof portfolio or file.

As you did last month with your vital papers, everyone in your family should have their own plastic envelope file, which will go into a duffel bag carrying your first aid and health supplies. I'd pick out a red duffel bag because you will recognize it immediately, and if you can get one with wheels, you'll be thankful.

First Aid Kits

In outfitting your first aid kit, it's much easier to start with premade, top-notch first aid kits, and I'd recommend an OSHA-approved workplace kit that can treat up to fifty people, which is available on Amazon. If you have a baby in your family, it's good to have a first aid kit for small children, too.

We all use over-the-counter health aids, such as pain reliever, bug spray (there are many natural insect repellents now), anti-itch cream for bites, sunscreen, blister remedies, blood clotting agents, and wound covers. But there's also cough medicine, cold relief, athlete's foot preparation, tampons, sanitary napkins, hand sanitary gel, and individual packages of tissues. After you've inspected your first aid kit, you'll know what else you need to fill in.

Don't forget rubber gloves, health masks, a splint, a sling, and a tourniquet. All of these are available online.

Finally, the Mayo Clinic reminds us: "Probably the only mistake a traveler can make with their first aid kit is not having one. There are many commercially available kits to be purchased. A bit of pre-planning can go a long way towards dealing with unexpected injury or illness" on an adventure or during an emergency.

Should you need to "borrow" supplies from the first aid kit, make a note and put it on the kit to flag your memory and replace it on your next trip to the pharmacy.

And don't forget the tick removal kit!

Joyful Simplicities for March

It isn't the great big pleasures that count the most, it's making a great deal out of the little ones.
—Jean Webster (1876–1916)
American novelist and playwright

☞ If you don't have them growing in your garden, bring home a bouquet of daffodils, now available in season. These beauties will brighten any space.

- Take a spring walk, scout your backyard, or visit a nursery and get some bare branches: cherry, crabapple, forsythia, birch. Cut the ends sharply on a slant and place them in a variety of attractive containers—large vases, colorful bottles, pottery jugs, even old milk cans—filled with tepid water. Use your imagination! Place your branches in a sunny spot and wait for spring to arrive indoors.
- Find a five-and-dime or dollar store. Cruise the aisles. You'd be amazed at what they still sell. Buy some old-fashioned terry-cloth dish towels to replace the ratty ones in the kitchen or get yourself the kind of mascara you put on with a brush. For a dime store website, check out www.thingsfromtheattic.com.
- Celebrate St. Patrick's Day (March 17). Wear green. Try your hand at baking a loaf of delicious Irish soda bread, along with a supper of corned beef, cabbage, boiled potatoes, and carrots. Serve with hot tea, cold beer, Irish coffee. For those who don't imbibe, there are marvelous nonalcoholic brews available that impart the taste but not the buzz of alcohol. Play some traditional Irish music and dance a jig in your living room. (I'm serious!) Get a small pot of Irish shamrocks or bells of Ireland at the supermarket floral department for your desk.
- Observe the vernal equinox on March 21 with a springtime dinner of salmon cakes, fresh asparagus, and new potatoes.
- Gather pussy willows, either on a walk or from a florist, and make a seasonal wreath for your front door. Get a circular wire base at a crafts shop and overlap branches of pussy willow, securing with florist's wire. Add a festive bow with long streamers to whip in the March winds.
- Collect your favorite affirmations and then record them on your phone or a digital voice recorder in your own voice. After you've recorded them, lie down on your bed, close your eyes, and play them back using headphones. Do this several times a week. This is a *very* powerful tool for transformation.
- The last week in March is the time to plant a living Easter basket. Find a pretty pastel-colored Easter basket, line it with pebbles (or a reusable plastic liner available at gardening centers), and add two inches of potting soil. Sprinkle fast-growing rye grass seed on top of the soil and then cover with another quarter inch of soil. Water well and cover with a brown paper sack for a few days until the seeds germinate. When the grass sprouts, place the basket in a warm, sunny window and continue to water. In a couple of weeks you'll have a basket of living grass. Add a bow to the handle and tuck in some painted wooden Easter eggs and a small

stuffed bunny for a charming springtime centerpiece. This is a delightful hostess gift to make if you're expected somewhere for Easter dinner.

☙ Have you outfitted a comfort drawer this month? If not, why not? If money is the reason, select one pleasure and begin slowly with one small symbolic item. The crucial point is to start self-care in a tangible way.

☙ How many creative excursions have you gone on this month? Remember, they don't have to cost a dime—just an investment of time—in order to be well-spent moments.

APRIL

April, the angel of the months.
— Vita Sackville-West, Lady Nicholson (1892–1962)
English poet, novelist, and garden designer

Perhaps it's because April is so full of dazzling sunlight. Perhaps it's because the earth seems greener. Perhaps it's because resurrection is this month's signature. Is this why our spirits start to soar? Now the season of darkness diminishes as the season of Light increases in strength. In the garden, primroses, pansies, violets, tulips, and lilacs burst with color. Each flower, plant, and bough bears profound witness to the power of authenticity. This month, on the *Simple Abundance* path, we continue to grow gracefully, creatively, and joyously into our Authentic Selves, awakening to our own beauty.

APRIL 1

Can You Remember?

*Can you remember who you were before the world told you who
you should be become?*

—Danielle LaPorte
Canadian best-selling author,
entrepreneur, and blogger

Do you know of Peru's "Queen of the Andes"? She's a seed-bearing
spiky, gigantic wonder that grows at the highest altitudes and in the
harshest conditions that no other plant on earth can survive and doesn't
begin her reproductive cycle until after she turns eighty! Think of that:
proof that eighty is the new thirty.

Or the African marvel, the Madagascar palm, which has been on the
earth for 80 million years? She was discovered for the first time in 2008,
because she blooms only once every century.

I want you to think of a woman's spiritual *moxie* as an indomitable
feminine strength, like the sap of these extraordinary botanical stun-
ners. All we need has already been provided for us, hidden in the secret
recesses of our hearts as small time capsules containing the seeds of
resilience, restoration, and self-reliance that grow best from the ashes of
our previous existence.

I love the fabulous word *moxie*. It's great American slang—a noun
that means courage, know-how, nerve, and verve. I love its exhilarating
combination. It perfectly describes our journey to find our Authentic
Selves. Originally coined as the brand name for a non-alcoholic health
drink in 1885, *Moxie* was good for whatever ailed you, especially if you
were shy and modest. And while we're both not coming to these pages
lacking anything, at times we can feel fragile and often frightened as we
begin searching for a splendid life to truly call our own. Divine Grace
always knew we would come to this turning point—giving up or going
forward. Accessing our own moxie was designed for this very moment.

Think of our moxie as a feminine force that only occurs when two
separate elements—inexhaustible courage and stubborn faith—are
mixed together. Through the spontaneous combustion of necessity and
passion they create an entirely new compound: steely determination.
Now ponder an irresistible force meeting an immovable object, and
you've got the spiritual moxie of your Authentic Self pushing through
everything standing in the way of your happiness.

Only after we have been broken and emptied of all pretenses; only
when we've faced heart-wrenching reckonings and impossible situations; only when the only opinions that matter are the Great Creator's

and our own; only when we remember who we were before the world told us who we should be, only then do we become our Authentic Selves.

Can We Have a Word?

We should have 70 lives. One is no use.
—Winifred Holtby (1898–1935)
English novelist, feminist reformer

*R*einvention.

If I hear that word again or read it today (and you can bet on it), I'll not be held responsible. I'll be driven to write another book.

Reinventing is the latest buzz. Retirement was for previous generations, but "reinventing yourself" has become the next big thing. At least that's what all the lifestyle editors tell us, spinning gray-haired Rapunzel fairy tales to keep us calm and working on. In magazine headlines and on websites—for example, "How Real Women Reinvent"—we're encouraged to reimagine our lives by creating new and radically different careers: the prosecutor converts to pastor; a hedge fund analyst distills small-batch whiskey; the forensic accountant becomes a financial astrologer; a pharmaceutical chemist transforms into a luxury chocolatier.

We must stop using this cockamamie cliché if we're ever to see our lives as a work of art. Inanimate objects can be "reinvented." The car now can be electrically charged. The plugged-in vacuum cleaner can now be powered by a cordless robot. That's "reinvented" or reconfiguring something that was initially introduced into the world in a different form. Plants have been "genetically modified"; animals have been "cloned." Fashion recycles hemlines, shoulder pads, and nipped waists every other decade. But Authenticity is *not* reinvention, modification, cloning, or recycling.

Authenticity is Divine growth; reinvention is substitution rather than evolution. Authenticity is a natural, organic flowing from your soul's inception to this moment and beyond, even if the branch you're trying to crawl out upon right now has been stunted through delay, disappointment, disuse, or denial. Authenticity is reimagining the spirit, style, and substance of how you'd like your daily round to unfold with beauty, charm, and grace.

Authenticity is considering what you need now in order to experience contentment. Authenticity is embracing what you want to do, want to have, or experience in your life regardless of anyone else's opinion of how sensible your choices are, because they are *your* choices. Authenticity is restoring passion, finding comfort, and being as prepared as possible for the unexpected.

Authenticity is recovering the part of yourself you might have abandoned long ago to be practical; perhaps you put other people's wants before your needs. We all have. Taking care of others before ourselves is a woman's default response. But Authenticity can also be discovering another woman within who is entirely her own person with an intoxicating optimism, exhilarating strength, and a radiant exuberance you never dreamed you possessed. It's your Authentic Self, and I'm staggered by her many accomplishments and emboldened by her *joie de vivre,* vitality, and vibrant visions of her future.

I'm dazzled by her courage and hard-won confidence that she can do whatever it takes to make these dreams come true. "I have a sense of these buried lives striving to come out through me to express themselves," the brilliant poet Marge Piercy confessed, surely an echo vibrating for all of us. Don't you want to meet her?

Then don't reinvent. Rediscover your Authentic Self.

APRIL 3

Verve: The Secret of Personal Style

The soul should always stand ajar, ready to welcome
the ecstatic experience.

—Emily Dickinson (1830–1886)
American poet

French women are famous for their verve, and Coco Chanel started it all by unlacing and tossing Victorian corsets out the window in 1910 when she opened her first shop in Paris.

Today when I think of verve, Amal Clooney leads the head-turning list because she showed us that an international human rights lawyer can rock the red carpet and the courtroom with style and substance. When asked by the paparazzi what she was wearing, Amal shot back, "I'm wearing Ede and Ravenscroft," the English legal robe purveyors since 1689.

Lupita Nyong'o, Jane Fonda, Cate Blanchett, Blake Lively, Helen Mirren, and Rihanna all know the ageless art of making an entrance. We can learn a lot just by observing how they smile, stop, turn, smile again. And their posture. What accessories are they wearing—or not?

Princess Diana possessed verve, and now her daughters-in-law, Kate, the Duchess of Cambridge, and Meghan, the Duchess of Sussex, have picked up her mantle; both have successful fan websites showcasing what they wore when and how you can get this look at more affordable prices. The British fashion industry has created a new category for the "Kate effect" and the "Meghan effect," and pulling up close behind is three-year-old style icon Princess Charlotte, whose regal look is a dress with smocking and a Peter Pan collar, a cardigan, matching shoes and hair ribbon in complementary colors.

So back to whose look do you want? Won't it be wonderful when we can say, "My own." Be assured, we'll get there together.

To give us hope while we learn the art of more dash than cash, let me comfort you with the knowledge that *every* famous name mentioned above also has a glam squad, headed up by a behind-the-scenes star whisperer stylist, who never appears and is rarely mentioned, probably because they signed a Non-Disclosure Agreement, but has the clout to borrow designer dresses—and jewels—for her clients.

A century before, Emily Dickinson showed verve by preferring to dress entirely in white, year-round, at a time when most Victorian women dressed in dark, somber colors. Perhaps Miss Dickinson knew that expressing verve through her clothing could jump-start the ecstatic experience she so fervently sought and encouraged others to seek as well.

Verve is focused creative energy, a sense of vitality or zest. Verve is the special ability or talent to pull something off with panache, from a fabulous outfit to a reimagined room, an exquisite couplet of poetry, or a meaningful presentation to a group. Who knew we could do that? We certainly didn't; that's why discovering secret pleasures is so much fun.

Often a craving for verve comes into our lives when we're discontented and discouraged; this is the Great Creator's prod to get us to lighten up, try something different, and begin trusting our instincts, no matter how much or little we have in our pin money jar. Verve is how passion plays, when we take a risk and to our delight it pays off. It's also the secret of personal style and a key to how to be happy for the rest of your life.

Be yourself, in a body that emanates verve, whether showcased in an outfit, a hairstyle, or in satisfying work that fits you from the inside out.

Wouldn't you want to be yourself at all times?

And how do we learn to develop a finely honed sense of verve? By paying attention to the details. By accepting each day's attempt to teach us more about our authenticity. By being constantly on the lookout for what excites us or moves us to tears, what makes the blood rush to our head, our hearts skip a beat, our knees shaky, and our souls sigh. "A market stall, a fine Bokhara rug, a scrap of Chinese embroidery—food for the eye is to be found almost everywhere," the British writer Jocasta Innes urges us to remember. This week let's take another look around what surrounds us.

APRIL 4

Playing Dress-Up: Empowering Your Authentic Self with Fun

Learn the craft of knowing how to open your heart and to turn on your creativity. There's a light inside of you.
—Judith Jamison
American dancer and choreographer

What interests us today is remembering the importance of lightening up. A lighthearted sense of spontaneity is closely aligned with Spirit. Think of the brother who makes you laugh or the friend who will call you up and ask you to meet her on the spur of the moment for a coffee. Don't you just love to be in their company? Lighthearted people possess the special gift, as dancer Judith Jamison tells us, of being able to open their hearts to life and turn on their creativity. Perhaps it is because these special people still honor the child within. This sacred craft of knowing is one that we can gradually learn to nurture on the path we have chosen.

Children love to play dress-up. Think of the excitement of a little boy putting together his costume for Halloween or a little girl lost in the pleasure of exploring her mother's closet and jewelry box on a rainy afternoon. Today we're going to play dress-up, too. I love to indulge in this pastime in the spring and in the fall when I change my seasonal wardrobe. It's fun to play dress-up by yourself or in the company of an accomplice, such as your daughter or a close friend. (Be forewarned, however, that with your daughter, you'll frequently hear inquiries such as, "Do you still want this?" Yes, you do.)

Look at your pared-down wardrobe with fresh eyes. Small changes can have a big impact on your look. Try jackets on with different skirts and pants and see if you can't put together new outfits. Try pairing a lean, tailored jacket with a flounced skirt and belting it. Instead of always wearing the print silk blouse you bought to go with your navy suit, try a white cotton one with a stand-up collar. If you normally wear your collars open, try wearing them closed with an oversized costume jewelry necklace.

A new you? Why not? Now pull your hair back and see what

statement or chandelier earrings look like. Get out your shoes. Do you always wear plain leather pumps to work? What about switching to the suede wedges you save for nights out? Work with whatever you've got in your closet. Have fun with this exercise. Think seven years old. Think "what the heck!" The American author and journalist Gail Sheehy tells us that "the delights of self-discovery are always available."

Let's make a new entry in the Gratitude Journal tonight. "I had fun today doing…" Now fill in the blank.

APRIL 5

Come Alive with Color

All my life I've pursued the perfect red. I can never get painters to mix it for me. It's exactly as if I'd said, "I want rococo with a spot of Gothic in it and a bit of Buddhist temple"—they have no idea what I'm talking about. About the best red is to copy the color of a child's cap in any Renaissance portrait.

—Diana Vreeland (1903–1989)
Legendary fashion editor

My first visceral experience of how color could change my life occurred when I was a teenager. We had moved from New York to a small Massachusetts town, and my parents had bought a beautiful New England colonial house built in 1789. Set back from one of the main roads and surrounded by a stone wall, the exterior of the house was white clapboard with traditional black shutters, like many of the houses nearby.

Shortly after we moved in, my mother painted the living room a vibrant shade of red. This was long before red became chic, and my teenage mind could not fathom what had possessed her. Neither could our new neighbors. But from the street the sight of the red living room through the windows framed by the white and black exterior took your breath away with its beauty. Mother hadn't consulted the family beforehand, she just followed her instincts, and the result was stunning, which is often the case when we seek and find our authenticity. Even though I had felt unhappy about moving, I always looked forward to walking through the front door of our new home. The red room transformed my attitude.

The colors you wear don't have to be the same colors you live with. I love to wear red and black, strong, creative, and dramatic colors, but I need to live with soothing pastels for comfort and joy. There are many facets to your Authentic Self, just as there are many facets to a beautiful diamond, and you can use color to express your many moods.

Think about the colors you love. Are you surrounded by them or wearing them? If not, why not? Look for more ways to come alive this spring with color. Too many of us are afraid of experimenting with color. Just keep this in mind: We are our own research and development team, and as with any science project, all we're seeking is information. Does this work or not?

Take a creative excursion soon to an aquarium or pet shop that carries tropical fish. When you get a glimpse of the Great Creator's color palette, it will astonish you. Today the design industries, all of whom work a year ahead, anxiously wait for the Pantone "Color of the Year" to be revealed. I wonder how many of the judges go on an exotic fish escapade beforehand.

What are the colors that speak to your soul? Head out to a paint store and look at the color spectrum among the sample paint chips; if you're like me, the variety will make your heart beat faster. You can even get small tester amounts of a few colors to try out inexpensively at home. Pick up some favorites.

Next, go to a fabric store (or online) and find a textile pattern that catches your eye. Buy a yard of it. Drape it over a couch or pin it up on a wall. Live with the colors for a month, then use the fabric to cover a pillow, or paint a room or a piece of furniture in that new hue. Brighten up your desk with colored files, paper clips, and note pads. Tuck in perky paper napkins when you pack your lunch. Display produce in a bright ceramic bowl on your kitchen counter so that you can see nature's vibrant spectrum. When next at an art museum, collect art postcards to post on a bulletin board or refrigerator, to place on a desk, and to send to friends. Allow yourself to be carried away by colorful impulses.

The nineteenth-century English art critic John Ruskin believed that "The purest and most thoughtful minds are those which love color the most." Let your love of color express the many hues and shades of your vibrant Authentic Self.

APRIL 6

More Dash Than Cash

Elegance is not standing out but being remembered.
—Giorgio Armani
Italian fashion designer

During the seventies I lived in London and worked as a fashion copywriter, earning fifty pounds a week, which was then worth about a hundred dollars. While I worked in a very glamorous profession, I lived in a dreary, cheerless cell euphemistically known as a "bed-sitter." It was one room. There was a hot plate to cook on, a sink, a two-shelf fridge, and about ten feet of space to do with what I liked. Basically, it was just four badly plastered walls, with an exposed lightbulb hanging from the ceiling. The communal bathroom was down the hall, and every time I wanted to take a hot bath, I popped a shilling into a meter to fire up the furnace for five minutes.

But my cell was located at the top of a stately Victorian building, overlooking a handsome private park off the King's Road in Chelsea. It had granite steps, a heavy wooden black door with a lion's head for a brass knocker, pristine white woodwork surrounding tall, elegant windows, and boxes overflowing with bright flowers. From the outside it looked regal, and I loved walking up to it because it made me feel "to the manor born."

Turning the key was another matter, for after I shut the door and trudged up four flights of stairs, Cinderella was at home from seven in the evening. But I was born a dreamer, and I dreamed of living in splendor.

At the time, England was trapped in a huge economic crisis over oil, and in London there were rolling blackouts, a three-day work week, massive strikes, doom and gloom. I considered myself very lucky to have any kind of a paying job. But there was little money for clothes and shoes—and I had to have both. (Think *The Devil Wears Prada*.) So I majored in the art of making silk purses out of sows' ears—seeking and finding inspiration everywhere.

Creativity is the love child of ingenuity and risk. English *Vogue* came out with a marvelous series known as "More Dash Than Cash," which seemed to sum up the decade. Vintage clothing started making a comeback; in Paris, the hallowed halls of haute couture or custom clothing for the very rich (Think *Phantom Thread*) were replaced by the new "ready-to-wear" or prêt-à-porter runway shows.

In London two global and iconic fashion phenomena took off—Barbara Hulanicki's sensational satin and slinky art deco dream clothing brand, Biba, and Laura Ashley's romantic Victorian-inspired floral dresses, pinafores, and petticoats started showing up everywhere. Like Marie Antoinette with her gorgeous little farm, sophisticated London women were wearing cottage sprig maxi rompers as if they'd just milked a cow. It was a heady, amazing time to be working in both London and Paris, and for a couple of years, I lived and breathed the fashion world.

Still, no matter how exhilarating the fashion shows, I ended up each night in a four-story walk-up with a bare lightbulb hanging over me. Hardly the place to entertain even myself. One Friday night on my way home, I passed the window of a large department store, Peter Jones, which anchored the King's Road and Sloan Square. A huge remnant sale was advertised, and the fabrics displayed in the window were dazzling. Curious, I went in, took one glance, and visions of grandeur came into view.

Mind you, I didn't own a sewing machine. I barely knew how to sew by hand. It didn't matter. The sight of table after table of the most beautiful bolts of fabrics I had ever seen was intoxicating, inspiring, and irresistible. Here was splendor, and it was affordable. At only one pound per yard, I splurged on an entire bolt—thirty-five yards of rust, hunter green, and saffron Indian paisley that was cotton with a glazed sheen. It took almost an entire week's salary, but it was worth every penny.

That weekend I cut, glued, stapled, draped, and hung fabric. I covered the walls with it, created a tented ceiling, sewed simple curtain panels by hand (where's there's a will, there's a way), covered my box spring, fashioned a bedspread, made pillowcases, and draped a canopied alcove to sleep in. By late Sunday night, both the room and I had been transformed. I could have been manic, but I prefer to think of that weekend as mystical. I was exhausted and exhilarated by my beautiful surroundings and my creative risk-taking. I was so proud of myself and bowled over by beauty that this probably could qualify as my first "ecstatic experience." But what's more, I had learned that I could trigger the ecstatic through my own creativity, instincts, and verve. Glory be, I wish I'd taken pictures!

I believe that lurking beneath every woman at her wit's end, whether she knows why or not, there's a woman needing to jump-start her courage and let loose her artist of the everyday. Let that artist out of the attic. Are you just itching to cut, glue, staple, drape, and hang something new and different on your walls or your body? Today I would love to convince you that there's no room in your home, nor outfit in your head, nor work in your heart, that cannot be transformed by using fabric, paint, a saw, a hammer, nails, needle and thread, a sewing machine, glue, the amazing staple gun, coupled with your own imagination, creative energy, and emotion.

Don't hesitate or second-guess the Divine spark. Charge ahead. Be on the lookout for the ecstatic experience. I know one is waiting for you.

Here's a hint: Triggering it will require more dash than cash. And you've got plenty of that—in fact, all you have is all you need.

You're Worth It

Some people think luxury is the opposite of poverty. It is not. It is
the opposite of vulgarity.

—Coco Chanel (1883–1971)
French fashion designer

Suppose your Authentic Self reveals that she'd like to be outfitted in a $1,000 cashmere blazer by Giorgio Armani, and all your budget can spring for is the J. Crew wool blazer on sale?

Often, on our unfolding *Simple Abundance* path, we need to come to grips with the fact that our material wants and our wallets don't match. This poses a delicate dilemma, especially if you're equally committed emotionally and intellectually to your spiritual growth and your checking account balance.

So here's a new thrill for the Gratitude Journal.

Have you explored designer resale rather than retail? The designer resale market—for clothing, shoes, and accessories—has reinvented itself. In fact, it is enjoying the most explosive growth in the entire fashion industry. eBay used to be our only choice when we thought of buying inexpensive new or used clothing. That game has changed with the emergence of resale designer goods. It's time to check out The RealReal, Poshmark, Vestiaire Collective, and Tradesy.

"It's not your mama's fashion industry anymore. Gone are the days of going to the mall to pick up the same clothes everyone else has. Style seekers want one-of-a-kind treasures and they want to experience the hunt for themselves. Resale satisfies those shopping desires where traditional retail falls flat," Nicole Lapin, a money expert and best-selling author, tells us. "Making smart and savvy life choices and financial decisions, the fierce female of today is choosing to be the Boss of her future...We've changed our mindsets from a place of deprivation to a place of aspiration and our finances and fashion sense have followed."

And guess who's leading this new-to-you resale resurgence: you, and then your mid-century modern mothers and grandmothers. These resale fashionistas are also selling their last season fashions very quickly in order to balance their wants and their needs. Or, as Marianne Williamson puts it, "Seek first the kingdom of Heaven, and the Maserati will get here when it's supposed to."

So will the Armani or Ralph Lauren. In the meantime, call on your creativity to compensate. Your creativity is a Spirit-given gift. Perhaps your frustration about not being able to buy what you want will become the catalyst that sends you to sewing classes and eventually has you designing your own clothes. Perhaps you'll learn how to become an educated, sophisticated, savvy shopper, or a stylist apprenticeship gets your well-clad foot in the door. Seek, we are told, and we shall find, be it a suit or our spirituality. Once we search within for our own special gift of Spirit, our material desires will diminish, whether through sewing or savvy seeking. We might be living in a material world, but thank goodness our Authentic Self is a well-dressed woman, and not a material girl.

APRIL 8

Affordable Luxury

Luxury need not have a price—comfort itself is a luxury.
—Geoffrey Beene (1927–2004)
American fashion designer

When women first heard of *Simple Abundance* they mistakenly thought it was part of the downshifting and frugality movement of the 1990s.

But this was never true. While thrift is a marvelous, creative home art, frugality is based on fear, and fear doesn't attract abundance, it repels it. Instead of practical wisdom, such as "A penny saved is a penny earned," the frugality movement gives us parsimonious exhortations to transform clothes dryer lint into Halloween costumes.

Simple Abundance is not about deprivation. Nor is it about spending more than you can afford in order to make yourself feel better. For me, *Simple Abundance* has become a daily meditation on achieving the true balance between comfort and joy, which is moderation. We also need to learn the art of receiving, gracefully and graciously. And the art of receiving has been a difficult one for me.

The Universe is not stingy. We are. In fact, some of us have very stingy souls. Perhaps not in how we treat others—our family, friends, and those less fortunate—but in how we treat ourselves. Yet how can the Universe give us more if our fists, hearts, and minds are clenched tight? *Simple Abundance* is about finally learning how to release feelings of poverty and lack and replace them with feelings of prosperity and affluence.

One of the ways in which we can start to experience more affluence in our daily lives is through pampering ourselves with affordable luxuries. Investing in a cord of wood for the pleasure of sitting before a blazing fire throughout the winter is one such luxury. Sipping a cup of cocoa with real whipped cream and shaved chocolate is another; it transforms a simple pleasure into complete contentment. Affordable luxuries awaken our awareness to the abundance that's readily available to us once we finally "get it."

Many people think that simplicity frowns on luxury. The Shakers led lives of utmost simplicity, but "the Believers," as they were known, also believed in the sublime luxury of eating well and the importance of using only the freshest ingredients, inventive spices, and herbs a century before Nouvelle Cuisine. In 1886 one visitor at a Shaker table pronounced his meal "worthy of Delmonico's," a famous landmark in New York City where the wealthy dined.

Consider affordable luxuries when you think about nurturing your personal style. What simple pleasures could make you feel more abundant? Perhaps wearing cashmere socks or scarf while you save for a long cashmere cardigan; indulging in the intoxicating pleasure of your favorite coordinated scent—perfume, body talc, and lotion; the sensuous feel of silk underwear and pure cotton pajamas against your skin; investing in a handsome leather bag in a hue that goes with everything; trading in paper tissues for white linen handkerchiefs (it's ecologically sound, too!); having your hair blown out once in a while between cuts, or investing in a quality hair dryer; encouraging your nails to grow with a weekly manicure; replacing conventional plastic buttons on clothing with beautiful vintage ones found at a flea market; enjoying a facial or luxuriating in a body massage; wearing "special occasion" jewelry like your prized diamond stud earrings on an everyday basis.

Today, declare to the Universe that you are open to receiving all the abundance it's waiting patiently to bestow. Each day offers us the gift of being a special occasion if we can simply learn that, as with giving, it is blessed to receive with grace and a grateful heart.

APRIL 9

Nurturing Your Authentic Flair

An interior is the natural projection of the soul.
—Coco Chanel (1883–1971)
French fashion designer

As you awaken to your authenticity, you may notice that bare walls, windows, and floors beckon invitingly like a new lover, while the stuff you've accumulated over a lifetime doesn't seem to even notice that you're in the room. It would be fun to eat dinner tonight on a wooden crate by candlelight eagerly awaiting a new interior—the authentic projection of my soul—to be delivered tomorrow morning. However, my bank account, probably like yours, won't permit this fantasy, and so I must proceed slowly. We need to view this as an opportunity instead of a stumbling block. Our real-life budgets may delay the process longer than our conscious minds might wish—especially when scrolling through Instagram—but it's the perfect pace to nurture our authentic flair.

To be honest with you, this morning I'm not exactly sure of how I want to express myself through my surroundings or what I want to wear. Are you? I thought I knew. I've loved some things passionately that have brought me great pleasure for twenty-five years. But I've also lived with other things I hated so intensely I became psychically numb to their presence. The *Simple Abundance* path is about transformation. However, transformation cannot occur without transition. This is a transitional period of liminality when things are barely perceptible—a personal rite of passage, from sleepwalking to awakening. The process is the reality, and it cannot be rushed.

So we learn the art of waiting patiently. To consider. Save. Reflect. Simplify. Embrace order. Get ready. Experiment. Observe. Embark on creative window-shopping excursions to antique and craft shows, auctions, renovator supply companies, thrift stores, flea markets, yard, tag, and estate sales, museums, interior design expositions, elegant decorative accessory shops, furniture showrooms, museums, and galleries.

If you see something you like, ask if there is to be a sale soon. Take detailed notes. See how other people live or have lived by taking jaunts to decorator showcases, historic homes, and all the wonderful house-and-garden tours that take place in the spring. Read books, browse online in measured time slots. How about fifteen minutes a day to peruse? Permission to print out images for your *Illustrated Discovery Journal*. If you like an image enough to print it out, then you're on to something. More scrolling than a quarter of an hour and we slip down the rabbit hole.

Continue to prime the well with visual images, collecting everything that you can on paper, from fabulous table settings to beautiful curtain treatments.

Mary Emmerling, the author and collector who was the catalyst for the American country design movement in the eighties, is a woman I absolutely love and admire. She has an incredible authentic style that's grounded in common sense. She recommends creating a personalized decorating notebook to help us keep track of our meditative musings. She uses a zippered, canvas, loose-leaf notebook (seven by nine inches) with plenty of pockets for such tools as a tape measure, scissors, pens, pencils, paper clips, sharpener, and calculator. She gives each room a section of its own, complete with a wish list, photographs charting changes, a floor plan, and an envelope for paint chips, fabric swatches, and receipts. In the back of the book she keeps a year's calendar noting sales and special events and a personalized resource guide with the names and phone numbers of stores, showrooms, dealers, contractors, and material suppliers. It's a dream archive that she can carry around with her so that she can catch inspiration as it floats by instead of letting it dissolve into the ether.

If you follow some of these suggestions, you'll be well on your way to developing and nurturing your authentic flair. Instead of being frustrated, you'll be grateful that you've been given the extraordinary gift of time—time to know what you love so you can love how you live.

APRIL 10

Trompe L'oeil: Thrift-Shop Pleasures

Beauty is altogether in the eyes of the beholder.
—Margaret Wolfe Hungerford (1855–1897)
Irish novelist

Jennie Jerome Churchill, the famous American beauty and mother of British prime minister Sir Winston Churchill, believed that "thrift and adventure seldom go hand and hand." Alas, poor Jennie, whose extravagant tastes led her to worry constantly about money, did not know where to shop.

Let us speak today of the rapturous joys of recycling. However, I refer not to bottles and cans, but to the Anne Fontaine iconic white shirt that's yours for two dollars and a trip to the dry cleaners. Or the gorgeous, genuine Gucci leather handbag that's a steal at twenty-five dollars, the black Yves Saint Laurent blazer they gave away for five dollars. (Cross my heart.) There are bountiful bargains with your name on them to be foraged from thrift shops, consignment stores, vintage clothing boutiques, and online designer resale treasures.

Every sane woman needs to have a tried-and-true new-to-you fashion source up her sleeve. There are four different kinds for you to cultivate. First, there are the thrift shops, such as Goodwill and Salvation Army. Because thrift shops sell merchandise donated to them, you never know the quality of what you might find, but it's always worth a look.

Upscale consignment shops differ from thrift shops because here's where wealthy women who aspire to be fashionable discreetly sell off last season's must-haves. This is where you can find designer suits, coats, dresses, evening wear, and accessories at a fraction of their original price. Vintage clothing boutiques stock one-of-a-kind classics from other decades—from white cotton Victorian petticoats to Carole Lombard salt-and-pepper tweed trousers from the 1930s. I'd recommend that you gradually work your way up to vintage clothing boutiques; they can be intoxicating, rather like drinking port in the middle of the afternoon.

And then there are the designer resale sites beyond eBay that are sources of great finds—as I mentioned earlier, The RealReal, Poshmark, Tradesy, and Etsy. Here top international designer pieces may still have high-bar prices, but it's worth a look because it can alert you to what you're drawn to right now. ThredUp is a great find, because not only do they sell a vast array of gently used clothes, if you scour your own closet for pieces to part with that are still in good shape, they'll sell them in exchange for credit against your future purchases on their site.

There are a few ground rules to the successful art of trompe l'oeil ("fool the eye") scavenger sorties. First you must be in the right frame of mind: Don't go when you're tired or stressed. You can't rush; you need to take your time and you need to keep your wits about you. Go alone so that the experience can take on a meditative quality. Take a certain amount of cash, which is preferred by sellers and also to set a limit on your spending; that's why if the cash is gone, it's time to come home. Have no expectations of what you're going to find. Just have a happy expectant attitude as if you were embarking on a treasure hunt. Because you are.

A favorite affirmation that I use is "Divine abundance is my only reality and Divine abundance richly manifests for me in the perfect item at the perfect price." It always does. Finally, you must haunt these hideaways regularly. New merchandise is always coming in. That black cashmere turtleneck on your wish list may show up next Tuesday.

This week indulge in a new pleasure: thrifting. The thrill of combining thrift and adventure makes it worth the search.

APRIL 11

Finishing Touches: The Art of Fashion Accessories

You can have anything you want in life if you dress for it.
—Edith Head (1897–1981)
Eight-time Oscar winner for Best
Costume Design

Women may be ambivalent about their clothing but they often form passionate attachments to their accessories: the gold monogrammed pin your best friend gave you for that landmark birthday, the opaque black hose that make you feel so sleek and sophisticated, the silver necklace you got on that fabulous trip to Santa Fe, the brilliant blue silk scarf your sister brought you back from Paris, the bright straw Nairobi bag that's the depository of your life.

Fashion accessories are the artifacts of our authenticity. They can have sentimental value, track our mood swings, endow us with a sense of security, let our personality shine forth, or sabotage our best efforts. Because of the emotion we invest in them, in many respects our personal accessories are even more important than our clothing—they are the finishing touches that define us, the punctuation of our personality.

Many famous designers think women overdo it with accessories. Coco Chanel always said we should look in the mirror before leaving and take one thing off. Sorry, this is one time I must disagree with Madame Chanel. I think many of us hold ourselves back with our choice of fashion accessories, conforming to what we think is acceptable or safe. It feels more comfortable when we color within the lines.

Chanel's rich American clientele would return to Paris twice each year to purchase their next season's haute couture. As the story goes, Coco forbade her staff from selling any more of the designer's clothes and accessories to one American client. Since this Texan grande dame was very rich and a longtime client, the Chanel staff could not understand this abrupt decision. At last, Mademoiselle Coco announced with frustration, "Because she wears everything together! She makes me look bad."

When a woman lets Spirit guide her as she seeks to discover and nurture her authentic style, fashion accessories can help her take small but important risks that increase her self-confidence. Clothes and accessories pulled together in unexpected ways can be empowering. Just think of how far Judy Garland traveled in blue checked gingham and ruby slippers when she was off to see the wizard of Oz.

Your selection of shoes, hosiery, belts, scarves, jewelry, hats, gloves, handbags, and fragrance can make a big difference in helping you announce to the world who you truly are as you unravel this mystery for yourself. Are you polished or playful? Sophisticated or quirky? Old-school or edgy? Your accessories give us a brief bio before we've even said hello.

"There are so many different factors that go into creating a best-dressed moment—the perfect dress, the hair and make-up, the accent jewelry," celebrity stylist Micaela Erlanger tells us in *How to Accessorize: A Perfect Finish to Every Outfit*. "Whether it's on the street or the red carpet, the best fashion moments happen when someone's personality shows through. Getting dressed should be done with a sense of playfulness, whimsy and joy, whether you're dressing for the most special day of your life, a Friday night date, a job interview or just a trip to the supermarket. I want you to feel and look your absolute best."

Finally, never forget that the most essential fashion accessories, the ones no woman can afford to do without, come from within. A generous heart, a spontaneous smile, and eyes that sparkle with delight can be part of any woman's signature look once she awakens to her authentic beauty.

APRIL 12

Learning to Love and Honor Your Body

The body is a sacred garment. It's your first and last garment; it is what you enter life in and what you depart life with, and it should be treated with honor.

—Martha Graham (1894–1991)
Dancer, choreographer, and American
modern dance creator

Which comes first, learning to love our bodies or possessing a positive body image? Either way, it works. If you don't possess a positive body image—and most of us don't—learning to love your body can help you develop one. "If you can learn to like how you look, and not the way you think you look," the pioneering American feminist Gloria Steinem assures us, "it can set you free."

The time has come for us to realize that until we work on increasing our self-esteem by loving ourselves in small ways, we can't begin changing ourselves for the better in big ways. We must start by choosing to break the self-destructive cycle of unrealistic expectations, especially our own.

Starting today, shun the world's ideal of beauty, because it's constantly changing. The great Egyptian queen Cleopatra longed to have varicose veins, Middle Age beauties padded their bellies. Queen Elizabeth I painted her face with white lead and vinegar. It's not a great look.

Don't wait for the world to celebrate you. Carve your own niche. Focus on what's great about you, forget what's not. Find joy in your own reflection. Instead of obsessing about a body that's impossible to achieve without a personal trainer, begin to discover how you can feel better about living in the one you now inhabit.

Learn firsthand the transforming power of nurture over nature. Nourish your body with healthy food and pure water. Slow down and remember to breathe before taking a bite. Breathe out stress and negativity, breathe in oxygen and positive energy. Rediscover how marvelous it is simply to move: stretch, dance, walk, run, jump, skip, play, embrace. Pamper your body with comfortable clothes, quiet moments, and soothing beauty rituals.

"A woman's relationship with her body is the most important relationship she'll ever have. More important than husband, lover, children, friends, colleagues. This isn't selfishness—it's just fact," health and fitness expert Diana K. Roesch tells us. "The body is, quite literally, our vehicle for being—for giving, for loving, for moving, for feeling— and if it doesn't work, it's fairly certain that nothing else in our lives will work, either."

Today, instead of hating your body, make peace with it. Choose to consciously love and honor the sacred garment Spirit provided for this lifetime's journey.

APRIL 13

The Only Weight-Loss Aid You'll Ever Need

Self-love is the only weight-loss aid that really works in the long run.
—Jenny Craig
Founder of Jenny Craig, Inc.
weight loss program

In the beginning, eating was meant to be one of life's sublime simple pleasures. Then Eve took a bite out of a forbidden fruit—an apple—and women have been at war with food ever since.

Food is not our enemy. If we're alive, we're supposed to love to eat. Food is the source of vital fuel our bodies convert to energy in order to survive. Not wanting to eat—as in anorexia, bulimia, or illness— is a signal that something's seriously wrong with us. Don't fight your hunger. Instead, respect it and respond to it with nutritious food that appeals to all your senses—not just taste but sight and smell as well.

Trusting our bodies to tell us what they need is scary for most women. We're afraid that if we throw out all the diets and eat when we're hungry, we'll never stop and end up in the *Guinness Book of World Records*.

However, the more we starve ourselves, the more weight we eventually gain, and then we end up hating ourselves even more. Any woman who has been on more than one diet in her life knows this painful truth. The only way to stop this heartbreaking cycle of self-loathing is to stop dieting and use our common sense. Eat in a way that's good for you, when you're hungry, drink when you're thirsty, sleep when you're tired, get in balance with your body through regular exercise, and nourish your soul through prayer or meditation.

"Be really whole," the Chinese sage Lao-Tzu told his followers, "and all things will come to you." Even how to finally make peace with our weight. Taoism—the Eastern philosophy of Lao-Tzu—teaches that the only way to be made whole is to yield. Yield to the fact that your body answers to a Wisdom that's higher than wanting to look like the waif on the cover of *Vogue*.

Every woman has a weight that's ideal for her as opposed to an ideal weight. This is the weight at which you feel the most comfortable, have the most energy, can stay well and feel good about how you look. We can achieve that weight when we begin to trust our bodies. Forget size and abandon the scale. Instead of weighing yourself, let your favorite clothes tell you how you are doing.

Above all, trust the guidance of your Authentic Self. Go within and visualize her. See what weight she carries. Ask her to help you achieve your perfect weight through the power of Love. Today, be willing to believe that self-love is the only weight-loss aid you'll ever truly need, because it's the only one that works.

APRIL 14

When You Hunger and Thirst

The body must be nourished, physically, emotionally and spiritually. We're spiritually starved in this culture—not underfed but undernourished.

—Carol Hornig (1959–2014)
Spiritual integrated nutritionist

Many women, including myself, swallow life in an attempt to keep it manageable. I mean this literally and figuratively. Whenever we're anxious, worried, nervous, or depressed, without thinking, we instinctively swallow food and drink in order to push away the uncomfortable negative experience we're feeling in our guts.

We hunger and thirst, but it's not for a bowl of ice cream or a glass of wine. It's for inner peace and deeper connection. Although to tell the truth right now, I could use both the ice cream and the wine as we ponder achieving a comfortable balance between love, hate, and our bodies.

Carl Jung, the famous Swiss psychiatrist, believed that alcoholism was a sacred disease. M. Scott Peck relates in his book *Further Along the Road Less Traveled* how it occurred to Jung "that it was perhaps no accident that we traditionally referred to alcoholic drinks as spirits, and that perhaps alcoholics were people who had a greater thirst for the Spirit than others, that perhaps alcoholism was a spiritual disorder or better yet, a spiritual condition." I believe this is also true about compulsive overeating, which is the addiction of choice for many women. We have such a passionate appetite for life, we just don't know what we truly need to satisfy our insatiable cravings for Wholeness.

When I first became aware that when I "swallowed" life I was really hungry and thirsty for joy and serenity, it became a turning point for me in learning self-nurturance. Finally, I understood that I wasn't underfed but spiritually undernourished. I realized I could go within and ask my soul—my Authentic Self—what I needed. I learned to stop and ask myself the questions "How can I care for you at this moment? How can I love you? What is it you truly need?"

The next time you reach to put something in your mouth, take one minute to focus your awareness on what you're doing before you do it. Are you eating because you are physically hungry, or because you are anxious? If you're anxious, a walk around the block instead of into the kitchen would be better for you and more loving.

At the end of the day, are you pouring yourself a glass of wine out of habit in order to signal that it's time to relax? Instead, why not take a few moments to slip into comfortable clothes, sip a glass of delicious fruit-flavored mineral water as you prepare dinner, and enjoy the wine with your meal? Learn to create ceremonies of personal pleasure that can nourish your deeper longings. As you nurture your spirit with kindness, your physical cravings will loosen their grip.

Realize today that you hunger and thirst for a reason. Ask your Authentic Self to reveal your deeper needs, so that Spirit can quench and satisfy your parched and ravenous soul.

APRIL 15

Discovering the Momentum of Creative Movement

The first time I see a jogger smiling, I'll consider it.
—Joan Rivers (1933–2014)
American entertainer

The world as I know it is divided into two types of people: those who exercise and those who don't. Those who do exercise seem to have more energy, less stress, fewer weight problems, and generally a more positive and optimistic outlook on life. Women who are fit will tell you that regular exercise is the single most important thing they have ever done to improve their life.

Women who do not exercise don't believe them and have every excuse in the world for why they can't or won't find out for themselves: They don't have the time, they're too out of shape, they're coming down with the flu, it's too cold or too hot, they're too tired, they're too depressed, maybe next week. I know all about the women who don't exercise regularly because for much of my life, I've been one of them, even after being scolded by my doctor and shamed by my family. We are kindred spirits of the author and philosopher Robert Maynard Hutchins, who once remarked that "Whenever I feel like exercising, I lie down until the feeling passes."

This is not good. This is not self-nurturing. This is not healthy. We *know* this intellectually. Since we are all brilliant women, there must be a way in which we can slowly convince our brains to take better care of our bodies. But this won't happen by imposing a strict new regime on the stubborn, conscious mind that always manages to outsmart us. It hasn't worked in the past, so why should it now?

We will change by seduction. Don't refer to the activity as exercise or fitness any longer. If you must call it something, call it creative movement. Forget about gyms, running, weights, and aerobic classes led by women with no bones.

Think about creative movement as a life-enhancing, enjoyable pastime, because it is. Just pause for a moment and imagine all the ways that you could move creatively that might bring you pleasure: dancing (ballet, tap, ballroom, hip hop, or Zumba), swimming, fencing, horseback riding, racquetball, tennis, golf, riding a bike. What about a mind-body-spirit form of movement such as yoga or the graceful ancient Chinese martial art tai chi?

Now think about taking a walk in the beautiful sunlight today. Walking is the best form of creative movement there is, and it doesn't cost a cent. Walking clears your head, fills your lungs with fresh air, lets off steam, builds up strength, and centers your spirit. Start moving, a step at a time, step after step. The positive momentum will take it from there.

Trust me, seduction works. Once upon a time I was kicking and screaming all the way to fitness. Now because my doctor told me I had to get stronger before I could partake in the two sports I do love, horseback riding and fencing, I'm doing deep breathing, stretching, and engaging in walking meditations. I feel better and I'm ready to move up to flights of stairs. Diana Roesch assures us, "With enlightenment and self-awareness, we can re-guide and realign our *whole* selves: our bodies, by finding new ways of moving and celebrating them and by adding good food in amounts they tell us they need; our souls, our sense of ourselves as good and worthwhile, by connecting them to the earth and to each other."

APRIL 16

Walking as Meditation

It requires a direct dispensation from God to become a walker.
—Henry David Thoreau (1817–1862)
American philosopher, poet, naturalist

As long as I approached walking as exercise, I never made it past the front door. But one day I was so anxious I felt as if I would jump out of my skin, and so I bolted out of the house at lunchtime as if I were leaving the scene of a crime.

Filled with disappointments, painful memories, and my own unrealistic expectations from the past—terrified of what the future held and the changes that were inevitable—the only safe place for me was the present moment: my foot against the pavement, the wind on my face, my breath entering and leaving my body. Forty minutes later I stopped, discovered to my amazement that I was on the other side of town, and headed back home, calm and centered. I have been in and out of walking ever since.

I say in and out of walking because my desire to walk increases a hundredfold by beautiful settings—particularly rural ones. For ten years I was frequently charmed by walking anywhere in the English countryside, and just the sight of Wellington boots, Barbour jacket, shepherd's crook, tweed cap and scarf at a mudroom door means a meander beyond the swinging farm gate. But what's out there? You'll never find out if you don't get going.

After I moved from England, when I walked in Taos, New Mexico, the enormity of the vast Western landscape, which was new to me, seemed as if it had been waiting for me all along. You could stand and twirl yourself around, arms extended, and whoop. The dogs could run circles around you and then sprint a quarter of a mile in front and back. Euphoria. I understood why pioneers pushed past everything to find their promised land. I also understood that the Great Creator wanted me to understand there was a landscape larger than the one I could see at the moment. I needed to trust and continue on in faith, one step at a time, until I arrived at wherever I was supposed to be.

I wasn't the only writer to feel this way. When D. H. Lawrence discovered New Mexico in 1922 he claimed "it changed him forever." He was to visit three times in eight years and in total only resided there for eleven months. Lawrence died in 1930 in France, but his spiritual awakening and longing for the Taos mountains was so profound that his wife, Frieda, brought back his ashes and buried him in a chapel at the small ranch where they had stayed.

There are different reasons for walking—to increase the heart rate and build strength, to solve a creative problem, to finish that argument with yourself or someone else, to saunter and wake up to the world around you, and to meditate. Julia Cameron, the creativity coach, suggests a twenty-minute walk a day and once a week walking for an hour. "Creativity is a spiritual process, one in which we speak of 'inspiration.' When we talk about inspiration, we are talking about drawing breath. Walking makes our breaking rhythmic and repetitive."

Most days I go on walks for a "moving meditation"—fitness of the spirit. I try to quiet the voices in my head, take long strides, and concentrate on the slow, steady rhythm of my breath, comforted by the interior silence.

Suddenly my reverie might be broken by the sound of birds singing, a dog barking, or the sight of a pretty garden. Thoreau complained of walking sometimes "without getting there in spirit...The thought of some work will run in my head and I am not where my body is—I am out of my senses." This happens to me as well, but I have learned to train myself to return my awareness slowly to the physical act of walking, for here in the present moment, one step at a time, I have found peace.

If you have had difficulty sitting down to meditate, you might like to give a walking meditation a chance, especially now that the beautiful weather has returned. Take into consideration your preferences: If you are not a morning person, take a walk at midday, in the late afternoon, or after supper under the stars. Even if you work in a city during the day, you can break at lunch and take a walk. No one needs to know that you've shut the world out and are meditating as you stroll down the street. I have found there is no wrong way to do a walking meditation. I now live in an urban setting surrounded by mountains and palm trees, and the view brings me much pleasure and peace here as it has anywhere else.

But I still don't walk for exercise. Instead, I walk to get into those riding boots and fencing mask as my soul tags along. I suppose it doesn't matter why we walk, just that we do.

APRIL 17

Making Peace with Your Hair

Genius is of small use to a woman who does not know how to do her hair.

—Edith Wharton (1862–1939)
First woman to win the Pulitzer Prize
for Fiction (1921)

A woman's hair has for centuries been called her "crowning glory," but every woman I know speaks of her intimate relationship with her hair as a nightmare. I don't know any woman personally who really loves her hair, just women who cope. Hair is a living, powerful, mercurial, metaphysical energy force to be respected, reckoned with, and reconciled to, but it cannot be controlled any more than atomic fusion.

Occasionally, hair can be cajoled into becoming conduct (we refer to these lapses as "good hair days"), but it can never be coerced. Think of all the money, time, creative energy, and emotion we invest in our hair. Yet most of the time it insists on expressing *its* authenticity, not necessarily ours. I don't know about you, but I'm exhausted from the mini skirmishes I wage with life every day, and the battle with my hair is not the least of them.

Most of us exist under a collective hallucination the American feminist writer Naomi Wolf calls "the beauty myth." We have all been brainwashed into believing that if we can just get the right shampoo, conditioner, perm, color, and cut, our hair will finally behave like that of the women in the display professions—television, film, and fashion—who, by the way, do not style their own hair. We would all have, if not fabulous, then at least presentable heads if we had a professional hairstylist on call every day, or at least whenever we appeared in public or in print. But that's not real life for me, nor probably is it for you.

At home, my hair never looks the way it does when I come from my appointment with the hairdresser. This is because I have yet to learn how to simultaneously hold a blow dryer and a curling brush in two hands and do whatever it is my stylist does as she swirls about me in the salon. So at home I have given up trying. I wash it, mousse it, let it dry, and then curl it with my trusty electric rollers. Some days it looks wonderful; other days it looks woebegone, and yet the process is virtually the same. Hair humbles us, and we need to make peace with it.

The way we do this is to accept it and acknowledge its personality: whether it's thick or thin, coarse or fine, straight or curly; the way it breaks when permed, is getting gray, or insists on parting down the middle. Getting to know your hair and working with it instead of constantly fighting it is the first step toward rapprochement and peace of mind. While my Authentic Self wears her hair in shoulder-length, Pre-Raphaelite blond waves, I've had to reconcile myself to the fact that I can't have wavy, blond tresses until they invent a perm that doesn't frizz color-treated hair (and they haven't). So I've chosen color over curl. Always it comes down to creative choice.

If you're currently unhappy with your hair, start patiently searching for pictures of hairstyles you like and bring those pictures to a hairstylist recommended by your friends for a consultation first. Have a conversation about the reality of your hair versus your fantasy about your hair. Consider the time you are willing to spend working with it every day. This is very important. See if you can't arrive at some middle ground that will make you happier.

If you're thinking of something drastic, such as going from long hair to short, place pictures of the new hairstyle on your mirror for a couple of weeks so that you're familiar with the change before it happens. It won't be so much of a shock then. Whether you believe in astrology or not, do not get any beauty makeovers while Venus, the goddess of beauty, is in retrograde. You have to trust me here, babe. You might not have a clue as to what I mean, but look it up; wisdom of the ages is meant to be shared, not hoarded.

Above all, try not to give in to impulse. We all have days when we scream, "I've got to *do* something with my hair," but those aren't the days on which to do it. Remember, the hair you know is easier to handle than the hair you don't. But be open to change, because there are few joys in life that can equal finally finding a becoming hairstyle. Thought that woman on the bus with the purple streaks looked great? Try it! Got a yen for a bob with bangs? Go for it! And if the worst happens, after you dry your eyes, remember it's only hair. It will grow again, and you will have become wiser.

Above all, learning to accept your hair is part of the process of learning to love yourself. The poet Marianne Moore believed that "Your thorns are the best part of you," and she was right.

APRIL 18

The Face in the Looking Glass

The most beautiful makeup of a woman is passion. But cosmetics are easier to buy.

—Yves Saint-Laurent (1936–2008)
French fashion designer

Who do you see when you look at the face in the looking glass? Are you beginning to see your Authentic Self? Are you becoming more comfortable with the uniquely beautiful face that stares back at you? I hope so. But this growth of self-acceptance and self-love is slow and very subtle, especially after years of benign neglect.

One of the ways that we can begin to love our faces is to enhance them with makeup. I have gone through many stages with makeup. There was a time during my twenties while I was working in fashion and theater, when I wouldn't have dreamed of walking out the door without my war paint on. For me, makeup was a sophisticated mask that endowed me with self-confidence.

In my thirties, after I had married, had my daughter, and spent so much time at home writing, I stopped wearing makeup except when I went out with my husband in the evening. It was a relief to stop wearing cosmetics because doing so gave me an opportunity to learn to feel comfortable with my features. The world I had come from had been so self-absorbed and obsessed by appearances. Now I was getting in touch with the inner woman and not concentrating on her outer packaging. But gradually, I noticed a difference in the way I felt about myself without makeup.

When I put it on, I liked the reflection in the mirror. When I didn't, I rarely looked. I began to become aware of the fact that looking your best, working with what you have, and bringing out your natural beauty with makeup was not as superficial a goal as I had originally thought. Makeup was simply a tool to help me look my best. When I looked my best, I felt better. When I felt better, I had more energy and accomplished more and was more outgoing. When I accomplished more and reached out more to others, they responded positively, and my self-esteem grew.

Making up my face again began a self-affirming cycle of acceptance. But more important, it began a ceremony of self-nurturing. I began to see that the ten minutes I took in the morning to put my best face forward for myself and not the world was a small but important way of nurturing my authenticity. Even the ritual of putting makeup on, when it comes from the heart, can be spiritual.

Today when you glance in the looking glass, bless the face that stares back at you. And if you feel like you need a little facial boost, try putting on some lipstick.

APRIL 19

Spring Rituals of Replenishment

Let your mind be quiet, realizing the beauty of the world, and the
immense, the boundless treasures that it holds in store.
All that you have within you, all that your heart desires, all that
your nature so specially fits you for—that or the counterpart of it
waits embedded in the great Whole, for you. It will surely come to
you.
Yet equally surely not one moment before its appointed time will
it come. All your crying and fever and reaching out of hands will
make no difference.
Therefore, do not begin that game at all.

—Edward Carpenter (1844–1929)
English poet

This is the season of renewal and replenishment. What better way to begin than to meditate on English poet Edward Carpenter's assurance that all our needs will be satisfied by the great Whole. Whatever we are waiting for—peace of mind, contentment, grace, the inner awareness of *Simple Abundance*—it will surely come to us, but only when we are ready to receive it with an open and grateful heart.

While you are waiting patiently, take comfort and joy in simple springtime rituals of rejuvenation. A favorite of mine is to search for a new sacred space out in the world. This reminds me that we carry our serenity with us. A shady grove of trees in an old cemetery, a beautiful public garden that's new to you, a museum gallery, the stacks of an old library, the hush of a quiet chapel where you can light a candle, even an outdoor café where you can sit basking in the sunshine can help you realize the boundless treasure and spiritual replenishment of a perfect solitary hour. The great mythologist Joseph Campbell, whose work on *The Hero's Journey* inspired and informed George Lucas's *Star Wars* saga, tells us that "Sacred space and sacred time and something joyous to do is all we need. Almost anything then becomes a continuous and increasing joy."

Taking the Cure: Bathing Pleasures

I can't think of any sorrow in the world that a hot bath wouldn't help, just a little bit.

—Ellen Glasgow (1876–1948)
American novelist who won the
Pulitzer Prize for Fiction in 1942

Every woman should be aware that there is a significant difference between bathing and taking a bath. Bathing is merely cleansing, but you can remove grime and sweat in a shower, for heaven's sake! Taking a bath, as the Victorian social critic Ambrose Bierce described it, is "a kind of mystic ceremony substituted for religious worship."

I believe in the rejuvenating power of hydropathy as a positive adjunct to psychotherapy. A century ago water cures were all the rage to combat the "new American nervousness" or "neurasthenia" that began to sweep the country as our great-great-grandparents adjusted to the relentless intrusion of technology into their lives and the resulting disruptions of "hectic modern living" in the form of telephones and electricity. Victorians would flock to spas to drink mineral waters and take medicinal dunks to cure the fidgetiness and racing pulses of anxiety attacks, insomnia, depression, and headaches.

Today, we can take the cure in the privacy of our own bathrooms. And being possessed of common sense, we should do it daily. Do not underestimate the blessings of a bath. It can calm your mind, relax your tired, tense body, and soothe your stressed spirit. It can help you drift off to the exquisite relief of sleep or wake you up and help you greet the day with enthusiasm.

My philosophy in life is very simple: When in doubt, take a bath.

Close the door, run the tap, pour in the bath salts or essential oils, lay out the fluffy towels, tie your hair back, and shut out the world by sinking into the tub. To my mind, baths are as necessary for spiritual replenishment and centering as is prayer and meditation.

In fact, a proper bath is one of the best ways of meditating; for once you're submerged in delicately scented warm water, where else would you want to be except in the present moment? Try bathing accompanied by candlelight, soothing music, a cold drink, or a good book (nothing too strenuous), or just let the silence envelop you as the ripple of more hot water splashes against your toes.

Begin to indulge in collecting accessories to make your bath more sublime: a long-necked scrub brush, an inflatable pillow, a bath tray. When people ask you what you want for your birthday, holiday, or

Mother's Day, tell them pampering bath products; that way you'll always have an assortment on hand. There is a dazzling array available: scented salts, oils, powders, bubble baths, and bath bombs (they fizzle quietly into the most delightful fragrances and colors). Start to find your favorites and think of them as affordable luxuries.

"A hot bath! How exquisite," the English novelist Rose Macaulay wrote in *Personal Pleasures,* published in 1936. "How luxurious, fervid and flagrant a consolation for the rigors, the austerities, the renunciations of the day."

APRIL 21

The Scent of a Woman

Smells are surer than sounds and sights to
make heartstrings crack.
> —Rudyard Kipling (1865–1936)
> English Victorian novelist and poet
> Nobel Prize in Literature, 1907

Among my hallowed haunts are visits to used bookshops. Unfortunately, this venerable pursuit has almost given up the ghost with the onslaught of online bookstores. But not in England's fair green isle, where any town large enough to have market days also has a tea room, a church, a pub, and a used bookshop.

A proper used bookshop comes with a little bell at the top of the door to let the owner know a customer has crossed the threshold. The intoxicating aroma of leather and paper foxed with age welcomes you for a browse. Books are piled higgledy-piggledy on the shelves and in looming towers on the floor. If you're a regular, the proprietor may offer you a drop of sherry to assist in deducing what it is you're really looking for, and you'll leave with old shopping bags filled to the brim, smiles all around, having just contributed generously to the bookshop owner's upcoming rent payment.

I was a stranger, just passing through Uppingham, when I happened upon such a promising shop. I asked the owner, a man I guessed to be in his forties, if he had any books on the five physical senses of sight, sound, smell, taste, and touch, and on the two mystical senses—our intuitive sense or "knowing" and our sense of "wonder." He led me to an area in the back, and I spent a pleasant hour rummaging through books for my project. When I was paying for my happy stack, the owner asked about my interest in this topic. I told him that I was writing a book on the spirituality of the senses—and that I believed the senses are our portals to the Divine.

"And the dead," he said softly. A look of incredible sadness came over him. He told me his wife had died quite suddenly the year before; they didn't have any children. "We were soul mates. We traveled the world together—life was a wonderful adventure with her." One of their favorite places was the garden at the Palace of Versailles near Paris, which they first visited on their honeymoon. After his wife's death he made a pilgrimage there.

"It was winter. The ground was frozen, the trees were bare, nothing was blooming. It was bleak, dishwater gray. I sat down on a bench and started to cry. We'd been inseparable for twenty years. I couldn't believe she'd abandon me so completely, even in death. I was so angry, I screamed at her, the sky, and at God. It was a good thing no one else was there or they would have dragged me away, not that I cared. Eventually I quieted down and began to walk slowly back to the front gate. Suddenly, I was surrounded by her scent. No woman ever smelled as good as my wife, or even like her. She smelled of lilacs, spring…and baking. My wife loved to bake. She smelled vibrant and happy. And all around me were fragrant wisps of *her*."

The image of this devastated man standing alone in a winter's garden, enveloped in a scent cloud of his dead wife's love, brought me to tears.

Now we were both crying.

"You probably think I'm crazy but I know she was there…with me." I reassured him he was not crazy but very lucky and blessed. He told me that this fragrant visitation lasted for about fifteen minutes, and then she was gone. Sadly, he's not "sensed" his wife again. But the memory of that mystical encounter will last his lifetime.

Every woman has her own scent, and I'm not talking about a favorite perfume. A woman's scent is a deeply personal bouquet of diet, heredity, hormones, hygiene, and health, an aroma as distinctive as her DNA. Napoleon famously sent a dispatch to his wife, the Empress Josephine, asking her not to bathe before he arrived home the next day. He adored her natural aroma. When my daughter was little and I went away on business trips, she would sleep on my pillow and underneath my down-filled comforter because they "smell like you, Mommy." After my father died, my mother gave me one of his handkerchiefs. I kept it in my bedside table drawer and when I pressed it up to my nose I was comforted once again by his immediate presence as scent memories conveyed his love across time, space, and eternity.

Many women shun even the thought of their natural scent. Instead, we spend a small fortune trying to mask our sensuality. Are we secretly afraid that we will offend? Perhaps because we secretly believe we "stink" at so many things we do, why would our *parfum d'une femme nue* be any different? But one of the miracles that occurs when we fall in love with Life is we begin to see ourselves through the lens of unconditional Love. We relax into the real. We stop hiding behind artifice. We embrace our Authentic Self.

This week try an experiment: Use pure soap and an unscented deodorant. Start in small steps to return to your authenticity.

Since Egyptian times, the feminine art of fragrance has been revered. Finding a perfume that complements and enhances your sense of well-being is a spiritual gift and sensuous pleasure. However, the crucial first step is discovering your base "note" before the layering of other fragrances. The true "scent of a woman" begins with you.

APRIL 22

Sensory Awakening

Nothing can cure the soul but the senses, just as nothing can cure the senses but the soul.

—Oscar Wilde (1854–1900)
Anglo-Irish poet, playwright,
and legendary raconteur

We were created to experience, interpret, and savor the world through our senses—our ability to smell, taste, hear, touch, see, and intuit. Although we are sentient beings with the capability "to perceive the world with all its gushing beauty and terror, right on our pulses," as poet, pilot, author, explorer, and naturalist Diane Ackerman tells us in her exquisite evocation *A Natural History of the Senses*, most of us journey in a dull trance, asleep to the mystery of everything about us.

In order for us to awaken and "to begin to understand the gorgeous fever that is consciousness, we must try to understand the senses," Ackerman urges. "The senses don't just *make sense* of life in bold or subtle acts of clarity, they tear reality apart into vibrant morsels and reassemble them into a meaningful pattern."

For the next week, I'm going to ask you to pause a moment each day with me and marvel at the natural gifts that have been so richly bestowed on us. George Eliot believed that "If we had keen vision and feeling for all ordinary human life it would be like hearing the grass grow and the squirrel's heartbeat, and we should die of the roar which lies on the other side of silence. As it is, the quickest of us walks about well wadded with stupidity."

Today, look at the blue sky, hear the grass growing beneath your feet, inhale the scent of spring, let the fruits of the earth linger on your tongue, reach out and embrace those you love. Ask Spirit to awaken your awareness to the sacredness of your sensory perceptions.

APRIL 23

Smells like Home

It's a funny thing coming home. Nothing changes. Everything looks the same, feels the same, even smells the same. You realized what's changed is you.

—F. Scott Fitzgerald (1896–1940)
American writer who captured
the Jazz Age in fiction

Our homes have their own particular scent, too. The aroma of fresh-baked bread, lemon-scented furniture polish, cat dander, damp dogs, mud on the doormat, laundry in the hamper. The scent of coffee, bacon, and ripening fruit in the kitchen; soapsuds in the bathroom; rumpled sheets in the bedrooms; fresh flowers, potpourri, burning logs, and newsprint in the living room.

"Nothing is more memorable than a smell. One scent can be unexpected, momentary and fleeting, yet conjure up a childhood summer beside a lake in the mountains, another, a moonlit beach, a third, a family dinner of pot roast and sweet potatoes during a myrtle-mad August in a Midwestern town," Diana Ackerman reminds us. "Smells detonate softly in our memory like poignant land mines hidden under the weedy mass of years. Hit a tripwire of smell and memories explode all at once. A complex vision leaps out of the undergrowth."

And if we lost our sense of smell, if suddenly we experienced *anosmia*, as do two million Americans? We would find ourselves bereft and cast adrift without the internal compass of scent.

Today, let us delight in the simple pleasure of our sense of smell. Indulge yourself with comfort aromas. Take a creative excursion to an Italian market; visit a Chinese restaurant for lunch; browse through a used bookstore; stop by the perfume counter of a large department store and inhale delight. Lie on the fresh grass in the backyard, turn over the earth in the garden, bury your nose in a bouquet of lilacs and lily of the valley (which should be blooming about now) and smell the sweetness of spring, all green and dew-dropped. Take a walk in the woods, a garden, or your neighborhood after it rains; go to a farmer's market and gather aromatic herb plants—rosemary, sage, lemon verbena, tarragon, mint, bay, and fresh lavender—for a kitchen-shelf garden; put a scented geranium in the bathroom.

Cook plum tomatoes, garlic, onions, sausage, and peppers in olive oil to crown the pasta for dinner tonight; simmer cloves, orange rind, cinnamon, and apples on the back burner for a delightful fragrance; experiment with blending your own potpourri; enjoy a scented bath and then a massage of a complementary body lotion.

"Smells spur memories, but they also rouse our dozy senses, pamper and indulge us, help define our self-image, stir the cauldron of our seductiveness, warn us of danger, lead us into temptation, fan our religious fervor, accompany us to heaven, wed us to fashion, steep us in luxury," Diane Ackerman reassures us.

The world around us possesses exquisite smells that can stir our memories, color our emotions, and transform our feelings and moods. So sacred was the power of scent that God instructed Moses to build an altar of fragrance and to burn sweet incense when he prayed. Today, when you inhale something wonderful, offer a prayer of thanksgiving for this marvelous, priceless gift.

APRIL 24

A Taste for Living

Life itself is a proper binge.

—Julia Child (1912–2004)
American chef, author, and television personality

Taste is the younger sister of our sense of smell, dependent on her sibling's guidance for a head start but eager to strike out on her own as soon as she's able. Diane Ackerman tells us in *A Natural History of the Senses* that a child has more taste buds than an adult (who has 10,000 taste sensors located in the mouth, primarily on the tongue but also on the palate, pharynx, and tonsils). Amazingly, our taste buds wear out and regenerate every ten days, although when we enter middle age they don't regenerate as frequently as we might wish. The idea that our senses become jaded as we get older—requiring new and fresh awakening—is, alas, correct.

The word *taste*, from the old English word *tasten*, meaning to touch and test, has always had a double meaning. In exploring and celebrating the simple pleasure of this intensely personal sense, we should look at both interpretations. The primary definition of *taste* describes the sensory faculty that enables us to distinguish substances dissolved in the mouth as sweet, sour, bitter, or salty. But the other definition of *taste* describes the mental faculty by which we discern or appreciate things for the joy they bring us.

Today let us explore ways to increase our capacity for pleasure—our taste for life—by delighting in this simple, yet highly sophisticated, sense.

Although many supermarkets now carry ethnic ingredients, it's much more fun to discover authentic tastes and aromas by hunting out unusual (for you) grocery stores in your neighborhood: Caribbean, East Asian, Indian or Pakistani, Italian, Cajun, German, French, Hungarian, Hispanic, kosher, or soul food. Just under the East Asian category alone you have Chinese (eight different styles of cooking), Japanese, Korean, Thai, Cambodian, and Vietnamese.

It wasn't until I was eighteen and out into the world that I discovered that all vegetables aren't gray in color when they arrive at the dinner table. What a life changer! And an artichoke—learning how to prepare and eat one. It was a thrill. So many of us just play it safe, re-creating the food we grew up with, but once we break out of that box, we have so many delightful dinners ahead of us.

There's a world of delicious morsels out there waiting to be found and savored. Inhale the vibrant aromas and bring home something wonderful, new, and different to cook for dinner this week. You could play a culinary game called "Around the World in Eighty Menus." To make it easier, invite friends to contribute potluck dishes. Who said we don't know how to have a good time?

Next, clean out your spice cabinet. This is both symbolic and necessary. Variety, after all, is the spice of life, and nothing broadens our sense of taste better than fresh spices do. After my daughter was born, I simply didn't have the time to clear out my spice cabinet. But once I embarked on the *Simple Abundance* path and was trying to introduce more order into my daily affairs, it was time to tackle the spices that had been there for years.

I reveal this pathetic, embarrassing truth in astonishment and wonder, primarily because, once I did, I was flabbergasted to discover that I possessed eleven cans of poultry spice and eleven cans of pumpkin pie spice. Do you have any idea how much space twenty-two spice containers occupy?

Now it doesn't take Miss Marple to deduce what had occurred in the life of the woman in charge of this kitchen. Every Thanksgiving since the baby was born, she had purchased new cans of poultry and pumpkin pie spice. Why? Was it because, as a renowned gourmet chef, she was extremely fastidious about the pungency of her spices?

I don't think so.

It was because she was frazzled and disorganized, trying to cope with the domestic chaos surrounding her. She had no clue that there were spices left over from the previous year and of course didn't want to be caught short.

Learn from this sorry story. Somehow, I suspect I am not the only woman in America with numerous souvenirs of Thanksgiving Days past. We need to clean our spice cabinets to make room for fresh ones (in case you're wondering, cardamom and coriander seed fossilize after a decade) because we're going to use them to reawaken our sense of taste. Think of Indian curry, rice, and mango chutney for dinner soon or a pan of lasagna redolent with basil, oregano, and garlic, or a pot of Southwestern chili. Supposedly the dying words of the famous nineteenth-century frontiersman Kit Carson were "Wish I had time for one more bowl of chili." Thank goodness we do.

Bon appetit! To the spice rack we go, large garbage bag in hand, once more with fervor.

APRIL 25

On a Clear Day You Can See Forever

The greatest thing a human being ever does in this world is to see something.... To see clearly is poetry, prophecy, and religion, all in one.

—John Ruskin (1812–1900)
Leading Victorian art critic

I've reached that awkward stage in my life when I can't see with my glasses on or with them off, so I constantly carry them around with me and momentarily panic whenever I've misplaced them. As my eyesight changes, I've become acutely aware of how precious our ability to see clearly is.

A friend of mine, Susan Abbott, is an extraordinary artist who creates panoramic watercolors that are breathtaking in their exquisite detail. Her eyes and hands apprehend a visual catalog of a woman's daily life with astonishing attention to the subtle nuances—nothing is too insignificant or uninspired for Susan's attention. Like a brilliant photograph, her still-life watercolor arrangements of meaningful mementos from a woman's life seize a moment in time to dazzling effect. Artists especially hold sacred the sense of sight.

Pablo Picasso once said, "If only we could pull out our brain and use only our eyes," we would be amazed at the world around us. Paul Klee, the Swiss artist, declared, "One eye sees, the other feels." As Paul Cézanne grew older, he doubted his powers of perception and worried that the authenticity of his art might be a quirk of nature. Because he had trouble with his eyesight he wondered if the unique way of seeing the world that he captured on canvas in painstaking single brushstrokes might be mere accident instead of genius. But perhaps Georgia O'Keeffe expressed it best when she observed that "In a way nobody sees a flower really, it is so small, we haven't the time—and to see takes time, like to have a friend takes time."

To see takes time. We haven't the time. Here is the unrelenting truth, and it's chilling to the soul. Most of us have been given a miraculous gift—the ability to see—but we don't take the time to do more than glance around. We take our sense of sight for granted. A dear friend of mine has been having some serious trouble with her eyesight, and as she shares her worries with me about losing it, I feel helpless. What she laments losing is being able to drive the car pool or take her children to the dentist, to do her grocery shopping, try out new recipes, read the newspaper, see the faces of those she loves, put on her makeup. Infinitesimal, precious moments that make up the days of our lives.

Today, really look around at your world—your family, your home, your pets, your coworkers, and the strangers on the street. Smile at everyone you meet because you can *see* them. Never forget that the gift of vision was so important that when the world was first created, the first command was for Light in order to see, and after finishing each day's task, the Great Creator glanced back and "saw that it was good."

We need to see how good it is, too.

APRIL 26

Major and Minor Chords of Pleasure

With stammering lips and insufficient sounds,
I strive and struggle to deliver right
the music of my nature...
— Elizabeth Barrett Browning (1806–1861)
Victorian English poet

Most of us who luckily possess all our senses think that if we had to lose one, the most terrible deprivation would be the loss of sight. But Helen Keller, who became blind and deaf after a mysterious fever at nineteen months of age, mourned the loss of her hearing more than her sight. The writer Hannah Merker tells us in her moving memoir on losing the sense of hearing, *Listening*, that "Psychologists say that deafness, or a severe hearing loss, acquired after a human being has known hearing, can be the single greatest trauma a person can experience."

Thirty years ago I was at lunch with my almost-two-year-old daughter in our favorite fast-food restaurant when a large ceiling panel fell and struck me in the head and sent me crashing into the table. I sustained a head injury that left me partially disabled for nearly two years. During the first three months of recuperation I was confined to bed and my senses were all skewed. My eyesight was very blurry, I was extremely sensitive to light, and even seeing the different patterns of the quilt on our bed disturbed my sense of equilibrium so much that we had to turn it over to the plain muslin backing. I couldn't read or comprehend words on a page. But the most disorienting disability was that my sense of hearing was affected. I could not listen to music because it made me dizzy. I couldn't even carry on a telephone conversation because, without visual clues such as reading lips, I could not process the sounds coming through my ears and rearrange them into meaningful patterns in my brain.

These unsettling side effects lasted for quite a while, but over a period of eighteen months my senses gradually returned—for which I'm deeply grateful. I share this story with you because I want you to consider how much we take for granted until we lose it, either temporarily or permanently. It deeply saddens me that many of us need to have pain as a wake-up call and it is shrill and sharp. Now I try my best not to stand on the sidelines of life with deadened, dulled, disinterested senses until another shock makes me suddenly aware of the magic, marvel, and the mystery of it all. And so should you.

The American Victorian author Kate Chopin wrote in 1900, "I wonder if anyone else has an ear so turned and sharpened as I have, to detect the music, not of the spheres, but of the earth."

Among my own favorites: the reassuring rhythm of a loved one's breathing in the middle of the night when I can't sleep; hearing "I love you" and "We're home," along with footsteps on the stairs; the voice of a good friend on the telephone; raindrops on the roof; cats purring; dogs thumping their tails; teakettles whistling; the melody of words strung together to form a sentence that stirs the imagination and illuminates the soul; the exquisite sounds of silence cascading over me when I momentarily let go and allow the Universe to proceed without my assistance or supervision; and music—music to soothe, inspire, and move me in unexpected waves of sublime pleasure. The concerto of real life is playing: delight with thanksgiving in the major and minor chords of its beautiful refrain.

APRIL 27

Reach Out and Touch Someone

Learn to get in touch with the silence within yourself, and know that everything in life has purpose. There are no mistakes, no coincidences, all events are blessings given to us to learn from.

—Elisabeth Kübler-Ross (1926–2004)
Swiss-American psychiatrist

Touch is the first physical sense we experience as strange hands pull us from the dark realm of the soul into the cold, harsh light of earth. After the security and warmth of the womb, frigid air assaults our fragile, naked bodies until we find comfort in our mother's arms with the sense of touch guiding our first few conscious moments.

For many people touch is also the last sense we experience as we depart this world—the squeeze of a loved one's hand. Sight, smell, hearing, and taste have gone before us. "The first sense to ignite, touch is often the last to burn out," the scientist Frederic Sachs tells us, "long after our eyes betray us, our hands remain faithful to the world."

We describe our mood swings as "feelings" and when something strikes a deep, sentimental chord in us we say we were "touched." When we feel alienated, fragmented, and adrift, we often refer to this estrangement as "losing touch with reality." Bumper stickers ask, "Did you hug your child today?" And did you? Because we all need to be hugged and touched, not just to thrive but to survive.

A good friend of mine, a hardworking single mother of two boys, regularly treats herself to a therapeutic aromatherapy facial and body massage. She budgets for it in her monthly expenses and thinks of it as preventive medicine—not covered by her health insurance but vital to her peace of mind and sense of well-being. She once explained to me that as her life is now—barren of intimacy—she's rarely touched, and she often felt overwrought, ill, and deprived until she realized that what she needed was therapeutic touching. Since she started her monthly massage treatments, she's hardly been sick and has enormous amounts of energy, which she needs for the extremely busy and demanding life she leads. She says that the healing effects of a massage can last up to three weeks and then it's time for another session. "You should try it," she urged me, but being practical and sensible (so I thought), I didn't, until she gave me a body and facial massage as a gift for my birthday several years ago.

Here's how I became a complete sensuist (someone who delights in sensory experiences, as opposed to a *sensualist*, someone who is excessively concerned with physical gratification). Take one stressed-out woman and isolate her in a tranquil massage room for one hour. Now, awaken her physical senses with the scent of aromatic essential oils; the hypnotic stroking of her face and body (especially the massaging of her feet and toes); the beautiful strains of Pachelbel's "Canon" playing softly in the background; the sight of shafts of sunlight dancing on the wooden floors; and the refreshing taste of sparkling mineral water and lemon in her mouth after the sublime massage session is over.

My first massage was a mesmerizing way to encounter the passage of time: when it was over, I felt such peace, joy, and relaxation it was as if I had been drinking champagne for breakfast or having a transcendental experience. This naturally–produced euphoria lasted for many hours, and that night I enjoyed the sleep of the innocent. The next day I felt ready to take on the world.

Today, reacquaint yourself with this powerful, life-enhancing physical sense so often disregarded. Embrace your children, stroke their hair, cradle them in your arms (no matter how big or squirmy they are), kiss your lover, caress your pets, experience the feel of different fabrics against your skin—do you prefer silk or fur or pima cotton? Enjoy a sensuous, warm, scented bath, then sleep in the nude on fresh flannel sheets in the winter and cotton or linen in the warmer months. (And if you don't sleep alone, be prepared for what might follow.)

Think about regularly treating yourself to a therapeutic body or facial massage. Don't feel guilty! Consider a massage the way you would getting your teeth cleaned, your hair cut, or a new pair of eyeglasses—occasional but necessary self-care expenditures to maintain your physical well-being.

The English poet William Wordsworth wrote of a woman, "She seemed a thing that could not feel/The touch of earthly years." Let us all become women who embrace our portion of earthly years with a passion by delighting in our sense of touch.

APRIL 28

The Intuitive Sense

Intuition is a spiritual faculty, and does not explain, but simply points the way.
—Florence Scovel Shinn (1871–1940)
American author, spiritual, and metaphysical writer
of *The Game of Life*, originally published in 1925

Intuition has been called our "sixth sense" and is often an ability ascribed to women. The English writer D. H. Lawrence believed that the intelligence that "arises out of sex and beauty is intuition," while anthropologist Margaret Mead concluded that feminine intuition was a result of our "age-long training in human relations." I'm not here to debate the existence of an intuitive power—the capacity to know something without rational evidence that proves it to be so—because I *know* that it exists. So do you.

However, the question that interests us today is: Do you use your intuition? Have you learned how to fine-tune the inner instinct that is constantly transmitting signals to you? Think of yourself as a radio. Is your dial set clearly on the intuitive station so that you can receive the information you need when you need it, or are you just picking up static?

Intuition is the subliminal sense Spirit endowed us with to maneuver safely through the maze that is real life. Wild animals rely on their intuition to stay alive; we should rely on ours to thrive. "It is only by following your deepest instinct that you can lead a rich life and if you let your fear of consequence prevent you from following your deepest instinct then your life will be safe, expedient and thin," Katharine Butler Hathaway wrote in 1946.

Intuition tries to communicate with us in inventive ways. One way is through what my friend Dona Cooper, the theater director and university drama professor, calls "the educated gut," which frequently slaps us to pay attention by triggering a visceral, physical reaction in our bodies. One such intuitive signal is the emotional trembling that accompanies creative discovery or warns us not to take a certain action. Another intuitive message breaks through when we suddenly grasp that to try something new might be delightful; we do so and are surprised by joy. A third intuitive nudge occurs through revelation; the inner *knowing* that helps us arrive at the right place at the right time so that we can be swept away by the benevolent flow of synchronicity that gets us where we're meant to be as easily as the Universe can arrange it.

Today, go within and seek the wisdom and guidance of your Authentic Self. She steadfastly waits to speak to you through the whispers of your imagination and the glimmers of your intuition. But if you want to learn to develop this marvelous power, you must first be willing to take a leap of faith and trust it. Put it to use in little ways. Use it every day, and eventually your sixth sense will flourish and enhance your life the way the other five senses do.

APRIL 29

The Feminine Allure

Taking joy in life is a woman's best cosmetic.

—Rosalind Russell (1907–1976)
American actress and entertainer

Ingrid Bergman had it in *Casablanca*. Fifty years later, Michelle Pfeiffer epitomized it as Edith Wharton's heroine, Countess Ellen Olenska, in the film version of *The Age of Innocence*. And Thandie Newton's graceful embodiment of the ravishing robot Maeve Millay in *Westworld* is subversive in its sentient sensuality.

What is this magnetic attraction? It is allure, the mesmerizing power to entice or attract through personal charm and mystery.

We're not much into mystery these days, which is a pity. These are the times of tell-all, tattletale, and tabloid truths. The playwright and spoken word artist Ntozake Shange (1948–2018) believed that "Where there is a woman there is magic," and I agree. But I also believe that where there is a woman, there *should* be mystery.

What intrigues me most is the mystery—the allure—of how some women seem to pull it all together so effortlessly. This is the aspect of the feminine mystique that compels and invites investigation. Who are these women and how did they evolve into these higher beings?

You see them in business meetings—confident, assured, and in command—or smiling serenely in the hallway at school while waiting patiently to pick up the afternoon car pool, a baby over one shoulder, a toddler in tow. These women don't look frazzled, fatigued, or fed up; they look fabulous. They are beautifully dressed, not a wrinkle or spot of drool on their shoulders. They do not simply juggle; they fly through the air with the greatest of ease. You wonder: What is their secret? Are they all on Prozac? Is it plenty of money, being well organized, or a full-time housekeeper and personal assistant? Maybe it's positive thinking or the favorable alignment of celestial bodies? Perhaps it is something more profound: a deep spiritual connection.

Does the computer ever crash when these women are on deadline, do the kids ever whine, does the car ever need to be towed, have they ever taken a dog who's just wrestled with a porcupine to the vet? You and I have, which is why occasionally Rio de Janeiro sounds appealing.

Then, without missing a beat, you wipe a snotty nose, change a dirty diaper, defrost the hamburger in the microwave, start the spaghetti sauce, sew a button on a coat, help someone with his homework. You pause for a moment, wondering what they would do if you weren't here and realize in the same breath that you're awfully glad you are. Much to your astonishment, it occurs to you that you must also possess some aspect of allure because everybody in the house gravitates to you. In the middle of the night they call your name.

And there's certainly enough mystery to ponder—such as the mystery of what will happen next. But instead of worrying or obsessing, you decide to just let go and see what occurs. You choose to take joy in your real life as it unfolds day by day, hour by hour, a heartbeat at a time.

Emily Dickinson confessed that "To live is so startling, it leaves little time for anything else." Your face may never end up on the silver screen. Nor will mine. But we can arrive at an inner awareness that just living and loving it all is alluring enough.

APRIL 30

Do Try This at Home: Water Supplies

In all the years when I did not know what to believe in and therefore preferred to leave all beliefs alone, whenever I came to a place where living water welled up, blessedly cold and sweet and pure, from the earth's dark bosom, I felt that after all it must be wrong not to believe in anything.
—Sigrid Undset (1882–1949)
Norwegian novelist and winner of the Nobel Prize in 1928

Much as Mrs. Miniver showed such valor and readiness in the film, how are you doing with preparing a Caution Closet? Sometimes when we really want to do something, real life gets tangled up in the loose threads of work, home, and routine. And to tell the truth, even the idea of stocking "just in case" provisions can make you anxious. It took me at least a year to get this done. And then I moved and had to redo it. So I'm with you and I completely understand the power of procrastination. How's this: All we're doing is reorganizing a closet, so if we need a flashlight, we know where to find it *with the batteries.*

And here's something we can add to our Closets that's worth its weight in gold: water, the magical elixir of life. It's not always available at a convenient faucet, but we forget this enormous daily gift until where we live is affected by a water crisis, from drought to floods, which are occurring more frequently each year.

Around the world, women bear the brunt of collecting water for their families. Kristen Kosinki traveled to Kenya and learned that in

Samburu, women and girls spend up to twelve hours a day foraging for water. Seeking to empower women, Kristen founded the Samburu Project, which has drilled a hundred local wells, bringing water to more than 100,000 families. It is this understanding of the profound relationship between women and water that inspires us to nurture and hydrate our loved ones.

Storing water brings a few challenges—from space to accessibility.

Emergency preparedness organizations recommend one gallon per person per day, and the emergency recommendation is at least enough for three days.

There is an online site, BePrepared.com, that is a commercial outfitter for both water and food, where you can see the different-size water containers, as well as tablets to keep water fresh. Amazon also sells water purification tablets. We simply don't know what the conditions will be like, so let's increase the water supply for each person with another five-gallon container or as much as you can do. If we're doing it, let's do it right.

You can store some water in the trunk of your car, but you need to be aware of the temperatures where you live. Plastic bottles can release chemicals in extreme heat, and water will freeze in cold climates. Storing water bottles or cans in a cooler in the trunk of your car will help protect them from changes in temperature. Water also comes packed in boxes, like juice boxes, which don't have any chemicals. While not always available in stores, online purchases make this a worry-free addition to your Caution Closet.

A tip from two hikers who were lost for five days on a one-day trip: They survived using a Lifestraw water purifier stick, which filtered out toxins and parasites from a stream. These are available online from Amazon and outdoors websites and are affordable necessities to slip into backpacks now, especially if you are an outdoor weekend adventurer.

Joyful Simplicities for April

There are no little things. "Little things," so called, are the hinges of the universe.

—Fanny Fern (1811–1876)
American domestic novelist

    🖋 Pick up a copy of Diane Ackerman's marvelous exploration *A Natural History of the Senses* and revel in an exhilarating reading romp that will intrigue and inspire you to become a sensuist.

    🖋 April is a wonderful month for all kinds of walks, whether in warm spring showers or balmy sunshine. The scent of the earth reawakening and the sight of Mother Nature's brilliant display of color will rouse and remind you how wonderful it is simply to be alive.

❧ Find a large fabric store for a creative excursion, even if you don't sew. Browse through the upholstery remnants. They make great inexpensive tablecloths or covers for furniture. Flip through the pattern book. Visualize the possibilities. Is there something you'd like to make for yourself? For the house? Then why not consider the possibilities? *It's never too late to learn how to sew.*

❧ Sort through your lingerie drawer. Discard ratty old bras and panties and reward yourself with a couple pretty new undergarments, bargains at discount stores like TJ Maxx and Marshall's. Lay down *colorful* paper and tuck lavender-scented sachets into your drawers.

❧ Go through your makeup and discard what's old and dried out. Replace darker colors with a paler palette for spring. Learn the secret of applying foundation lightly so that it seems natural by blending with cosmetic sponges and brushes instead of your fingers. Or try tinted moisturizers. Visit the cosmetic counters of a large department or cosmetics stores like Sephora or Ulta and discover who's offering free makeovers. (Many cosmetic companies introduce their new spring line of makeup at this time of year.) You don't have to buy anything! When the beauty consultant is finished, thank her enthusiastically and tell her you want to walk around with your new face and see how it feels before investing in new makeup.

❧ Collect rainwater to wash your hair. Victorian women believed rainwater made their hair softer.

❧ Find a refreshing new scent for spring—try rose water, lilac, or lily of the valley. Wear a scent you love every day.

❧ Resume the restorative pastime of weekend roaming; be on the lookout for vintage linens at estate sales and for plants and herbs at farmers' markets.

❧ When it showers, curl up under a blanket in the afternoon and listen to the raindrops on the roof. Keep a packet of crumpets or scones in the freezer, so you can enjoy these only on rainy days. Earl Grey or Darjeeling are both lovely afternoon brews.

❧ Bake a batch of hot cross buns.

❧ Do you have a pretty umbrella and rain boots? Why not?

MAY

All things seem possible in May.
> —Edwin Way Teale (1899–1980)
> American naturalist, photographer,
> and writer

The month of May casts her magic spell as spring's promise is finally fulfilled. This month we turn our attention homeward, as we continue to weave Simplicity into our daily round while reacquainting ourselves with the transformative power of the third *Simple Abundance* Grace—Order—which bestows balance into our hectic lives. As we learn what we want to keep in our daily round, especially the boundaries around our precious personal space, we discover what we're ready to let go of. With fresh eyes and a loving, appreciative heart, we learn to savor everyday epiphanies as we encounter the Sacred in the ordinary.

Sacred Partnerships

Between the Home set up in Eden, and the Home before us in Eternity, stand the Homes of Earth in long succession.
—Julia McNair Wright (1840–1903)
The Complete Home, 1879

Sacred partnerships arrive in our lives in many forms. Sometimes they're of wood and stone instead of flesh and bone. Unexpectedly, a blind date becomes a vision of domestic bliss. The French call this astonishment a *coup de foudre,* an intense and immediate attraction— love at first sight—which conveys as much shock as desire.

The House of Belonging is ancient Celtic metaphor for the body as the earthly home for our souls, as well as for the deep peace and feeling of safety, joy, and contentment found in intimate connections with people, places, and homes. The Irish poet, scholar, and mystic John O'Donohue exquisitely explored these beautiful themes in his book *Anam Cara: A Book of Celtic Wisdom.* "When you learn to love and to let yourself be loved, you come home to the hearth of your own soul. You are warm and sheltered. You are completely at one in the house of your own longing and belonging."

I truly believe that there is a House of Belonging waiting for each of us at different times in our lives; sacred homesteads waiting to wrap us in comfort and solace. Waiting to be found, waiting to be built, waiting to be renovated, waiting to be cleaned up. Waiting to *rescue* us, even as we lovingly *restore* its wooden floors with our time, emotion, and creative energy. But most of all, there is a House of Belonging waiting to be *recognized,* even as it surrounds us. The blessing of *recognition* is priceless. Ask for this Grace today.

I used to believe that we all had a "forever" home. But now I know, that like love itself, there are no "forevers" in our stories. Life has taught me there is also the here and now home, which can take care of you, no matter what your circumstances might be here and now. And making a home for yourself is the greatest act of self-care you can provide for your soul.

We feel so lost and alone in these in-between stages of life. But like little hermit crabs on the beach that move into a succession of borrowed, abandoned shells large enough for them to grow into, we always have a choice. "One is free, like the hermit crab, to change one's shell. Or carry it on their backs," Anne Morrow Lindbergh reminds us, which begs the question: Which will it be this year? Change or carry?

Every relationship you have—with other people, your work, your art, your passionate yearnings—reflects in some way your soul's intimate relationship with you. Nowhere is this spiritual truth more apparent than in the relationship we have with our homes.

This emotional attachment—good, bad, or indifferent—is a spiritual daily tutorial in Love. "Everyone longs for intimacy and dreams of a nest of belonging in which one is embraced, seen, and loved," John O'Donohue reassures us. "Something within each of us cries out for belonging. We can have all the world has to offer in terms of status, achievement, and possessions, yet without a sense of belonging, it all seems empty and pointless."

When I glance back through years of my Gratitude Journals, I'm surprised by how often "my beautiful home" appears. I was giving thanks for different dwelling places at various stages of my life's journey. Along the way, I've discovered and *accepted* the truth that we're meant to move in and out of time, space, and place as well as change, circumstance, and choice. How gracefully we learn to accept our cycles of life and their different scenic designs *is* the spiritual lesson. For when it comes to the difference between houses and homes, as it is with true love, outward appearances are often deceiving. It's what's inside that counts.

MAY 2

Changing Places

Your home should tell the story of who you are and what you love most, collected and assembled in one place.
—Nate Berkus
American interior designer, author,
television personality

There's a fair chance that by the time a woman is forty she will have moved at least seven times during her life. And the prediction for a lifetime of moves now is eleven. Some moves will be considered "happy" ones, such as your first apartment, setting up house with your "intended," or getting married. Some moves will be circumstantial—a new job, the rent goes up, or you're downsizing. Some moves may be forced upon you by catastrophic change beyond your control—from an unexpected divorce to natural disasters.

A lot of moves are considered temporary, or so you think, until a decade later, you're bursting from the seams in a place you never particularly wanted to live in at all. That is, until the walls of adjoining apartments start to collapse around you. I greet change with as much enthusiasm as the brick wall has for the wrecking ball, but when a dwelling is declared uninhabitable it's time to go. I'm not psychic, but if this is your current living situation, as it was mine, then, sweetie, let me rent you a van.

Still, there's a good reason why moving wins the grand prize as the number one stressful rite of passage ahead of death, divorce, or debt. Maybe it's because no matter what the reason, moving is all these things simultaneously.

And then there's the dream house, which is never about moving but rather about romantic obsession. We've all been vulnerable to that subversive but imaginative personal catalyst for change: the passionate love affair that sweeps us away from all rational thought.

Interestingly, did you know the name of the greatest lover of all time, *Casanova*, means "new house."

Oh, the thrill of it all: the finding, first sighting, the offer, the rival, the wooing, the winning. Then the engagement period: the bliss of designing your new nest to perfection; until the hullabaloo of builders, plumbers, electricians, paint chips, fabric swatches, and cooking on a hot plate for months drives you stark raving mad. But at last, when all is done, our happily-ever-after commences—whatever that looks like or however short-lived it might be—until the inevitable parting.

I remember when I was looking at houses in England, I was shown a gorgeous Georgian manor that had been completely restored to its flawless Jane Austen ideal. It was listed as a "turnkey" property because you didn't have to do anything except turn the key and unpack your suitcases.

However, viewing this beautiful house was very unsettling; from the moment I entered I began shivering because the vibrations were so intense. It felt as if the walls were weeping. Had someone died here? Did a tragedy occur here? As I was led from one exquisite room into another, I started to get heart palpitations. The physical distress I felt as my chest tightened became so severe, I had to go back outside to catch my breath.

But this wasn't a haunting. I've been in haunted houses before, and these vibrations weren't old, creepy, or menacing. This was fresh sorrow. Raw. Inconsolable. I felt as if I needed to scoop something invisible, intangible, and bereft into my arms and whisper, "There, there…"

Finally, I decided to ask the estate agent. "This is some woman's cherished home and it's as if she and the house have been torn away from each other. Can't you feel it? What's the story here?"

Only then did the real estate agent explain, rather reluctantly, that, indeed, a couple had spent several years restoring the house and the gardens from an eighteenth-century wreck to movie-set perfection, worthy of Mr. Darcy's fictional estate Pemberley in *Pride and Prejudice*.

But suddenly, a few weeks before my visit, the family had left England abruptly to escape an Inland Revenue raid for tax avoidance.

They'd left in the night, hurriedly abandoning their dream house, hangers still swaying in the closets. All I could do was bless the house and the woman who had loved it so and had decorated it with such impeccable taste.

The hangers, by the way, were a padded taffeta plaid in salmon pink, green, and blue. I've been looking for that fabric ever since; I even carry a swatch in my handbag. But I digress. I usually do when I'm telling stories about women and dream houses because I find them irresistibly romantic, riveting, and the decorative details delicious.

A love affair with a house is the most spellbinding and hypnotic tale that can be told. Whether a woman is single, divorced, married, or widowed; age eighteen or eighty; there's no passion as perfect as the dream that someday, some way, somewhere she will inhabit her own cozy nest.

Because there's nothing more enchanting than planning her home's beautiful décor; and no illusion as seductive as the fanciful notion that once she crosses the threshold, she'll stay there "forever," which is a difficult fantasy to dismantle. "I am as susceptible to houses as some people are susceptible to other human beings. Twice in my life, I have fallen in love with one," the early twentieth-century English writer Katharine Butler Hathaway confessed. "Each time it was as violent and fatal as falling in love with a human being."

From the scented linen closet to the built-in kitchen pantry, from the window seat, plump with decorative pillows, to the rose-covered arbor leading to the backyard, each nook and cranny of this fantasy has been lovingly imagined since we were little children playing house. No doubt the magic spell was cast when Mother draped a blanket over the dining room chairs, and we crawled underneath to put our dollies to bed or to engrave into our memories the beguiling rug pattern.

"Even though your dream house is at the end of a long, long road, your head may be buzzing with plans for that home you will have someday. Already you probably have a stack of clippings, sketches and what not—ideas you want remember for your own house," Elinor Hillyer reassured the young woman who purchased *Mademoiselle's Home Planning Scrapbook* in 1946. "You can't keep all those house plans in your head—keep them in here."

The scrapbook she referred to was twelve by fifteen inches, silver-gray cardboard, spiral bound with big envelopes—one for every room—for stashing paper dreams. I'm amazed by the similarity between it and my own *Simple Abundance Illustrated Discovery Journal*, which is also a spiral-bound journal with envelopes. But long after I designed the *Illustrated Discovery Journal*, I found Mrs. Hillyer's scrapbook while antiquing, which is my favorite pastime and meditation. Somehow sifting through the domestic shards of women who no longer can bear witness to life's glorious mystery helps me ransom, reclaim, and redeem what's truly precious in my own existence.

However, I'm stumped by Elinor Hillyer's first rule for successful dream house planning. "Have a fair picture in mind of the kind of house you want and the kind of life you and your young man want to build for yourself." To be perfectly honest, my first *Illustrated Discovery Journal* came about because I couldn't visualize either the life or house I wanted. And certainly, neither the life nor the house came with a spouse.

Besides, during different phases in my life, my dream house has run the gamut from a Victorian gingerbread to Frank Lloyd Wright prairie style; a Tuscan villa with a vineyard to an artist's pueblo in Taos and a ranch in Big Sky country in Montana.

So why don't we just play spin the map? Because my actual dream house purchase wasn't on any of my personal wish lists. It was a sixteenth-century English stone cottage, with only two rooms, an ancient apple tree in front, sheep grazing outside the kitchen window, and the sound of horse hooves on the lane. Be still my beating heart. How's that for practical? Oh, yes—and it was in another country.

But, just one look, that's all it took. Just one look and the earth tilted on its axis. I seem to recall swooning, with the same witless intensity usually reserved for completely unsuitable men. "Whoever loved, that loved not at first sight?" the sixteenth-century playwright Christopher Marlowe wondered, and rightly so.

Ten years into my "forever" I was also forced to leave my home unexpectedly, hurriedly, wrenched away with my clothes still hanging in the closet, under the cloak of an American business trip, taking only a suitcase and my aging cat. I'd discovered I'd married an English con man, a convicted fraudster, and needed to file for divorce as soon as I could make it safely across the Atlantic. However, not for an instant did I fathom I'd never be coming back to Newton's Chapel.

We think forever is endless, but every dream comes with an expiration date. Forever can vanish in the blink of an eye, which is why we must cherish each day while we're living it. One of Heaven's greatest blessings is that we can't see far up the road, so meting it out in twenty-four-hour parcels is just about what we can handle.

Still, with the passage of time, your backward glances provide memories to sift and sort, and they shape your personal Woman with a Past story, however you choose to tell it. Because we can't go forward until we're willing to go back.

"You need to claim the events of your life to make yourself yours. When you truly possess all you have been and done, which may take some time, you are fierce with reality," the extraordinary Florida Scott-Maxwell reassures us, and she ought to know.

Born in 1883 to British ex-pats trying to establish a citrus growing colony in Florida (and hence named after their unsuccessful attempt), she was educated at home, went on the stage at sixteen, and began writing short stories at twenty. After her marriage in 1910 to John Scott-Maxwell, she moved to her husband's native Scotland, where she worked for women's suffrage, wrote plays, and raised a family. At fifty-six she divorced and cared for her four children by working as a journalist. Later, she completely started over by studying under the noted Swiss psychiatrist and psychoanalyst Carl Jung, becoming a female pioneer in psychoanalysis, practicing in clinics in England and Scotland.

I love how Florida Scott-Maxwell describes the comfort of her first home following her marriage's end. "After a time of trouble, I found a likeable flat which was to be my home. I had had a long need of one, so it was also my dear shelter. My daughter and I moved in one evening with two suitcases, two beds, three pots of bulbs, a kettle and tea things. We lit a brilliant fire in the seemly little grate with the dry slats the builder had left after making a big opening between the two public rooms. I lay listening to pigeons on the roof...I listened, looked out on the trees beyond both windows and I was free and happy...It was already so precious to me that its surface was almost my skin."

Almost her skin. A home so alive and protective, it's as close as your own skin. She was, of course, describing a House of Belonging, though to an outsider she was exchanging a large Scottish country house for a tiny apartment. She would go on to have other homes, but she knew that night, as I've learned now, that any shelter bringing contentment and refuge—however temporary they might be—is your House of Belonging.

So I want to wrap you in my arms and reassure you that it doesn't matter *where* you live today or the *why* behind your leaving it tomorrow. You may be rooming in a motel or seeking sanctuary in a safe house halfway between your past and your future. You may be without a roof to call your own, camping out on a friend's couch, in your sister's bedroom, or on a community cot. You may be locked in a tower until you can grow your hair long enough to make a fairy-tale escape or pitching a tent on the dark side of the moon. Heaven knows, I've lived in some of these settings at one time or another. What makes any dwelling place worthy are the dreams you cradle close while you're sheltered, temporarily, in this transitional terminal toward tomorrow.

You deserve to live in a home that embraces, nurtures, delights, and inspires you. And if you haven't found your House of Belonging yet, remember this, darling girl: All that you are seeking is still seeking you. Pull the Master Builder's blueprint down to shelter your soul. I promise, you are closer than you think.

MAY 3

On Holy Ground

I have no home but me.

—Anne Truitt (1921–2004)
American sculptor

The moment I wake up, I say this little prayer for both of us.
Today, shall we say it together?

*Piercer of Doubt and Kindler of Courage, bless this woman, my
dearly beloved Reader. Thank you for your clarity and compassion.
Thank you for Divine Completion. We ask for the gift of Grace today
to finish whatever we started and abandoned so long ago; to let go of
the ghosts that harass our days and haunt our nights.*

*We ask to return in safety and strength to the ruins of our regrets, to
ransom what can be rescued and release what begs for rest. Help us, we
pray, to make the transition from fear to faith, to make peace with our
past, so we might live this day with the astonishing wonder of our first
and the wisdom of our last. Encourage us to claim all the events of our
lives so that we might become fierce with our own exquisite, incomparable reality.*

*Shape, from all our sighs, a shelter of serenity; design, with all that
delights, a dwelling place of contentment. Return to us the repose of
our ravished souls.*

*Grant us safe passage from our turbulent endings, through a
Divine transition to our tenuous but true new beginnings. Please lead
us to the threshold of our own understanding. Welcome this woman
to her House of Belonging. Come, celebrate her home. Thank you
that it is now and shall always be, three times three, Past, Present, and
Future.*

Gratefully, Amen.

Now, take a deep breath and let today unfold gently, with the new
awareness that all you have is all that you need for today.

A Home for the Soul

The ordinary arts we practice every day at home are of more
importance to the soul than their simplicity might suggest.
—Thomas Moore
American psychotherapist, former monk,
and spiritual writer

In places and people, we seek that elusive feeling of being welcomed.
We want our houses and apartments to be warm and nurturing and
beautiful, but they are sometimes territories of chaos and confusion,"
the architect and author Anthony Lawlor ruminates in his luminous
book, *A Home for the Soul: A Guide for Dwelling with Spirit and
Imagination.* "Yet the haven the soul seeks is close at hand, within the
stove and the cupboard, on the bookshelf, and in the closet. With the
eyes to see it, and the hands to create it, we can recover the home that
the soul desires."

In other words, let's reach for the broom. How we care for our homes
is a subtle but significant expression not only of our self-esteem but the
contentment of our soul.

Soulfulness is not necessarily linked to religion. As Lawlor points
out, "Someone may access soul through the prayers, ritual, and scriptures of their faith, but they can also encounter soul in a flavorful stew,
the caress of a lover, or the textures of a pine floor. A chapel within a
cathedral may be a shrine of spiritual peace, but a window seat within
a living room can offer a haven of quiet renewal." Especially if you can
see out of it.

"The most immediate way of deepening soulfulness in a home is
through cleaning and repair. Housework, however, is denigrated in our
society," Anthony Lawlor admits. But cleaning is an "act of discerning" what will benefit not only our homes but ourselves. "In the rush
of modern living, cleaning can be a technique for settling down and
engaging in the simple pleasures of bringing order to our personal corner of the world...Cleaning blesses our houses and apartments with
care," allowing homemaking to become "a pathway for soul making."

MAY 5

Living in the House of Spirit

*How to be happy when you are miserable. Plant Japanese poppies
with cornflowers and mignonette, and bed out the petunias among
the sweet peas so that they shall scent each other. See the sweet peas
coming up.*
*Drink very good tea out of a thin Worcester cup of a colour
between apricot and pink...*

—Rumer Godden (1907–1998)

Anglo-Indian author

It was the small things that helped, taken one by one and savoured,"
the Anglo-Indian author and dramatist Rumer Godden recalls in her
mesmerizing memoir of an authentic life, *A House with Four Rooms.*
"Make yourself savour them," she told herself when life was not tidy.

Life is not tidy around here today: Schedules are colliding, needs
are conflicting, and the house is strewn with real-life refuse, reflecting outwardly the disarray of my mind at this moment. My natural
inclination—which I am thwarting with a tremendous act of will—is to
start cleaning. But if I stop to clean, I'll interrupt the rhythm of the day.
I only have a few precious hours to work uninterrupted before the clam-
oring of the world resumes. A few precious hours to hold one thought in
my head and follow it word by word to its completion, even if it takes all
morning. Then get it on the page.

One of the reasons I love Rumer Godden's writing is that she stitches
the colorful threads of her extraordinary life—domestic, creative,
and spiritual—with such deftness; the hem that seems to hold her
life together rarely pulls or gapes the way mine does more often than I
care to admit.

Born in 1907 to English parents who lived in India, she was a true
child of the Raj in the days when the British Empire spanned the globe.
And though she would return to England at various times, she lived
most of her life in her cherished India. She began her career in 1936 and
published seventy books, her last novel written as a young slip of a girl
of ninety, and she mastered every literary genre: novels for both children and adults, nonfiction, short story collections, memoirs, poetry,
and dramas. Nine of her novels were made into films.

Many of her renowned novels, which are very mystical, celebrate
the fruitfulness of real life: the magic, the mystery, and the mundane.
The *New York Times* noted that she was a writer who "belongs in that
small exclusive club of women—it includes Isak Dinesen and Beryl
Markham—who could do pretty well anything they set their minds to,

hunting tigers, bewitching men, throwing elegant dinner parties, winning literary fame."

Of all her books, however, it is her memoirs that are my favorites. I am captivated by how she lived, nurtured a family, and pulled together many homes out of shells of houses all over the world, while writing almost continuously. She is a glorious storyteller, but no story is as riveting as her real life. Or ours, for that matter.

The soul-craft of establishing safe havens set apart from the world, in which to seek and savor small authentic joys, is a recurring theme in her work, whether the haven is behind convent walls or in the nursery at the top of the stairs. No matter where she kept house, Rumer Godden's secret to living an authentic life seems to have been dwelling in the House of Spirit as she tells us: "There is an Indian proverb or axiom that says every person is a house with four rooms: a physical, a mental, an emotional and a spiritual one. Most of us tend to live in one room most of the time, but unless we go into every room every day, even if only to keep it aired, we are not a complete person."

MAY 6

Being Home

August 1945: There was a time before the war—it seems in another world. Where has it gone? Am I the writer who wrote Black Narcissus? *Has she gone, just as the money's gone? Is it possible I shall write again? First, I must cope with England...which has never seemed so alien.*

—Rumer Godden (1907–1998)
Anglo-Indian author

When I want to be brave and I'm feeling anything but, I turn to my favorite comfort ritual: reading about other women's lives, especially those from the past that have slipped through the cracks of social and domestic history; women from all walks of life who were flesh, bone, and blood before they became icons and archetypes, whether famous or forgotten trailblazers. There is so much wisdom, contentment, and delight to be found as a literary adventuress and a time-traveling domestic explorer. From them I gather cautionary tales, astute observations, affectionate advice, surprising confessions, and sensational strategies to help me figure out what comes next.

"What were they thinking?" is an Internet headline often used as a commentary over funny or bizarre photographs. But I use it as a personal prompt to discover what my cherished Women with a Past were thinking as they faced the heartrending challenges, crossroads, changes, and choices that shaped the trajectory of their lives.

These are stories of women who cried themselves to sleep, women who raised a fist to Heaven and swore that as God was their witness they would never be hungry again, women who howled at the moon in righteous fury, women who fiercely protected their homesteads with heroic mettle and spiritual moxie. Watch out for a woman who's paid her dues and has something to prove. Women with a Past should come with a warning label, but then we'd miss the fun of hanging out with them. Throughout the rest of the book I'll be sharing some of my favorite Women with a Past with you for a dose of spiritual moxie when we need it most.

I search through vintage memoirs, biographies, letters, diaries, and especially auction house catalogs of women I admire who seemed to play out charmed lives in the public gaze and on the pages and canvases of their art. In fact, their lives became their art, and that's the True North for our compasses as well.

I have a tremendous admiration for women who have experienced significant reversals of fortune in between the lines of real life with dignity and grace. How did they recover when sorrow slapped them down? How did they feel after achieving a long-desired dream, only to find that friends were too jealous to share their joy? How did they cope when suddenly their success turned to ashes? Where were they when they discovered that all the money they'd entrusted to their husbands was gone, including earnings from future obligations? As I search, the same four-letter word always finds its way into their stories and into my heart: home.

My favorite revelation, among many, is in Rumer Godden's memoir *A House with Four Rooms* concerning the years between 1945 and 1977 after the huge success of her third novel, *Black Narcissus*. By the time it was made into a breathtaking Academy Award–winning film (1947) starring Deborah Kerr as the Mother Superior of a small group of Anglican nuns trying to establish a mission in a remote Himalayan outpost, Rumer was in despair caused by her husband Laurence's fiscal philandering. She recognizes (as must we all) her own naïveté and wishful thinking at having granted him carte blanche over their finances, even though she was the primary wage earner.

"Wanting for him to truly be head of the house I had left our expenses to him, making over money when he asked [writing checks from her account to cover his debts]...but nothing had been paid. Sometimes I still cannot believe it; Laurence had stood by while I sold the furniture, knowing that he had already sold it twice over to different people. He had sold the car. When I went to the bank to try and cash the children's policies they had already been cashed; our joint account was empty."

When Rumer was handed a list of the debts her husband owed to his brokerage firm and was asked by the managing director, "What are you going to do?" she said, "Pay them."

Of course, this is the first response an honorable woman would have—isn't it?

But it shouldn't be.

"No" is the correct answer, in case you're wondering. These were not her debts. I sense you're mulling over the situation, as I once did.

That's because *No* is such a foreign word for so many women, Rumer didn't find it in her vocabulary. What a steep learning curve is the wisdom to say no in order to take care of ourselves. Learning to take care of yourself first is hard because it goes against the grain of our nurturing nature.

Here's the difficult lesson Rumer Godden shares with us as we come to terms with gaining authentic balance in our lives, which includes clarity, safety, and solvency. "Of all the silly things I have done in my life I expect that was the silliest; it took almost all the *Black Narcissus* money I have saved. In those two words I threw away what would have been some security for myself and the children."

But still, she had to go on, and she did, writing another sixty-seven books with grit, grace, and moxie. "To despair is traitorous to your gift," was her message to me many mornings, virtually pulling open the curtains and setting a cup of tea on the nightstand. "To wake for the first time in a new place can be like another birth," so let's recognize each morning that the gift of *today* is wondrous.

"Every book I write, a novel, a memoir, that is even remotely connected with our family begins the same way, with a landfall, an alighting in a strange place to start a new life, probably in a new way," Rumer Godden shares. "The first thing I try to do anywhere, in any house is to make it into a home; slowly the deserted house becomes alive."

Perhaps I feel such a cherished kinship with her because my life seems to have mirrored the upheaval she also endured in seeking and finding her Houses of Belonging. But it is Rumer Godden who has taught me that "forever" begins and ends every twenty-four hours—a priceless discovery and treasure beyond measure, once you get over the shock of it. You have no idea of the sheer relief that comes when you simply delete the word *forever* from your vocabulary and stop trying to fit every dream into a cubbyhole of eternal impossibility.

Instead, let us awake fresh to each individual day in our newly imagined House of Belonging.

Home Alone

Too many of us don't know how to treat ourselves well, almost as if we feel we don't deserve to, don't have time to, don't want to feel guilty about doing so.

—Dominique Browning
American writer and editor

You can have a wonderful partner, a happy marriage, and a loving family and still feel estranged from your surroundings. Somehow you know you're not living in your House of Belonging.

Why is that, do you think? Because the House of Belonging is not just a place. It is a *presence*—your authentic presence in your own life and your own home. One of the ways we take care of ourselves is by creating a home for ourselves, no matter how basic it is in the beginning, and especially if we're single. And yet many of us hold back because, for some faulty wiring, unconsciously we think we don't deserve it.

In her inspiring and poignant *Around the House and In the Garden: A Memoir of Heartbreak, Healing, and Home Improvement,* Dominique Browning tells the story of a friend that is a powerful cautionary tale for all women of a certain age who haven't invested emotionally, psychologically, spiritually, creatively, or financially in feathering their own nest. "What she wanted—and what she had planned on—was to fall in love, get married, and make a home with someone. It wasn't happening, though."

Although this woman "was a person of accomplishment, fortitude, and sophistication" as she entered her forties, she began to feel increasingly uncomfortable in her living space. This was because the woman—who could be any of us—"was having a tough time giving herself permission to go ahead, buy a place, decorate, live well. She who never took no for an answer at work seemed paralyzed when it came to telling herself yes."

And why did she have this difficulty? Because she felt uncomfortable in her own skin. And is there a woman among us who doesn't? In fact, in so many ways, we are composite echoes of each other sharing one malady; when we don't feel comfortable in our own bodies, it's so easy to extend this sense of exile to the houses we inhabit. This sad, sorry, silent, secret, and heartbreaking truth is the reason we can't receive the gift of comfort—or belonging—when we cross our own threshold, even though we are able to bestow it lavishly upon others.

And why? Probably because we don't believe we deserve it. Like many women, I was raised to believe that the good things in life—the roaring fire, the beautifully set table, the delicious food, the good wine—are meant to be shared. However, in the span of every woman's life comes a solitary season or two—or even a decade—through choice, change, or circumstance. Why bother preparing the fire, cooking the meal, laying the table, opening a good vintage, if you're going to sip and sup alone? If no one is going to praise your apple pie, why bother making it?

These are difficult truths for us to read, hear, or share. But once we do, my darling, this wounding, this psychological self-harming, this private shaming can end and our sophisticated self-sabotage can be called out for what it is. Then slowly, moment by moment, day by day, you can begin to heal one entry at a time in your Gratitude Journal, for you'll be writing the most heartwarming story you'll ever hear: your own.

Please don't waste the time that I did or feel embarrassed or hesitant about committing to establishing your House of Belonging and enjoying the best vintage—wine, food, furnishings, art—you can afford *now*.

"Even if we're not flapping about with mates and chicks and all the little wormy things of life, we are still nesting," Dominique Browning reassures us. "We are giving ourselves shelter. Our work may be harder, but it is not less loving for being done alone." Going ahead on your own does not mean you're "shutting the door on the hope of finding true love," she says. In fact, it's the complete opposite. You're opening a new door to Love: the front door.

There is a splendid French fable, *La Petite Maison,* about a clever man who builds a house as a secret weapon for his seduction of beautiful women. He lavishes so much passion and attention on his house that women swoon upon entering. You should know that feeling as well. And you will—by consciously choosing to be gratefully and graciously home alone, dwelling in your House of Spirit.

MAY 8

A Welcome Retreat: Home as a Haven in a Hectic World

I believe I know the only cure, which is to make one's center of life inside of one's self, not selfishly or excludingly, but with a kind of unassailable serenity—to decorate one's inner house so richly that one is content there, glad to welcome anyone who wants to come and stay, but happy all the same when one is inevitably alone.
—Edith Wharton (1862–1937)
American novelist, interior and landscape designer

The nineteenth-century novelist Edith Wharton, who captured the Gilded Age of New York society so brilliantly in her subtly nuanced novels *The House of Mirth* (1905) and her 1921 Pulitzer Prize–winning *The Age of Innocence* (the first female author to be awarded the honor), began her career writing about houses.

In fact, she published America's first best-selling interior design book (co-authored with the architect Ogden Codman), *The Decoration of Houses*, in 1897 and would become renowned for the interior of her thirty-five-room mansion—the original designer showcase—in Lenox, Massachusetts, known as The Mount. However, despite her ability to afford the best art and possessions, Edith never experienced or expressed a depth of emotion or bonded with her homes until, at the age of fifty, she fell passionately in love with a house in the south of France.

"I feel as if I were going to get married—to the right man at last!" she wrote about her beloved Hyeres and indeed, she spent the rest of her life there—twenty-five years—for she had found her House of Belonging in this modest French villa and the stunning gardens she would design surrounding it.

I find it fascinating that all her life Edith Wharton would use the metaphor of houses and architectural references to explore feminine belonging and sense of entitlement when describing a woman's nature. A woman was like a huge house with rooms set aside for visitors, and other rooms—the more comfortable ones—meant only for family and friends. "But beyond that, far beyond, are other rooms, the handles of whose doors are never turned...and in the innermost room, the holy of holies, the soul sits alone and waits for a footstep that never comes."

Many people associate this longing with a lover, but Wharton wasn't looking for just a lover, and her track record with the men in her life, while familiar to many of us, was certainly not the ideal. She finally divorced her philandering husband after he started squandering her money earned from the great success of her novel *The House of Mirth*, and she endured a tortured affair with a married English scoundrel who repeatedly broke her heart.

I believe Edith Wharton finally recognized that the footstep her Soul was waiting for was her own, when she confided that "To be able to look life in the face, that's worth living in a garret for, isn't it?"

It doesn't matter when we arrive at the same conclusion, but sooner will make us happier than later.

MAY 9

Everyday Edens: Spending Another
Day in Paradise

Home is the definition of God.

—Emily Dickinson (1830–1886)
American Victorian poet

Eden is that old-fashioned House we dwell in every day," Emily Dickinson reminded me as I wandered around my Takoma Park living room years ago picking up a purple hairband, colored markers, a young artist's sketchbook, a tennis racket, the minutes from last week's city council meeting, a stack of *Beckett's Baseball Card Monthly*, assorted CDs, one viola, various mail-order catalogs, three days' worth of newspapers, two pairs of shoes, an empty Doritos bag crumpled up next to the couch, and a hairbrush (mine, but probably used by the owner of the purple hairband).

This is Eden?

Poets, it seems, have waxed lyrical about the joys of domesticity for centuries, no doubt because they lived with loving, patient, and nurturing women who created havens of tranquil order in which they could work in peace and comfort.

But did you know that the recluse Emily Dickinson—who rarely left her home after she was thirty-four—was also very domesticated? In fact, her greatest ecstasies were said to be cooking and writing poetry. And since the bulk of her poems—1,775 of them—were only published after her death in 1886, it was her cooking skills that first won the Belle of Amherst, Massachusetts, her fame for (among other culinary delights) a moist, dense black fruitcake served at afternoon tea and scrumptious parcels of gingerbread lowered in a basket from her second-floor bedroom sanctuary to hungry neighborhood children.

Separated from us now by the chasm of more than a century, her contented and self-contained confinement seems to me to be the perfect antidote to our abrasive twenty-first-century existence. "I don't go from home unless emergency leads me by the hand," she wrote to a friend in 1854, "and then I do it obstinately and draw back if I can."

How I long to draw back, too. To simply sit still for twenty minutes in the backyard basking in the sunshine, watching the birds build their new nests, watching the cats watching the birds, greeting the new blossoms in the garden, and enjoying a fresh cup of tea and Miss Dickinson's letters to the world, as she called her poetry.

However, before this idyllic reverie can commence, I must clean. I must pick up the debris of our daily life and bring order to this room, for I cannot stand the chaos, clutter, and confusion here for another single moment. There is simply no time for poetic musings.

Or is there?

Perhaps now—of all times—when I am nearly bowed under physically, emotionally, and psychologically by the minutiae of the mundane, is the very moment I need the reverence of poets who bear witness to the sacredness of the ordinary. Then perhaps I shall see, not just other people's belongings, but all the beauty, joy, and abundance that literally lie at my feet. If I can be still for a moment and fully enter the experience of bringing Order and Harmony to my home, perhaps I can discover that the poetry of this afternoon is to be found in the perception of my tasks.

For what is the purpose of cleaning this room? Is it simply to pick up trash and dispose of yesterday's newspaper? Or is some inspired action at work here? In the process of transforming this room into a safe and serene haven where my family can come together to enjoy the comfort of each other's company, am I not changing the perception of my work?

We are all given a choice each day. We can react negatively to the demands made on us or we can choose to live abundantly, to transform the negative into the meaningful. Attitude is all. If I do not endow my life and my work with meaning, no one will ever be able to do it for me. If I don't recognize the value of what I am doing here in this living room, certainly no one else can. And if home-caring is not sacred, then forgive me, for I truly have no conception of the Divine.

And so, to lift my spirits and celebrate my choice, I listen to a Bach concerto as I clean. I put on the kettle to make myself a fresh pot of tea. I throw open the windows to catch a spring breeze.

Emily Dickinson never received an email or text. Never knew what a telephone was, a personal computer or a television. She became rich in all that truly matters—family, friendships, food, home, nature, ideas, literature, music, and her art—discovering that "To live is so startling, it leaves little time for anything else."

If only we could gratefully receive this gift of wonder and recognition, we could become the heiresses of happiness, wealthier beyond our wildest dreams.

How lovely the living room now appears and how ready it is to affectionately receive once again hats and coats, backpacks and briefcases, and today's ephemera wrapped in an everyday epiphany that Miss Dickinson shares with both of us: "Forever—is composed of Nows."

MAY 10

The Personality of Your Home

A house is who you are, not who you ought to be.
—Jill Schary Robinson
American novelist

Like it or not, the personalities of our homes are accurate barometers that reflect, through our surroundings, where we have been, what's going on in our lives, and who we are—today, this moment—although not necessarily where we're heading.

Admittedly, this is not the most reassuring thought for a meditation, especially if you could see the state of my home as I write. Nevertheless, it's true. "You will express yourself in your house whether you want to or not," said the mother of modern style, Elsie de Wolfe, who transformed the way America decorated for half a century with her book *The House in Good Taste*, written in 1913.

Your response is probably: "If I had the money to redecorate, you'd see the real me." No doubt. I don't entirely disagree. But we can't afford to put our lives and creativity on hold until there's more cash, because we only end up shortchanging ourselves and those we love. Today we can use the *Simple Abundance* steps—acceptance, blessing our circumstances, and discovering our personal preferences—to jump-start the expression of our authenticity through the way we care for and decorate our homes. When we do, the Graces of Gratitude, Simplicity, and Order will begin to transform the places where we live into hallowed havens of comfort and contentment—with or without the new slipcovers.

After my first book—*Mrs. Sharp's Traditions: Revising Victorian Family Celebrations of Comfort and Joy*—was published, a sleek, glossy magazine known for its lush pictorials (which I adore) wanted to pay me a visit for an intimate glimpse of "the woman behind the book." So successfully, it seemed, had I evoked the Victorian era in my writing that the magazine assumed I lived in a perfectly restored nineteenth-century home. How could I not?

Alas, I didn't. And I panicked.

"Calm down," a longtime friend who works in Hollywood consoled me. "Pull focus and take another look." In the movie business, "pulling focus" occurs when the camera lens slowly changes its distance for the sharpest clarity of image. "Your home is warm, charming, cozy, interesting, inviting. There are fabulous shots all around you. Don't be so hard on yourself."

But as a journalist, I knew what this magazine expected, and I didn't live in it. If my home was going to be on public display, I wanted it to be perfect; I desperately wanted to live up to the expectations of others instead of realizing that living up to my own was difficult enough. Instead, my publicist arranged for the interview to take place over afternoon tea in a hotel.

While money certainly helps us express ourselves through our surroundings, creating a warm, inviting home that reflects our own personality doesn't have to begin with clicking the "buy" button for online shopping. If you must, add your "can't live without" item into your basket and then take a walk around the block, clean off a kitchen counter, or throw a load of wash into the machine. Sleep on it. Give yourself a time-out between seeing, clicking, and buying. This is how we build personal boundaries that sustain and protect us.

Today, no matter where or how you live, look upon your home through the eyes of Love. Walk around the rooms and offer thanks for the walls and roof that safely enclose you and yours. Pause for a moment to consider all the women who have lost their homes through death, divorce, debt, or natural disaster *today*. Be grateful for the home you have, knowing that, at this moment, all you have is all you truly need.

MAY 11

Eminent Domain: Whose Home Is It, Anyway?

Your house is your home only *when you feel you have jurisdiction over the space.*

—Joan Kron
American author and film director

Unless you live alone, is your home your own? Yes, we're talking about the idea of personal "eminent domain." We've all followed it since our Goldilocks days: Papa Bear's chair, Mama Bear's chair, and a chair just for me. Well, do you have one? A chair just for you? I hope so, and if you don't, that personal need moves right up the list for "must have"; with proper lighting so you can read, and an ottoman sized just perfectly for your tired legs. You can't relax if you don't have the necessary instruments for relaxing, just as we wouldn't expect Yo-Yo Ma to play his cello without a bow.

Very often personal eminent domain extends to other people because it's been requisitioned by them. That's why your small city apartment living room is also your writer-partner's study during the day. Or why the dining room table and chairs do double duty as a castle fortress. Your crafts studio once again becomes a bedroom for a grown child who has returned home. Or why your guest room has been transformed temporarily into a sickroom for your ill mother-in-law. Perhaps this explains why your basement family room has been revamped into a hideaway to suit teenagers craving their own space in the house.

Recognizing and acknowledging the needs of those you live with as well as your own is the first step toward making everybody's habitat happy and harmonious, the way a home is meant to be.

For nearly four years after my daughter was born, the tables in our home were bare (if you don't count crayons or Legos) until she became old enough to appreciate looking at beautiful objects without playing with them. This was for her safety and my sanity. Gradually, Waterford crystal wedding presents started to coexist cozily with her toys as our belongings became intertwined, reflecting the personalities of everyone who resided there. Then, a young kitten named Mikey, who wasn't bound by the laws of eminent domain or gravity, came to live with us and some of our cherished breakables were once again packed away until he learned not to take flying leaps onto the fireplace mantel. He did, which is why he lived to the sweet age of seventeen and traveled with me to my home in England and back to California.

Space is often an unaffordable luxury for many, but does this mean we have to put off indefinitely the transformative work of authentic home-caring? A home's tranquility always comes from within no matter what the circumstances. The space one's soul requires cannot be measured in inches, feet, or dollars.

Don't be discouraged by practical considerations, even if right now you might not be free to truly express yourself through your surroundings. Begin to work with, instead of fighting against, your limitations. Never forget that your life and decorating styles are works-of-art-in-progress and will be all your happy days.

Interior decorator and writer Alexandra Stoddard, whose style and grace I adore, believes that "where we are in our lives and our relationship *with others*" must take precedence over our decorating choices, and she's right. "Sometimes what *we* want just isn't practical or right for us now. A home with small children *should* be set up differently than one with grown children. If you're divorced or remarried and stepchildren visit you often, you'll want to make appropriate arrangements for them. These are not so much questions of lifestyle as of life *passages*...An honest home that rings true to the lives of the people who occupy it will always be disarmingly refreshing to visitors." And with the right perspective, it can be for those who live there as well.

A Life of One's Own

Face it, Lady Slane. Your children, your husband, your splendor, were nothing but obstacles that kept you from yourself. They were what you chose to substitute for your real vocation. You were too young, I suppose, to know any better, but when you chose that life, you sinned against the light.

—Vita Sackville-West, Lady Nicholson (1892–1962)
English novelist, poet, and garden designer

One of the most delightful novels about a woman's fierce determination to enjoy her own thoughts, desires, wants, needs, choices, and simple pleasures before ending her days with a long sigh of resignation is Vita Sackville-West's *All Passion Spent,* published in 1931.

The novel opens with the announcement of the death of a "Great Man," Lord Henry Slane, former Prime Minister, and Viceroy of India, who has been around for so long, everyone thought that he was immortal.

So did his wife of seventy years, Deborah, Lady Slane—who married in the 1850s barely out of her teens. She had once dreamed of being an artist, but instead deferred to what was expected of her, which was an aristocratic marriage, social duty, and motherhood. Her six children, now all in their sixties—who were probably spoiled rotten while growing up—are now disagreeable, greedy, and pompous in their dotage. Like a wake of vultures, all of them, dressed in black crepe, are gathered together in the drawing room with their equally repulsive spouses having the lively conversation, "What shall we do about Mother?"

They decide that "Mother" shall spend part of the year with each of them, paying for her own upkeep out of her considerable fortune. However, Lady Slane has a shocking plan of her own. Lady Slane has just discovered that a charming little cottage she's loved for the last thirty years is available for rent. She's going to move from the luxurious family mansion in Mayfair to that cottage in Hampstead, a very unsuitable and unfashionable suburb of London where artists and riffraff reside. And so, along with her aged French maid, Genoux, she moves in and starts over. Her rules are very simple—no one under the age of forty is to visit apart from her cherished great-granddaughter, and if any of her children want to visit, they need to make an appointment.

We are privy to Lady Slane's feminine delights: picking out new wallpaper and the color of paint, the curtains, the plants in the garden, the happy anticipation of a small stack of new books, the renewal and acknowledgment in an old friendship that might have been romantic before it slipped away beneath decades of duty.

It is a rare thing, a story that reveals a woman's discovery of her inner life, even as we do. I think that Lady Slane would wish for each of us that we not hide behind our obligations to others before we throw another log on the passionate embers of our lives.

MAY 13

After the Fact: The Art of Decorative Detection

*When friends enter a home, they sense its personality and charac-
ter, the family's style of living—these elements make a house come
alive with a sense of identity, a sense of energy, enthusiasm, and
warmth, declaring, "This is who we are; this is how we live."*
—Ralph Lauren
American fashion designer

Shortly after my husband and I were married, my parents moved to a smaller home in a different state and began divesting themselves of furniture and belongings. Because of my love of Victoriana at that time, my mother gave me my grandmother's nineteenth-century front parlor suite—a love seat and two chairs—which she had purchased at an auction in 1921 at the Ritz Hotel in New York City. She also gave me a pair of turn-of-the-century china lamps. Shaped like urns, the lamps (which sat on brass pedestal bases and were nearly four feet high) were forest-green with gold leaf trim and featured a huge pink calla lily in the center.

The lamps were hideous. But it took me years to open my eyes and realize it.

This authentic awareness came as I was attempting to bring Order, the third *Simple Abundance* Grace, into our lives. I began to do this by wandering through the rooms of our house dispassionately observing our patterns of living: how we stored things (or didn't), what areas became catchalls, where we succumbed to the tendency to take things out but not put them back because it wasn't convenient.

During this investigation I turned my attention, like a detective perusing a crime scene, to examining decorative objects that surrounded me daily, especially noting their presence and validity. "Who lives here?" I asked as I began searching for myself. Every time I came into the living room, I found myself recoiling from those lamps. "God, they're horrible," I would mutter under my breath and move on. Finally, one day, Heaven's interior decorator said in desperation, "Well, get rid of the damn things and stop whining."

What can I say? Some of us are heavy sleepers and rouse very slowly.

Twenty years can go by before you realize one bright sunny morning that your mother's grand piano doesn't really fit into your city co-op or lifestyle, especially since you don't play the piano. Or perhaps you've outgrown the veneer bedroom set that you got from a thrift shop for your first apartment and have repainted three times. If the thought of picking up the brush again makes you want to cry, don't do it, even if it's practical. Instead, look for another bargain that you'd like to live with.

During the 1870s and 1880s, a philosophy known as the Aesthetic Movement sprang up on both sides of the Atlantic and began to focus on beautifying every aspect of Victorian life. The heart of the movement was realizing the importance of nurturing the soul through beautiful surroundings.

This week I'd like you to wander slowly through your home, one room at a time, and glance at the objects that surround you daily. Are you truly comfortable with them and what they whisper about you? Do you love them or just live with them? It doesn't matter how you acquired these objects. It doesn't matter how much you paid for them. No immediate decisions need to be made as to whether you should keep them. Awareness is all we're seeking.

Above all, don't be embarrassed by how long you may have waited to start searching for your authenticity. "To one who waits, all things reveal themselves," the nineteenth-century English poet Coventry Patmore reassures us, "so long as you have the courage not to deny in the darkness what you have seen in the light."

MAY 14

Rediscovering the Sacred Soul-Craft of Home-Caring

A well-run home is a microcosm of sanity in a world that is plainly mad. If a home doesn't make sense, nothing does.
—Henrietta Ripperger (1890–1974)
American literary domestic author

For centuries young women have learned how to run a home, how to cook, and how to raise a family by tying themselves to their mother's or grandmother's apron strings. George Eliot (the pen name of Victorian writer Mary Ann Evans) tells us in her novel *The Mill on the Floss*: "There were particular ways of doing things in the Dodson family— particular ways of bleaching the linen, of making the cowslip wine, curing the hams and keeping the bottled gooseberries, so that no daughter of that house could be indifferent to the privilege of having been born a Dodson, rather than a Gibson or a Watson."

Unfortunately, I wasn't born into the Dodson family. Nonetheless, when I was a senior in high school, I won a Homemaker of Tomorrow award. This greatly amused and perplexed the nuns who taught me, considering that home economics was not even part of our curriculum. It also absolutely stunned my mother, who knew the state of my bedroom and her continuing struggle to get me to clean it. But I had won the contest—which was based on an essay and not on a bake-off—by writing about the importance of homemaking as an endangered calling.

Many Mid-Century Modern women were raised with mixed messages, especially by the time we were graduating from high school and beginning college. The great majority of our mothers were full-time homemakers, but they wanted us to have careers. However, in 1965, when the rumblings of the feminist movement were starting to be heard, our mothers felt reading *The Feminine Mystique* (after they have finished it, of course) was better preparation for a woman's adult life than teaching us how to make a bed, sort white from colored laundry, organize a closet, or make a meat loaf.

If you were lucky, your mother helped you understand you could do both—enjoy a life that balanced home and meaningful work in the world. But most of us were not that lucky, or as George Eliot puts it, born a Dodson.

Today, it's not so much one or the other—women start successful companies, launch banks and media empires, explore space, trade securities on Wall Street, close million-dollar movie deals, get elected to national office, anchor the nightly news, write Supreme Court decisions, and win Nobel Prizes. They also regularly run to the grocery store on the way home from work, wash the laundry when everyone in the family has run out of clothes to wear, and search for a comfortable place to sit at the end of a long day amid overwhelming pandemonium.

Now what used to be called homemaking is referred to as "adulting." This tickles me, because every day there are plenty of adult chores that need to be done around here, and I'm the only adult in this apartment. Meals need to be made, laundry washed, garbage put out, cat litter changed, and dishes cleaned. Believe me, this drudgery is desperately seeking adulting, but I don't want to be the one doing it. Of course, because we now live during an era of complete convenience, there are many ways one can outsource these domestic burdens. And at times in my life, I certainly have. It's expedient, but it's also expensive. That's why I think we need to call a truce with ourselves and suspend the hostilities between our argumentative shrews and our Authentic Selves.

The time has come for us to look deep within. Reconsider how caring for our homes can be an expression of our authenticity. We may not necessarily know how to bleach linen, make cowslip wine, or bottle gooseberries, but it's not too late for us to rediscover the sacred soul-craft of home-caring.

Let's start by what we call taking care of ourselves and our homes: Change a chore into a task. Creating a comfortable, beautiful, well-run home can be among our most satisfying accomplishments as well as an illuminating spiritual experience. I can't promise you that overnight we can change "adulting" into "child's play." But like sweat equity, channeling your time and creative energy closer to home will produce a big emotional return for you and those you love.

MAY 15

Getting Your House in Order

My life will always have dirty dishes. If this sink can become a place of contemplation, let me learn constancy here.
—Gunilla Norris
American author on household spirituality, and psychoanalyst

Because we dread it, we put it off for as long as possible until we must dig ourselves out.

Many women approach the unrelenting, repetitive, exhausting, and unproductive work known as housekeeping like the torture of Sisyphus. After offending the Greek god Zeus, Sisyphus was punished by having to roll an enormous stone to the top of a steep hill. Every time he managed to pull off this feat, the stone would slide back down, and the poor soul would have to start over again. Women do the same thing, the French feminist Simone de Beauvoir observed in her book *The Second Sex*: "The clean becomes soiled, the soiled is made clean, over and over, day after day."

That is, of course, assuming we get around to it daily. For two-thirds of American women who also work outside their home, this means working a second shift tackling household jobs between the hours of seven p.m. and seven a.m.

And you wonder why the soiled stays soiled until you can't stand it?

When I discovered—to my dismay—that Order was the third Grace that needed to be gently explored and embraced on the *Simple Abundance* path, I balked. Although I frequently felt frazzled and adrift, especially when trying to find something or ignore the disarray around me, the virtue of Order seemed very old-fashioned, unimaginative, and uninspired—as dreary and cheerless, in fact, as the word *chore*. What I longed to bring into my life was something more uplifting.

But as I reflected on the simple, uncluttered, *serene* lives of the Amish, the Quakers, and especially the Shakers, I became struck by their seamless stitching together of life, work, and art through the thread of Divine Order.

Order shaped every part and nurtured every nuance of Shaker life, from their daily schedule of tasks to the way they expressed themselves authentically through their surroundings. Mother Ann Lee, who founded the United Society of Believers in the First and Second Appearance of Christ in 1774, instructed her followers to remember that Order was heaven's first law. "There is no dirt in heaven," she counseled her charges.

Members of the Shaker "family" were to keep their personal belongings and tools in such perfect order that they could be found at a moment's notice, day or night. To accomplish this, the Shakers elevated Order to a sacred art: Just to gaze at the exquisite beauty and brilliance of Shaker built-in drawers and cupboards is to know that in the House of Spirit a sublime pine cubbyhole awaits with your name on it. The Shakers believed that their daily work, including housekeeping, was a personal expression of worship.

"Prayer and housekeeping—they go together. They have always gone together. We simply know that our daily round *is* how we live. When we clean and order our homes, we are somehow also cleaning and ordering ourselves," the sublime writer on household spirituality Gunilla Norris tells us in her modern book of hours, *Being Home.* "How we hold the simplest of tasks speaks loudly about how we hold life itself."

MAY 16

A Place for Everything: Preserving Your Sanity with a Personal Plan

If you want the honest spiritual truth, my prayer is this:
Dear God, get me out of this mess.

—Rita Mae Brown
American author

We long to make sense of the work we do in our home, to master the sacred art and craft of doing it and to establish a microcosm of serenity, security, and sanity for ourselves and those we love.

But how and where do we begin, especially if we never were taught to put our things away so that we might find them on another day? And if we did not learn the rudimentary lessons ourselves, how can we possibly teach our children the life-sustaining skills they need, from cooperation to cooking? Getting our houses in order and endowing our children with a respect for, and appreciation of, order and work is one of the most precious gifts we can give them and ourselves.

What kind of a homemaking relationship did you have growing up? Who taught you to cook? Some of the best chefs in the world learned to cook with their fathers. Did someone patiently show you how to fold clothes, iron a blouse, make a bed, or knead bread? Did a grandparent demonstrate how to polish a table, or refinish a floor, fix a loose light fixture, put up preserves, prune a rosebush, hang a curtain, or hem a skirt? Some lucky women grew up with family members who taught them the art of home-caring, not just sharing recipes and household hints but instructing them on how to cream the butter, fold fitted sheets, thread a needle, make a quilt, passing on a priceless domestic dowry that money couldn't buy. Traditionally these home tutors were mothers "performing the rituals of the ordinary as an act of faith," Marilynne Robinson tells us in her exquisite novel *Housekeeping*, mothers knowing that the "dear ordinary heals" and imparting this sacred truth to their daughters.

After searching a century's worth of housekeeping advice found in domestic manuals, from Mrs. Isabella Beeton's classic *Book of Household Management*, published in 1861, to *Martha Stewart's Homekeeping Handbook*, one thing is clear: Sanity is preserved with planning. Always remember that *plan* comes before *work* in the dictionary and with good reason. But before planning, you're going to have to *think* your way through housework, just as you'd approach an overwhelming project at work.

Now none of us would dream of plunging in without thinking when working at a job for which we're paid. Why should we do any less for a job that compensates us with room, board, love, and contentment? By thinking first, instead of just reacting to the chores, interruptions, and demands that are made on us, we can reclaim control over our daily lives. We need to learn to run our homes instead of letting the housework run roughshod over us.

First, figure out what your standard of ideal housekeeping is. Remember, it *doesn't* have to be the same as your mother's or the Dodsons'. Close your eyes for a moment and imagine that you are walking through your front door. In your ideal version, what does the room look like? Your personal standard of ideal home-caring is the minimum you can live with and still feel content.

For example, I can personally live with dust (though I do draw the line when I can write my name on the bedroom bureau), but clutter drives me crazy. It's more important for me to have the common rooms of our home and my bedroom tidy than to have them pass a white-glove test. So, given the demands on my time, I will be content if the house can, on a consistent basis, remain reasonably straight instead of being ready for a magazine pictorial. Determine your livability quotient. It's the first step toward devising a personal plan that will work for you.

Next, you need to figure out what needs to be done, who can do it, and when. The simplest way is to break your housekeeping demands into categories: daily duties, weekly chores, monthly jobs, and seasonal tasks. See on paper how much you really do. You will be astounded. Now, who lives with you and can share the load? Once you've identified the jobs for your home and the workers available, write them down. What you're creating is a *Simple Abundance* strategy that brings Order and Harmony to your home, while providing you with enough time and space to savor the journey.

To jump-start the bringing of Order into your home, here are four old-fashioned rules that can change the quality of your daily life beginning today. Repeat this recipe for contentment out loud every morning and evening for twenty-one days. Let it become your personal mantra to maintain serenity. Write these instructions on index cards and post one in every room of your home. Teach these words of wisdom to your children; whisper them into your partner's ear:

1. If you take it out, put it back.
2. If you open it, close it.
3. If you throw it down, pick it up.
4. If you take it off, hang it up.

MAY 17

The Tao of Home-Caring

Time to dust again.
Time to caress my house,
to stroke all its surfaces.
I want to think of it as a kind of lovemaking
...the chance to appreciate by touch
what I live with and cherish.
                              —Gunilla Norris
                              American author on household spirituality,
                              and psychoanalyst

As the story goes, the Chinese sage Lao-Tzu (who was born five hundred years before Christ) decided to leave the province where he lived because he became disillusioned with the corrupt and decaying dynasty that ruled it. When he arrived at the border, a guard asked the wise old man if he would write a book before he left, instructing seekers in "the art of living." Lao-Tzu willingly agreed. He called his book the *Tao Te Ching*. When it was completed, he departed China, never to be seen again.

The *Tao Te Ching* is the sacred text of the Chinese religion known as Taoism and one of the most widely translated books of all time. Its followers strive to live according to the principles of the Tao (pronounced *doh*), which they believe governs the order of the Universe. Like Zen, Tao, or the Way, is a spiritual path; it must be intimately experienced instead of intellectually comprehended if insights are to be discovered. One of its main themes is unity, based on yielding rather than resisting. ("Tao is eternal without doing, and yet nothing remains undone.") When a seeker commits to the Way she sheds her expectations, becoming an empty vessel to be filled to the brim with both the yin and yang, the opposite male and female energies of life—career and home, dark and light, sorrow and joy, intimacy and solitude, aggression and passivity.

How can the enigmatic advice of an ancient Chinese philosopher help us get our houses in order? If our souls are so preoccupied with undoing, how does anything ever get done?

Inexplicably, it gets done by pausing. By reflecting on the way in which our life proceeds day in, day out. What works, what doesn't. As we pause to reflect before doing, we come to an awareness of how the nature of all things—even the minutiae of the domestic sphere—contributes to the Harmony of the whole. One of Lao-Tzu's illuminating lessons is that "naming is the origin of all particular things" and that "mystery and manifestation arise from the same source."

I have taken this wisdom to heart, especially in how I perceive the work I do at home. Drudgery can be transformed, through a willing and open heart, into labors of love. I've mentioned it before, but it takes a little time for us to understand the profound power we have over any situation by the words we use to describe it.

Start with the words that describe, or name, your efforts. The biggest catalyst for change at home was when I started calling "chores" my "tasks." Instead of calling your daily round "housework" why not call it "caring for my home." This completely elevates our perspective. Redefining our work casts a subtle but powerful spell over the subconscious mind. And after all, *caring*—for yourself, your loved ones, your pets, and your home—is truly what you are doing when you dust, change the kitty litter, sort the laundry, prepare the meals, and work in the garden. Just a few days ago we were ready to outsource the whole kit and caboodle to the first willing adult we could find, and we might tomorrow. The essential balance occurs when we understand that while we can pay somebody to help us, the caring has to come from our hearts.

Domestic theophanies are visible manifestations of Spirit in the home. We find them by looking for Mystery in the mundane, seeing the Sacred in the ordinary. For me, this is the heart of the Way, the Tao of home-caring. Lao-Tzu urged seekers to "regard the small as important" and "to make much of the little." Today, try to glimpse everything you do in your home, no matter how insignificant it may seem, as part of your authentic path to Wholeness, and it shall become so.

MAY 18

What Lies Beneath

Freshness trembles beneath the surface of everyday, a joy perpetual in all who catch its opal lights beneath the dust of habit.
—Freya Stark (1893–1993)
English-Italian explorer and travel writer

Inside your home, you keep mementos of your past that help or hinder your movement into the future. You keep the articles of warmth and refuge that help you weather the storms outside and within you," Kathryn L. Robyn gently comforts us in her amazing book *Spiritual Housecleaning: Healing the Space Within by Beautifying the Space Around You.* "You should be able to expect this space to provide you with the means to cleanse and feed yourself, to rest your body and your mind, to engage in quality and intimate times with your friends and loved ones, to entertain and stimulate you. You may take it for granted that you can unlock the door and receive these gifts of shelter every time you come home."

But the heartrending truth is that many women—women just like you and me—don't receive these gifts when we walk through our doors. And so, because they can't come home to a house that shelters their own body and soul, they run away into the shelter of superficial addictions—food, drink, shopping, smoking, sex, social media, workaholism, and perfectionism—where the spiritually homeless gather.

"We move in and out of our homes as if they mean nothing to us, as if we mean nothing to them, as if that glorious feeling of *being alive* had nothing to do with living each day. Only now and then does something happen that causes us to comment with profound astonishment, 'That got me where I live,' " Kathryn Robyn admits (surely for most of us).

Perhaps it's time to take another look at where you really do live, *as if you have never seen it before.*

"Whatever the size and scope of it, you doubtless have a kitchen, a bathroom, a place to sleep and a place to sit. You may do all this living in a one-room studio or in a towering estate with dozens of rooms," Kathryn reassures us. "The size of your house is not related to the size of your soul, but the condition of your dwelling does present a picture of the conditions of your being—body, mind and spirit."

She suggests what habitual patterns we should be searching for, in order to bring both our outer wants and our inner needs into balance.

"Is it chaotic, spare, colorful, an afterthought? Are you a person who needs an unstructured environment, a clear routine, reminders of joy, space to feel? Does your house reflect or provide you with your needs? Could it do this better? Do you know what those needs are? Or are you ignoring that knowledge, restricting your ability to respond to the requirements to your being? Have you followed somebody else's rules and abandoned your own before you even knew what they were?"

Don't feel bad if you can't answer these questions right now. By the end of a little spiritual housekeeping, you will.

MAY 19

Sacred Space

When we walk through our front door we should be able to leave the stresses and strains of the outside world. A home should provide us with a sanctuary for the soul, a haven for the senses.
—Jane Alexander
English author of books on well-being and
spiritual homemaking

For ten years Kathryn Robyn helped support herself by cleaning houses while she was studying energy healing and transformational theater. In her extraordinary book *Spiritual Housekeeping*, she fuses her expertise in both healing and home-caring into a passionate and practical spiritual practice that is bound to speak to many women where they live. It certainly does for me.

"Your home is sacred space, a sacred space with your address. Most people think of these places as mundane. Pity. If we ever needed them to be sacred, we need it now," Kathryn tell us. Unfortunately for us all, the expression *sacred space* is becoming as clichéd as the use of the word *soul*.

What does the expression *sacred space* mean to you? Hallowed, holy, blessed, sanctified? Why, yes, according to the dictionary and common usage. But how about happy, enchanted, wondrous, magical? Not really?

Well, let's think again. Unfortunately, holier-than-thou words "can be so loaded with religious teaching they make us think of things saintly, moralistic, righteous, pious, devout. These words hold pressure to be a certain kind of 'good' that scares many people away. And so they should," Kathryn Robyn believes. Instead, she would like to expand the expression *sacred space* to mean "something much more innocent, more clean, more *possible*.

"*Sacred* comes from the root word meaning whole: To be your own sacred self, wholly you, then, is to be connected to that divine spirit— God, Mother Earth, the Universal Life Force—however you perceive it. When you say something is sacred to you, you mean it is special to you in an intrinsic way; maybe it helps you feel more whole. Depending on where you're coming from, you may discover sacred space in a church, a temple, a mountain grove, a rocky beach, an art museum, or even the historic home of Elvis, Virginia Woolf, or Jackie Robinson."

Admit it, you're smiling. This thought is so smile provoking, so hold it today as you walk around the rooms where you live. Where are you the happiest in your home? Then that spot is sacred to you. "Sacred space feels inspiring, peaceful, comforting, or healing to body, mind or spirit," Kathryn Robyn reminds us. "Healing also comes from the word for whole, of sound body and mind. When that space is your own house, it is easier to feel whole and connected in your daily life."

MAY 20

Real Life Begins with Reverence

I don't believe; I know.

—Carl Jung (1875–1961)
Swiss psychiatrist and psychoanalyst

By this time you may have picked up that the *Simple Abundance* path is spiritual as well as creative and practical. But *Simple Abundance* will work for you even if you're ambivalent about whether Spirit exists. If you consciously work to bring more Gratitude, Simplicity, Order, Harmony, Beauty, and Joy into your daily life, your world will be transformed whether you believe a Higher Power is guiding you or not.

But if you commit to your spiritual awakening and discover that there is a benevolent Life Force as the most important part of the process, something marvelous will happen. Life will not feel as fraught, as frazzled, or as fragmented as before, because you'll realize that the spiritual, the creative, and the practical can't be separated. They can't be separated in quantum physics and they can't be separated in your home life.

You think you are only making a casserole, when really, you're ministering to hungry bodies and weary souls in need of love and nourishment. A friend is hurting, so you spend a lunch hour searching for the perfect card to send her. Months later she tells you how much comfort you conveyed across the miles. A woman emails your small and struggling business looking for a certain item that you are out of temporarily.

She can't wait for you to reorder because she needs it for her daughter's birthday party. Instead of sending her away disappointed, you give her the name of a competitor's website.

In the past, you might not have done this, but now you're learning, there is no competition in the spiritual realm. You were not aware that every choice you make every day is part of the Sacred Whole. But as Christina Baldwin writes in her inspiring book *Life's Companion: Journal Writing as a Spiritual Quest,* if we "ready ourselves with spiritual openness," eventually we will come to the awareness that "Spirituality is the sacred center of which all life comes, including Mondays and Tuesdays and rainy Saturday afternoons in all their mundane and glorious details."

A few months ago, you might not have believed this could be true. But with each day on the *Simple Abundance* path, you have become more open to the mystery, the magic, and the majesty of the Master Plan because you are committed to your spiritual awakening. You don't have to just believe anymore, because you know.

MAY 21

Our Mother, Ourselves

You might not have thought it possible to give birth to others before giving birth to oneself, but I assure you it is quite possible; it has been done; I offer myself in evidence as Exhibit A.
—Sheila Ballantyne (1936–2007)
American author

Many women I know share a seldom-expressed yearning to be comforted. To be mothered. This voracious need is deep, palpable—and often unrequited. Instead, we are the ones who usually provide comfort, caught between the pressing needs of our children, our elderly parents, our partners, our friends, even our colleagues.

Though we are grown, we never outgrow the need for someone special to hold us close, stroke our hair, tuck us into bed, and reassure us that tomorrow all will be well. Perhaps we need to reacquaint ourselves consciously with the maternal and deeply comforting dimension of Divinity in order to learn how to mother ourselves. The best way to start is to create—as an act of worship—a comfortable home that protects, nurtures, and sustains all who seek refuge within its walls.

Gloria Steinem has written movingly of the need to reparent herself after she began exploring, in midlife, the issue of self-esteem. Because her parents divorced when she was ten and her mother suffered from a debilitating depression, the legendary editor of *Ms.* magazine assumed the role of family caregiver.

Decades later, as a leader of the feminist movement, she organized, traveled, lectured, campaigned, and successfully raised money for causes, but she didn't know how to take care of herself—emotionally, psychologically, physically—even though she had spent her life taking care of others. Nowhere was this truth more apparent than in her home. She reveals in her book *Revolution from Within: A Book of Self-Esteem* that her apartment was little more than "a closet where I changed clothes and dumped papers into cardboard boxes." Gradually she came to the belated awareness that one's home was "a symbol of the self" and in her fifties began to enjoy her first real home.

Today, as you walk through your own home, think about ways that you can start to mother yourself—every day, not just once a year—in small but tangible ways. There should be comfortable places from the living room to the bedroom that invite you to sit, sleep, relax, and reflect. There should be small indulgences from the kitchen to the bathroom that pamper and please. There should be sources of beauty throughout that inspire, order that restores, and the quiet grace of simplicity that soothes.

The poet Ntozake Shange wrote, "i found god in myself & i loved her/i loved her fiercely." There is no more beautiful way of honoring the love of the feminine divinity waiting to mother us than by celebrating the temple where her Spirit dwells on earth.

MAY 22

Clearing Out What Isn't Useful or Beautiful

Have nothing in your homes that you do not know to be useful and believe to be beautiful.
—William Morris (1834–1896)
Nineteenth-century British textile designer,
author, and artist

In England during the 1880s, a breath of fresh air blew through stuffy Victorian parlors when poet, craftsman, and designer William Morris founded the influential Arts and Crafts movement. Morris and his associates crusaded against the cheap and shoddy furniture and decorative accessories that were then being mass-produced and crammed into middle-class homes in a frenzy of excess.

Morris urged Victorians to rid themselves of the ugly, the useless, and the uncomfortable in favor of simple and "honest" furnishings. The Irish poet W. B. Yeats termed Morris's call for the aesthetic alchemy of beauty and function in the home "the long-waited-for deliverance of the decorative arts."

On the *Simple Abundance* path, our authentic decorative deliverance arrives when we begin to appreciate and use the Morris rule—ridding ourselves of anything we do not believe to be beautiful or useful—as we restore order to our homes and simplify our lives.

Begin this week with a pad and pen. Browse through the rooms of your home meditatively. Let the Divine Graces of Simplicity, Order, Harmony, and Beauty accompany you. Really look at your surroundings—your furniture and decorative accessories. Give thanks for your home exactly as it exists today.

Now begin the inquiry. Ask each possession, are you beautiful? Useful? Is it time for you to move on? You will undoubtedly come to an object that is neither beautiful nor useful but has sentimental qualities. Begin a new category (sorry, Mr. Morris) on your clearing list. But use restraint. Does it really tug at your heartstrings? Would you mourn if it disappeared? Be truthful. No one is privy to this exercise except your Authentic Self, and she's trying to tell you something. Listen. (If it tugs at someone else's heartstrings, send it to his or her room.) Write all this information down. Always allow yourself time to think on paper before you act.

The next step in the process is to make a commitment, in *writing*, on your calendar to do one room a month. On the appointed day, plan to spend a few hours (as you did when you weeded out your wardrobe, remember?). Be sure you have plenty of boxes and garbage bags available. Now, start to sort: If it's not beautiful, useful, or sentimental, it goes. One pile is for items to give away or sell at a local charity resale shop, or on one of the many online sales tools like eBay, Everything But the House, and Let Go, just waiting for items such as Great Aunt Gladys's vase with the nymphs or the Japanese sake set you received as a wedding present and hated on sight. The other pile is for perfectly good objects of previous infatuations that no longer make your heart beat faster. This pile can be recycled as future gifts or be resale bound. The third pile is for things you can't stand or are old and broken, and these are just to be trashed.

There is an ancient metaphysical law that says if we desire more abundance in our lives, we must generate a vacuum to allow ourselves to receive the good we seek. How can better come into our lives if there's no room for it? The way we provide the vacuum is by giving away what we no longer need or desire but what can serve others.

We all change as we grow (that's how we know we're growing). This includes our personal style. If you no longer love your Fiesta cereal bowls and now want to collect Joanna Gaines's Magnolia's Hearth & Hand stoneware, or if the Limoges luncheon plates left to you by your grandmother don't really suit your style of entertaining, sell them on an online auction site, because they're quite valuable, and then replace them with something valuable to you because you love it.

But it is a wonderfully abundant and simple pleasure to bring a friend a hostess gift of homemade banana bread beautifully wrapped up on a platter that never really suited you but is one that she's admired.

Deciding to simplify our lives and bring order to our homes by sending on the objects we no longer love to new, happier incarnations with people who will genuinely appreciate them is the way to open ourselves up to receiving an abundance that will perfectly suit us.

MAY 23

The Ruskin Spring Ritual of Restoration

In order that people may be happy in their work, these three things are needed: They must be fit for it. They must not do too much of it. And they must have a sense of success in it.
—John Ruskin (1812–1900)
Leading Victorian art critic

The sun is shining, the windows are streaked, the white curtains seem more than just a tad dingy. Could this house need a spring cleaning? But the windows and curtains can wait because the sofa and a new book beckon.

So do the junk drawers. You know, those black holes lurking beneath the tidy surfaces harboring clutter and God only knows what else. Lost objects. Found objects. Objects somebody in the family might use in another lifetime. Or the unrecognizable. You name it, it's in there.

Now I don't know about you, but I have junk drawers in every room of my house, and I've only recently moved into this apartment. But I didn't have time before I moved to clear my junk drawers, so they were just emptied into a brown box and taped shut and marked "Bedroom," "Kitchen," "Living Room." All the stuff that was in the old junk drawers is now in the new junk drawer boxes.

So you might understand the dilemma I face. However, as I've been relearning the lessons of *Simple Abundance*, I have faced my compulsion. I was becoming orderly on the surface, but seething underneath was absolute domestic anarchy. I knew it. My Authentic Self knew it. It made and continues to make me very uncomfortable. "To be buried in lava and not turn a hair, it is then a man shows what stuff he is made of," wrote the Irish playwright Samuel Beckett in *Malone Dies*. For grown women the same challenge comes when we rally enough courage to face up to clearing out the junk drawers. Take a deep breath. I've got the garbage bags.

Having acquired great and profound experience in the once-every-decade junk drawer approach, I recommend that we clear out the junk drawer clutter of a lifetime this spring in manageable increments, following John Ruskin's advice. Don't do too much of it at once; that way, you can feel successful about your efforts. Each month tackle just one room or storage space in your home. Then break the room down: The first week, clean out the junk drawers, then the closets, then any other specific storage areas such as under the beds, the linen closet, the bathroom cabinets, the pantry. Above all, don't attempt to do too much at once or you'll sabotage yourself. The family room game closet hasn't been organized in five years? Don't worry, it can wait another two months, or however long it takes you to get to it. Carefully consider the areas of your home that are causing you the most frustration today and then prioritize them in order of annoyance.

Although I believe very firmly in sharing work around the home, I have come to the reluctant conclusion that clearing out clutter has to be a solitary occupation. *You must do this alone.* I cannot stress this point enough. Spouses or partners and children will never let you throw anything away. "Oh, that's where *that* was," they will say, picking up virtually every object you're trying to throw out (including the Lion King finger puppet) then leaving the stuff somewhere else in the house for you to trip over. Forget it. If they've lived without it for five or ten years, they can do without it forever. Trust me, you must clear away clutter alone or you will lose your mind in the attempt.

One last clutter clearing caveat: what to do with the "I don't know what this is, and I don't know where it belongs" box. If any item can't be identified by a member of the family, it gets tossed. Here is the only aspect of clearing out where I invite consultation. But remember, you must be ruthless. When in doubt, throw it away. You don't need it. You don't want it. You forgot you even had it, so don't keep it. No, it will not come in handy someday. Furthermore, you do not, under any circumstance, want the contents of your junk drawers ending up being thrown into "junk boxes" and then producing another genus of clutter, as I did (and a very real possibility for chronic hoarders), which will then only disappear down to that subterranean landfill known in the common vernacular as the basement (or the attic or the storage shed). But that is, as they say, another story for another day.

Every cleared junk drawer, each closet, each successful attempt at organizing only reinforces your feelings of taking back control of your life. I had never really considered how being disorganized beneath the surface had weighed upon my mind. But once I cleared away the clutter,

I felt a wonderful sense of renewal, joy, and inner peace. Here was the essence of *Simple Abundance*, and it had cost me only time (to plan), courage (to show up for work), and physical energy (to do it).

Don't be surprised if one fine spring day you suddenly feel the urge to wash the curtains and clean the windows. The Light is beautiful and you can see clearly now.

MAY 24

The Spark Joy Intervention

The space in which we live should be for the person we are becoming now, not for the person we were in the past.
—Marie Kondo
Japanese organizing consultant and
best-selling author

Recently my daughter Kate, now grown up and just married, asked if she could help me get my new apartment organized. Her wedding, my moving, and an exciting new writing project all converged in the same month, so there's been little time to spare for getting organized. Her company and her offer to clear some space in the bedroom where I'm writing were completely welcomed.

Kate was eager to put some of Marie Kondo's organizing theories to the test in my house. Like many women I, too, was inspired by Kondo's advice. I particularly love that her approach begins with gratitude.

"There's an opportunity to learn from all the things in your life, including the ones you discard," Marie tells us. "Thinking deeply about each item you discard will affect how you live and acquire new things moving forward." I'm in complete agreement with her—on the page.

However, I'd read that quote before I'd personally experienced her KonMari technique, which takes no prisoners. I do still believe that William Morris's two-point rule (Is it useful? Is it beautiful?) is a great positive motivator for helping us to clear clutter. If you add John Ruskin's advice to always do a little at a time—a drawer, a dresser, a closet—you will eventually get everything done, without doing yourself in.

So the first clear-out day arrives, as does my KonMari disciple. While I make tea for us, the dearly beloved zealot is in the bedroom from which I can hear strange noises. She has now pulled EVERYTHING out of my closet and piled it on my beds. Drawers and boxes emptied, shoes, hand-bags, sweaters, coats, dresses, tops, trousers, bras, scarves, belts.

"What are you doing?" I was thunderstruck with horror as a

mountain of stuff grew before our eyes. Kate explained, "You don't have to get rid of anything you really love. We're sparking joy!"

Are we now? Because I'm wondering what the difference is between a full-blown panic attack and Marie Kondo's brand of joy. And so, held hostage for hours, we processed our piles of Keep, Give Away, or Sell, and the famous I'm Not Sure pile, as in "I'm not sure what I want to do with that."

"Why do you have two of so many things?"

"Because that blouse looks good on me and I needed one for New York and one for England."

"Well, you're in California now, so you only need one."

Oh, mercy. I'm amazed I lived to tell the tale.

What I will admit is the more we did KonMari, the more I reconsidered the middle I'm Not Sure category and winnowed it down.

Hours passed and garbage bags kept leaving the apartment. Finally, at seven p.m., the bed was cleared, and my daughter was getting ready to go home. There really was fresh energy flowing in the bedroom.

But to me, the funniest moment came when Kate caught me furtively retrieving the two identical blouses, and she reprimanded me in the voice she reserves for when her dogs play all casual after they've wreaked mischievous mayhem. There I was, nonchalantly trying to hide the two blouses until I burst out laughing as I realized I'd joined the defensive canine pack.

If you want to spark a little joy in your home or apartment, a few gentle suggestions—unlike other clutter-busting clear-outs, don't do the KonMari alone. Have someone spot you (particularly a KonMari disciple) just like you do in a gym when you're increasing your free weights. The size of the pile that will amass on your bed is overwhelming, but any venture that begins by offering Gratitude must be good for you. So I leave you today with Marie Kondo's wisdom to ponder in your heart. It makes so much sense.

"By handling each sentimental item and deciding what to discard, you process your past. If you just stow these things away in a drawer or cardboard box, before you realize it, your past will become a weight that holds you back and keeps you from living in the here and now. To put your things in order means to put your past in order, too. It's like resetting your life and settling your accounts so that you can take the next step forward."

And I so want to know the balance of Divine Completion in my life, don't you?

"It is not our memories but the person we have become because of those past experiences that we should treasure. This is the lesson these keepsakes teach us when we sort them. The space in which we live should be for the person we are becoming now, not for the person we were in the past."

The person we are becoming. Now *there's* something to spark joy.

A Sense of Charm

Why do we love certain houses, and why do they seem to love us? It is the warmth of our individual hearts reflected in our surroundings.

—T. H. Robsjohn-Gibbings (1905–1976)
British-born architect and furniture designer

The minute we walk into a home, we know whether it has charm. There's a coziness that attracts us with cheerful hospitality. The warm resonance of a charming room beckons us to sink into comfort to our heart's content.

Simple beauty delights. Serenity, harmony, and order soothe. Touches of whimsy amuse. Personal memory reacquaints the present with the past. All's right with the world in such an engaging and inviting home. Think of the homey settings in the wonderful black-and-white movies of the 1940s, such as *The Ghost and Mrs. Muir, Bringing Up Baby, Christmas in Connecticut,* or *The Enchanted Cottage.*

Consider the film director Nancy Meyers's fabulous scenic design and the authentic beauty of the houses in her different films such as *What Women Want, Father of the Bride, Something's Gotta Give, It's Complicated,* and *The Intern.* These incredible homes are individual characters in the plots of her romantic comedies, and they always belong to the heroine. Her love/work balance may be chaotic, but her home is serene and we collectively wish it were ours.

It's no surprise that Nancy admits that she does love decorating. "I must say, it's a world I find tremendous fun. I can't redo my own house every three years, so I put all that energy into a movie. I start like any homeowner would. We bring in fabric samples, look at construction drawings. We really do build the house from scratch. I get to be the homeowner without any of the bills."

She's given us a secret strategy that we can borrow. Even if your dream house is in your heart but not on the horizon, imagine all the steps you'd take as if you were really building it. That's the bridge spanning the spiritual and material world. One caveat: You must believe that this home is absolutely real, as real as any of Nancy Meyers's movie set marvels.

"If you have it," the English playwright Sir James M. Barrie wrote about charm in 1907, "you don't need to have anything else; and if you don't have it, it doesn't much matter what else you have."

Money can purchase beautiful furnishings and decorative accessories, but it cannot ensure that charm abides with us. I believe this is because charm seems to be a quality of the soul that cannot be bought or sold. But charm can be channeled from the Divine Interior Spirit. It is accessed through our authenticity, expressed in our personal flair and our appreciation for the sheer loveliness that's all around us.

"Beauty doesn't lie in the expenditure of much money, but in the artistic disposition of little," says a reassuring article entitled "The Charm of the Unexpected" published in the August 1917 issue of *The Mother's Magazine* during World War I, when making do with less was a necessity. A century later we know what women want because we all share this yearning. Today, realize that "the desire to make the home dearer and sweeter to those who live in it" is still the enduring secret of endowing our homes with charm.

MAY 26

Progress, Not Perfection

Perfectionism is self-abuse of the highest order.
—Dr. Anne Wilson Schaef
Spiritual author and addiction expert

It was a beautiful Sunday afternoon in May—sunny and warm with a refreshing breeze. Just perfect. The kind of day you dream about in the depths of winter. That morning my daughter and I had enjoyed a pleasant outing at a farmers' market where we purchased baby lettuces, basil, tomato plants, nasturtiums, and marigolds. The week before we had successfully searched for a lovely terra-cotta urn in which to plant a French salad *potager*. I had discovered this marvelous idea for a container garden in a lifestyle magazine article and thought it sounded like fun. So did my daughter. We plotted, planned, and planted with great enthusiasm and pleasure.

When we had finished planting, we had trouble getting some loose, wet potting soil off the sides of the potager. I used a sponge and smeared it with mud; Kate doused it with a watering can, getting better results, but it still wasn't picture-perfect. I'm embarrassed to tell you how long we fussed with perfection, but finally I'd had enough. "Okay, we're done. It's beautiful."

"But it doesn't look like hers," an exasperated voice complained, pointing to the article.

"No, it doesn't. It looks like ours. Ours is great. Fine. *Close enough.*"

"But hers is perfect. Everything she does is perfect. I want ours to be perfect, too," a determined young lady of eleven fumed in frustration.

Time out. Serenity 101: Progress, Not Perfection. The glamorous lifestyle gurus who have advised us through books, magazines, and television shows starting in the 1980s and have crescendoed in popularity via the blogs, Instagrams, and photo sharing sites we all see now haven't really been honest with us. They have full-time professionals working for them, including stylists—stylists who wave magic paintbrushes dipped in burnt sienna over mud smears on terra-cotta potagers before the flash pops or the camera rolls.

I tried to explain this to my daughter. "It's image, illusion, make-believe. It's a million-dollar industry. What we're seeing isn't always the real McCoy. Now this," I pointed out with satisfaction, "is real, mud and all. It's real and it's wonderful."

Eventually I convinced my cherished skeptic to wait and see (Mother Nature did not fail me, and spring showers became our stylist). We spent the rest of the afternoon happily turning over earth as hard as granite for an old-fashioned fragrant cottage garden with English roses, lavender, hollyhocks, and delphiniums. Nearby the cats were delirious over the newly installed catnip plot.

How much of our lives is frittered away—spoiled, spent, or sullied—by our neurotic insistence on perfection? And the story I just shared took place during the prehistoric era before the internet. I'm afraid it's only gotten worse since then. Out of curiosity, I just went to Pinterest to see how many photos of potagers have been posted; I've found 452 of them, and each one is more perfect than the next. Even though I'm currently living in an apartment with no garden, patio, or balcony, I want them all! Right now!

Perhaps we were pushed into perfection because our parents expected us to live up to a standard they knew they themselves could never achieve. It wasn't enough in my family to win first place, we also had to *make it look easy.*

Certainly, our parents wanted more for us. But more of what? Misery? Haven't you had enough? Today, accept that perfection in any field is unattainable. In real life we should strive to be our best—not the world's. Still, there always will be a misspelled word, a stain on the carpet, a terra-cotta potager with streaks of mud.

Perfect women do not manifest on this plane of existence. Celebrities who sell perfection are more to be pitied than censured, envied, or emulated. Why? Because, despite their fame and bank accounts, they rarely know a moment's peace; the whole world is watching, waiting for a misstep. And then, when it happens, the collective glee of strangers and the social media backlash is horrific to live through.

Thank you, no. I'll pass. Won't you? Perfection leaves so little room for improvement. So little space for acceptance—or joy. On the path we have chosen, progress is the simple pleasure to be savored. Daily. Of course, perfect *moments* are sure to be ours, such as spending a sunny afternoon in May gardening with a daughter. Life and potagers don't have to be perfect to be pleasing.

MAY 27

Simplify, Simplify, Simplify

Out of clutter, find simplicity.
—Albert Einstein (1879–1955)
German-born Nobel Prize–winning
theoretical physicist

After a morning spent sifting and sorting through the beautiful, the useful, and the useless, I glanced around our living room floor. It resembled an archaeological dig with small stacks of artifacts all separated according to their domestic categories. I wondered what an anthropologist considering the juxtaposition of junk and precious mementos (such as my grown daughter's last pacifier from when she was a baby) would tell the world about the woman whose life was now reduced to a series of neat and pleasing bundles.

Soon it came time to return what was being kept to where it belonged, and the rest to labeled garbage bags for removal. This, believe it or not, was a source of great contentment.

As I wandered through other rooms of the house I considered the common thread in the lives of the world's great spiritual teachers and traditions: Jesus Christ, Mohammed, Buddha, Lao-Tzu, the Hebrew prophets, the Moslem sufis, the Catholic saints, the Hindu rishis, the Shakers, the Quakers, the Amish. *None of them had junk drawers.*

That's because they all embraced simplicity. Spirituality, simplicity, and serenity seem to be a sacred trinity; three Divine qualities of the orderly soul. The nineteenth-century American essayist, poet, and philosopher Henry David Thoreau believed "our life is frittered away by detail."

Sorry, but I disagree, Mr. Thoreau. I think our lives are frittered away by lack of focus. But how can we focus our attention on what's truly important when we're half crazed because we can never find anything? However, Thoreau's remedy for the frittering frets still works today: "Simplify, simplify, simplify."

This week consider that with a little bit of courage and imagination you can find the breathing space you crave. You may think you're only clearing clutter from a junk drawer or juggling commitments to find a few hours to get your house in order. But your soul knows better.

Order Within

What a gift of grace to be able to take the chaos from within
and from it create some semblance of order.
—Katherine Paterson
Chinese-born, award-winning
American writer

While spring is the traditional season for bringing order to our homes, it is also the perfect opportunity for seeking order within. "Spring cleaning can also be psychological, a time-out to confront the emotional clutter that has accumulated in your mental closet," writer Abigail Trafford recommends. "It's a pause for introspection—a midcourse correction for ordinary people in ordinarily stressful lives."

One way to begin seeking order within is to come to grips with what drives you crazy but you've been too distracted to do anything about. Run a video of your typical day through your mind and view with compassion the woman hanging on at the end of her rope. What makes you cringe? It could be anything from rushing off to work convinced that you've forgotten something you need for the day, to never finding anything to wear that's unwrinkled, to discovering as you're cooking dinner that you're out of a necessary ingredient. All these situations cry out for order, just as your fragmented soul does.

There is a better way to live. It begins when we establish order within, so that order will become a visible reality in our daily round. Start by bookending your day with reflection first thing in the morning and last thing at night. This quietude will remind you that you *can* make the choice every morning to live in the world but not be caught up in the frenzy of it, especially a frenzy of your own devising. Your bookends can take as little time as ten minutes each. I know I've suggested private interludes before (and will continue doing so). You just don't think you have the time. You may not, today. But snatch time tomorrow. Allow yourself just ten minutes before anyone else is up and after everyone else is settled in.

What to do when you first awaken or before drifting off to sleep? Quiet your mind, lift up your heart, muse, mull over, make discoveries. Consider, conceive, create, connect, *concede that it all starts within*. Pray, read the Scriptures, sacred poetry, or a meditation from an inspirational book. Think about the day ahead and how it might unfold more smoothly. Invoke Divine Order, asking Spirit to take charge of your life today and every day. Visualize yourself at the end of a happy, stress-free, productive day, relaxing and enjoying the well-deserved leisure of the evening.

Stroll into the backyard, onto a balcony, sit on the front porch or front stoop with a cup of coffee and wait for the sun to rise. Observe how gently but surely the natural world renews itself daily. You may not believe this, but Mother Time does not rush; seven o'clock does not tell six o'clock, "Get a move on, there are places to go, people to see, emails to send."

If you have children, commute ninety minutes to work, or need to reach European clients on the telephone, what I am suggesting probably seems impossible, a suggestion from someone who obviously hasn't a clue as to how you really live. But I've occasionally experienced these scenarios, and even though you need ten minutes to start and end your day more than the rest of us, let your Spirit be your guide.

Bookending your day by nurturing your Spirit can mean rousing your body even earlier than usual on a morning when you're too exhausted even to crawl out of bed. And it might mean spending an extra moment with yourself at night when you're so ready to collapse into a deep slumber. But trust me, it is well worth taking that time.

Here's what I do many mornings and evenings to ease myself into these calming moments: a half hour before I have to rise and just before I go to sleep, I lie snuggled in bed and listen in the dark to Gregorian chants—the sublime, ancient Latin invocations sung by Benedictine monks for the last 1,500 years. It's a pity I don't understand every word the monks are singing, but it doesn't really matter. All I know is that the soft, rhythmic chants reassure and soothe me on a very deep level. Sometimes I pray with the monks, other times I like to imagine they are praying *for me*. It's a gentle, centering, and comforting reminder that another, truer reality exists, something I'm apt to forget in the middle of a busy day—as you probably are, too.

Today, seek order within, so that Divine Order may be manifest outwardly in your daily round.

MAY 29

The Art of Puttering

Puttering is really a time to be alone, to dream and to get in touch with yourself... To putter is to discover.
—Alexandra Stoddard
Author, interior designer, lifestyle
philosopher

In my mind there are significant distinctions among straightening, tidying up, cleaning, and "puttering." The first three home-caring tasks are the underpinnings, providing the order necessary for ritual. Puttering is the intersection of introspection and inspiration. It's not on our to-do list, therefore it charms, centers, and cajoles stressed spirits. But I can't begin to enjoy rearranging personal mementos or a beautiful vase of flowers with clutter all around me and cobwebs in the corners. Surely, I'm not the only woman in the world who has ever glanced up at a corner of her living room and found a masterpiece worthy of *Charlotte's Web*? So I usually set aside late Saturday afternoon for puttering, after I've primed the house as a fresh canvas inviting me to paint beauty in my surroundings.

Unlike cleaning, which can be a group activity, puttering is a solitary pursuit, to be approached with an unhurried pace for maximum metaphysical benefits. The essence of puttering is rearranging, although I also consider polishing silver, washing china and crystal, displaying flowers, even moving furniture to be part of the puttering genus.

Part of the pleasure of puttering is free association. Think of puttering as a domestic Rorschach test. Instead of interpreting inkblots, we muse on the hidden meaning of personal possessions until we flow on to dreams, choices, risks, pleasures, authentic preferences. You think you're just rearranging favorite things on a mantel, bookcase, or tabletop, but in fact you're really designing a fresh interior lifescape. "Creative puttering is actually one of my favorite things to do at home," writer and interior designer Alexandra Stoddard reveals. "It helps us to become aware of what's still important to us, what continues to have meaning. This quiet, private act can...bring the different aspects of your life into sharp focus—and identify your needs."

Music plays an important part in my puttering ritual. I love to listen to music while home-caring, and my selections, depending on mood and task, range from Bach to Broadway. But for the most introspective puttering, I'll choose a movie soundtrack, such as *Out of Africa* or *The English Patient*. As I listen to a haunting score while rearranging family pictures or my small collection of Irish cut glass, or while replacing winter's dried boughs with fresh flowers, I understand better just what these cherished possessions mean to me. Whether your home is in the city, country, or suburbia, each in its own way offers fertile ground upon which to sow your dreams. Puttering scatters the seeds of what we love. In due time we shall reap an abundant harvest of contentment.

A Nest of Comforts

Ah! There's nothing like staying home for real comfort.
—Jane Austen (1775–1817)
English novelist

Jane Austen's novels are known for their witty, ironic, and perceptive slices of eighteenth-century English family life. But they also reveal, between the lines, their author's love of cozy "nest[s] of comforts." Miss Austen, who wrote at a little desk drawn close to her hearth, describes such a haven in her novel *Mansfield Park*, in which her heroine, Fanny Price, can retreat "after anything unpleasant...and find immediate consolation in some pursuit, or some train of thought. Her plants, her books...her writing desk, and her works of charity and ingenuity, were all within her reach...she could scarcely see an object in the room which had not an interesting remembrance connected with it."

No matter what our decorating style—realized or aspired to—the essential spiritual grace our homes should possess is the solace of comfort. As we discover and express our authenticity through our surroundings, comfort becomes our priority. After I began the *Simple Abundance* path, it shocked me to discover that there were very few places around my home where I felt truly comfortable. The search for authenticity is like living on a fault line; you never know when the earth is going to move beneath your feet.

Today, think about your own nest. Is it so cozy that you never want to leave? It should be. Do you have the comforts that you crave? Do you even know what they are? When was the last time you gave *your comfort* the thought it richly deserves?

Today, make a wish list: soft, snug places to sit; plump pillows to support or encourage you to take a nap; a place to put your feet up; proper reading lamps; plenty of bookcases; something always on hand that's interesting, illuminating, or irresistible to read; places to display favorite things; convenient tables for refreshments; a well-organized and well-stocked desk from which to run your life; as decent a sound system as you can afford; a good coffeemaker, a pretty teapot, or juicer; plants and flowers to delight; backyard furniture that beckons you to linger; and a pretty garden or terrace to linger in.

Everyone's list will be different. Take the time to figure out what you need. Think about rooms in which you have felt instantly at home throughout your life, even if they weren't yours. What appealed to you and made you want to stay? Comfort was probably the key. Today, consider what you need to build a personal nest that comforts body and soul.

Do Try This at Home: Having Something to Wear

Clothes and courage have so much to do with each other.

Sara Jeanette Duncan (1861–1922)
Canadian journalist and author

Soon after *Simple Abundance* took off like a firecracker, I was teaching a seminar at Disney World, and we were able to attach a family vacation to the trip. I had one day free and so we did some of the other Orlando attractions because Katie and her dad were going to have several days of Disney and Epcot magic.

On the free day, we got caught in the worst thunderstorm and couldn't get a ride to our hotel, so we gave up trying and walked back. We were wet for hours. After hot showers we went downstairs to get a pizza for dinner. That night when I was writing in my Gratitude Journal, I put as number one being in warm, dry clothes. When I was moving, I sorted through a box of old notebooks and came across 1996's Gratitude Journal, and when I saw the entries that day, I really laughed out loud because my number two was the hot shower. And number three? Landing on *USA Today*'s best-seller list in the top slot. We think it's the big moments and achievements we'll never forget, but truly it's the small and overlooked blessings that tell the narrative of our lives.

The big moments are life's punctuation marks.

One of the joys of keeping a Gratitude Journal is you discover what truly matters, day in and day out. And clean, dry clothes is certainly up there, especially if you're caught out in an unexpected storm. Tide has a disaster relief program called Loads of Hope, which brings portable laundry equipment in trucks so that people caught out in an emergency can feel comfortable as they recover. "At Tide, we believe in the power of clean and in times of crisis, hope can come from the look, smell and feel of clean clothes." Amen to that.

So why don't we pack some fresh, clean clothes in case we have to leave suddenly; two complete outfits for each family member. One outfit should be for hot weather such as short-sleeve T-shirts, and another for cold weather, including warm cold-weather underwear. Here's a list to help you get organized.

2 T-shirts

2 long-sleeve polo shirts or turtlenecks

2 pairs of slacks or jeans

2 sweatshirts, one lightweight, one heavier hoodie

7 pairs of socks: 4 cotton pairs and 3 woolen pairs

1 pair of hiking or all-weather boots, warm enough for walking through snow and rain

2 pairs of sneakers with good support

Hat, scarf, and 2 pairs of gloves, one for work, the other for freezing temperatures

1 waterproof lined parka

1 heavier jacket with removable liner

After you've gathered everyone's clothing, each person should have their own clear plastic storage container to keep their clothing separate with labels on both the sides and top.

As you prepare your clothing container, ask yourself if there's anything else you need such as sunglasses or an extra pair of eyeglasses, maybe an extra baseball cap, and place them inside, too. The entire point of this exercise is that the moment you open the closet door, you can say, "Thank goodness, I'm ready."

Joyful Simplicities for May

It was one of those beautiful lengthening days when May was pressing back with both hands the shades of the morning and the evening.

—Amelia Edith Huddleston Barr (1831–1919)
British-American novelist

May Day morning awakens the ancient Celtic season of Beltane. Traditionally this is the time to embrace all of Mother Nature's bounty. Open all the windows of your home this day and let the balmy breezes freshen your intimate spaces.

- On May Day, hang a basket of flowers on your front door and your next-door neighbor's. A breathtaking May bouquet that is the essence of *Simple Abundance* can be created with small stems of pink dogwood blossoms, lilacs, and white parrot tulips that have frilly blooms. Share a bouquet with a friend or colleague.
- May honors Flora, the Goddess of Flowers. Early morning sojourns in your backyard or garden (if you have one, it should appear often in your Gratitude Journal) are perfect for reawakening a sense of wonder. Leave a handkerchief out at sunset and let the dew soak it

overnight. For an appearance "younger than springtime," dab your face with drops of dew for an everlasting radiance.

ॐ For Mother's Day, give yourself a small token of esteem (*you* know what you really want) to honor the Great Mother within. See if it can be something from your comfort wish list. Do this whether you have children or not. Do this if you have pets, which are the fussiest of kids. If you do have children, forgive yourself for not living up to your own expectations (who could?), mentally toss out last year's accumulation of guilt, and start off fresh. If your own mother is still alive, take the time this year to write her the long letter you've often thought about writing, sharing all the loving things you want her to know. If your mother is not in this world, talk to her in your heart. She'll hear you.

ॐ Tackle just *one* junk drawer each week. Throw away more than you keep. You can follow organizers like @thehomeedit, @horderly, and @lifeinjeneral on Instagram for inspiration on reorganizing your drawers (and other areas of your house, too).

ॐ If you've a sweet spot for vintage homemaking, British style, have you found Alison May's scrumptious BrocanteHome.net? I've been one of Alison's fans since she started her blog in 2004 and I was living in England. She continues to fulfill my nostalgic need for my English home rituals. I never leave her website without learning something charming.

ॐ This month brings a desire for deep spring cleaning—emotionally and home-keeping—as our reawakening feminine creative energy slowly increases along with sunshine, birdsong, apple blossoms, budding lilacs, and crisp lavendered linen. Brocantehome.net has a marvelous Order of Works for "bottoming out a room," which is what English homemakers call spring cleaning.

ॐ And I've discovered The Laundress (www.thelaundress.com), a New York shop and website for eco-friendly laundry products (including hand washing and taking care of your loveliest lingerie). Remember how we used to play house when younger, and we'd pull out our washing tub and supplies? It's no different when we're grown. With the correct tools, we can transform a chore into a soul-caring task.

ॐ For a well-spent interlude, completely clean one part of your house each week of May—the kitchen (fridge, pantry, under the sink, junk drawers, and cabinets), the bedroom (nightstand and closet), bathroom (check expiration dates, organize backstock, create storage systems that work). Breaking big jobs down into manageable tasks is really the secret to getting things done. If you want further help and inspiration, the organizational company Life in Jeneral has a thirty-one-day challenge saved in their Instagram stories that I've found particularly helpful.

ॐ Our closets are one of the toughest parts of the home to tackle for countless reasons (emotional, financial, quantity). Make sure you do a proper purge and sort—and consider the hanger swap that every professional organizer recommends. Use the same hangers throughout. It does wonders for making the closet space feel neat and orderly and pleasing to the eye. If you can afford new hangers, Joy Mangano Huggable Hangers are the professional go-to, but Amazon has some great ones too in their basic collection.

ॐ One Saturday afternoon after cleaning, putter for an hour to your favorite music. Rearrange your favorite collection of personal mementos and pictures. Savor the sweet memories. Enjoy traveling back in time in your mind.

ॐ Hooked on Houses (hookedonhouses.net—you can follow her on Instagram, too) is a website I love because Julia Sweeten adores houses that have appeared in films and on television, and her website takes us behind the scenes of many of them. As soon as I see a black-and-white film, particularly from the thirties and forties, I let out a sigh of relief because the set designs are revelatory. I always look for domestic details, the trim of upholstery, the curtains, the period details in the kitchen. Consider why these charming, cozy sets draw us in to stay a while.

ॐ If you have a cherished collection, do you display it? Think of new ways to surround yourself with the things you love.

ॐ Decorate your mantel and table or desk with boughs of greenery for your home and workspace. Make a simple wreath from twigs and leafy branches blown away from spring storms or simply display them in your favorite vases or holders. Thank the trees for their offerings. Ancient wise women during the Arthurian era believed the simpler the wreath, the greater the power. Twigs of the blessed hazel tree were much sought after, and one hair from each resident of the home was included in the weaving to provide further protection.

ॐ We, too, should give thanks to the Celtic Mother of Abiding Shelter, praying that you and yours be spared weather and harm in and to your house from unforeseen accidents, the storms of life, and Nature's fury. Bless the walls that surround you, the roof that protects you, and floors that you stand upon. I have always had the Biblical verse on an entrance wall of my homes that reads: "As for me and my house, we will serve the Lord." (Joshua 24:15) Did you know that you can get virtually any quote today on a removable backing? Search for "Custom Removable Decals for Walls" online.

ॐ Is it May thirty-first yet? If it is, it's time to make the potato salad! Or whatever dish means "summer" to you. For me, that means Southern potato salad, which is only prepared or served in June, July, and August. Yes, I wear white shoes only until Labor Day!

JUNE

I wonder what it would be like to live in a world where it was always June.

> —Lucy Maud Montgomery (1874–1942)
> Canadian author of the Anne of Green
> Gables series

Thirty days hath perfection, she calls herself the month of June... In case you haven't noticed, there's splendor in the vase and a riot of color in the garden. The roses and peonies are in bloom, and it's time to feast on strawberries and cream. The fresh fragrance of freedom is in the air and nobody's paying attention to what we're doing. School is over, summer camp begins, and visions of vacations dance in our heads. Our smiles deepen, our laughter increases, our hearts open. This month we rediscover that it is life's enrichments rather than the riches of life that bring us true contentment.

JUNE 1

She Is There

*House ordering is my prayer, and when I have finished my prayer
is answered. And bending, stooping, scrubbing, purifies my body
as prayer doesn't.*

Jessamyn West (1902–1984)
American Quaker author

You clean a cluttered closet, slowly sorting through clothing, considering what is to be saved, stored, or shared with others. She is there. You gather together the fruits of the earth on the altar of your kitchen counter, baking not a blueberry pie but a benediction, invoking an unspoken blessing for those who will partake of your love offering. She is there.

You ready the guest room to welcome friends to your home, dressing the bed with your best linens, laying fluffy towels on the chair, arranging a small bouquet of flowers next to the reading lamp along with a few of your favorite books. She is there.

You polish the silver, fold the laundry, iron the tablecloth, wash the dishes, replace the candles. She is there.

She is Hestia, the venerable domestic spirit. We may not have known her name, but we have felt her move through us when we experience pleasure in our daily round.

Three thousand years ago in ancient Greece, Hestia was the goddess of the hearth, guardian of family life and the temple. It was to Hestia that women turned for protection and inspiration so that they might, as an act of worship, transform their dwelling places into homes of beauty and comfort.

Hestia was one of the twelve Olympians in classical Greek mythology. But she is the least known of all the deities, and there are no legends about her, even though Zeus granted her the privilege of sitting in the center of their celestial home so that she might receive the best offerings from mortals.

While the other gods and goddesses were personified in sculpture and paintings, Hestia was not rendered in human form. Instead, her spiritual presence was honored as an eternal flame burning on a round hearth. Jungian analyst and author on women's spirituality Dr. Jean Shinoda Bolen tells us in her book *Goddesses in Everywoman* that Hestia's sacred fire provided illumination, warmth, and the heat necessary for food. Despite her anonymity through the ages, "The goddess Hestia's presence in the house and temple was central to everyday life" in ancient Greece.

Today, as in ancient times, reflecting on Hestia "focuses attention inward, to the spiritual center of a woman's personality," according to Dr. Bolen, enabling us to tap into an inner harmony as we go about our daily round. Hestia is not frazzled, hanging on by a thread. Instead, Hestia is "grounded in the midst of outer chaos, disorder, or ordinary, everyday bustle." Everything that needs to get done in the home is accomplished with ease and grace. By knowingly seeking encounters with Hestia in our daily life, by letting her quiet, calm, orderly presence influence our behavior, we can come to the awakening that there is sacred mystery in the mundane.

And just how do we do this? Sometimes I'll invoke Hestia's help as I work around my home. Or I'll ask myself, is this how Hestia would approach this task? Of course, if I must ask that question, I know the answer, but the asking of the question brings my awareness back to the contemplative nature of home-caring.

Most of all, Hestia gently reminds me, as Dr. Bolen points out, "[T]ending to household details is a centering activity equivalent to meditation," if we want to make it so. If you feel you have no time to sit down to meditate, that you have a valid excuse for not seeking communion with Spirit because the floor must be swept, realize that if you approach your tasks with reverence, not just your home will be transformed. The Goddess knows what it takes to run a household and She has deemed it holy. So should you.

JUNE 2

In Praise of Modesty

Style is to see beauty in modesty.
—Andrée Putman (1925–2013)
French interior and furniture designer

Modesty isn't a very exciting virtue. A sparse or stark style can be sophisticated and dramatic, but modesty seems dull, too often confused with the girl in the muslin dress sitting on the side of the gymnasium who's never asked to dance. However, the French designer Andrée Putman, who reinterpreted everything from hotel interiors to pencils, believed "unless you have a feeling for that secret knowledge that modest things can be more beautiful than anything expensive, you will never have style."

Perhaps as a child you were told not to toot your own horn, even when you accomplished something amazing. Or maybe you were told to stop dreaming of setting the world on fire, and "have more modest aspirations, so you won't be disappointed." Maybe even now when you try to express your Authentic Self, you may hear an old voice berating you for "being a show-off."

Yet at the same time, out of the corner of our eyes we see it's the *big* gestures that get all the attention in life. Glamour. Fame. Wealth. The trinity of what's considered good taste worshiped by the world. Or at least that's the way it looks from here.

It's always the wealthy women or celebrities (who don't even pay) who make it on to the international best-dressed lists. Whose homes do we want to see? Why, the movie stars' mansions that are glorified in glossy layouts of print and digital dreams.

It's *not* enough to write a finely honed first novel; it has to be a best-seller, or you'll have difficulty publishing a second one. You can't just be a talented actress, you must win an Academy Award to be considered a bankable investment. When was the last time you heard of an Olympic bronze medalist signing a million-dollar endorsement deal? That's because the gold goes to the champions. Being a modest success just doesn't make it. We hear "modest" and think "mediocre."

So let's meditate on Modesty for a moment. What if she isn't the self-effacing, shy, retiring, nerdy virtue we've thought she is? What if Modesty is really passion restrained? What if Modesty is a virtue so full of her own smoldering sense of self that she isn't distracted by the glitz?

The American writer and illustrator Oliver Herford believed that modesty was "the gentle art of enhancing your charm by pretending not to be aware of it." People with an authentic style know who they are but, even more important, *they know who they are not.* They don't care about labels. They care about personal expression. Frank Lloyd Wright never would have allowed his house to be decorated from Urban Outfitters, even though both modes have their fans. The trick is to go deep enough to mine the core of your authenticity, because when you love everything that surrounds you, the room loves you back.

JUNE 3

An Interior Vision Inventory

We shape our dwellings, and afterwards our dwellings shape us.
—Sir Winston Churchill (1874–1965)
British Prime Minister and painter

The fantasy is that you simply start with a color, a couch, or a pine sideboard that you absolutely adore. So far, so good. What next? Now you effortlessly pull the room together, expressing through your dazzling decorative choices—the carpet, the curtains, the crockery, the coffee table—the woman who loves art deco, cozy English cottages, or mid-century modern.

But what if *today* you suddenly don't know what you want to hang over the couch, lay on the floor, or put on the shelves? What if the couch came from your partner's first marriage, the carpet from your mother, the coffee table from Goodwill? What if you know what you want but must choose between that antique pine sideboard and a down payment on that much-needed new car?

Then it's time for an interior vision inventory. One of the benefits of sorting through your belongings and identifying what's beautiful, useful, or sentimental is that clarity emerges. You probably will be surprised by how much you already own that is simply waiting to be reconsidered, rearranged, reupholstered, refinished. Just don't be surprised to discover that even if what you live with is beautiful, it might no longer suit you.

A dear friend of mine collected kilim pillows with a passion for years. But one day it occurred to her that she hadn't been spending as much time in the living room as in the past, even though she'd invested lots of money and energy to decorate it and loved the look. She finally realized that the patterns were too busy to come home to after the rigors of a long day and that the dark colors, while dramatic, depressed her.

Torn between being practical—just letting the room stay the way it was—and discovering what truly pleased her now, she opted for pleasure. She not only wanted to bring the room to life, she needed to be able to live in it. Her new passion became peace of mind. The first step was to empty the room, leaving only the couches, which she recovered with plain white slipcovers. She painted the walls and bookcases white and eliminated the pillows. But since the pillows are still beautiful, she's storing them until another setting invites their presence. The only color in the room comes from her beloved books. Her new personal flourish is restraint. Now when she comes home, she feels contented instead of uncomfortable, which, after all, is what authentic decorating should be about.

Decorating shouldn't be about how a room looks in a magazine or Instagram feed as much as how *you feel* in that room. If you are to create rooms with an authentic view, self-exploration must come before paint chips and fabric swatches.

Personal flourishes can bridge the gap while we wait for our interior vision to find outward expression in our surroundings. Maybe you can't manage the cost of a new sofa just yet but could afford a new scatter rug to place nearby to give it a lift. Maybe you could give a lamp a fresh look with a different shade, arrange flowers in a teapot instead of a vase, find a pretty porcelain cup to hold pens, position a picture on a small easel instead of a wall, take the doors off the kitchen cabinets, and most important, learn what you can live without.

Personal flourishes can be had for little or no money if you are willing to invest passion, perseverance, patience, and a fresh perspective.

JUNE 4

Let Passion Be Your Decorator

It seems to me we can never give up longing and wishing while we are thoroughly alive. There are certain things that we feel are beautiful and good, and we must hunger for them.
—George Eliot (1819–1880)
Author of *The Mill on the Floss* (1860)

One of my favorite pastimes is reading novels that celebrate domestic delights. The pages of the 1930s short story writer Kathleen Norris, authors Laurie Colwin, Rosamunde Pilcher, and Nora Ephron reveal not only passionate love affairs, but delectable descriptions of food and furnishings that capture my imagination even more than the plots.

Another favorite literary domestic is Daphne du Maurier. Here is her rendering of the first Mrs. de Winter's study from her novel *Rebecca*:

"This was a woman's room, graceful, fragile, the room of someone who had chosen every particle of furniture with great care, so that each chair, each vase, each small infinitesimal thing should be in harmony with one another and with her own personality. It was as though she who had arranged this room had said: 'This I will have, and this, and this,' taking piece by piece from the treasures in Manderley each object that pleased her best, ignoring the second-rate, the mediocre, laying her hand with sure and certain instinct only upon the best."

Achieving authentic Harmony through our surroundings—laying our hands with sure and certain instinct on that which best expresses our sense of self—begins to occur as Order is gradually restored to our lives and our homes. But even if you have not yet found the time to clear closets and drawers of clutter or sift and sort through your belongings to decide what is beautiful, useful, or sentimental, don't be discouraged. Important inner work is taking place that will soon become visible.

Probably because I am a writer, I think discovering your authentic style is very similar to the creative stages of writing a book. A book may look inanimate, but like a home, it lives, breathes, and expresses your being.

As a writer, the gleam of inspiration comes first; similarly, your decorating discoveries might begin with a picture of a living room that makes you sigh. To flesh out my initial idea for a book I need to do research; that's what you're doing on your inspired excursions and with your decorating archive.

Next, I need a working table of contents or an outline; you would develop a plan or budget. At this point, I'm usually overwhelmed by the enormity of the project; you may be, too. For me, this feeling only subsides after I plunge in and start to write my rough draft; perhaps you're now pulling up the old carpet to refinish your floors, or you've begun stripping wallpaper or painting.

Usually after I've finished the rough draft, there's an initial sigh of relief followed by another wave of panic. (Does this really work?) However, once I step back and begin to edit, a sense of calm is restored. Ideas come fast as the book—or the room—begins to take shape.

Now the real fun starts: revising. This is the stage in which you make the room come alive with personal flourishes, adding the decorative details and accessories that have special meaning. Or editing them out. I love the flourish of revising because you get to fix what doesn't work, making what does work even better. But we're still not finished: The first draft is always followed by another and another, with more revising until my agent or editor tells me it's time to stop. I wouldn't exactly describe the conveyance of a writer's manuscript to her agent as a tug of war, but it's close. "If I only had more time," the writer says, which could be ten days, ten weeks, or ten years.

However, here is today's happy thought: You do! You do have more time!

When you're creating a visual memoir through your surroundings, it's a never-ending story. You don't have to stop. In fact, you really can't. You'll always be revealing a new aspect of your personality as you discover it. You'll constantly be editing, weeding out what you outgrow, making both subtle and significant decorating changes as the chapters of your life allow for, or demand, rewrites.

But whether we're giving birth to a book or a home, we need to bring a sense of passion to our work. Let passion be your muse, the authentic decorator. Let her guide and teach you to trust your instincts. Aspire to live surrounded only by those things that you passionately love. Be patient: A magnum opus can take a lifetime to create.

The famous interior decorator Elsie de Wolfe admitted, "I can't paint. I can't write. I can't sing. But I can decorate and run a house, and light it, and heat it, and have it like a living thing..." With passion as your authentic decorator, every room in your home can tell a riveting tale about the extraordinary woman who graces it with her presence.

Coming Home to Yourself

There are homes you run from, and homes you run to.
—Laura Cunningham
American novelist and playwright

We all do it, however neat and clean our home may be. As soon as we learn company is coming, we rush to straighten the pictures, fluff pillows, buff mirrors, sweep away cobwebs, and desperately camouflage any rumple or pile of untidiness. In other words, hide all evidence of our day-to-day existence. Suddenly we not only want to welcome our guest but welcome them into a home that reflects our inner ideal.

Strange in this journey of life, how Destiny keeps bringing us back upon ourselves, rather like a circular stairway, to face lessons we've not yet mastered. Our spiritual lessons are the myriad life experiences that come our way, especially the ones we don't understand. How long have I written about domestic bliss—the passion for it, the cherishing of its ordinary daily round, the ache when it is gone, the gnawing to bring it back. These days my constant craving is once again being able to come home to myself.

What do you usually do as soon as you walk through the door? Glance through the mail? Listen to your phone messages? Check your email? Turn on the evening news? Do you feel disappointed if nothing urgent is happening? Oddly, now that communications have become instantaneous, it's incredibly difficult to wean ourselves from the sensory overload of the outside world, unless we do it by indulging our physical senses instead.

What about creating an unwinding ceremonial for your common days? Grant yourself a half hour spent downshifting. Take your time as you change your clothes, put the kettle on, or pour a glass of wine, caress your pet, water the plants. Play some special music that induces serenity or smiles and listen to it only when you come home in the evening. Putter around the different rooms. Can you go out to the backyard and cut a small bouquet of flowers or seasonal branches? Could you bring some flowers home with you once a week? Enjoy arranging them. Can you hear a clock ticking? If your heart races, a sure way to calm it is the soothing rhythm of an old clock. Let the rooms you'll be living in tonight welcome you home.

In the past, it was customary for people to "freshen up" before the evening with a shower and then a change of clothing. On those nights when you're so tired you just want to drop, a quick shower before slipping into something comfortable will give you a new boost of energy to enjoy a pleasant evening—doing whatever it is you want to do.

Now, what about that something comfortable to wear? While it's tempting to change into old sweats, tatty jeans, or the nightgown you've had since high school (even if lights-out is hours away), don't be ashamed of your own company. Create a more positive, self-aware presence with something loose and soft—fresh knitwear, an elegant caftan, a striking kimono, a vintage dressing gown. If you're more comfortable in pants, a pair of soft yoga pants and a brightly colored T-shirt does make you feel better. Clothes don't make the woman, but what we wear at home—even if we're alone—is a subtle but telling indication of where our self-esteem is now. Women tend to have public clothes and private threads. In public we appear pulled together physically and emotionally; in private we're falling apart and let it all hang out. This truth might make us laugh—but when I wonder why I'm not the most spontaneous woman in the world I realize it's that once I cross the threshold, I'm hanging by a thread, literally.

After you've reconnected to everything living in your environment (and that does include you), get the evening meal started. When it's under way, sort the mail (next to a wastepaper basket), tossing the junk mail into the trash without opening it. Should you be so fortunate as to have gotten some personal letters, save them until you can give these rare pleasures the attention they deserve. And here's a radical thought: Set a time when you'll check your email and another when you'll answer it, as well as a time to return phone calls (preferably tomorrow).

If you only do one new thing between now and the end of the year, strive to make at least three evenings a week as personal as possible. Come home to yourself.

JUNE 6

Ask, Ask, Ask

Ask, and it shall be given to you; seek, and ye shall find; knock, and it shall be opened unto you.

—Matthew 7:7
New Testament

When was the last time you felt comfortable asking anybody for anything—for advice, for help, or even for directions? I've spent a considerable portion of my adult life asking questions as a journalist, so you'd think that asking on my own behalf would come easily.

It doesn't. Nevertheless, I've recently discovered something that's brought a sense of adventure to my daily round. It's so simple, it's scary.

It's *asking* for what we want. Help. Advice. Wisdom. Guidance. Information—especially information.

Information is what led me to a delightful local coffee bar. As I write, I'm enjoying a delicious glass of iced café latte at an outdoor table, shaded by a bright red-and-white-striped umbrella, surrounded by charming white pots of geraniums. Every few minutes I peek with pleasure into the shopping bag at my feet to look at my new summer linen separates. They pass the *Simple Abundance* test: They look great, feel wonderful, and were on sale.

After clearing closets and drawers, I was down to one outfit I could wear on the street (you think I'm kidding?). But everything I saw at the stores was too expensive, didn't look or feel right. So for months I avoided buying. Then I ran into a woman I know who possesses a sure sense of style. Her wardrobe is terrific, but she could pull off wearing a burlap sack with panache. When I've seen her in the past, I usually ended up sighing wistfully. This time I cut to the chase. Where does she shop? She graciously detailed not only the stores but the different fashion lines she prefers. Then she recommended I visit one great shop soon; they were having a fabulous sale. *Ask* to get on their mailing list, she advised, because they'll let you in on unadvertised specials.

"It is a long time since I have asked heaven for anything, but still my arms will not come down," Spanish poet Antonio Porchia mused, giving voice to the profound paradox of asking. We want, we need, we desire, we yearn, but we don't ask. Still our arms stay up in the air. Longings cross our mind, but we don't really commit ourselves. We don't lay it on the line. We don't ask because we're afraid somebody will say no. Who? It doesn't matter. It could be Spirit, our spouse, or our supervisor. But when wishful thinking doesn't magically manifest what we want, we feel as if we've been turned down or a dream's been denied. So, in future, we choose not to ask, but continue to wish, existing in a constant state of deprivation.

Asking comes with no guarantees. "I ask for things that do not come. I urge you for things that do not happen," writer Marjorie Holmes confides in her wonderful book of prayers, *I've Got to Talk to Somebody, God.* "Though my knuckles are bloody from knocking, and my voice is hoarse from asking," she writes, the door remains fast and there is only the Great Silence. In the Great Silence of unfulfillment all that you can hear are your own sobs. I know. But I also know if we don't ask, we haven't got a prayer getting our needs and wants fulfilled.

Today, start asking. You see a woman with a great haircut? Ask where she got it. Ask for the name of a great paint color in a home accessory shop, a fabulous recipe from a hostess, the name of a piece of music you hear over the speakers at the hair salon. Ask your partner to take the kids for the afternoon to give you some time to yourself. Ask the kids to pick up their toys so that you don't have to do it. Ask for a deadline extension. Ask for the day off. Ask for a raise. Ask when the next sale will be. Ask Spirit for a daily portion of grace. Ask Divine Wisdom for operating instructions. Ask your guardian angel to manifest holy assistance. While you're at it, ask for a deeply personal miracle—you know, the one you need so much you're afraid even to pray for it.

Ask for what you need and want. Ask to be taught the right questions. Ask to be answered. Ask for the Divine Plan of your life to unfold through joy. Ask politely. Ask with passion. Ask with a grateful heart and you will be heard.

Just ask.

JUNE 7

Favorite Things: Enjoying Cherished Collections

Each item in a collection has its own story, its own memory—the search, the day you bought it, who you were with, the vacation...
—Tricia Guild
British interior and textile designer

Do you remember the movie *Titanic*? Well, in one of the last scenes in the movie there's a wide shot of vintage photographs in frames surrounding the aged Rose sleeping that show us how Rose went on with her life after surviving the harrowing sinking of the great ship and the loss of her cherished Jack Dawson.

Or to be more precise: how Rose *chose to live* each day. Personally, I wouldn't have been surprised to hear that she spent the remainder of her life wrapped in a blanket in the corner of her bedroom with the curtains closed, because that's where I'd have been.

Instead, there are photos of Rose horseback riding, playing polo, fencing, flying an airplane, deep sea fishing, going on safari, waving aloft from top of a camel near the pyramids, mountain climbing, racing cars—in other words, living life at full throttle and with the biggest smiles. It makes me grin just to think of how happy she looks in those vintage photos.

This is my favorite scene in the film; it might have been ten seconds long. But from the moment I saw it, a profound enchantment came over me; I realized that this fictional woman's amazing life came only when she *made the choice to live again* after surviving the darkest soul-crushing tragedy. And so for the last few years I have collected vintage photographs and albums of women explorers and adventuresses and their period travel ephemera.

I also collect the stories of their lives, my cherished Women with a Past, weaving their lessons into the fabric of my daily life. It's probably the most marvelous collection I've pursued since I began collecting quotes, which cost me nothing except time, imagination, emotion, and energy and led me to the path of *Simple Abundance*. As daughters of Eve, there's such joy in sharing our incredible feminine lineage and legacy with these extraordinary Women with a Past.

What do you collect? What favorite things have you accumulated over the years that you now lovingly display around your home? I hope you love whatever it is with a passion, for there are few pleasures that can compare to browsing in little, out-of-the-way shops and flea markets, searching for that mysterious object of desire, the value of which you alone know in this world.

There are wonderful things to be found online, too, particularly on eBay, Etsy, and the marvelous estate online site Everything but the House (EBTH). I regularly check my well-curated wish and watch lists, even if it's just to browse. However, sometimes these online auction sites can really sting like a paper cut, though, when something you've tracked for nine days goes in the last four seconds to another buyer.

Still, it's the thrill of the in-person hunt that holds our interest today, the glimpse in real time of the undiscovered. You see it—over there—its beauty beckoning you to come closer for a better look. Quietly it whispers, "Take me home." Heart pounding, you turn it over for its price, hoping you can afford to do just that. Success! Casually, for you wouldn't want to give away your secret, you pay for it while exchanging pleasantries, then slowly walk out the door, smiling. Gloating is considered bad form and might even cause a canny shopkeeper to raise the price when she realizes how badly you want it.

I was once in a New Mexico ghost town with one woe-begotten shop and found a Fred Harvey milk bottle for a dollar, and like a lunatic, I couldn't stop rattling on about it to my daughter, Kate. Well, don't you know the miserable git behind the cash register took it out of my hands, gave me back my dollar, and said that it was a museum piece and was mistakenly put out in the front of the shop. It took Kate years to find another one online, which she gave me triumphantly one Christmas, and I was thrilled. But I'd also learned a valuable lesson. Zip it!

So now you've found your treasure, but don't utter yippee until you're safely in the car. Then comes the joy of bringing it to its new home and rearranging its companions to show off your prize. You stand back. It's perfect: the moment *and* your collection. It is now a tangible reminder of how surprising and wondrous life is, or can be when choices made from the heart make you smile just thinking about them.

Finders, Keepers: The Fun of Foraging

*The whole thrill of junking is that you just know the next table will
have what you've been looking for all your life.*
—Mary Randolph Carter
Author, photographer, and artist

This time of the year you can usually find me foraging on weekends.
Rambling and roaming, I rummage, following handwritten signs
posted on telephone poles. Searching for nothing and everything in general. Why should I limit my expectations of fun?

The sun is shining, I've got a full tank of gas, ice-cold lemonade in
a Hydro Flask, and just enough money to have some fun, but not go
nuts. Sometimes a sidekick rides along, other times I'm footloose and
fancy free, just moments away from finding what I've been looking for
all my life, though Heaven only knows what that is. Maybe today I'll
find out.

Now is the season of yard sales, garage sales, tag sales, and weekend
flea markets. It's time to trade online for the lure of outdoor tables.
Foraging is good for the soul. Often after we've made a major change in
our lifestyle by tightening the purse strings—whether it's voluntary or
necessary—a deprivation detox is required. The world hasn't stopped
selling, we've just stopped buying.

When this happens, it's easy to start feeling a little self-pity, especially when we're bombarded on all sides with the kind of slick advertising that pushes all our emotional buttons to convince us that more is
what we need, not less. You may intellectually want to divest yourself
of the desire for worldly goods, but the material girl in all of us still can
suffer from the "gimmes." The best way I've discovered to hush her up
is to take her out more often to outdoor stalls and sales.

I lump all outdoor shopping under the heading of flea market finds,
but there are a few distinctions worth noting. Yard and garage sales
mean someone else hopes their trash will become your treasure. It
might, but you've often got to sort through various items to find it. Still
it can't hurt to look.

Estate and moving sales offer the best assortment of recycled furniture, household goods, even clothing. Estate sales are often run by
professional dealers, so they're more organized and usually start on a
Friday running through the weekend. Plan on getting there early for
the best selection, but at the end of the day or on Sunday afternoon
you'll get the best deals. Weekend flea markets are where professional
dealers—many from hundreds of miles away—gather to sell their wares

outdoors. You can find virtually anything, from antiques to junk, and the prices will reflect this.

"The strategy of flea market shopping is simple, yet complex," reveals interior designer Charlotte Moss in her book *A Passion for Detail*. "If you go in search of a particular object your eye will 'edit out' other very suitable objects. This method sets you up for disappointment. However, if you go for the pleasure of it, for the mere hunt, you are bound to see something to come home with...Don't forget that objects are not the only benefit to shopping a flea market. Your curiosity will be rewarded, and you may come home with some great ideas—and the exhilaration is free!"

JUNE 9

Show and Tell

Create a home that gives something back to you.
—Zandra Zuraw
Founder and cohost of The Little Yellow
House Blog

Remember the weekly ritual of show-and-tell in grammar school, when we'd bring something in and then, standing in front of the entire class, tell them about it? Those were the days. Wouldn't it be great if every collector had a captive audience with which to share her treasures?

As you launch your next adventure as a domestic explorer, I have four *Simple Abundance* suggestions to contribute that can help make your outings more pleasurable:

1. *Always* remember and *assert* that Divine abundance is your *only* reality and that Divine abundance will richly manifest itself in the perfect purchase at the perfect price if it's for your highest good.
2. *Always* ask, "Is this the best you can do?" It's a friendly way of bargaining, and you *never* know.
3. *Always* know what you're going to do with the item when you get it home. I know a woman who needed to have a yard sale to get rid of all the things she'd accumulated in a decade of compulsive garage sale bingeing. Just because it's cheap doesn't mean it's meant to be your bargain.
4. *Always* set yourself a fixed limit of what you're going to spend for guilt-free shopping. I usually allow myself twenty dollars per weekend in the summer for foraging. (Anything over this amount is not an imaginative impulse but a choice requiring

careful consideration.) Always bring cash; it helps to control your spending, and most outdoor sales don't take checks or credit cards anyway. The amount you set doesn't matter as much as your psychological limit. Many weekends I end up not buying anything at all, so that money stays in the flea market wallet for next week. Patience brings pleasure.

Most of all, just enjoy the chase. And since, of course, you've decided to buy only what's useful or beautiful (preferably both), you're not wasting money; you're investing in your resourcefulness. After all, you can experiment with a new painting technique, such as sponging, stippling, or spattering, on a ten-dollar bureau, and if it doesn't work, you won't feel guilty.

"It's not about cost or provenance," Mary Randolph Carter, the brilliant author, photographer, artist, and creative director of Ralph Lauren, reminds us about the beauty of found objects. And if anyone knows how to find buried treasure it's Carter, who has written twelve books on collecting, including the Junk series of decorative details. "You make a connection with something. You want to give it a home and a new life."

Foraging gives us the ability to view the old and abandoned in a new light—reclaiming them from oblivion with creativity and choice, just as we redeem the days of our lives with imagination and love.

JUNE 10

You're My Thrill 101

Style has nothing to do with money. Anybody can do it with money. The true art is to do it on a shoestring.
—Tom Hogan
Collector and retail entrepreneur

There are five *Simple Abundance* strategies that are essential to elevating secondhand skills to new-to-you savvy:

1. Save. Seek. Find.
2. Understand scale and proportion.
3. Trust your instincts.
4. Train your eye.
5. Take your time.

1. Save. Seek. Find. Or, as the ancient Vulcan sages put it, "Live long and prosper." If you save money while seeking what you really love, you will eventually find it *and* have the cash to pay for it. (This *is* how the Universe decorates.) It may take longer than a week, but it will happen. Years from now, we'll meet, probably in a thrift shop, and we'll know each other by the gleam in our eyes. We'll acknowledge each other with the secret slogan, "Save. Seek. Find." I just hope your hand isn't on the mirror I've been eyeing for over my mantel! Oh, go ahead and take it, if it's perfect for you. I've learned spiritually that when I let go with a smile, something even better for me shows up. Remember the Universe needs a vacuum to fill, and I'm happy to oblige.

2. *Understand scale and proportion.* The real reason that your room or outfit doesn't look like the pictures in a magazine or on Instagram has less to do with your choice of fabric, color, or style than with its scale and proportion.

Tom Hogan, co-owner of the former sassy, thrift-shop-chic home furnishings shop Chartreuse (which sold out of their entire inventory the day after a *New York Times* rave review in the nineties) believes the secret to a great-looking room comes down to striving for balance. Not symmetry, so much as the visual weight of scale and proportion.

For example, if you have one big, heavy piece at one end of a room, you need to balance it with another bulky shape at the other end. If you want to mix modern and rustic for an eclectic look, go ahead, just make sure each style is represented in the same proportion. I like pairs of things—pillows or lamps.

3. *Trust your instincts.* You know what you love. Don't be guided by "friends, fads and fashion," advises Tom Hogan. If you do, six months from now you'll be so tired of the item, you won't want to walk into the room or your closet. "That is money wasted."

4. *Train your eye.* "Your eye is used to a certain look, so anything different is going to look funny," says Tom. Before you order twenty yards of a new fabric, live with a sample draped over the furniture for a couple of weeks. If your eyes don't adjust, you know it's not for you.

5. *Take your time.* "Don't be in a hurry to pull it all together. People make the mistake of doing it too fast and then they end up hating it," Tom Hogan counsels. The best rooms and wardrobes seem to evolve gradually. They don't spring from your head or a store in finished form. And always leave room for inspiration. You may never know what "find du jour" you'll discover tomorrow.

Next time you head out the door on a shopping expedition, just remember authentic style has nothing to do with money and everything to do with trusting your instincts.

Class dismissed.

You Say Bedroom, I Say Boudoir

*There is hardly anyone in the civilized world—particularly those
who do just a little more every day than they really have strength to
perform—who has not at sometime regarded bed as a refuge.*
—Annie Edith Foster Jameson (1868–1931)
English Edwardian novelist known as
J. E. Buckrose

Of all the rooms in her house, a woman's bedroom is the most personal expression of the state of her soul. For her bedroom reflects a woman's truth—her past, present, dreams for the future, or lack of them. Her hopes, her sorrows. Her passions, pleasures, peccadilloes. What she believes about herself, what she thinks she's hiding, and, obviously, is not.

Just as *night* and *sleep* are not synonymous, neither are *bedroom* and *boudoir*. By the way, what are you actually doing in your bedroom? Don't tell me you're sleeping because I won't believe you. If you've managed *that* miracle, you certainly don't need my advice. So let's think of other reasons for having a bedroom. Repose, rest, relaxation, reading, and, of course, romance? We live in hope.

I fear that the bedroom is no longer the refuge it was intended to be. Instead, I'm sensing a communal home ec center has popped up in its place—which is why we end up ironing; folding clothes; trying on clothes for tomorrow; bill paying; exercising; catching up on the news or finishing work we've brought home, before we turn in. And when we finally do plop down on a pillow, we're dead as a stoat, until the alarm goes off like a starting pistol for the next twenty-four-hour shift.

Now, back to the bedroom we don't have. Believe it or not, it isn't a bedroom we crave, it's a boudoir. A place to beat a classy retreat, where you retire instead of unraveling.

The marvelous writer Judith Thurman tells us that the boudoir was literally "a room in which to sulk, for *bouder* in French means 'to sulk.' This is a wry and rather elegant way of signaling a need most women share but don't in reality admit to: the need to be invisible."

She continues our French lesson: "You can hide in any room with a good lock on the door. But the boudoir is to a spare bedroom what a peach silk peignoir is to a terry cloth bathrobe (which turned pink when you washed it with your daughter's gym uniform)...The sumptuousness of a boudoir is essential to its nature. It's a form of nourishment, or respectful self-indulgence."

Can you think of any reason a woman might want to be invisible in her own home? Time alone or off for good behavior doesn't just mean taking a nap.

Judith Thurman offers us some amazing boudoir suggestions: "[S]taring at a fire, watching the rain, listening to music through a set of earphones, reading catalogs, stenciling a picture frame, fantasizing about an old flame, doing a double-acrostic while drinking an entire pot of espresso, trying to explain oneself telepathically to one's mother, writing a seductively critical letter to a famous novelist that will never get mailed, sorting one's panty hose by color, studying palmistry or ancient Greek, making an evening purse from the scraps of some old silk ties..."

In other words, doing something that's not important to the rest of the world, but is vital for your own sanity and survival.

True, not many of us have separate rooms for our boudoir, but creating one is more a state of mind than of space. Perhaps the computer, exercise equipment, or ironing table can't be moved somewhere else (if they can't, don't give up trying!). However, it might be screened or curtained away from your sleeping area.

I believe that we look at a room in a different light when it's truly our personal domain. You probably don't spend as much time in your bedroom as I do, because that's where I usually write, but yours should be your domain as well. Over the next few days let's ponder four personal spaces that might be pure fantasy for the moment but will help us recognize the happy roles they could play in our daily round. Humor me, for I have deemed these essential for our future thriving—a boudoir, a vanity, a scented linen closet, and a proper pantry. Personally, I've never had all four at the same time, so I'm delirious at the very thought of it, even if its reality is in my future.

As for turning your bedroom into a boudoir, here's where we have fun. You already have things that you love but don't trot out too often, right? How about silk scarves or shawls as table covering? Hang a fluttery negligee or evening wrap over the edge of a closet door or on the back of a chair; prop a feather concoction over the corner of the mirror. Arrange tiny clear Christmas lights around the outline of your headboard. Replace your practical curtains with sheers of fabrics—a double layer of tulle or chiffon becomes cascades of moonlight or streams of sunlight to dance on your floor.

I think a woman should be rapturous about her bed coverings and obsessive about what lies beneath them. How do your sheets *feel* against your skin? Are they stiff, unforgiving, worn thin, or ratty? Silk sheets cost the earth, but they wear well and last for years without showing their age—keeping you warm in the winter, cool in the summer, and perhaps encouraging you to adopt Marilyn Monroe's advice to wear only Chanel No. 5 to bed.

Pillows. I've rarely passed a beautiful one by, and if I did, then I regretted it immediately. Ruched, tasseled, tufted, silk, velvet, embroidered, trimmed, beribboned, festooned—the imagination boggles. You can move a matching pair (for symmetry!) anywhere in your home and delight in how they perk up a corner.

No, it is not possible to be too extravagant when it comes to designing your boudoir.

As often as you can indulge in a bouquet of fresh flowers, please do; even if they're small or fragrant seasonal plants, like jasmine and angel's trumpet, which blooms at night. We must keep something living in our bedrooms, so the room realizes the cycle of life is continuing even during the night. And no, the hours that we're up in the dark scrolling and clicking, clicking and scrolling do not count!

Seek until you find the most gorgeous scented candle or diffuser fragrance reeds that you only use in your boudoir. Take the time to find a cozy soft throw to toss over the end of your bed to encourage naps. Group your perfume bottles on a pretty mirror, silver, or decoupage tray. Ransom gorgeous candleholders on your flea market adventures. Plant a window box inside whether you overlook your own backyard or a brick building. This is a simple indulgence you'll come to love.

Find the prettiest "do not disturb" sign and hang it on your doorknob, and if you live with a cast of thousands, then supplement your boudoir door with an inside chain lock. Take those oversize coffee table books and stack them on a chair near your bed. Reading them at night can feel incredibly indulgent.

Yes, self-indulgence is the mood we are trying to conjure.

And finally, have the following phrase made into a clear removable sticker for your boudoir wall. I found it twenty years ago on a Tao tea box, which just goes to show you that inspiration is all around us. I had it stenciled and framed for over the bed. Here is my new life philosophy:

True passion is intoxicating and invigorating,
soothing and sensuous,
magical and mystical.
I just thought you should know what you're in for!

JUNE 12

Vanity of Vanities

At the dressing table, every woman has a chance to be an artist.
—Sophia Loren
Iconic Italian film star

Every woman deserves one place that can serve as an altar to her vanity, because really, are we ever vain about any part of our physical being?

Ah, the dressing table, that seemingly forgotten footnote of a bygone era, a space where a woman could sit down and lavish herself with attention and care. A respite, where she could apply her makeup, or style her hair, or practice her skincare routine—with all those lotions and potions—before heading to bed. A spot where she could be renewed.

"The lure of the dressing table is its promise of transformation. We come to it nose shiny and hair awry, a fright, and rise up powered sleek, a sight for sore eyes," the American poet Cynthia Zarin tells us. "In addition to its transforming powers, the dressing table is a place of rapprochement. We fall out constantly with our own faces. We despise our noses, despair over our chins. But with blushes and shadows we make up."

Perhaps you've never had an argument with your natural beauty. However, it has taken me a lifetime to learn how to befriend myself. But I know I certainly feel better when I take care of myself, and somehow I think having a comfortable, designated beauty spot would help. While I'm at it, a kidney-shaped table with a billowing skirt, a beveled-glass top, and a beautiful tripart mirror.

"Your opinion of yourself is based on a remarkable extent on your care of your body," Margery Wilson wrote in *The Woman You Want to Be,* published in 1942. "To keep up your courage, keep up your grooming. Nothing aids morale so much as a feeling of physical freshness—and nothing damages it so much as a little neglect."

Even though dressing tables, or vanities as they are also called, are seen less and less in our homes, it doesn't mean we can't recapture the essence of what they were. Start as small as a vanity case, then, if possible, move to a dresser top or a top shelf on a low bookcase. Make room for a small table. Set up a tabletop mirror and beautifully display your brushes and products in attractive containers. If you simply don't have the space designate a shelf or drawer in your bathroom—lazy Susans are great for easy product access on a shelf and stackable clear bins are godsends for any drawer. Just seeing your feminine tools neatly arranged in a clearly visible, easy-to-reach, designated space will bring more thoughtfulness for your own self-care. A visual reminder to take more time with things that make us feel good.

"This is what rituals are for. We do spiritual ceremonies as human beings in order to create a safe resting place for our most complicated feelings of joy or trauma, so that we don't have to haul those feelings around with us forever, weighing us down. We all need such places of ritual safekeeping," Elizabeth Gilbert tells us in her memoir *Eat, Pray, Love*. "And I do believe that if your culture or tradition doesn't have the specific ritual you are craving, then you are absolutely permitted to make up a ceremony of your own devising, fixing your own broken-down emotional systems with all the do-it-yourself resourcefulness of a generous plumber/poet."

And that is why a woman needs a proper vanity space, to celebrate as you grow into your stunning authentic beauty.

JUNE 13

You, Me, and Vivien Leigh

Not very many women expect to attain mansions. All that most of us ask of Providence, husbands and architects is a house just big enough for our families, properly arranged to make good house-keeping possible.
—*House Beautiful*, February 1932

Is there a woman alive with as much storage space as she really needs, or as many closets as she truly wants? Of course not.

" 'I don't want a lot of rooms in my house,' they tell each other over their tea and cucumber sandwiches. 'I want a few nice rooms, and about fifty closets,' " the *House Beautiful* architectural editor wrote in 1932 pleading for "long-suffering but hopeful Housekeepers" across the country. That sounds about right, a few nice rooms and fifty closets.

See, it's not in our imagination that we're the only women in the world who don't have enough cupboards or closets. Eighty-seven years ago, over cucumber sandwiches, our great-grandmothers were confessing to this confidential need. *House Beautiful* lets the secret out of the bag:

"Clothes closets have, in the past few years, become something of an art. In the large cities shops exist which makes a business of tacking glazed-chintz frills on the edges of shelves, of building a complicated edifice which reminds one, somehow, of a dovecote, to house the innumerable hats, shoes, and frocks of milady's wardrobe. Of course, for most of us, these closets exist only in advertisements or in magazine articles."

Remember my house-hunting excursions in England? Well, during my search, I discovered that Notley Abbey, the former home of Sir Laurence Olivier and Vivien Leigh, was up for sale. I went to look at the shambled wreck it had become since their highly celebrated romance and marriage, which began in 1937 and lasted until their divorce in 1960.

You could see the former beauty in the bones of the house, and it was easy to imagine how much fun it would be restoring Notley to its passionate perfection—complete with faded and peeling Sybil Colefax rose chintz wallpaper in the foyer and up the sweeping staircase.

But again, as I wandered from public rooms to the private part of the abbey there was a distinctly unsettling feeling. The sensations were old and clammy, as if you needed to put on a sweater or turn up the heat. Then I entered Vivien Leigh's bedroom suite, which included a little sitting room for the boudoir and a bathroom with dressing area on either side of the bedroom. But something was missing. After a few minutes I was stunned to realize that she didn't have a closet to her name! Vivien Leigh, with not one closet!

According to her biographers, Vivien spent many long periods confined to bed suffering from both bipolar disorder and tuberculosis, from which she would die at just fifty-three years old. In my own life, I've learned to live with bouts of clinical depression successfully treated with medication, but, sadly, such breakthroughs were unavailable to Vivien Leigh. However, it didn't escape my notice that her intimate surroundings couldn't have contributed to her well-being. No woman, especially one who is ill, whether it's from a bad cold or a chronic debilitating condition, can ever hope to find respite or recover in a clammy, cluttered bedroom.

Just as emotions trigger our spending patterns, storage space determines our ability to create a comfortable home for ourselves. It's funny what weird personal prompts can set us off, but the thought of the exquisite Vivian Leigh (and, of course, Scarlett O'Hara) without a decent closet triggered a visceral reaction in me.

The English estate agent explained that Vivien Leigh probably had a huge armoire to hold her negligees, day dresses, and evening gowns (remember women dressed up in the thirties, forties, and fifties), but it couldn't assuage my disappointment at this domestic oversight. Where did her shoes go, and the hats, the handbags and gloves?

When a woman is in an emotional crisis, she won't feel better to see piles of clothes strewn all around the room. I'm very serious about this. A woman's welcoming home goes a long way toward alleviating her discomfort, and closets are the first step toward recovering a sense of balance and inner equilibrium, especially when the world is out of control daily.

So, it would seem, no matter how rich and famous a woman might be, if someone else picks out the house (and Notley Abbey was Sir Larry's first love) she could come up short in the closet and cupboard department. Regrettably, for you, me, and Vivien Leigh, the closets women still lust after only exist on the pages of glossy shelter magazines, dazzling Instagram feeds, and in closet stores. Which probably means that most of us are still making do.

After all, no matter what shape your house is in today, no matter how much money you have in your checking account, no woman—and that includes both of us—wants to be overwhelmed by chaos. You just don't have enough room for everything. I know how frustrating and exasperating this feeling can be, so we must become cleverer about how we use the space we do have. Life is infinitely better with proper cupboards and closets. Nothing could be simpler or clearer.

JUNE 14

How Do You Define Her Space?

Essentially any space can be viewed as an opportunity to cultivate a haven…Personal space is as necessary as air and water… Every woman deserves one place that is unapologetically hers. With a style that defines her. Where she sets the rules.

—Jacqueline de Montravel
Writer, editor, stylist

In this lifetime, hopefully, I'll have a boudoir, a vanity, a scented linen closet, and a fancy pantry. All in the same home. However, having happily winnowed down the spaces of my desire, I'll begin with a fully functioning closet or two.

"There is nothing like fixing up closets to give you a feeling of complete satisfaction," Henrietta Ripperger wrote in *A Home of Your Own and How to Run It*, published in 1940. Likewise, few things are as frustrating as searching for something you know should be in there and not finding it because it shares a hanger with something else. "The real waste in clothing comes not in the buying, but in not using it," Mrs. Ripperger reminds us, and we know she speaks the truth

So whether you're using the Morris method or Marie Kondo, here are a few gentle suggestions. Start with an easy task by taking everything out of *only one* closet and sorting it all into two piles—the immediately wearable and the not.

Let's look at the second pile first. You'll be amazed at how much of your wardrobe is not being worn because pieces are irrevocably torn, stained, or never was altered to fit. Now, unless something has such sentimental value that you'd grab it in case of fire, toss it. (If it were that important, you would have repaired it years ago.) I once kept a green satin evening suit from the forties that was two sizes too small and zipperless. I'd held on to it for more than a decade because it represented both a memory and a fantasy—the babe I'd been in my twenties when I'd lived and wrote about fashion in Paris, and the spirit of the woman I wanted to become again, including learning dressmaking skills. As soon as I made the connection, I gave it away to a friend who wore it with glee as soon as she replaced the zipper, which she did in about a week. She looks fabulous in it, and her gratitude is enduring.

Now evaluate the importance of the wearable clothing by asking each piece these four questions:

When were you last used or worn?

Did I feel beautiful or comfortable in you?

When and how could you be used or worn in the future?

If I were moving instead of cleaning, would I take you with me?

This last question elicits your true feelings. There are bound to be items of clothing that you've not worn because they don't fit anymore (and don't fool yourself into thinking that losing a few extra inches or pounds will make a difference, because we both know it won't). I keep two sizes, and if I'm getting tight in the bigger size, I know it's time to exchange the wine with sparkling water until I can fit back in the smaller size.

More to our point (I think that we all forget this qualifier), do the clothes hanging in your closet fit your *present* lifestyle? Or has it changed without your closet catching up with you? Do the clothes you reach for every day fit your daily round? What about the becoming reflection you yearn for in the mirror? Perhaps you traded in working in an office and now work from home. Or hiking has become your new passion instead of golf. If the shoe continues to fit the current you, wear it. But if not, recycle.

We think that it's dresses, skirts, and pants hanging in our closets, but really, it's our past, for most items of clothing are associated, for good or ill, with people, places, and periods in our lives. Laura Ashley for me will forever be a backward glance to glimpse one more time the wife and daughter of a small-town mayor, identically dressed in white sailor dresses, red-ribbon straw boaters, and parasols for the annual Independence Day parade. It doesn't matter how far removed either

Laura Ashley (who tragically died in 1985) or I have become from her first cottage sprig print—we women twist our heartstrings in emotional memories.

I once fell in love with a black lace cocktail dress that cost more than I ever thought I'd earn, but I envisioned wearing it for a special, hopefully romantic occasion, and I was willing to pay the price for both fantasies. I may have looked gorgeous in that dress (and luckily, I have the photographs to prove it), but that didn't alleviate the evening's distress when it turned out to be a romantic disaster. Long after I parted from the man, the dress remained on its black lace padded hanger. Every time I cleaned the closet, I convinced myself that it had been too expensive to give away. But what was hardest to abandon was all the pent-up emotion, frustration, disappointment, and anger that I hadn't been able to express all those many years ago.

Finally, Heaven helped me, and yes, I do believe a stuffed closet and living in chaos is within the reach and power of prayer. Eventually I truly was ready to move on, but the fancy threads were binding me to a part of my past best left behind. So I decided to create a ritual romantic exorcism. Once again, I got all dolled up in the dress, poured myself a glass of champagne, and sat down at the dining room table for a little uncensored conversation with the greatest love I never had. It was very therapeutic. Then I blessed it, had it dry-cleaned, and passed it on to another good friend of mine who looks terrific in my former misery; in fact, it's become her "lucky in love" outfit. Go figure.

It's easier for us to get rid of clothes we've physically outgrown than the ones we've spent a lot of money on or invested with our hopes. But severing the emotional threads that bind us, whether they're silk, wool, gossamer, or regret, requires unconditional commitment to our future happiness, and sometimes that desire takes longer than we'd like to make its way down to the soul level. But, trust me, when the soul divests for the heart, you'll wonder in amazement and true gratitude why it took you so damn long to clean out that closet.

JUNE 15

The Home of Your Dreams

If I were asked to name the chief benefit of the house, I should say: the house shelters daydreaming.

—Gaston Bachelard (1884–1962)
French philosopher

Did you ever see the witty and winsome 1948 movie classic *Mr. Blandings Builds His Dream House*, starring Cary Grant and Myrna Loy? This charming cautionary tale is about a successful New York advertising executive and his family, who live in a cramped city apartment and long for their own home in the suburbs. They embark on an expensive adventure to build the perfect rose-covered cottage in Connecticut. Each day the modest house grows larger and so do their bills. It's a saga anyone who has ever bought a house knows only too well. But at the end of all the Blandings' tribulations their dream comes true, even if their nerves are frayed and their bank account is overdrawn. I hope they lived happily ever after; it turned out to be a wonderful house.

It takes literally years to birth a dream, whether it's a family, a career, a home, or a lifestyle. Dreams also extract a price. An ancient proverb puts it this way: "Take what you want, says the good God, but be prepared to pay for it." Dreams cost money, sweat, frustration, tears, courage, choices, perseverance, and extraordinary patience. But birthing a dream requires one more thing. Love. Only love can transform a houseful of needy, self-centered individuals into a loving, close-knit family, a passion into a livelihood, or a mere dwelling into a home that perfectly expresses your authenticity.

Even when money is not a consideration, love and time are still necessary to turn a house into a home. Samuel Clemens moved into his dream house with his beloved wife Livy and their three daughters in 1874. It was an imposing, nineteen-room, red-brick Gothic Victorian mansion in Hartford, Connecticut. Over the next thirty-five years Mr. Clemens devotedly decorated, renovated, and lavished so much expense on his house that his passion drove him into bankruptcy. (Which he resolved by writing books as "Mark Twain.") Because of all the love he and his family bestowed on their home, "it had a heart and a soul, and eyes to see with; and approvals and solicitudes and deep sympathies; it was of us, and we were in its confidence and lived in its grace and in the peace of its benedictions. We never came home from an absence that its face did not light up and speak out in eloquent welcome—and we could not enter it unmoved."

Is there a woman here who doesn't long to live in such a home? A home that embraces, nurtures, sustains, and inspires? Still, many of us think this will only happen when we've got the money to move someplace else. Surely, it can't happen here. I mean, just look at this place! But let's take another look. "I dwell in possibility," Emily Dickinson confided. We can, too. Don't look at the problems. Search for the possibilities. It doesn't matter where you live at this moment. You may be in a trailer, an apartment, or a house. You may even be rooming in a motel. It may not be your dream, but it does shelter your dreams. Those dreams can transform it into the home for which you long. Love knows how to paint, refinish, plaster, wallpaper, stencil, plant, sew, and build, even on a budget. Love knows that whatever you lack in your checking account can be made up by investing time, creative energy, and emotion. We need to learn Love's decorating secrets.

But before we pick up a hammer, a paintbrush, or the real estate ads, we need to daydream. Walk through the different rooms where you eat, sleep, and live. Bless the walls, the roof, the windows, and the foundation. Give thanks as you sift and sort, simplify, and bring order to the home you have. Realize that the home of your dreams dwells within. You must find it in the secret sanctuary of your heart today before you can cross the threshold of tomorrow.

JUNE 16

Secret Anniversaries of the Heart

The holiest of all holidays are those
kept by ourselves in silence and apart,
The secret anniversaries of the heart...
—Henry Wadsworth Longfellow (1807–1882)
American poet

There are days of oldness, and then one gets young again," the writer Katharine Butler Hathaway observed in 1930. "It goes backward and forward, not in one direction." She was musing, I think, not about the circuitous passage of time, but of memory.

This is the traditional month for orange blossoms, lace, and rice, but wedding anniversaries aren't on my mind. Today I am thinking of singular rites of passage. June is the month of secret anniversaries of the heart. These are the anniversaries we never talk about, keep in silence and apart. You might remember a first kiss, while I can't forget the last time I held my father's hand.

Many of my June memories involve summer pastimes I enjoyed as a little girl—summer theater performed on the patio while the grown-ups sipped their cocktails, the tinkling of the ice cubes along with the applause; pony rides; the splash of water at a pool or the gleeful dash through the sprinkler on the lawn. Those are followed in rapid succession by the indelible memories of June with my own little girl. Midsummer's Night Eve and preparing a tea party for the fairies; then the excitement of running into the backyard the next morning and finding presents suspended in colorful netting and ribbons.

This week I was doing errands and passed a large middle school where all the families were having picnics in their own small clusters of happiness. Suddenly, a big sigh of recognition traveled from my heart to my breath: "Oh, look, it's the end-of-year picnic. I always loved the end-of-school picnics." In a moment I was back in Takoma Park, picking up the best tuna sandwiches in the whole world, brownies, and mini fruit tarts at Everyday Gourmet to take to the Washington Waldorf School for the last day of school and our collective summer picnic on the playing field.

Secret anniversaries often reveal, in mystical ways, our place in the world and our sacred connections. They can be joyful or sad or, surprisingly, both at the same time; major turning points or minor epiphanies. You might remember the day you got your first position after years of study or received a special love letter. As you pull his beloved but ratty T-shirts from the dryer are you reminded of sending your child off to his first overnight camp? He's thirty now and in town for a visit, but where did that sentimental potpourri of fresh air, pine needles, calamine lotion, roasted marshmallows, and ghost stories around a blazing campfire come from?

Or you might recall a painful loss you can't share with others; the due date of a baby who was never born or only lived for a few days. The way the garden withered on the vine when your husband of thirty years told you casually one night, as you prepared his drink, that there was someone else taking over your position. Maybe it's time to end that long-standing breach with a friend because it doesn't matter who was right at the time; the only thing that matters is how you can make all right today.

Sometimes it takes long years to recognize the importance of such secret anniversaries—or to even know that you have one to acknowledge or commemorate with a silent pause and prayer, so that the past can move on with dignity. The past asks only to be remembered. The past wants us to move on more than the present can ever imagine, because until it does, we can't have the future that's waiting to unfold. The sacred contract and prime directive of the past is to get you to your future.

Our senses are the conduits of these soul memories. The song does remember when, as do the lilacs that bloomed every spring on your mother's dressing table among the crystal bottles of fragrance and the soft light behind billowing organza curtains; the old baseball glove; the sheer ecstasy of the outside shower at your best friend's beach house; Nana's potato salad and the sour cherry pie from the farmers' market. The dead cat's collar, his favorite blanket, how he took his last moments on earth with you cuddling him as he licked the tears off your cheek.

These things matter—they are the soul's touchstones of truth; *memento mori* (translated from the Latin "remember that you will die" but more importantly, "remember to live"). It's taken my entire life to understand that we can't receive the blessing or the bounty if we're not willing to acknowledge the benediction hidden behind every letting go. If I can cut you a little slack from the cosmic curriculum to speed your journey, then you can do the same for yourself.

Our senses are spiritual code breakers ready to reveal what's been pushed down or hidden from view as we stumble through our days; exhausted by the frenetic pace and sheer expense of time, exertion, and emotion required just to make it through our daily round. Technology has run roughshod over our lives. Which do we pay attention to first: the text, the call we're on, or the one on call waiting? Maybe it's the email or the beep from our new smart watch. Each encounter brings with it a sense of false urgency. Yes, I realize that instant communication is a critical component in our world, and change is life's only constant. But secret anniversaries of the heart are ancient, primal pathways sent to lead us to connections more powerful than we can even imagine.

Sometimes we dismiss the tugs of recollection as sentimental, impractical, or unimportant. Unruly, even. You might be blindsided by the green bud that astonishingly sprouts on a dead rosebush you began watering "just to see" what might happen. We often confuse the dormant with the dead; we'd like to be rid of painful memories and "move on" before the memories are ready to bid us adieu and depart on their own. But honoring the personal passages that altered the trajectory of our lives (especially if we are the only one who does remember) is how we grow, change, and eventually heal. We find the strength to continue our journey to Wholeness with morsels of our soul's manna: remembrance.

As Amy Tan suggests in her novel *The Joy Luck Club*, "I can never remember things I didn't understand in the first place." Perhaps this is true for all of us, and our secret anniversaries of the heart are meant to be our spiritual go-between, messengers of understanding sent to nudge us two steps back so that we're at the right time and place for the next giant leap forward.

JUNE 17

A Nook of Your Own

In solitude we give passionate attention to our lives, to our memories, to the details around us.

—Virginia Woolf (1882–1941)
Influential twentieth-century modernist
writer

In October 1928, the British novelist and literary critic Virginia Woolf gave two lectures on women and fiction at Cambridge University in England. In her talks she publicly voiced for the first time what women had quietly shared among themselves for centuries: For women to create, they needed privacy, peace, and personal incomes. The following year these lectures were published as *A Room of One's Own*, which was Woolf's recommendation if women were to honor and hone their creativity and not become "crazed with the torture" of silences.

The American writer Tillie Olsen exquisitely explored the creative voice when it is muffled, muzzled, and mute—"the unnatural thwarting of what struggles to come into being, but cannot"—in her book *Silences*, published in 1962. Olsen herself was silenced for twenty years while she raised and supported four children through menial jobs that left her no energy to write; she was nearly fifty when she published her acclaimed first novel, *Tell Me a Riddle*.

Many of us today experience creative silence. Not the hush of the heart necessary to bring forth the unexpressed from Spirit, but the creative silence brought about by circumstances we feel are beyond our control: lack of time, and/or lack of space or a place to create. Perhaps we also suffer from a lack of clarity, a failure to realize how necessary it is to nurture our sacred creativity daily. And, of course, the lack of money to pursue our creativity on a larger scale—or so we think. If you have a story to tell and you won't or can't because you're working to pay the rent or care for your children, the passion will burn from within, branding the words on your soul until you let them escape, even if it is for only one hour each Saturday afternoon.

Many of us, unless we live alone, don't have a room entirely our own. But that does not mean we cannot carve out a small psychic space— even a nook—to call ours alone. I have a friend who created a personal space in the corner of a city apartment with a floral folding screen from the 1930s that she found at a flea market. Behind it she angled a small desk and a chair near a sunny window for a restorative retreat.

No room for a screen, a desk, and a chair? Then start with a bookcase all your own. Here's where you will keep sentimental items, like a crystal paperweight a friend gave you "to help you see your future," a beautifully bound leather notebook, perhaps a cup filled with luxurious colored pencils, all the little things you love but haven't gathered together. And to commemorate your being an Artist of the Everyday, have a cup with different-size paintbrushes. The important thing is that the bookcase be yours: a psychic space that offers passionate reminders to attend to your private, artistic impulses, a place to encourage you to reclaim your creativity, and every time you pass, it shall bear silent witness that you are an Artist of the Everyday. And I promise, the day will come that you'll recognize this truth and honor it.

JUNE 18

Kitchen Confidential

This is not my recipe. This is a memory, retrievable only as memories are, by evocation and gesture and occasional concreteness that is not factual. And I resist making it a recipe. This is art and love, not about technique. Some things need to be learned standing beside someone.

—Elizabeth Kamarck Minnich
Educator and author

My mother shared some recipes with me, but I can't really say she taught me to cook. I don't have any memories of standing beside her at the stove, a confession that brings tears to my eyes. All I know about cooking I learned from other writers in the kitchen. The late, dearly missed, and much loved Mary Cantwell taught me how to cook in the early 1970s when she wrote a cooking column for *Mademoiselle*.

Mary would later spend sixteen years as an editorial writer at the *New York Times* and helped create the influential "Hers" column that appeared at the back of the Sunday magazine. And Mary wrote a three-volume memoir that makes the reader feel as if you were her closest friend. Standing next to Mary at the stove in my single-girl kitchen, I mastered the mysteries of the perfect macaroni and cheese and gained a personal sense of pride from knowing that, if pressed, I could throw together a creditable Christmas pudding.

Later in the 1980s, after I was first married to Kate's father, my cooking mentor and much-loved writer in the kitchen was the novelist Laurie Colwin, who also loved to cook. She taught me how to make gingerbread—and that good olive oil, sweet butter, and organic chickens were affordable luxuries, even when the wolf was at the door. Our lives were very similar—we were close in age, each had one daughter, and both of us wrote for a living. But most of all, Laurie Colwin and I were dedicated homebodies who found delight and excitement right here at home. Both of our days were structured around scribbling things down on paper, after-school activities, pot roasts, and the shared belief that good cooking is a high art—the holy trinity of love, security, and food.

Another thing we shared was an infatuation with cookbooks. "No one who cooks cooks alone. Even at her most solitary, a cook in the kitchen is surrounded by generations of cooks past, the advice and menus of cooks present, the wisdom of cookbook writers," she reminded me as I thumbed through my dog-eared, grease-stained collection of her cooking essays, *Home Cooking: A Writer in the Kitchen* and *More Home Cooking: A Writer Returns to the Kitchen*. And how dearly present she remains in my kitchen though she died in her sleep, at forty-eight, nearly three decades ago.

I have had since my mother's death a flowered accordion file containing her recipes, which I was not able to bring myself even to untie until years later. Corn bread, seafood cocktail (only as an appetizer for holiday dinners), Mom's mouthwatering Kentucky sage dressing (not stuffing!), spaghetti sauce (not pasta!). But here is a recipe I don't believe ever was served at our table: Cream Mongole with Sherry, serves four. Basically, it's two kinds of soup, tomato and pea—with light cream, sherry, and Worcestershire sauce. My basic instinct to continue living healthfully raises doubts about trying it now, but who knows? Mother has neatly typed out this mixture on a formal recipe card for a reason.

Maybe Mother had writer's block. She'd always wanted to be a writer, but never submitted anything for publication and never lived to see my success as a published author. Perhaps she thought she'd bring order to her mind and kitchen with typed recipe cards. Was this soup to impress guests? My imagination is drawing a blank. When we had company, Mom made clams casino and oysters Rockefeller. How proud I was to offer them, beaming in the praise she wouldn't accept for herself.

"The kitchen is about the re-creation of childhood the way you wanted it to be, keeping all that was wonderful in your own early years, while weeding out those things that caused pain. We remember the hubbub of women, the warm sweets and hovering smells, the unction of food and love, the wrapping hug of the wainscoting of counters and ovens around the walls, the inkling that one might always find a mother there," Nora Seton reminds all of us in her luminous memoir *The Kitchen Congregation*.

"The kitchen slips noiselessly into the dreams of our children before they are conscious of it, before they have children of their own and wake up," Nora Seton tells us: "Mothers and daughters share the kitchen with a common knowledge of women passing their lives there—at the sink, the stove, scanning the shelves of the pantry. The walls are our backsplash. Our laughter glazes the countertops. Here and there are the scratches that mark out moments of anguish. We cry at the sink, blotting our tears with damp dishtowels."

Nora Seton believes it's very important that we don't confuse kitchens with food, and I couldn't agree more. "Kitchens are about process, about the making of the meal, those hours, a quiet retreat or a din of beloved voices, this preparation of a favorite or sacred recipe, like the staging of a private play."

So about that recipe for Cream Mongole with Sherry. You're on your own with that one. I've still not made it, so proceed with caution.

JUNE 19

Secret Passions: The Fancy Pantry

The array of pots rather amazed her at first, but John was so fond of jelly, and the nice little jars would look so well on the top shelf.
—Louisa May Alcott (1832–1888)
American literary domestic who created
the Little Women series

Today we shall indulge in the perfect summer fantasy: the time-honored tradition of "putting up" elegant edibles. What would summer be without the contemplation of the preserved, the pickled, the potted, the candied, the brandied—the fabulous foodstuffs of fancy pantries?

Like scented linen closets, well-stocked pantries have long been a feminine passion. Were there shelves carved out of stone in the prehistoric caves at Gargas in the French Pyrenees? Undoubtedly. Where else to store the shanks of salted wild boar? Twenty thousand years later, Victorian women elevated the stocking of a pantry to an esoteric art, inspired by nineteenth-century literary domestics' luminous descriptions of deep drawers, cubbies, and bins big enough to hold cornmeal and graham flour; of spacious shelves on which to store turkey platters; and of row upon row of the prettily packaged and deliciously displayed.

There is something so nourishing and nurturing about the notion of proper pantries and well-stocked larders—a continuing link of reconnection and restoration with preservation, the comfort of all that was good in the past, and the reassurance we need so much today.

A century ago women didn't agonize over food the way contemporary American women do; sadly, we rarely take pleasure in eating, and this emotional flatline is evident in the way we store our food. If you are a fan of *Downton Abbey*, then you will have met the formidable cook Mrs. Patmore, a tiny woman with a huge presence who presides over the great house's kitchen, larder, pantry, and reputation among the English aristocracy because of the sophisticated entertaining that was expected and required for a titled family like the Granthams.

Most of the *Downton Abbey* scenes with Mrs. Patmore showed her only at work in the kitchen. Ah, but what we didn't see were the specially designed rooms off the kitchen—the larder—which had one outside wall and ventilation, and groaned with shelves of meat, fish, and fowl—not only baked or roasted but potted, brandied, and smoked; cheeses stored on cold slate shelves; freshly churned butter and eggs and dry ingredients—flour, sugar, salt, rice, oats, and bran—stored in burlap sacks.

In another room was her pantry—a cook's pride and joy. Mrs. Patmore's pantry shelves held glistening jars of jams, jellies, conserves, fruited honeys, marmalades, mustards, chutneys, pickles, nuts, and herbal marinades and remedies. There were tins for bread, cakes, pies, scones, and biscuits. Willow baskets would hold apples, pears, and seasonal fruit, such as apricots, peaches, and plums, as well as root vegetables with the goodness of the earth still clinging to them.

Every modern woman should know the sublime pleasure of gazing on glistening jars wearing tiny floral scarves and white crochet caps. But how to begin? Look no further than Helen Witty's indispensable, irreplaceable, irresistible primer, *Fancy Pantry* (1986). Now I know this book is out of print, but if you look online you can find it, and believe me, this book is worth the search. Written for all those who believe that genuinely delicious food is an affordable luxury, *Fancy Pantry* shows you how. I can't even browse through this delightful book without wanting to jump up and start playing in the kitchen.

However, I do not mean to suggest you should put up a hundred jars of zucchini marmalade in a sweltering kitchen the size of a shoebox (in between finishing next year's projected office budget, attending your child's softball championship game, and packing for a week at the beach).

I *am* suggesting that you might find as much delight as I do in homemade caraway rusks, essence of sun-dried tomatoes, spiced blueberries, fruit-flavored vinegars, and my favorite, fruit honeys, which aren't honeys at all but a beguiling cross between syrups and preserves and are scrumptious over pancakes, desserts, or by the spoonful.

What I am suggesting and what I do is visit farmers' markets and stock up on comestibles that other enterprising women with home-grown businesses have preserved especially for souls such as ours. If you want to go one step further, you can even get pretty, small-patterned fabric already cut out in circles to fit on top of your jams, jellies, and chutney, tying with ribbon, raffia, or twine. Pretty labels are available online. (Check out Etsy and try not to go wild.) I also like to pick up preserves from other parts of the country when we go away on vacation.

Still, perusing *Fancy Pantry* might be enough to convince you to try your hand at your own put-ups. Helen Witty believes that all "souls should have a pantry, however modest," and I heartily agree.

JUNE 20

Secret Passions: Scented Linen Closets

And still she slept an azure-lidded sleep
In blanched linen, smooth, and lavender'd.
—John Keats (1795–1821)
English Romantic poet

If all the world were mine—from the sea to the Rhine—I would happily give my love all—in return for a large, walk-in, fragrant, and expertly organized linen closet.

Close your eyes for a moment and let an azure-lidded fantasy flood your mind. You are led to a door and enter to find a small room filled floor to ceiling with built-in storage. Cupboard doors with glass knobs. Drawers that glide open with a simple touch. Inside are linens of every muted shade your heart desires, and in every fabric—Egyptian cotton, percale, linen, and silk—all triple folded and perfectly arranged by type and color. On the shelves are matching, labeled white baskets with the finest Turkish towels in all shapes and sizes. You touch them reverently and marvel at their impeccably coordinated beauty. Not only are they everything your heart ever wanted, but you can easily find them now, too. The air is perfumed with an intoxicating fragrance of French lavender, Bulgarian rose, and calming Tuscan bergamot. A sigh of exquisite pleasure escapes your lips. This dream can last as long as you desire or as short as you need to regain your balance. You can return to this setting frequently now that you've discovered what "serenity" looks like, a quiet sphere away from the frantic world. It will be yours. It will be…

Well, it might be yours, but after years of conjuring up this feminine reverie, it still isn't mine. Not for the lack of trying, and yet my closet still more resembles a yard sale than this perfection—full of mismatched, well-worn sheets, an odd assortment of towels (one or two may have bleach stains on them), and a handful of old blankets the cats have long since made their own. If this image reminds you of your own closet, perhaps it's time for us to both move on to a more accommodating and achievable fantasy, *ma chérie*.

The delightful writer Mary Cantwell (to whom you've just been introduced) once mused about the elegant lives lived by contemporary domestic gurus, who naturally had scented linen closets. She recalled that once she, too, was tempted to create a proper linen closet for herself, but alas, did not achieve her quest because "I am a lazy woman and bad at tying bows."

While tying silk ribbons on linens to keep things orderly *and* pretty may no longer be the trend *du jour*, the idea of marrying the aesthetically pleasing with the practical will likely never go away. The pull of perfection is and will always be profound. "Ordering my linens into ranks would have been a form of defense in a world I found disorderly," Mary confided wistfully. "There was not, is not, a thing to be done about pestilence, death and the bad dreams that sneak up on us when we're not sleeping. But I would have had that cupboard, that proof positive that I could make tidy my minuscule corner of the universe. Seeing Wamsutta, Martex and Cannon neat and cozy in their ribbons might even have afforded me a Fantin-Latour moment."

Henri Jean Théodore Fantin-Latour was a nineteenth-century French artist famous for his beautiful paintings of flowers, and frequently referenced by domestic goddesses in the past. However, even Fantin-Latour could not render a Fantin-Latour moment out of the closet in my hall. Here, there are no Instagram-worthy angles of my perfectly folded organic bath towels, or my color-coded 1,200-thread-count sheets. No, here on five shelves, crumpled sheets fight for space with washcloths, while cold remedies, toilet paper, tissues, and soap battle it out with lightbulbs and extension cords.

But where there is life, there is hope. And while there is hope, there is life—we just need to know how to begin. In looking back at Mary Cantwell's words, I'm most struck by her use of "minuscule," as in small masterpiece, something attainable. You may not be able to dash to the Container Store and drop hundreds on matching bins and dividers right now, but you can weed through what you currently have, refold it neatly, and arrange by type and color. And if the whole closet feels overwhelming, begin by organizing one drawer or isolated shelf—as my daughter Kate did when she recently tackled her own linen madness. It may have taken her a few weeks to slowly get through it, but she now takes great relief in knowing which sheet set goes to which bed.

It is important to do this, because in my opinion, a linen closet is not a frivolous indulgence. No, no, no. It's an essential. Soul nurturing, sanity preserving, homeopathic medicine for frazzled nerves. We are grown women; we know the difference between a passing whim and a true need. For what is the harried feminine heart seeking in stacks of the scented, orderly, and pristine? A vision that refreshes and restores. A solitary sensory delight of sight, and fragrance that soothes as it energizes.

Think of an aromatic, well-stocked pantry (didn't I just convince you?); a beautiful vanity for our makeup (haven't I made our case?); a cozy book nook (needs no more explanation); and a mudroom, just because there must be somewhere to deal with dogs, mud, and boots, even if it's just a rack at the back door. How differently might we feel to know such balance in our daily round? "Our feelings are our most genuine path to knowledge," the poet Audre Lorde tells us.

Let's introduce such pleasures into our homes, perhaps by starting with the linen closet. When our own small domestic gestures—our everyday epiphanies—act as visual oases throughout our daily round, we are nurturing our dormant selves with love and care.

JUNE 21

Our Secret Gardens

I am sure there is Magic in everything, only we have not sense enough to get hold of it and make it do things for us.
—Frances Hodgson Burnett (1849–1924)
British-born American novelist

When I lived outside of Washington, D.C., during the nineties, I had a secret garden, which I shared with the Episcopal Bishop at the Washington Cathedral. Known as "The Bishop's Garden," it was a walled combination of an herb and rose garden, which you entered by pushing a heavy wooden door through a stone arch. Although it was a "public" garden, I rarely encountered another soul there. Throughout the spring and autumn, I would frequently go there to enjoy a picnic lunch followed by a quiet writing session before the afternoon car pool.

Twenty years later I would live in Newton's Chapel, surrounded by a wall and a gate and a beautiful garden. It's no wonder that the Bishop's Garden, which was such a part of my daily meditation during the long writing of *Simple Abundance,* eventually led to my own secret garden.

I've always found the backstories of writers—especially if their work has met with some success—so fascinating because like them, I, too, live in between the lines.

The backstory of Frances Hodgson Burnett's creation of *The Secret Garden* long after she had to abandon the English sanctuary she'd so loved and rescued at Great Maytham Hall on the Kent seaside is a powerful and poignant personal story for me.

It was 1898, the twilight of the Victorian era. Finally, after years of magazine serial and children's story writing during a difficult decade that included poverty, the death of a child, a nervous breakdown, a long-standing marriage ending in divorce, and a tumultuous second marriage to a scoundrel young enough to be her son, Frances had an unexpected hit on her hands with *Little Lord Fauntleroy* (1886). Suddenly the money started rolling in, and the Little Lord Fauntleroy "brand" became one of the first examples of a successful product extension based on a book. There were toys, games, a clothing line, plays, sequels, and eventually when Hollywood could catch up, movies. Imagine Harry Potter and the celebrity of J. K. Rowling without the internet.

But even back then, with an international best-seller came public fervor, professional demands, lack of privacy, and increased scrutiny. Discouraged and shocked because of the public outcry over her divorce and remarriage to an actor (which she knew was a mistake as soon as she said "I do"), she needed a quiet place to beat a retreat, collect herself, and rebuild her life. She was a bundle of nerves, deeply depressed and unknowingly ill with the early stages of tuberculosis. She had no strength, breathed with difficulty, and struggled with exhaustion, just as her publisher was demanding more of her. Since Frances was the sole support of an entire retinue of people, it seemed she had no choice but to go on. And so she retreated to the mild southern English seaside of Kent.

Although eight miles from the coast, you can practically hear the waves beating against the shore at Great Maytham Hall, a giant wreck of an imposing Georgian house, which was just about caving in on its knees when Frances rented it. There were a series of walled gardens, she was told, but the outdoor space had become so overgrown it resembled Sleeping Beauty's castle during its hundred-year sleep. Frances's future and the world's "Secret Garden" was so covered in thick and thorny vines, it couldn't even be seen.

Have you ever felt really burned out? When just the thought of going downstairs to make yourself a cup of tea requires the effort and strength of a mountain climber? That's how spent Frances was by that time. But every morning outside her bedroom window a robin sang on a branch. Her curiosity was aroused, and then slowly, as her physical energy increased, Frances finally managed to take walks outside. Soon she had the strength to pull back and cut away the dead growth of what had once been a rose garden. Next, she discovered a heavy wooden door and pushed her way through it to what would become her private outdoor sacred sanctuary. Step by step, day by day, she transformed the garden by planting more than three hundred coral pink rose bushes and ramblers.

Here Frances spent contented days, alternating between gardening and writing, shadowed by a large floral Japanese parasol. On chilly days she would wrap herself in a large lap rug and only retreat to the Hall when she was forced to. Over the next nine happy years she would write three more books and a play. But in 1907 her lease at Great Maytham Hall was not renewed and, heartbroken, she returned to America. Immediately she started planning and planting a replica rose garden on Long Island, but more importantly, she began work on what would become her most renowned accomplishment, *The Secret Garden*, published in 1911.

The Secret Garden is the story of the redemption of two lonely children, a sick boy and an orphaned girl, who are encouraged and nurtured by Mother Nature to bring back to life an abandoned overgrown garden hidden behind stone walls. Its miraculous revival becomes an inspiring metaphor for their own rescue and resurrection, as well as for that of the author herself.

Toward the end of her life, Frances recalled how working in the garden at Great Maytham Hall had restored her own will to live and sense of self. The fond memories of "a softly rainy spring in Kent when I spent nearly three weeks kneeling on a small rubber mat on the grass edge of a heavenly old herbaceous border bed" remained vivid in her imagination as well as "the plants which were to bloom in loveliness for me in the summer."

I believe we all have a "Secret Garden" in the depths of our soul and the state of that garden depends upon the health and vitality of our inner life, not our outer one. When, through death, debt, divorce, or illness, we are abruptly pulled away from the life we expected to be living, planned for and dreamed about, and suddenly find ourselves in an alien landscape, it is staggering to all our senses: the five physical senses as well as the two spiritual senses—intuition and wonder. What's so shocking is that this new reality has no timetable. There can be a lengthy state of grief and dismay—even a form of amnesia. Others may think we're back to normal, but in fact we might as well be living in a hologram—suspended in neither the past, nor the present, nor the future.

So how do we move from shadow to sunlight? Through asking for one day's Grace and expressing gratitude. Through choosing one morning not to keep our head turned to the wall but to get out of bed. Step by step, we enter our daily round to find that our faded dreams move from pastel hues to vibrancy, in the same way that an overgrown and abandoned garden returns to life. We cut away one hurtful vine at a time and refuse to replay those miserable memories for one entire day. Then two. Then a week. And one day, you discover that you've been moving forward, which had been impossible a month ago. The seasons change. And you go on.

Today revisit the secret garden in your soul; push open the heavy wooden door. Put on your spiritual gardening gloves and get your sharpest clippers. Each day, clear one vine, cut away one thought of the past that's holding you back. Have you ever had a woman-to-weed wrestling match? That's what it's like, and that's what it takes.

Every day we determine our destiny by what we think about. Nobody knows how inconvenient I find this truth to be. But the only thing you or I can do about it is change our thoughts. Weed out our disappointments, frustrations, diminished ambitions, unfulfilled expectations, sorrow, and frustration about what has gone before or for what has not yet come. Emotional underbrush and weeds only choke our days, and our days become our destiny. Bless your imagination, pray that a new idea will be planted by the Sower of dreams. Then let passion tend the garden with patience and perseverance. For, as Frances Hodgson Burnett discovered, and we can, too, "When you have a Garden, you have a Future and when you have a Future, you are Alive."

JUNE 22

Stilled Life

Art must take reality by surprise.
—Françoise Sagan (1935–2004)
French novelist, playwright, and screenwriter

The painting is small enough to cradle in your hands. Incredibly simple—an isolated white cup, saucer, and silver spoon. But the astonishing power of its quiet restraint never fails to move me. The first time I saw the French painter Henri Fantin-Latour's still life *White Cup and Saucer*, painted in 1864, I turned to a stranger and said, "How dear!" The startled man looked at me, then the painting, smiled, and said, "Yes, you're right. It is quite *dear*. Isn't that a lovely word to describe a painting?"

For whatever reason, *dear* is the word I associate with still-life paintings—groupings of common objects such as fruit, flowers, dishes, and books, which I collect. Perhaps it is because the still-life artist bestows such affection and reverence on the trivial, the ordinary, the everyday. This loving exuberance always leaps off the canvas and grabs hold of my heart. Attention must be paid. Life says, *"Look at me!"* through the artist's brushstrokes. *"Look at me, for the love of all that's holy. Look at me and live in me today."*

One reason I'm magnetically drawn to still-life paintings is that they're an antidote to my usual state of perpetual motion; sitting still is difficult if I'm not writing; standing still is virtually impossible, unless it's in front of a painting. These quiet moments of contemplation are a salve for the soul; when I turn away, not only does my sense of sight seem more acute but my sense of place has returned to its sacred center. I feel balanced once again, by what I love—the ordinary.

Creating your own still-life compositions provides a delightful and calming time out. You may not be a painter, but as an Artist of the Everyday, you still have the artist's tools to help you see the mundane in a new way—color, light, arrangement, and observation. The painter Paul Cézanne loved creating kitchen still-life paintings—a yellow pottery bowl with a few apples, a loaf of bread, a colorful blue napkin. The next time you're feeling frazzled or fragile, take ten minutes and putter.

For the living room, pull down a vase that has been empty for too long and fill it with a budding branch. One of Vincent van Gogh's most beautiful paintings is *Sprig of Flowering Almond in a Glass*. I always associated dark moods with van Gogh, but this small, exquisite rendering of hope is a poignant testimony to isolated moments of serenity— even brief ones.

In your bedroom, why not gather together on the top of a dresser those black satin evening shoes you love (but rarely wear), a perfume bottle, a necklace, and a scarf? Pull a favorite hat out of its box and prop it on the bedpost. (Should someone ask, "Why is that there?" tell them it reminds you of how much you love hats and how rarely you wear them. But that's going to change, isn't it?)

Above all, play with arranging your belongings. Let the juxtaposition of the ordinary objects surrounding you speak a truth about you. Life expresses much in the juxtaposition of a bowl of cherries, a few flower stems, a cup and a saucer. The gift of the everyday *is* very dear.

JUNE 23

Phantoms of Delight

And now I see with eye serene
The very pulse of the machine;
A being breathing thoughtful breath,
A Traveller between life and death.
The reason firm, the temperate will.
Endurance, foresight, strength and skill
A perfect Woman, nobly planned...

—William Wordsworth (1770–1850)
English Romantic poet

You probably looked at your phone before settling down to read this. That's how we react to the possibility of "Breaking News"—and lately, breaking news seems to be a constant all day, every day, gluing us to our phones, blinding us to the beauty that surrounds us in an instant.

I try hard to build antidotes to that impulse into my day, and today I managed to tear myself away from the present to meditate on the English poet William Wordsworth's poem about his wife, Mary Hutchinson, called "A Phantom of Delight." I was struck by the thought that we need to know that we are already "a perfect Woman, nobly planned." We don't know this about ourselves, and we need to nourish ourselves and remind each other of it every day, in every way possible.

Most days are so out of kilter—a profound imbalance between handling whatever today brings and a deep yearning for foresight and strength to see our way out of the world's commotion. This alone is hard enough. Is it impossible to think that we could move beyond that to resurrect our dreams?

We need three ten-minute time-outs daily for body, mind, and soul restoration.

Think of the word *meditation*. Unless you regularly meditate, two clichés come to mind: being uncomfortable and breathing calisthenics. So let's do the reverse today—get comfortable and then start considering breath's true nature—as does the Traveller in Wordsworth's poem, the thoughtful breather hovering between life and death.

"Breath is sensuous, rhythmic, and always with us, as long as we are alive. Also, breath is a gift to us from the larger world...an intimate exchange with the entire cosmos in which we live and move and have our being," Camille Maurine and Lorin Roche remind us in *Meditation Secrets for Women: Discovering Your Passion, Pleasure and Inner Peace*. "Breath is intrinsically full of grace."

So is their wonderful book, which celebrates the truth that what women look for in meditation differs radically from that of men. "For thousands of years monks have been the primary custodians of the knowledge of meditations and the creators of its techniques, so naturally it has been designed to meet their needs. Consequently, most teachings on meditation are still shaped by attitudes that worked in the distant past, in the Far East, for reclusive and celibate males." Camille Maurine points out, "Most teachings just do not comprehend the female body and psyche."

Because I can't really sit in a lotus position, back aching, mind racing, and hyperventilating (my typical reactions to a day of writing), I've always had the problem of answering the question, "Do you meditate?" But I do try to luxuriate in my senses, indulge my yearnings, rejoice in my desires as I work and wait patiently to see them grow in reality. I certainly long for the Divine and pray each day to be delivered to my passion.

"This is meditation—luxuriating in the sensory world, resting in the simplicity of your own being, enjoying yourself shamelessly," Camille Maurine reassures us. Using our senses as a guide to rediscover the joy of breathing is a way to stretch our capacity for pleasure. Now, you may ask, what delights are waiting to be found in something as ordinary as breathing? (This question would never cross your mind or lips if you've just recovered from a nasty bout of bronchitis or any condition of the lung.)

Save a bit of today's portion of endurance, strength, and skill before drifting off to sleep. Use it to listen to some relaxing music, to ease you into riding the gentle wave of inhaling and exhaling until the sound of your breath becomes a sigh of grateful contentment.

And may you awaken to see yourself as Wordsworth did. "A Spirit, yet a Woman too...A perfect Woman, nobly planned."

JUNE 24

The Fragrant Home

I wish that life should not be cheap, but sacred,
I wish the days to be as centuries, loaded, fragrant.
—Ralph Waldo Emerson (1803–1882)
American philosopher and poet

From the moment man, woman, and child first began to follow their noses, scent has been an irresistible magnet drawing the heart and imagination home. "There's no place like home," the nineteenth-century actor and playwright John Howard Payne wrote in 1823, recalling the woodsy fragrance from the cheerful hearth of an old, shingled cottage in East Hampton, Long Island, where he spent his early childhood. Perhaps there's no place like home because no place else on earth smells quite like home. Your home.

As far back as ancient times, people sought to sweeten their surroundings, as often for medicinal purposes as it was for aesthetic ones. Greeks and Romans used fragrant woods, such as cedar, for storage cabinets and chests, scented their clothing and bedding with herbs and flowers, and perfumed the air of homes and temples with aromatic candles. Floors were covered with herbs and grasses as a hallowed greeting; the strewing of palms before Jesus is a source of the observance on Palm Sunday.

Until the turn of the twentieth century people carried pomanders, not the clove-studded orange of today but decorative, pierced cones of metal for men or ceramic posy holders for women that also could be pinned as brooches. Worn close to the neck, with fragrant flowers and herbs replaced every day, they were known as "tussie mussies."

When ladies went out into public, they wore cloth "sweet bags" to ward off germs and shield sensitive nostrils from the stench of the great unwashed neighbors. Even the Bible contains (Exodus 30:23–24) a recipe for "a holy anointing oil" of spices mixed with olive oil—with precise measurements, as dictated by God to Moses, including instructions on how to apply it throughout the house of worship, to purify virtually every surface. "God is in the details," the famous German-American architect Ludwig Mies van der Rohe tells us. And according to precise Biblical reference, it seems so.

Now the next time you return home from a day out, I want you to try a little sensory perception project: Take a deep sniff as you enter your front door. What's your first impression? Furniture polish, ammonia, a flowery carpet cleaner? Your pets? What you cooked last night?

How appetizing does your kitchen smell between meals? How refreshing is your bathroom scent? Your bedroom? Is your laundry room redolent of dirty gym clothes? How many uncoordinated perfumes, candles, and cleansers are masking each other's effects, or producing an unintended sensory fog? Does your home smell like *you*, or is there competition from your neighbor's barbeque or secondhand cigarette smoke?

Many modern products attempt to imitate what our ancestresses used to clean and scent their homes. Our modern lemon disinfectant wipes, pine-scented cleansers, and waxy spray polishes, for example, trace back to past centuries when the *real* substances were put to such uses. Floral carpet powders attempt to replicate but bear little resemblance to the fragrance of a carpet swept with a sprinkling of dried lavender (which still works beautifully today). And let's not even get into the nasty pungency of commercially made insect repellents, especially as compared with age-old and effective rosemary or thyme. Who, exactly, are we trying to get rid of, anyway?

There are so many wonderful ways to release gorgeous scents that are good for you: fresh fruits, living or dried herbs, essential oils, fragrant woods, ground spices. A few drops of essential oils can be simmered in water, carefully warmed over a burner or in a diffuser made especially for aromatherapy oils. But reed stick diffusers, with liquid or without, are marvelous, too, and as easy as opening a box.

However, when you have a free fifteen minutes at home, treat yourself to this well-spent recipe for a beautifully scented kitchen counter: Place the peel of citrus fruit (mix, if you can, orange, lemon, and lime) in a large salad bowl; finely chop stalks of your favorite fresh herbs (fresh or dry), add some dried potpourri (even a stale one you were going to throw out) and a few drops of essential oil in your favorite scents (rose is my basic). Tossing the ingredients together as if it were a salad is all it takes to release a welcoming fragrance.

"You'd be so nice to come home to," Cole Porter wrote in a song he penned for the 1943 film *Something to Shout About*. With a little self-care, you'll be able to hum that tune when you turn the key.

JUNE 25

Choosing to Blossom

And the day came when the risk [it took] to remain tight in the bud was more painful than the risk it took to blossom.
—Anaïs Nin (1903–1977)
French-American novelist, poet, and diarist

How much time, passion, energy, and emotion do we expend resisting change because we assume growth must always be painful? Much personal growth is uncomfortable, especially learning to set boundaries in relationships. When we commit to nurturing our Authentic Selves, people close to us are going to start noticing that changes are taking place. This is the season when growth in the garden, which had been gradual, now accelerates. It's that season for us as well, now that we're six months into the journey toward Wholeness.

It can be difficult to express your authentic needs by saying "Sorry, I can't" when everybody else assumes you can because you always have. But it's worse to thwart the ascent of your authenticity. The day comes—maybe it's today—when "remaining tight in the bud" is more painful than blossoming. "Garden-making is creative work, just as much as painting or writing a poem," the Victorian writer Hanna Rion tells us. "It is a personal expression of self, an individual conception of beauty." Gardening is also a wonderful way to gently explore some of the personal growth issues raised by authenticity. Mother Nature is a patient mentor.

Can you find one perfect rosebud, either in your garden or at a flower shop? Place it on your desk or night table. The Talmud tells us that "Each blade of grass has its Angel that bends over it and whispers, 'Grow, grow.'"

So do we.

JUNE 26

Onward and Upward in the Garden

Gardening is an instrument of grace.
—May Sarton (1912–1995)
American poet, novelist, and memoirist

Gardening was one of the first gifts *Simple Abundance* bestowed on me after I embarked on the authentic journey. I had never really gardened before because it seemed like too much mind-numbing, back-breaking work. (Notice that no one ever says *playing* in the garden. It's always *working* in the garden.) I was already working too hard in the house and at my writing to work in a garden as well.

However, when I moved to the rural English countryside, authentic longings began surging to the surface, for the English are passionate gardeners. From postage stamp plots to large country houses, all of England is blooming. And I was seized with the determination not to greet another spring without snowdrops, crocuses, primroses, bluebells, daffodils, and tulips in my yard. There was already a lovely lilac tree in the front of the cottage. Since I knew absolutely nothing about gardening, I sought the advice of famous women gardeners: Gertrude Jekyll, Vita Sackville-West, Celia Thaxter, and Katharine S. White.

Katharine White was an editor at *The New Yorker* from its early days, in 1925, until her retirement in 1958. She was also an avid gardener. Her husband, the writer E. B. White, recalls in the introduction to his wife's book *Onward and Upward in the Garden*, "She simply accepted the act of gardening as the natural thing to be occupied with in one's spare time, no matter where one was or how deeply involved in other affairs."

Katharine White also adored shopping in mail-order catalogs. "Hour after hour, she studied, sifted, pondered, rejected, sorted in the delirium of future blooming and fruiting," writes E. B. White. This insatiable passion for gardening catalogs prompted her to take up writing after decades of editing. Her first feature was a critical review of seed catalogs and nurserymen that launched her famous garden writing series "Onward and Upward."

To my mind, there are two types of gardeners. There are those extraordinary women who not only know every flower but know each one by its Latin name. They keep meticulous gardening journals, plot plant placements on graph paper, and never break into a sweat when wielding a trowel and a spade. Katharine White belonged to this gardening genus.

"Grunge" accurately describes the other group. We are always hot, smelly, and sweaty in the garden, boasting not so much a green thumb as dirty fingernails because we forgot where we put our gardening gloves. We speak of "that little yellow flower" and point. We also tend to be manic about gardening, seized not only by visions of earthly Paradise but also our vivid imaginations.

How else to explain why it never occurred to me when I ordered fourteen rosebushes in February that they would all arrive on the same May morning, necessitating two days of frenzied labor? Unfortunately, no gardener accompanied them. Before rosebushes can be planted, very deep holes must be dug. Still, into the ground they all went. They became the love children of my middle age, conceived during passionate afternoon perusals of glossy gardening catalogs in winter's inclement weather.

Gardening came easily to Katharine White, but writing was "slow and tortuous going," her husband noted. Creating phrases is far easier for me than double-ditching a flower bed. Still, I think of my adventures in the garden as a trajectory of forward motion, an evolution of soul.

Gardening has become an unexpected instrument of Grace, for I've discovered hours of inner peace on my knees, digging in the dirt. Here is the one place I don't think about work or worry about whatever it is that I can't control. The complete absorption, the sacrament of the present moment I experience when planting or weeding, brings exquisite contentment. My mind is stilled, and my heart expands. Now I know why the Great Creator intended for woman to flourish in a garden. So much for second-guessing the wisdom of Spirit.

A beautiful dusty rose named "Pleasure" beckons me. Onward and upward. It's time to play.

Late Bloomers

Bloom where you're planted.

—Mary Engelbreit
American artist and designer

I was considered a late bloomer for my generation. I married at thirty-two, became a mother at thirty-five, published my first book at forty-three, and planted my first real garden when I was forty-five. I feel shy about admitting all this, as if it's a cosmic flaw, but May Sarton, who wrote, gardened, and lived each day with an enviable passion, reassures me that "Gardening is one of the rewards of middle age, when one is ready for an impersonal passion, a passion that demands patience, acute awareness of a world outside oneself, and the power to keep on growing through all the times of drought, through the cold snows, towards those moments of pure joy when all failures are forgotten and the plum tree flowers."

The plum tree isn't blooming today, but there is much to recommend late blooming. Especially if we're all doing it with every breath we take, in our own authentic style.

But sometimes we're afraid or think we're just not ready. So here's something to contemplate as you consider the blooming process. Are you ready to stop pursuing other people's dreams? Can you identify whatever's been holding you back—particularly if you're the one doing the holding? Living is not a passive spectator sport. Are you ready to enter that new, colorful territory ahead?

Shortly after I began exploring and experimenting with the Graces of *Simple Abundance* as a creative conduit for contentment, I had a wonderful dream.

I was led to an old walled garden and shown a golden key that was lying on the path. As I turned the key, a heavy wooden door easily swung open to reveal a dark, dismal wasteland of dead and overgrown plants. Everything was dark. But once inside, I could see an archway leading to the most beautiful garden I had ever seen, bathed in warm sunlight.

Still, I was unwilling to leave the desolate garden behind to step into Paradise. Something invisible held me back, tangled in the underbrush. Finally, I struggled through the archway. When I did, the wasteland disappeared. I was surrounded only by beauty and abundance and experienced great joy and serenity.

When I awoke, I knew exactly what the dream meant. The lush garden was the awareness of abundance in my life, and the wasteland was the manifestation of my thoughts of lack.

Both abundance and lack exist simultaneously in our lives, as parallel realities. It is always our conscious choice which secret garden we shall tend. The invisible underbrush holding us back is our own thoughts. When we choose not to focus on what is missing from our lives but on the abundance that's present—love, health, family, friends, work, and personal pursuits that bring us pleasure—the wasteland falls away and we experience joy in the real lives we live each day.

So first let's try to outfit an outdoor sanctuary for you. If you have a backyard, could you place a comfortable chair and a small table in a shady nook? Hang a hammock? Arrange some furniture at the end of the front porch or on a patio where you might beat a retreat when you need a respite?

And while you're at it, don't forget to tend your interior secret garden, because the seeds that will blossom in outward expression are always first scattered within. Weed out disappointments, frustrations, diminished ambitions, unfulfilled expectations, and anger about what has gone before or what has not yet come. These emotional weeds only choke your creativity. Let an unfettered imagination sow the seeds of possibility in the rich soil of your soul. Then let passion tend the garden with patience and perseverance. Or as Jane Fonda (gorgeous in her eighties) advises, "It's okay to be a late bloomer, as long as you don't miss the flower show."

JUNE 28

Repotting: Giving Roots and Yourself Room to Grow

Repotting means accepting that the way is forward, not back. It means realizing that we won't again fit into our old shells. But that's not failure. That's living.
—Heather Cochran
American novelist and television producer

Uh-oh. Dropping leaves. Whatever can be the matter? The plant has been watered; it basks in the light; it's neither too hot nor too cold. I pick up the pot and look at the small drainage hole in its underbelly. Tiny white roots are frantically pushing through in a futile attempt to escape confinement or at least find a little more breathing space.

Pot-bound. Did you know that plants need to be repotted at least every two years? This has not been a problem for me in the past, since plants rarely made it that long around here. But as I become a better caretaker of myself, I care better for everything. However, even if the roots don't need more room to grow, the old soil should be replaced because all the nutrients have been consumed. The interior of the pot is a wasteland.

"I don't know when I myself am too pot-bound," Gunilla Norris confesses in her numinous devotional, *Being Home*, "lacking courage to be replanted, to take the shock of the new soil, to feel into the unknown and take root in it."

We, too, need to consider repotting for growth. But when? When we wilt even before the day begins. When we can't seem to visualize or dream. When we can't remember the last time we laughed. When we have absolutely nothing in the next twenty-four hours to look forward to. When this happens, week in, week out, we need to realize that we're pot-bound. We need to gently loosen the soil around our souls, find something that sparks our imagination, quickens our pulse, brings a smile or a giddy lilt to our conversations.

Repotting doesn't mean we have to leave the marriage or quit the job. It just means we need something *new*. Why is it too late to go back to college if you do it one course at a time online? Maybe this is the summer to learn to speak French or to start your own gift basket business? Perhaps you can get the sewing machine fixed, try making blackberry cordial, or take up fencing, which is a thrilling sport and always looking for new enthusiasts. What's stopping you from applying for that grant or fellowship, pulling together that one-woman show, attending that lecture series, publishing your own newsletter, or just sending for that intriguing mail-order catalog? What about that novel idea? Page one will stay blank until you put something on it.

As I work with my plants, I see that the roots are just stunted. Gently, with my fingers, I untangle them.

Leaf. Stem. Root.

Mind. Body. Soul.

Three in one. Spirit's seamless thread of mystery. I have often thought that if I could just discover where one strand left off and another began, I could understand it all. As it is, I understand little, yet somehow, I know.

I set the plant into a slightly larger pot. Not too large; we must not overwhelm but encourage. So, too, I must not take on the world but simply each task before me. Now I add rich potting soil. Water. Slowly I take the plant to a shady spot for a day so that it can adjust to its new environment. But even at this moment, the stem seems straighter, the leaves uplifted.

Root and bud bear silent witness to the restoration.

Real Life Has a Steep Learning Curve

I would like to learn, or remember, how to live.
—Annie Dillard
American Pulitzer Prize–winning author

Now the revelations come very quickly and from all quarters because you're ready to start making connections. In the Old Testament, God uses donkeys, rocks, and burning bushes to deliver Divine messages, so don't question the validity of what you hear or how you hear it *if the truth resonates within.* You might be reading a story, watching a movie, or chatting casually with a friendly grocery store clerk. Don't cut yourself off from sources of inspiration.

One of the quantum leaps that comes about on the *Simple Abundance* path is the sudden awareness that you've spent your entire life going backward instead of forward. You may have believed that seeking a spiritual path was all about submission, sacrifice, and suffering and that only the worldly path could provide freedom, fulfillment, and good fortune. Then, one morning—maybe even this morning—you make a connection. And when you do, you realize that you have to unlearn practically everything you've taken for granted: chapter and verse.

Don't panic. This really isn't as hard as it sounds. Has the other path worked? Have any of the world's gifts blessed you with authentic happiness? Has the perfect job, relationship, house, money, or anything else you thought would do it for you fulfilled you for longer than a week? So trust your experiences and impulses; you've had them for a reason. Real life has a steep learning curve, but once you respond from personal knowledge instead of by rote, it's easier than you might have thought. What's more, real life actually becomes fun.

Here's what I think happens. Just before we come to earth to begin this life, we are given a photograph of our futures—the Cosmic Plan—to get us excited about the great adventure ahead. As the photo pops out of the celestial camera, we're in such a hurry to get on with it, we grab the negative instead of the photograph. Now we've got the pattern of a fabulous life, but the perspective is reversed. What's white looks black. What's black appears white. We've got the big picture, but it's backward. So we cry when we should be laughing, are envious when we should feel inspired, experience deprivation instead of abundance, do it the hard way instead of the easy way, pull back instead of reaching out. And worst of all, we close our hearts, so we won't get hurt, when opening them is the only way we'll ever know joy.

How many times have we waited for Spirit to move for us, when in fact, Spirit is waiting to work *with* us? Today, take the negative of your Cosmic Plan and let Love develop it so that you can begin living the life for which you were created.

It's time to move forward.

JUNE 30

Do Try This at Home: Keep Calm and Carry On

She reached her doorstep. The key turned sweetly in the lock. That was the kind of thing one remembered about a house: not the size of the rooms or the color of the walls, but the feel of the door-handles and light-switches, the shape and texture of the banister-rail under one's palm; minute tactual intimacies, whose resumption was the essence of coming home.

—Jan Struther, *Mrs. Miniver*

One of the reasons I admire Mrs. Miniver is that she moves so deftly through her ordinary tasks while facing the jobs of extreme days, such as fitting the family for gas masks, with such repose of the soul. Great Britain had declared war on Germany on September 3, 1939, and the first bombs were dropped on London September seventh. By the end of that month all British residents had been supplied with personal gas masks to be carried in a paper box with a shoulder strap. There were tiny helmets for babies. And it was a penalty offense for anyone outdoors not to be in possession of a gas mask.

In her essay simply titled "Gas Masks," Mrs. Miniver quietly confides, "but bearing no signs of apprehension... 'If the worst came to the worst' (it was funny how one still shied away from saying, 'If there's a war,' and fell back on euphemism)—if the worst came to the worst, these children would at least know that we were fighting against an idea, and not against a nation... It was for this, thought Mrs. Miniver as they walked towards the car, that one had boiled the milk for their bottles, and washed their hands before lunch, and not let them eat with a spoon which had been dropped on the floor."

Gratefully, the gas masks were not needed. But, until America entered the war two harrowing years later, when the English government feared a massive Nazi invasion, the Ministry of Information commissioned a series of simple but striking red posters to reassure and rally the British people, like this one:

YOUR COURAGE, YOUR CHEERFULNESS,
YOUR RESOLUTION WILL BRING US VICTORY.

Another poster read FREEDOM IS IN PERIL. These posters appeared all over the country on billboards and at train stations. Another poster was prepared, and more than two million copies were printed, but these were to be distributed only should the *worst* happen. It read simply:

KEEP CALM

AND

CARRY ON

Despite living through air raids, the bombing of Britain, the evacuation of 1.5 million children and pregnant women from London to rural towns to escape the Blitz (which was ten months of nightly bombing raids), the evacuation miracle of Dunkirk, the drastic rationing of food and other essentials from eggs to thread to stockings—the worst actually *never* happened. The poster was destroyed.

Then a decade ago, an English bookseller found one of these posters in the bottom of a box of old books he'd bought at auction. He framed it and put it beside his cash register. There were so many requests to buy the poster that he had it reproduced. Now, eighty years after the invasion never happened, the slogan has taken on cult status. The reassuring message speaks volumes to all of us, about any situation.

Keep Calm and Carry On.

I have this profound personal prompt framed in my kitchen and printed on couch pillows. Its quiet confidence never fails to bolster my spirit. No matter what may happen in the course of today, if you keep calm and carry on, then give thanks that you made it through the day, and know there is nothing you and Spirit can't handle together after asking for grace.

So far our Caution Closet has taken care of important documents, first aid, water, and a change of clothes.

Now we're going to start to focus on food for you and whoever lives with you, and for pets. The goal is to get you out of the door as fast as possible with the necessities, so we'll carry our emergency sustenance planning into July as we explore the world of victory gardens and cooking.

Food preparation really depends upon the old journalism formula of the five Ws: who, what, where, when, and why.

Who do you live with, and do they include children and pets? Start with assembling in bulk different flavored protein bars and shakes—three bars a day per person, three powdered or long-life packaged protein shakes a day (which don't need refrigeration), and boxes of cereal, again in different flavors. For beverages, freeze-dried instant coffee and tea bags. If you use milk, or there are children in the family, there is powdered and instant milk, as well as boxed long-life milk, which tastes best but is heavier to carry.

For your pets, fresh, unopened bags of their favorite food. Collapsible pet bowls are available for both water and dry food.

Finally, be sure to check the expiration date on the protein bars and shakes, milk, and pet food. Again, you're going to store everything in a large, clear plastic storage container, light enough for you to lift on your own when filled. This is very important. When I was first arranging my own Caution Closet, I had everything I needed but I couldn't even lift the backpack. If that's the case, then a large duffel bag with wheels would be preferable.

After finishing this month's preparation, aren't you amazed at how serene you feel? You've done something amazing and practical. You're taking care of yourself and those you love by systematically preparing for the unknown and life's uncertainties.

Now, if you haven't started, or started and stopped, please know, so did I. Start, stop. Start, stop. For all kinds of reasons or daily life. But the last thing in the world that I want is for you to feel pressure from this activity. All you need to know is how much I care about you—and when you feel like doing this, I've listed the order that worked for me and it might for you, too. You can even think of my "old-fashioned" advice, as a poster found in the bottom of a box of old books—which made sense and cheered you up.

Joyful Simplicities for June

I believe the nicest and sweetest days are not those on which anything very splendid or wonderful or exciting happens, but just those that bring simple little pleasures, following one another softly, like pearls slipping off a string," the Canadian writer Lucy Maud Montgomery reveals through her heroine, Anne Shirley, in the Anne of Green Gables series:

When Midsummer arrives, it's a time to look ahead and dream. Perhaps, if one is lucky, the days ahead will unfold as a "never-to-be-forgotten summer—one of those summers which come seldom into any life, but leave a rich heritage of beautiful memories in their going—one of those summers which, in a fortunate combination of delightful weather, delightful friends, and delightful doings, come as near to perfection as anything can come in the world."

When was the last time you tasted something so delicious it made you giddy with pleasure? How about a few new summer taste sensations?

- Enjoy a frosty pitcher of lemonade and conversation when you come home from work. While the premade generic brand is fine for most days, why not treat yourself to an old-fashioned nectar made from fresh lemons and simple sugar syrup? Here's how: Boil two cups of granulated sugar and one cup of water with the rinds of three lemons cut into thin strips for five minutes. Let the syrup cool and add the juice of eight lemons. Strain and store in a covered container in the refrigerator. Use two tablespoons of the syrup for every glass of ice or carbonated water to make a fizzy lemonade.
- Remember that ice cream is good for the soul. Go to the market and bring home a new and different assortment. Freeze a home-made batch, treat yourself to a cone for lunch, visit your local specialty store.
- One June weekend buy a whole watermelon and keep it in the refrigerator for at least a day so it gets ice-cold. Cut it in large pieces and sit on the porch, back deck, or front stoop eating watermelon with family or friends, spitting out the seeds. Have a contest to see who can shoot the farthest. But don't hit any passersby!
- If you have two trees, hang a hammock. Or if you're lucky enough to have a hammock with a stand, get it out of the garage and set it up. Now lie in it, with a pillow, soft throw, and anything else you fancy.
- Take a trip down memory lane by catching lightning bugs or fireflies on the lawn at twilight. Prepare an old-fashioned hotel for them in a clean mayonnaise jar with holes punched in the lid and layered with grass (remember?). Be sure to let them fly away home after a brief visit!
- Celebrate the summer solstice on June 21 by camping out in the backyard. Pitch a tent, bring out the sleeping bags, build a campfire in the grill. Serve hot dogs and the original s'mores for dessert. To make s'mores (in case you don't know how), take two graham crackers and sandwich a thin chocolate bar with a toasted marshmallow. Eat one. Eat some more! Tell ghost stories, then sleep in the moonlight.
- Create a cocktail garden by growing herbs specifically for creating fresh, artisanal cocktails in your home. Put freshly harvested mint in your mojito or use thyme in a tequila fizz. The cocktail garden brings renewed and complex flavors to your drinks.
- Treat your Authentic Self to the most stylish straw hat you can find.

꙳ Paint your toenails red.

꙳ You might not be able to create a real secret garden, but a secret spot in which to sit can be yours by creating a living tepee in the backyard with a wooden stake and string, then planting scarlet runner beans, morning glories, or sweet peas. When the vines appear, guide them up the strings. Retreat to your tepee frequently to contemplate the meaning of life. If there are "littles" in your life, they will be overjoyed with this summer project. So will you, because it really doesn't take much to make us happy and grateful.

꙳ Even if you're convinced that you don't have the space for a garden, container gardens will inspire you to get in there with a spade and a pot. There are so many different types, beginning with window boxes. And now container gardens are blooming vertically for the apartment dweller. There are plenty of books on container gardens in bookstores and on Amazon. They contain fabulous suggestions and instructions for planting window boxes, barrels, tubs, urns, baskets, adorning garden walls, and much more.

꙳ If gardening really isn't your thing (there are many of us who struggle to keep plants alive) but you still want to surround yourself with plants, don't despair! Succulents like jade, aloe, and snake plants are low maintenance, modern looking, and will brighten any space.

JULY

Lovely July...with the evocative murmur of honey bees on the wing and the smell of sun tan cream.

—Cynthia Wickham
Gardening author

Sultry, steaming, sweltering. July. Slow down. Or stop. It's time to shed ambition and expectation, along with commutes, clothing, cell phones, and calendars. Now our wants seem to diminish. Is it because our needs are met? A shady nook, a cold drink, a cool breeze—whether indoors or out. A respite from the rigors of the day. Time off for good behavior. Summer is not so much a season as a melody, that tune of contentment we hum as the days begin to beautifully blur. The pursuit of happiness becomes our personal priority this month, as the sweet strains of the fourth *Simple Abundance* principle—Harmony—start to be heard in our hearts.

JULY 1

Constant Craving

I have learned, in whatsoever state I am, therewith to be content.
—St. Paul (Philippians 4:11–13)
New Testament

In my twenties, I thought fame would do it. In my thirties, I became convinced that a comma in my checking account balance was the answer. In my forties, I finally figured out that all my seeking can be summed up in one word: contentment.

I was grateful to realize that fame comes at too high a price. Being considered an "accomplished" woman who shepherds successful creative projects from conception to completion is much more appealing than being famous. And in the deepest recesses of my soul, I know that money cannot guarantee happiness. I realized this with certitude the summer morning I read that a famous and wealthy author, whose books hover on the best-seller lists for months, had lost a beloved child to a freak accident. While washing the breakfast dishes, I glanced out the kitchen window to see Katie bouncing a tennis ball against the back of the house—happy, safe, alive. I knew that famous author would trade all her worldly success in a heartbeat to know again the blessing bestowed on me that morning. After I prayed for her, I prayed for myself. Please let me never forget how rich my wonderful life is right at this moment. Please let me never forget that all I have is all I need. Please let me never forget to give thanks.

But I know that I am a much happier woman when I can pay my bills with ease, take care of all my needs, indulge a few of my wants, and have a comfortable cushion of savings in my Margin of Happiness account.

Still, these days contentment is my constant craving. So much so that I have begun asking each twenty-four golden hours stretching before me, luminous in their potential for pleasure, what might be mine for the taking. Sometimes it's as simple as making a delicious tuna fish sandwich with celery and tarragon mayonnaise on buttermilk honey bread for lunch—the way I do for guests and for my family but rarely take time to do for myself. Or as easy as sitting on the beach, not with work in my lap but a great book.

Just as negative addictions sneak up on us a day at a time, so do positive cravings. Meditation, creative movement, moments of self-nurturance that bring contentment—all can become positive habits of well-being. I find that when I take twenty minutes to get quiet and go within, work with the visual images in my *Illustrated Discovery*

Journal, take a walk, or ask how can I make the next task more pleasurable, my wants diminish.

Today, consider the desires that really count—what you really need to be content. Then make sure there's at least three moments today that fulfill mind, spirit, and body with what you alone must have.

JULY 2

The Simplest of Pleasures: One Good Thing That Is

Each moment in time we have it all, even when we think we don't.
—Melodie Beattie
American author

Some days are shaped by simple pleasures, others are redeemed by them. Today—a beautiful summer's day at the beach—was shaped by joyful simplicities. Idylls on a screened porch, roaming in interesting shops, an afternoon on the shore with family and friends, irresistible reading, confidences exchanged while the waves lap at ankles, an ice-cream cone for lunch, strolling the boardwalk, playing amusement park games, winning a prize. Then back to the house, a refreshing outdoor shower, cocktails and conversation, the conviviality of cooking dinner with a dear friend, an abundance of delicious food, delightful wine, laughter, and good cheer—and so to bed, happily.

An Irish proverb tells us, "Better one good thing that is, rather than two good things that were, or three good things that might never come to pass." Today there was no need to glance wistfully at the past or project anxiously into the future because the present was fully lived and simply abundant. Today was rich with one good thing after another until it literally overflowed with pleasure.

But not all my days are beach sojourns. Not too long ago, an eight a.m. phone call announcing a major change in plans sent my day careening out of control. I hung up the telephone, my heartbeat accelerating. In one stroke, my carefully arranged coping strategy was out the window and my host of commitments had been made almost impossible to meet. This was too much, I thought, as I paced back and forth, muttering and moaning under my breath. I had three choices before me, but only one real-life solution: scream with rage at the top of my lungs, put my head in the toilet, or take a deep breath and redeem the day with Plan B.

Since I have an understanding in my home not to do anything that might alarm children or animals, screaming was out. The toilet bowl was out as well. If you're really going to drown yourself, you can't do it in a bucket of water. So I poured myself a cup of tea and recalled the Hasidic prayer, "I know the Lord will help—but help me, Lord, until You help."

The reality was that the day would be as hard as I made it. Or as pleasant. There was nothing I could do about my circumstances but accept them. "It's always my choice," I reminded myself. Not necessarily *to like* whatever life throws at me, but to try to catch the ball. After all, success in life is not how well we execute Plan A; it's how smoothly we cope with Plan B and did I mention Plan C? For most of us, that's 99 percent of the time.

I considered Plan B: redeem the day with simple pleasures, some good things to look forward to. At first, learning to mentally shift gears down to Plan B takes some attitude adjustment, but, like driving a sports car with a stick shift, it becomes an automatic reflex with practice.

First, I took my tea out into the garden to calm down. I pulled a few weeds, picked some flowers. After arranging them, I looked at cookbooks. Should I prepare something new for dinner tonight or a comforting favorite? The peaches on my table at home were perfectly ripe, so I could make dumplings for dessert. Why not stream a period film on my watch list as a treat after supper? In the meantime, I decided to make the most of an hour of uninterrupted work before I had to leave the house. Better a golden hour that is rather than two that never were or three that obviously will not come to pass today.

The day stretched before me—not as I had hoped. But not, thank heaven, beyond redemption.

JULY 3

The Hungry Soul

I cannot count the good people I know who to my mind would be even better if they bent their spirits to the study of their own hungers.

—M. F. K. Fisher (1908–1992)
Preeminent American food writer

"When Eve bit into the apple, she gave us the world as we know the world—beautiful, flawed, dangerous, full of being. She gave us smallpox and Somalia, polio vaccine and wheat and Windsor roses," Barbara Grizzuti Harrison tells us in the illuminating and provocative collection of essays *Out of the Garden: Women Writers on the Bible*. "Eve's act of radical curiosity" also gave us desire, appetite, and hunger.

Without Eve, I wouldn't be wondering what to cook for dinner tonight. Nor would you. Without Eve, I wouldn't be cooking up creative projects that often seem simple but are complicated in reality, rather like preparing a new dish for a dinner party without completely reading the recipe beforehand. I also wouldn't know the earthly pleasures that I love, as well as the intense desire for mystical morsels that only Spirit can provide: inner peace, joy, harmony.

Most of us eat three times a day (at least), but how often is our hunger really satisfied?

Many of us constantly hold ourselves in check—about food, relationships, careers—stuffing our desires down deep into the self, as if sheer determination can keep the lid on longing. But I am gradually coming to an awareness that hunger is holy. We're meant to be hungry every day and to satisfy that hunger every day. Why else would the first petition in the Lord's Prayer be for daily bread, even before Divine assistance?

Our souls know many different kinds of hunger: physical, psychic, professional, emotional, creative, and spiritual. But the Great Creator gave us the gifts of reason, imagination, curiosity, discernment; we possess the ability to distinguish between our hungers. Are you really hungry this morning for a breakfast biscuit or a break? Is it passionate kisses you desire or pasta? Or a good night's sleep? Then don't sit up watching reruns with that third glass of wine. Turn the television off and tuck yourself in, and if you're not alone, invite someone to join you.

"When I write of hunger, I am really writing about love and the hunger for it, and the warmth and the love of it," the great gastronome and poetic food writer M. F. K. Fisher confessed in 1943. "And then the warmth and richness and fine reality of hunger satisfied...and it is all one."

Don't despise desire, daughter of Eve. Within your desire is the spark of the Divine. Spirit desired to be loved. A woman with a lusty appetite was created to satisfy that longing.

Love. Hunger. Appetite. Desire. Holiness. Wholeness.

It is all One.

JULY 4

Getting Real and Personal in the Pursuit of Happiness

> Expect nothing; live frugally on surprise.
> —Alice Walker
> American Pulitzer Prize–winning novelist
> and poet

We had just come back from watching a wonderful, old-fashioned parade. There's been an Independence Day parade in Takoma Park for one hundred and thirty years; it's the oldest continuous parade on the East Coast, and they take the pursuit of happiness very seriously. This year, I hope you do, too.

In 1890, philosopher, psychologist, and spiritual pioneer William James, the brother of the famous American novelist Henry James, set off his own fireworks with the publication of a landmark exploration on human happiness, *The Principles of Psychology*. Twelve years in the writing, two volumes and fourteen hundred pages long, it boldly went where no book had ever gone before, investigating the mind-body connection, the impact of our emotions on behavior, and the importance of nurturing an inner life instead of concentrating on the outer trappings to achieve personal harmony. With this book, Dr. James became the father of the American self-help movement.

William James was also an eloquent and persuasive champion of a philosophical school of thought known as pragmatism. He argued that the world already exists when we are born, and we must accept it as it is. But our ability to create our own inner reality can determine if we view the Universe as friendly or hostile. "Be willing to have it so," he urged, because "...Acceptance of what has happened is the first step in overcoming the consequences of any misfortune."

Being a pragmatist, Dr. James believed that personal happiness hinges on a practicality: If your reality lives up to your expectations, you're happy. If it doesn't, you're depressed. This is as real, personal, and simple as philosophy and psychology get, and it makes perfect sense. Of course, this means we have a creative choice to make if we want to be happy. Do we consciously and continually strive for more accomplishments and accumulations? Or do we lower our expectations, live with what we have, and learn to be content?

Many of us mistakenly think that lowering our expectations means we must surrender our dreams. As one friend put it, "Sorry, Sarah, but this sounds like giving up to me."

Absolutely not.

Dreams and expectations are two very different things. Dreams call for a leap of faith, trusting that Spirit is holding the net, so that you can continue in the re-creation of the world with your energy, soul gifts, and vision.

Expectations are the emotional investment the ego makes in a *particular outcome:* what needs to happen to make that dream come true. The ego's expectations are never vague: Oscars, magazine covers, the *New York Times* best-seller list. Your dreams must manifest *exactly* as the ego imagines or someone isn't going to be very happy. And guess who that is? The ego! Since none of us can always predict either the future or the best outcome for our authentic path, this kind of thinking is self-destructive. Because if we don't live up to the ego's expectations, we've failed again. And at some point, we really *do* give up.

The passionate pursuit of dreams sets your soul soaring; expectations that measure the dream's success tie stones around your soul. I don't think we should just lower our expectations; I believe if we truly want to live a joyous and adventurous life, we should relinquish them.

Living your life as a dreamer and not as an "expecter" is a personal declaration of independence. You're able to pursue happiness more directly when you don't get caught up in the delivery details. Dreaming, not expecting, allows Spirit to step in and surprise you with connection, completion, consummation, celebration. You dream. Show up for work. Then let Spirit deliver your dream to the world.

After a lifetime of setting myself up for heartache, the way I now try to approach the delicate balance of dreams versus expectations is to dream, do, and detach. "When once a decision is reached and execution is the order of the day, dismiss absolutely all responsibility and care about the outcome," Dr. James tells me. I approach my work with a passionate intensity, acting as if its success depends entirely on me. But once I've done my best, I try to let go as much as possible and have no expectations about how my work will be received by the world. I have consciously chosen to be surprised by joy. It's a choice you can make as well.

Today, try to get real and personal about the pursuit of happiness. Oprah Winfrey once said that God's dreams for her were much more than she could ever have dreamed for herself. I don't think any of our dreams begin to come close to the dreams Spirit has waiting with our names on them. I also believe we'll only find out once we start investing our emotions in authentic expression, and not in specific outcomes.

JULY 5

Cooking Companions

Yes, there was a trick to it. You inherited your life, or you invented
it. You figured out what you wanted life to be and then somehow or
other you made it that way. Then, miracle of miracles, you liked it.
— Laurie Colwin (1944–1992)
American writer and food essayist

In the 1980s, I became best friends—again through the printed word—
with Laurie Colwin, who captured the ups and downs of domestic bliss
with a pen and a fork. I introduced you to Laurie last month. Laurie
taught me that gingerbread triggers rapture (when following her recipe),
and when your heart is breaking, put on an apron and rustle up something delicious.

Laurie wrote five novels, three collections of short stories, and two
books of kitchen tales that are compilations of her food essays and recipes. She also seems to have loved striped Picasso-esque French T-shirts
because in nearly every picture of her, she's wearing one, grinning.

I longed to write as beautifully about food as Laurie did, but it wasn't
my métier. Still, we became close even though we'd never met, through
that intimate, mystical bond that grows stronger over the years between
writer and reader. This occurs when the reader's grateful heart realizes
to her astonishment that the writer knows her in a way that even her
family and close friends do not.

And while I loved Laurie's novels and short stories, I adored her
cooking essays. (Now they are gathered in two delectable collections,
Home Cooking: A Writer in the Kitchen and *More Home Cooking:
A Writer Returns to the Kitchen*.) The day was always richer when I
had Laurie to read and a new recipe to try. It was as if a close pal had
dropped in for a cup of coffee, a chat, and, of course, a big piece of cake.

Another thing Laurie and I shared was an infatuation with cookbooks. Regular cookbook adventures are a perennial pleasure, and I
can't recommend them enough. I read cookbooks the way many women
read fiction—in bed at night or while watching the potatoes boil. This
probably explains why my favorite fiction is always stronger on domestic details than sex. I can imagine how two people make love, but I want
to *know* what they ate before and afterward!

Of course, I haven't cooked much of anything from all my cookbooks. Yet. I simply love to flip through them and stick little yellow
Post-it notes scribbled with "sounds good" on their pages for "tomorrow." Cookbooks aren't so much about what's for dinner as they are
about a world of abundant and creative choices. With cookbooks our

options are always open; we may not be able to fly to Paris this afternoon, but we can open a book and rustle up a gratin de poulet au fromage if we're so inclined.

One terrible October morning in 1992, I came downstairs to make breakfast and get Katie off to school. In between packing lunch and urging her to get a move on, I glanced at the newspaper and was stunned to learn that Laurie had died in her slumber of a heart attack at just forty-eight. How could the buddy who urged me to make the most of each meal and every day be gone? I didn't start crying until everyone left and have never really stopped. I spent that morning making—and eating—an entire pan of gingerbread, in between blowing my nose, rereading her reminiscences, praying, and mourning the loss of an extraordinary woman and writer who celebrated the Sacred in the ordinary.

"I know that young children will wander away from the table, and that family life is never smooth, and that life itself is full," Laurie tells us, "not only of charm and warmth and comfort but of sorrow and tears. But whether we are happy or sad, we must be fed."

This is why I love cookbooks, especially hers.

JULY 6

Home-Grown Bliss: The Romance of Kitchen Gardens

For what was Paradise but a garden and orchard of trees and herbs.
Full of pleasure and nothing there but delights.
—William Lawson (1553/4–1635)
English clergyman and gardener

Of course, it would all end and begin again in a garden. Love. Admiration. Adoration. Celebration. Devotion. Frustration. Obsession. Relinquishment. Redemption. Renewal. Restoration. The Divine and perennial passion to be reignited annually as long as humans live and lust on this earth. Not between Adam and Eve, mind you, but between Eve and Eden.

Even women like myself, whose horticultural knowledge is limited to planting with the green bit on top, are apt to stir with basic instincts that can leave us feeling like natural women when the sun shines, the earth grows warm, and the air becomes moist and soft with promise. Once more, we say with great conviction, "*This* is the *year* I shall *have* a garden." And again, with great feeling, *fortissimo*. I don't know about you, but this year I mean it. Shall we go forth—with pen and spade?

Equal parts flower, vegetable, fruit and herb, the romance of kitchen gardens—and the passions they inspire—transports culinary history from the whispers of the past, through your back door and onto your plate within minutes. The first time, or every time for that matter, that you bite into something you've grown, a little bit of Paradise is restored. You say to yourself, this is right, this is good, this is life as it can be, this is food as it was created in the beginning. It's a shivery, thrilling moment when you personally understand why the Psalmist wrote, "Taste and see how good is the Lord."

When I was living in England, I treated myself to a birthday weekend at French chef Raymond Blanc's exquisite hotel, Belmond Le Manoir aux Quat' Saisons in Oxfordshire. Every detail—the ambiance, décor, fragrance, and, of course, the food at this two-star Michelin hideaway—was sensory, scrumptious, and sublime. But my favorite remembrance is wandering through Raymond Blanc's two-acre kitchen garden, where he organically grows more than ninety vegetables and fruits and seventy herbs. As I stood there in euphoria, I made a promise that someday I'd be standing in my own walled kitchen garden, and this dream is more precious than diamonds.

"In France the kitchen garden or potager, has for centuries been a cornerstone of the country way of life," Georgeanne Brennan tells us in her books *Potager: Fresh Garden Cooking in the French Style* and *In the French Kitchen Garden: The Joys of Cultivating a Potager*. "Much more than a vegetable patch, the French Kitchen Garden is a communion between the indoors and the outdoors—a means of living in harmony with the earth...Growing a potager is a life-affirming, enriching pursuit that can easily be adapted to almost any climate or lifestyle."

I know, the conundrum of where to begin. I don't have two acres now. But then neither did Raymond Blanc twenty years ago. So it's really a choice between a little plot of land or a big pot for our experiment. Personally, I think a half whiskey barrel painted green, as the sorely missed garden writer Suzy Bales used for her "salad bowl," is a brilliant way to begin with baby lettuces (cos; mesclun, which is a mixture of salad leaves; and my favorite, lamb's ear—*mache* in French), then add watercress, spinach, no-fail cherry tomatoes (the Italian cherry tomato pomodoro and the yellow pear), spring onions, miniature French cornichon cucumbers. Now add a barrel for herbs: Genovese basil, Italian parsley, rosemary, dill, oregano, and a little bay tree.

Well, you see where all of this leads: to home-grown bliss. If you've never had a vegetable potager, you could even scale it back to red and yellow tomatoes, basil, lamb's ear lettuce, and spring onions in one pot. To make it pretty around the rim, plant an edible flower, such as the Empress of India nasturtium, which gives a spicy bite to your salad and looks divine.

You will be so happy starting with even the tiniest plot or the biggest pot. And if you live in an apartment, then an indoor window box with white lattice in place of a curtain to catch and train vines are for you because you can't fail—and really, the first couple of seasons of growing and gardening need successes, don't they?

What comes next, of course, will be ordering heirloom vegetable catalogs next winter, stockpiling treasured gardening tomes, foraging for the prettiest floral gardening gloves, a fetching, big-brimmed straw hat, and good tools that "feel" right in your hands. Oh, and let's not forget the affordable necessity of a generous knee pad for weeding, a brightly colored enamel watering can, and a gardening notebook with graph paper so that you can draw your everyday Eden in detail.

You may not have a French walled kitchen garden this summer or even a small one behind a little white picket fence, the more traditional but still delightful perimeter. Neither do I. Gardens, like our lives, need to be plotted, planned, and planted before they yield their harvest. But you can, along with me, sow the seeds of this bountiful and joyful simplicity into your imagination today. "The first gathering...of salads, radishes and herbs made me feel like a mother about her baby—how could anything so beautiful be mine?" Alice B. Toklas, the American art collector of the Parisian avant-garde during the twenties, reminisced. "And this emotion of wonder filled me for each vegetable as it was gathered every year. There is nothing that is comparable to it, as satisfactory or as thrilling, as gathering the vegetables one has grown." She went on to write a cookbook, *The Alice B. Toklas Cookbook*, in 1954, and it remains one of the best-selling cookbooks of all time.

JULY 7

Cooking for Comfort

It seems to me that our three basic needs, for food and security and love, are so entwined that we cannot think of one without the other.

—M. F. K. Fisher (1908–1992)
Preeminent American food writer

Comfort food: quirky and quaint. For Beyoncé, it's that chicken from Popeye's. Chrissy Teigen, anything you can do with Velveeta. Jennifer Lawrence wants Cool Ranch Doritos, and for Blake Lively, it's Kraft Macaroni & Cheese.

Really? Can't we do better than that? Except Chrissy, who has serious comfort food cred with me because she's written two funny *and* delicious cookbooks, *Cravings* and *Hungry for More,* and actually uses Velveeta in some of her recipes.

But where are the mashed potatoes, the brioche French toast, the fettuccine Alfredo? Where's the pizza and the entire pint of salted caramel ice cream? Where are the brownies? Or Kit Kat bars?

Comfort food, personal patterns of consolation, encoded on our taste buds past all forgetting, as unmistakable as greasy fingerprints. When the miseries strike and you're down in the dumps, food transformed by love and memory becomes therapy.

Comfort food is one of six basic food groups: haute cuisine, lean cuisine, comfort food, soul food, nursery fare, and chocolate. Now there are some who lump the last four into the same category. However, domestic explorers such as ourselves, in search of the sublime, appreciate the subtle nuances of succor.

Comfort food is hearty. When hearts are heavy, they need gravitational and emotional equilibrium: meat loaf and mashed potatoes, macaroni and cheese, chicken potpie, red beans and rice, creamy risotto. Food that reassures us that we will survive. With such sustenance we can keep on going and going, especially when we don't want to take another step. Soul food takes us back to our roots, nursery fare tucks us into bed, and chocolate alters consciousness. Different foods for different moods.

It's important to realize that comfort food is not haute cuisine. You won't find it in a four-star restaurant, but you might get lucky in a diner. The more you pay for your meal, the less likely it is to bring you comfort. Pleasure can be bought, but comfort must be given. Even if you give it to yourself.

Comfort food is also not lean cuisine. Perhaps you've wondered why lettuce—even radicchio drenched in balsamic vinegar—doesn't satisfy the way lasagna does. There is a perfectly wonderful scientific reason for this physical phenomenon. Consider this: Certain delicious foods—carbohydrates—make us feel calm and content because they literally change our brain chemistry by increasing the levels of serotonin, the *natural* feel-good enzyme. In other words, pasta and potatoes are Mother Nature's Prozac. Are you starting to feel better already?

Here is a *Simple Abundance* plan for making cooking for comfort a joyful simplicity: Start a file just for comfort food recipes. When you prepare hearty comfort foods, double your pleasure by doubling the recipe to freeze for another meal. Near your refrigerator door keep track of what you've frozen, so that you know what's available when black clouds hover. It's such a simple pleasure knowing that there's something delicious and comforting in the freezer for dinner, especially when you've been working hard all day long and no one appreciates it.

"Since we're forced to nourish ourselves, why not do it with all possible skill...and ever-increasing enjoyment," the marvelous M. F. K. Fisher asks. And when we sit down not only to eat, but to be cheered and comforted, let us do so "with grace and gusto" and a grateful heart.

JULY 8

In Search of Soul Food

Soul food is just what the name implies. It is soulfully cooked food or richly flavored food, good for your ever-loving soul.
—Sheila Ferguson
American singer, actress, and author

Soul food is our personal passport to the past. It is much more about heritage than it is about hominy. It's Grandma's beaten biscuits or Nana's borscht. Sheila Ferguson tells us in her cookbook *Soul Food: Classic Cuisine from the Deep South* that it's "a legacy clearly steeped in tradition; a way of life that has been handed down from generation to generation."

And while the expression "soul food" is typically used to describe traditional African-American cooking, this emotionally evocative cuisine is universal to all races and cultures. Real soul food only knows the borders of the heart. Soul food is cosmic culinary memories, stories, and recipes. It's how to fry the chicken or the wonton, shape the noodles, simmer the brisket, roll the tortilla, sweeten the iced tea.

Whenever I went home to visit my parents, who are now both dead, the first and last meal my mother always prepared for me is my favorite: soup beans, a tangible time transporter to her old Kentucky home and mine. Soup beans are pinto beans that have simmered slowly for hours, until they create their own soup. Ladle soup beans over mashed potatoes. Serve with coleslaw, hot cornbread slathered with real butter, and an ice-cold beer.

During the last summer of my mother's life, Katie and I traveled north for a family reunion of all my mother's children and grandchildren. There were conversation, cooking, comfort, closure. Although I knew intellectually how to prepare my favorite meal, I didn't emotionally. I couldn't think about my mother dying; I thought about my last helping of *her* soup beans. There are many ways to grieve.

When preparing soul food, we can't cook by the book but rather by instinct, by using our senses. "You learn to hear by the crackling sound when it's time to turn over the fried chicken, to smell when a pan of biscuits is just about to finish baking, and to feel when a pastry's just right to the touch," Sheila Ferguson tells us. "You taste, rather than measure, the seasoning you treasure; and you use your eyes, not a clock to judge when that cherry pie has bubbled sweet and nice. These skills are hard to teach quickly. They must be felt...and come straight from the heart and soul."

This summer, collect soulful recipes, or let someone you love but don't see very often cook for you. Better still, try taking a personal cooking lesson. You might think you know how to make jam cake with caramel icing, but do you?

JULY 9

Nursery Fare for Children of All Ages

Animal crackers, and cocoa to drink,
That is the finest of suppers, I think;
When I'm grown up and can have what I please
I think I shall always insist upon these.
—Christopher Morley (1890–1957)
American novelist and journalist

The first Christmas I spent away from home was in London in 1972. A few days before December 25, a big box arrived with gifts. Among them, from my mother, was a pair of red flannel pajamas-with-feet. Where she ever found them in my size I can't imagine, but now that I know about these things, I'm sure she spent hours planning and searching for my surprise.

At the time, however, I didn't appreciate either the gift or the gesture. I was twenty-five, thought I was sophisticated, and was insulted that she still thought of me as a baby—which, of course, is exactly what I was. My mother, who had been stationed in England during World War II as an army nurse, knew that London could be cold, damp, dismal, and, at its worst, numbing. Since I knew zip, I promptly discarded the pajamas, preferring to shiver in a black silk kimono.

What I wouldn't give for those pajamas now! They would perfectly set the mood for a nursery supper, which is what grown women, like you and me, sometimes need in order to "make it all better," at least for a little while.

When you're cranky and cry easily, when you are so tired that your eyes burn from keeping them open, when you need hugs and someone to rub the top of your head and whisper "Shh...There, there..." and no one is around, you need nursery fare. Nursery foods are the well-loved recipes from childhood that conjure up the happy, innocent moments when all was right with the world because we knew our place in it, dressed in our flannel pajamas with feet, as we sat down for supper before a story and bed. "Nighty-night," we'd say as the door slowly closed until there was a slender sliver of light from the hallway. "See you when the darkness goes…"

Once, at the end of a delicious sophisticated dinner party attended by smart, successful forty-somethings, the witty banter came to an abrupt halt when our hostess brought out dessert. In front of each guest, she put a bowl of rice pudding, covered with warm cream and sprinkled with cinnamon and nutmeg. After the first tentative mouthfuls came squeals of delight and, in unison, "I haven't had this in years!" The pleasure at that table was palpable.

"Nursery food is the supreme comfort. No wonder, because however abysmal it really was, childhood looks so appealing the farther away it gets," write Jane and Michael Stern, authors of a wonderful collection of yesterday's taste thrills, *Square Meals*. "You remember warm farina served in a bowl decorated with dancing bunnies, or the ritual cup of cocoa after school." For those of you who have never enjoyed the sublime delights of warm farina, it's milled wheat that's cooked and served like porridge.

Now that we've all grown up, the nursery at the top of the stairs remains a sepia-colored photograph, or even a past fantasy, for many of us. But since we can have what we please for supper, we shouldn't forget that we're never too old to discover nursery fare, especially if we never heard of it or tasted it before. Good heavens, who raised us? Certainly, not Mary Poppins!

Here's a Nursery Fare Menu:

- Welsh rarebit (toast with melted cheese on it).
- Milk toast (toast in a little warm milk in a skillet. Sprinkle with a dusting of sugar, cinnamon, raisins, and cocoa).
- Beef tea (think bone broth or the most delicious consommé).
- Coddled eggs (a soft-boiled egg in a cup).
- French toast fingers (crustless rectangular strips of toast).
- Baked bananas (Peel and cut bananas in half. Place in baking dish, add honey and cinnamon, bake at 400 degrees F for fifteen minutes).
- Egg custard…and that includes everything from crème brûlée to flan!

If you can't remember when you last indulged in something smooth, comforting, and delectable, something that made you smack your lips, then it's been too long. To refresh your memory, the Sterns have devoted an entire chapter to nursery food in *Square Meals*. And a wonderful book I cherish is *Molly Keane's Book of Nursery Cooking*, which is an Irish memoir plus recipes from the Anglo-Irish novelist and playwright born in 1904.

The next time you're on edge, stop for a moment to concoct something creamy to soothe your jaded palate and jangled nerves. And if that doesn't work, there's always a blanket and your thumb. So wash your hands, pull up a chair, and let's read about animal crackers.

The kitchen's the coziest place that I know;
The kettle is singing, the stove's aglow,
And there in the twilight, how jolly to see
The cocoa and animals waiting for me.

Don't worry, there's enough for both of us. I'm a big girl now. I know how to share. And if you see that adorable Chrissy Teigen before I do, tell her we need to have our nursery fare, reimagined for children of all ages in her next cookbook.

JULY 10

Kitchen Mysticism

After all, it is those who have a deep and real inner life who are best able to deal with the irritating details of outer life.
—Evelyn Underhill (1875–1941)
English-Anglo spiritual author and mystic

Woman's normal occupations in general run counter to creative life, or contemplative life, or saintly life," Anne Morrow Lindbergh, the author and aviatrix, consoled me as I ricocheted from summer camp drop-off to computer, to summer camp pickup, to computer, to kitchen, and back to computer at eight in the evening. The summer I came across that quote my life, by necessity, was broken up into two-hour increments, which is not the most conducive way to create or contemplate.

It is a subtle irony, but one not lost on my Authentic Self, that while writing a book of meditations—a work that you might imagine springs from the author's deep spiritual reservoir of calm—I seemed to be in perpetual motion. This was either a cosmic joke or a cosmic lesson, to be learned the easy way or the hard way. I couldn't just write about

Simple Abundance; I had to live it, or I might as well have been writing science fiction.

I desperately needed to restore harmony in my life, to find balance again between the inner and the outer, the visible and the invisible. The writing didn't seem to be coming *from* me as much as *through* me, almost *in spite* of me. The strings on this instrument had become very taut, and desperately needed to be loosened to keep from snapping. Maybe you feel the same way. Maybe the pitch of pressure is too high, the tone in your voice too sharp, the decibels of the demands on you deafening.

It's best to explore the fourth *Simple Abundance* Grace—Harmony— most deeply when life is out of tune. I'd recently read a lovely book, a spiritual journey written by a gifted woman writer, who actually went to a monastery in order to concentrate, create with clarity, and complete her book on time. You can imagine what part of her journey made the strongest impression. Since I obviously couldn't follow her example without abandoning husband, child, and animals, all of whom were waiting, as I wrote, to be fed, my only option at the moment was to stop working and head into the kitchen. I might not be able to say mass or meditate, but I could make a meal.

"The home is a sacred place where you can communicate with the four elements of the universe: earth, water, air and fire," says writer and kitchen mystic Laura Esquivel, author of the luminous novel *Like Water for Chocolate*. "You mix it with your love and emotions to create magic. Through cooking, you raise your spiritual level and balance yourself in a world that is materialistic." In a world that is frequently out of kilter, the kitchen is as mystical as a monastery.

Slice red and yellow bell peppers, tiny eggplants, and zucchini into strips. Chop red onions, fresh basil, oregano, and Italian plum tomatoes. Sauté slowly in good olive oil and minced garlic until the vegetables are soft. Take a sip of wine. Add penne pasta to boiling water for twelve minutes. Grate fresh Parmigiano-Reggiano cheese. Warm storebought rosemary and ricotta focaccia in the oven. Toss the pasta and vegetables together. Sprinkle with cheese. Call everyone to the table. Stop to give thanks. Offer a toast and a thanksgiving for good health, love, companionship, delicious food, and a moment of contentment. A day fully lived, simply abundant.

Evelyn Underhill, an English mystic and writer of the early twentieth century, believed that women mystics with worldly responsibilities often became "visionaries, prophetesses" because they were able to combine "spiritual transcendence with great practical ability." Be they poets, saints, or cooks, they "remained all their lives the devout lovers of reality" while seeking the Divine.

Now *that* is music to my ears. Want to hum along?

JULY 11

Cooking as Art: Creative Discoveries
in the Kitchen

The discovery of a new dish does more for the happiness of the human race than the discovery of a star.
—Jean Anthelme Brillat-Savarin (1755–1826)
Epicure and first influential writer about food

Few of us have enjoyed the thrill of mounting a one-woman show of our art. But we can all cook a meal. Most of our meals are prepared by rote and the easier the better. However, tonight, instead of thinking of dinner as just another obligation, think of it as an opportunity for jump-starting your creativity. Cooking is one of the best ways for your Authentic Self to remind your conscious self that you are an artist. Like the union of canvas and pigment, cooking is alchemy, a work of Wholeness-in-progress.

A paring knife can be as creative as a paintbrush. Scraping, slicing, shredding, stirring, simmering, sautéing are all sleights of hand that switch your conscious mind onto artistic, automatic pilot.

Once the conscious mind is distracted, the creative mind takes over, even if you aren't aware of it. Whenever I don't know what to do—whether it's writing or living—I seek discoveries in the kitchen, such as trying to re-create a great dish I enjoyed somewhere else. The worst that can happen is that the experiment's a flop and we end up eating sandwiches before bed. The best is that my pleasant brainstorming and the supper that results provide a new taste sensation, reminding me that nothing need be taken for granted—especially moments of doubt, frustration, and hunger.

"If your regrets linger, if you cannot find inspiration in solitude, then you still have much to learn from the writers and the poets and the cooks on becoming the artist of your own life," Jacqueline Deval reflects in her tantalizing novel *Reckless Appetite: A Culinary Romance*. "…You can never re-create the past. But you can shape your own future. And you can make a cake."

This week try making a cake from scratch as a meditation. Think of the most luscious cake you can imagine, the cake of your dreams, the cake you've always wanted to eat but never had the time to make. The cake that has always seemed too daunting. Take time, make time, make your cake. Declare the kitchen off-limits. The artist is at work. Slowly, carefully, and mindfully gather together the raw materials for your creation: flour, eggs, milk, baking powder, baking soda, salt, spices, and sugar.

If something is perplexing you now, see the situation as simply an ingredient in the great recipe that's real life. Each ingredient makes its own authentic contribution to the whole, yet each ingredient changes— the salt and the sugar become one—transformed by the four elements of the Universe: fire in the oven, water from the tap, earth in the grain, the air embracing all. Do not discount the fire that burns in your soul, the water of your sweat and tears, the earthiness of perseverance, and every breath you take as you struggle to master the art and unravel the mystery of an authentic life.

And when your cake emerges from the oven, fragrant and full of flavor, consider for a moment the difference between creating a cake—or a life—from scratch and one that's thrown together with a ready-made mix. Convenience foods may save us time in the kitchen, but the cook always knows, just as the artist does, what is the genuine article and what merely passes for real.

JULY 12

How to Cook a Wolf

There's a whining at the threshold—
There's a scratching at the floor—
To work! To work! In Heaven's name!
The wolf is at the door!
—Charlotte Perkins Gilman (1860–1935)
American author, journalist, and social
reformer

Who's afraid of the big, bad wolf? We all are. Because sooner or later he's whining and scratching at everybody's door. When the wolf arrives, "Our texture of belief has great holes in it," M. F. K. Fisher recalls. "Our pattern lacks pieces." Mary Frances Kennedy Fisher was arguably America's greatest food writer, and she knew all about lean times. In fact, one of her early books was entitled *How To Cook a Wolf,* which was published in 1942 during the worst of the wartime food shortages.

Like the best cookbooks and memoirs, she wrote from personal experience. During much of her life, M. F. K. had to keep the wolves at bay. Although she was well known, writing for *The New Yorker* as well as many other publications over many years, she was never well paid and continually had to scratch out a freelancer's hand-to-mouth lifestyle to help support herself, two daughters, and, at various times, three husbands. I say "lifestyle" rather than "existence" because

M. F. K. Fisher knew how to live well despite her bank account. She never reduced herself to mere existing, whatever her circumstances. Poverty is always experienced in the soul before it is felt in the pocketbook.

In fact, it seems incredible to think of M. F. K. Fisher as lacking for money, because she never lacked a simply abundant life. Perhaps she enjoyed "the good life" we all long for because she embraced it with a grateful heart. She traveled, lived in France and Italy, wrote many magnificent books, knew passionate love, enjoyed a wide circle of friends and admirers, and always savored the everyday epiphanies of eating and drinking well. M. F. K. Fisher's Authentic Self found outward expression in exuberance.

For those of us who would like to follow in her footsteps, she recommends weeding out desires, leaving only holy hungers, "so that you can live most agreeably in a world full of an increasing number of disagreeable surprises."

How did she do it? By not running scared when the wolf arrived, by not giving in to her fears that he would blow her house down. She knew that the twists and turns of fate came in cycles. By concentrating on the good at hand—today—a good glass of wine, a ravishing tomato, a loaf of warm bread, cheese, and the best butter you can spread—any hunger can be sated. A beautiful sunset, a lively conversation, a loving relationship, music, a deep breath, and a grateful sigh for what is make up the moments we remember. The good life does not depend on extravagant indulgences. The good life does not deprive. It expands as it exults. "You can still live with grace and wisdom," M. F. K. encourages us—if you rely on "your own innate sense of what you must do with the resources you have to keep the wolf from sniffing too hungrily through the keyhole."

JULY 13

Stocking the Larder

Cooking—yes, and living become simpler rites this month. I have made a list of satisfactory meals planned around only one cooked dish. This list is hung on the door of my kitchen cabinet for reference. When I am lacking in ambition, I do not wonder what to have for dinner.

—Nell B. Nichols
Woman's Home Companion, July 1925

One of my favorite literary domestics is Nell B. Nichols, a columnist for *Woman's Home Companion* during the 1920s, 1930s, and

1940s. Before Gwyneth Paltrow, Nigella Lawson, and Martha Stewart, the world had Nell Nichols. There was nothing she couldn't do. But Nell's great gift was that she never made you feel inept; you knew if you followed her blithe instructions carefully, you could also experience domestic bliss.

Nell cooked, canned, cleaned, organized from broom closet to basement with cheerful élan; she tried out new gadgets like the vacuum cleaner and deemed it a "valuable friend," but she also cherished old traditions like bleaching white linens by drying them in the summer sunlight. Reading her columns is like being spoon-fed black-cherry pudding: soothing, comforting, completely satisfying, yet a bit piquant. After an hour with Nell I always want to bob my hair, slip into a simple drop-waist cotton chemise, tie on a checked apron with a bow, as I tap my feet listening to Scott Joplin's ragtime or syncopated rhythm on the wireless (radio to us) as I dye unbleached muslin curtains "to pretty up the attic windows."

During the decades that Nell Nichols reigned as queen of the home front, "efficiency" was the buzzword in women's magazines. Women were exhorted to consider homemaking not only as an art the way their Victorian mothers had, but as a science—home economics. One bit of wisdom for which I'll be eternally grateful to Nell is her plea that women "plan more to work less in the kitchen."

Two home-caring tasks that consume a great deal of creative energy each week are grocery shopping and meal preparation. I've created *Simple Abundance* strategies for stocking the larder that can help you reclaim a sense of control when cooking. The first is to create a master grocery list. This task will take you only about an hour and will return an abundance of time in the future.

Divide your grocery list into different categories, such as fresh produce, dairy, meat, fish, staples, paper, and personal care products. These will serve as automatic reminders. I have my master list on my computer, and every Friday I print it out and check off what I need, or you can save it to a notes app and work from it off your phone. There are also many fantastic grocery list apps that can do everything from comb your grocery list and provide the best available deals at local supermarkets, synch among multiple users so family or roommates can add to it, and help with meal prep and planning for the week.

Before I can make out an efficient grocery list, I need to devise menus, so I know what I'll be cooking and what I need to shop for. Again, there are currently several great apps (and more to come) for this.

A few to consider are:

Paprika Recipe Manager: Browse recipes online, download the recipe, and save with the click of a button. You can also easily create grocery lists from your recipes, too.

Yummly Recipes + Shopping List: It is touted as having the most recipes of any app; you can also input your zip code, and your chosen recipe's ingredients are generated into a list that is sorted by aisle for the store of your choosing. Click any applicable coupon links and the app will apply those savings directly to the order, too.

Mealime Meal Plans & Recipes: Pick a diet plan, ingredients to exclude, and serving size, then build a meal plan for the week from a curated collection of recipes.

By planning your meals in advance, you'll avoid forgetting any necessary ingredient at the market—which we've all done countless times over the years—plus you'll reduce waste and care for Mother Earth.

A *Simple Abundance* strategy is to sit down and write out your family's favorite meals; you might even ask for suggestions. Be sure to include side dishes, vegetables, and desserts. Then create a master menu file. Again, you can do this on an app, use recipes stored in your computer, or even write out your repertoire of menus on index cards. A core of at least a dozen meals enables you to create a sense of variety at dinnertime. Eating the same thing repeatedly can get awfully dreary, but it's so easy to get into a rut!

Many of us simply don't have time during the week to experiment in the kitchen. To keep your beloved "customers" coming back to your restaurant (or even just yourself), try to include two new recipes a month. Save them for weekends, when you have more time and can enjoy the simple pleasure of cooking something new and different.

"Just one word more—please steal time every day, if you cannot find it in any other way, to lie on the grass, or in a hammock, under a huge tree this lovely month…and relax. What a tonic this is for the soul! What a rest for weary nerves! The greatest need today is for calmer homes, and no fireside can be calm unless its guardian is at peace with the world," Nell B. Nichols reassured readers in the summer of 1924.

"Won't you agree with me, as you lie looking up at the leafy canopy above you, that a home now and in every other month must be a haven to the spirit as well as a place in which the physical needs are supplied?"

Yes, Nell. Yes. Thanks for reminding us.

The Celebrating Table

The table is a meeting place, a gathering ground, the source of sustenance and nourishment, festivity, safety, and satisfaction.
—Laurie Colwin (1944–1992)
American writer and food essayist

Whether we're single, in a relationship, with or without children, we all must eat dinner. The evening meal should be the highlight of the day. If the day has been peaceful, pleasurable, and profitable, it's time to celebrate. If the day has been difficult and discouraging, it's time for comfort and consolation—blessings by themselves and reason to celebrate. Either way, the celebrating table beckons.

Just as there are different food categories, there are different types of dining in: takeout, home cooked, and full-on feasts. All of us make do sometimes, but as a lifestyle choice, rotating frozen meals can quickly lead to psychic starvation and dietary deprivation.

Takeout cuts corners miraculously, but done on a regular basis is extremely expensive. So is dining out a lot, which also can make you feel as if you're endlessly on the road and not connected to home at all. Cooking at home can be wonderful, and with meal kit companies like Blue Apron, Hello Fresh, and Plated, it's never been easier or more attainable for any level of chef. Or you can also brave it the home-style way, which is what I like to call homemade Monday-to-Friday suppers. With planning, these meals can be easy, fast, and delicious.

There was a time when I wouldn't begin to think about what to have for dinner each day until four o'clock that afternoon. Today this thought makes me shudder. Planning, shopping, and cooking for a crowd in the space of an hour is self-abuse, pure and simple. Fear not: With resources online and a plethora of apps there's no end of easy ways to plan your meals and do weekly grocery shopping.

If you're a bit more old-fashioned and prefer to work from a book, a long-standing favorite of mine is the *Monday to Friday Cookbook* by Michele Urvater. Michele's a professional chef who created this cookbook because, at the end of a long day cooking for other people, she wanted simple but savory, no-fuss suppers for her family. She'll teach you how to stock the pantry with staples, what to fix when schedules clash, and how to avoid Mother Hubbard's empty cupboard syndrome with style.

"We need time to defuse, to contemplate. Just as in sleep our brains relax and give us dreams, so at some time in the day we need to disconnect, reconnect, and look around us," Laurie Colwin reminds us. "We must turn off the television and the telephone, hunker down in front of our hearths, and leave our briefcases at the office, if for only one night. We must march into the kitchen, *en famille* or with a friend, and find some easy, heartwarming things to make from scratch, and even if it is but once a week, we must gather at the table, alone or with friends or with lots of friends or with one friend and eat a meal together. We know that without food we would die. Without fellowship life is not worth living."

Come, the celebrating table beckons.

JULY 15

Are We Having Company Tonight?

I learned early on that setting a table is so much more than just laying down knives and forks. It is creating a setting for food and conversation, setting a mood and an aura that lingers long after what was served and who said what was forgotten.

—Peri Wolfman
Tabletop designer and author

When preparing a meal, the last thing many of us think about, except when we're expecting company, is our table setting. For guests we'll bring out the good china, stemware, and linens, but for ourselves, the everyday, no matter what shape it's in, will have to do. Yes, it will be fine, if it's all you have. But if you continually choose the chipped over the beautiful china behind the glass doors when you don't have to, then making do is not enough.

The rituals of nourishment cry out for the communion cups, the special plates on which to break bread, the candle flame, the circle drawn in the dirt. Ritual protects and heals; ritual symbolizes to all who come to your table seeking rest and renewal that they are enclosed within a Sacred space.

You may think you're only laying a place at the supper table, but when you trust and follow your creative impulses to bring forth something beautiful, you experience the Sacred in the ordinary. Moses looked for God in the burning bush. We need look no further than our tables, the tables that the Hebrew Psalmist tells us have already been prepared for us so that our cups might runneth over.

"When I think back to our family meals, it isn't the taste or smell of the food that I recall as much as the way the scene looked," reminisces Peri Wolfman, coauthor with her husband, Charles Gold, of *The Perfect Setting* as well as other entertaining titles. "The ambiance of the table, the patina of the wood, the candlelight, the colors, the sense of harmony and order."

Today our style of entertaining has become more casual than the starched linen and polished silver of past generations, yet the sense of harmony that can be conjured up with an inviting table setting has not changed. Nor has the need. If anything, we hunger for Harmony more than we do for sustenance. But we don't need to feast from fine Italian linen every day: a beautiful wood table set with simple white napkins, pottery plates, oversized water goblets, votive candles, and a small bouquet of flowers or centerpiece bowl of fresh fruit is a simply abundant setting that elevates eating into the exquisite pleasure of dining.

When you take extra moments to prepare an attractive table, you're really performing an invocation, welcoming Spirit to be present in recreation and remembrance. Choosing to dine rather than just eat is a small but significant step toward self-nurturance, and one to savor if we live. Creating an inviting table is possible more nights than you think, especially if you approach it as another venue of artistic expression in your daily round and confine your efforts, as Peri suggests, to "the simple, the doable, and the affordable."

Today, start using and enjoying the beautiful things that already surround you in your home. Don't save their loveliness only for other people to recognize and appreciate. Using them, you will become aware that authentic aspirations—from setting a pretty table to finding your life's calling—are legitimate longings.

Company *is* coming for dinner tonight. Guess who? It would be a quantum leap in abundance consciousness, if, when your Authentic Self graces your table, she finds generous portions of the love, respect, and welcome she so richly deserves served up on the most beautiful plate you own.

JULY 16

A Seasonal Feast: The Joy of Anticipation

Why is any day better than another, when all the daylight in the year is from the sun?
By the Lord's decision they were distinguished, and he appointed the different seasons and feasts;
Some of them he exalted and hallowed, and some of them he made ordinary days.

—Ecclesiasticus (Also Called Sirach) 33:7–9

The joy of seasonal cooking is the simplest of pleasures, but one of the most overlooked. It brings balance, harmony, and rhythm to our days, demonstrating with gentle wisdom that simplicity and abundance are soul mates. The joy of seasonal foods transforms even the ordinary days at the table into hallowed moments, calling to mind the Book of Proverbs' wisdom that "the cheerful heart has a continual feast."

Cooking with the seasons is also more affordable. We often think that using the freshest foods possible, at the peak of their flavor, is a luxury, but seasonal cooking is the best way to eat *well* and eat whole foods, on a budget. What's more, if your frugality is so subtle and sophisticated, your material girl can't begin to feel deprived—not when she's enjoying a dinner of grilled vegetables with marinated goat cheese, bruschetta (toasted Italian bread topped with tomato and garlic), and a berry crumble for dessert.

Summer is when Mother Nature shows off, proving that the Universe is not stingy. Gardens and farmers' markets now overflow with the goodness of the earth. Now, while the summer is offering bountiful home economics lessons, is the perfect time to reconsider how you cook throughout the year.

One of the most wonderful cookbooks for seasonal feasts I have ever discovered is *Judith Huxley's Table for Eight.* Judith Huxley was a superb writer, cook, and a gardener, and her love of all three authentic arts is evident on every page of this marvelous book. It is out of print, but you'll feel that searching for it is time well spent. (Used editions of it show up on Amazon, so you might get lucky!) There are fifty-two sensational menus—a week-by-week walk through the year celebrating the pleasures of the table. I return to this beloved cookbook again and again, usually on Sundays, when I prepare our family feasts.

"There is no season such delight can bring," the English poet William Browne believed, "as summer, autumn, winter and the spring." The simply abundant joy of seasonal foods will convince you that life can be a continual feast at Mother Nature's table.

JULY 17

Loaves and Fishes, Part I

We have here but five loaves, and two fishes.

—Matthew 14:17
New Testament

Do you know the story of Jesus feeding the crowd of five thousand believers, seekers, skeptics, and the simply curious who had come to hear him teach? At the end of the long day, when the disciples wanted to send everybody home, Jesus told them not to be ridiculous, that the people were tired and hungry. "But we only have five loaves of bread and two fishes, barely enough for ourselves," the disciples argued. "How can we feed that many?"

"Give me what you have," Jesus told them. Then Jesus looked up to Heaven, offered thanks, blessed the food, and gave it back to the disciples to distribute. Miraculously, after everyone had finished eating as much as they wanted, twelve baskets of leftovers remained.

I love this story because it's such a powerful illustration of abundance consciousness, providing us the model for simply abundant living. The gospels of Matthew and Mark report that Jesus performed this simply abundant miracle *twice*. On the second occasion, four thousand people were fed with seven loaves and a few fishes. By this time the increasingly threatened high priests had started stirring things up. They demanded that Jesus demonstrate more signs and wonders to prove his divinity. He dismissed their taunts and walked away, cautioning the disciples to "beware of the yeast of the Pharisees and Sadducees" (referring, I imagine, to traditional religious hot air). But the apostles took Jesus's warning *literally* and assumed that the bread in that town was spoiled. So they decided not to buy any local bread and planned to eat when they got to the next town.

Hours later they found themselves crossing a lake in a boat, with the journey taking much longer than anyone had expected. The disciples began complaining about not having any bread because of the yeast being tainted. Ravenously hungry, they asked, "What will we do? How will we eat?" Jesus, clearly frustrated at their failure to fully grasp His message, berated them with these words: "You of little faith—why are you talking among yourselves about having no bread? Do you *still not understand?* Don't you remember the five loaves for the five thousand, or the seven loaves for the four thousand? And how many basketfuls you gathered? How is it you don't understand that I was not talking to you about bread?...Do you have eyes but fail to see, and ears but fail to hear?"

This is great stuff, because the delicious morsel hidden beneath the story of abundance and lack is that the apostles just *didn't get it*. Miracle after miracle kept occurring before their eyes, but they didn't see what was really going on. That's because they were ordinary human beings, even though their spiritual tutorial was being given by a Master. It still wasn't enough, because they had not personally experienced an inner shift.

The same thing happens with us. How often in our lives do we still *not get it?* The "it" could be a power struggle going on in an important relationship; an inability to control our spending; a career problem undermining our self-esteem; the beginnings of addictive behavior in ourselves or our loved ones; or an unconscious form of self-sabotage that has us bouncing from one self-inflicted crisis to another. The "it" doesn't matter. Some such scenario is occurring in most of our lives and will continue, *again and again and again,* until the moment we begin to see the pattern. Perhaps we should start paying attention. It doesn't always have to be "déjà vu all over again."

When we don't get it, it's usually because we can't interpret the outward experience as it is relayed through our internal speaker system. We can't process it in our souls. What's really happening in our outward lives is somehow taking place in a foreign language that we don't understand. So we either assume that the outward manifestation is reality (which it isn't necessarily), or we keep having to repeat the experience until it starts to make sense—rather like learning a foreign language by total immersion. The poet Edna St. Vincent Millay put it this way: "It's not true that life is one damn thing after another—it's one damn thing over and over."

But speaking in tongues is a gift of Spirit. The language of the heart is longing; the language of the mind is rationalizing; the language of emotions is feeling. Spirit speaks them all. Today I would love for all of us to get it at last and that includes me (what can I say, inspiration ebbs and flows around here). I want both of us not to focus on what we don't have today but to be grateful for what we do. For us to accept, give thanks, bless, and share. For us not to hoard or hold back for fear that there won't be enough. Because Spirit lacks for nothing.

As long as you have a few loaves and fishes, and know what to do with them, all you have is all you need.

JULY 18

Loaves and Fishes, Part II

Hospitality is one form of worship.

—The Talmud

Like other simple pleasures in our lives—decorating, gardening, cooking—many of us put off entertaining because we make it such a big deal. We fix more elaborate and expensive meals for guests than we do for ourselves, taking both extra money and extra time to plan, shop, and cook.

We make a special effort to create the perfect atmosphere, beginning with a blitzkrieg of housecleaning and ending with a table setting worthy of a photo shoot. The family rhythm is often disrupted for days and includes everything from moving furniture to abandoning regular routines. I have known women who get so rattled that they're swearing "Never again" as they open the front door to greet guests. It's no wonder that the thought of entertaining overwhelms us. And so it often remains just that—a thought—until a special event is thrust upon us and we must rise to the occasion.

I was heartened to discover that during the Depression the good times didn't completely disappear. Instead, domestic pleasures were scaled to a comfortable dimension. Parties were pared down. Instead of multicourse meals, there was one course that became the theme, such as drinks and finger foods, soup and sandwiches, pancakes or spaghetti, dessert and coffee. Parties moved from the dining room into the kitchen; at kitchen parties a new recipe would be chosen and its preparation was part of the fun. Savory potluck dinners became fashionable, with each couple or guest providing a course until the meal was elevated into a feast.

Potlucks are a marvelous simple pleasure worthy of revival. When invited to a party, most people will ask if there is something they can bring. When everybody brings a special dish, time and cost are kept manageable and the menu can go gourmet even if the party is down-home.

In France, the weekly feast for family and friends is based on *cuisine de femme*, "the food of women," which has taste and soul and meaning. For a delicious way to begin a new ritual where classic French cuisine meets healthy meals, take a look at Béatrice Peltre's *My French Family Table: Recipes for a Life Filled with Food, Love, and Joie de Vivre.*

One of the most important lessons of the miracle of the loaves and fishes is that the bounty was shared. We need to remind ourselves that good times need to be shared as well, especially if we want more of them in our lives.

JULY 19

Carving Out Time for Personal Pursuits
That Bring Contentment

It is the soul's duty to be loyal to its own desires.
It must abandon itself to its master passion.
—Dame Rebecca West (1892–1983)
British author, journalist, and literary critic

After putting down her pen, the Florida novelist Marjorie Kinnan Rawlings (who won the Pulitzer Prize for *The Yearling*) cooked up plots as she baked pies. Isak Dinesen arranged flowers. Susan Sarandon plays

Ping-Pong (yes, Ping-Pong). Katharine Hepburn whiled away the long stretches on movie sets by knitting, and Mary-Kate Olsen is an equestrian who regularly competes in show jumping. Even Queen Victoria filled dozens of sketchbooks with charming watercolors of her children that reveal a glimpse of the real woman who delighted in holding a brush when not ruling an empire.

"We are traditionally rather proud of ourselves for having slipped creative work in there between the domestic chores and obligations," the American writer Toni Morrison, who won the Nobel Prize for Literature in 1993, observed. "I'm not sure we deserve such big A-pluses for that."

But the house calls to us. The children call to us. The work calls to us. When, then, does the painting or the poem call to us?

Probably every day. But we're too busy listening to everybody else instead of to our Authentic Selves. Maybe it's because we've convinced ourselves that we really don't have the time for personal pursuits that bring us contentment if they take longer than fifteen minutes. Perhaps we don't hear the whispers of authentic longing because we don't *want* to hear.

If we hear, we might have to acknowledge, even respond. We're afraid to hear the promptings of the woman who wants to learn how to draw, dance, raise orchids, reupholster a chair, and make sushi. We might have to take a class or buy a book, a pad and pencils, leggings, a plant, fabric, and a rice cooker. No time to be passionate, we have to be practical. Essential, uncompromised longings will have to wait until there's more time: when the children are back in school, when Mom's feeling better, when things let up at work.

How about an answer we haven't heard before? How about, "My authentic passions will have to wait until I'm ready to admit that pursuing them is essential for my happiness?" How about, "I haven't learned yet how to put myself on the list of priorities?" Please notice I didn't suggest putting yourself first; I just want to get you on the list.

The Victorian writer Mary Ann Evans knew how to be practical about her passion for writing. She assumed a man's pen name, George Eliot, so that her novels *Middlemarch*, *Silas Marner*, and *The Mill on the Floss* would be published in an age that discounted the authentic longings of women. This is what she says about master passions: "It is never too late to become what you might have been."

Space and time to nurture our creativity may be one of our authentic hungers. Perhaps we think that only food, alcohol, work, sex, shopping, or social media can reduce the gnawing to a dull throb. But maybe if we took an hour a day to paint, to plot, or to throw pots we wouldn't be in pain—physical or psychic.

Just maybe.

True North

It is good to have an end to journey towards; but it is the journey that matters in the end.
—Ursula K. Le Guin (1929–2018)
American science fiction/fantasy author

I used to believe that happiness could only be found after arriving at my heart's destination. Explorers call it "True North"—the fixed point in the sky that never changes in a spinning world. For me True North was enough success to ensure that there was plenty of money to control my own creative destiny, to allow me the luxury to pursue my passions.

Now that I have spent far longer on the road from here to there than I could have ever imagined when the adventure began, I have come to an awakening. I've always controlled my own creative destiny, though not always its course. I simply didn't have the common sense to realize it until now.

But more to the point, I've learned that the spirit of our journey is as important, perhaps even more important, than the arrival at our destination. In order for us to realize genuine happiness, we must be willing to court contentment every step of the way. For after all, the journey is really all that most of us will ever know. Day in, day out. The journey is real life.

One day in 1923, the artist Georgia O'Keeffe came to the same conclusion. "I found myself saying to myself...I can't live where I want to...I can't go where I want to...I can't do what I want to. I can't even say what I want to. I decided I was a very stupid fool not to at least paint as I wanted to...that seemed to be the only thing I could do that didn't concern anybody but myself."

We may not all be able to paint like Georgia O'Keeffe, who found splendor in bare bones and desert sands as well as flowers, but we can certainly learn to follow her example, one day at a time, to carve out time for rewarding reveries that acquaint us with our Authentic Selves and give us glimpses of our True North.

For it's during our expectant hours—those hours that might once have been called "idle"—that we are most pregnant with our own potential. The English writer Rupert Brooke, who perished in 1915 and became known as the Great War poet, celebrated quiet joys so eloquently. He spoke of those few lucky souls who could "store up reservoirs of calm and content...and draw on them at later moments when the source isn't there but the need is very great."

This skill—the soul-craft of devoutly caring for our Authentic

Selves—rarely comes naturally or easily. But with practice, with patience, with perseverance, and prayer it does come. At the very least, we can ask for it.

JULY 21

The Importance of Solitude

If women were convinced that a day off or an hour of solitude was a reasonable ambition, they would find a way of attaining it. As it is, they feel so unjustified in their demand that they rarely make the attempt.

—Anne Morrow Lindbergh (1906–2001)
American pioneering aviatrix and author

I am convinced that when the end of the world comes it will arrive not as two clashing armies on the brink but as a "last straw": the email that unravels six months' work in a single sentence, the telephone call that sends us reeling across the room, the seemingly innocent request to perform yet another task. Can we attend one more meeting? Write an additional memo before we leave the office? Bake another batch of cookies? Do one more errand? Suddenly, without warning, women will rush screaming into the night, leaving men and children shaking their heads in amazement wondering if it was something they said. Always remember, Greta Garbo never declared she wanted to be alone. She said: "I want to be *left* alone." There is a significant difference.

I believe that it's essential for busy women, by which I mean all of us, to pause a moment—this moment—to reconsider the entire subject of solitude. Too many of us approach time alone as if it were a frivolous, expendable luxury rather than a creative necessity. Why should this be so?

Could it be that by shortchanging ourselves, the only thing impoverished is our inner life? And after all, if the lack doesn't show on the surface, if we can pull it off one more time with smoke and mirrors, why, then, of course it doesn't count. Or does it?

"Certain springs are tapped only when we are alone. The artist knows he must be alone to create; the writer, to work out his thoughts; the musician to compose; the saint, to pray. But women need solitude in order to find again the true essence of themselves," Anne Morrow Lindbergh urges us to remember. "The problem is not entirely in finding the room of one's own, the time alone, difficult and necessary as this is. The problem is more how to still the soul in the midst of its activities. In fact, the problem is how to feed the soul."

Neglect Not the Gifts Within You

*She endured. And survived. Marginally, perhaps, but it is not
required of us that we live well.*
—Anne Cameron
Canadian novelist, screenwriter, and poet

Oh, yes, it is! We may come back to enjoy another life—and I'm open
to that possibility—but until I know for sure, I don't want to waste the
one I'm living right now. I've endured. I've survived. And I've lived marginally, but living well *is* all it's cracked up to be.

Over the years, particularly as I have *gradually* tried to honor Spirit's
unfolding in my life by not neglecting the gifts within me, I have meditated long and hard about this inner directive, this craving for solitude.
For I love the company of my loved ones and I'm excited by brainstorming and creating fabulous projects with a professional team, but what
I have discovered while composing my authentic concerto is that my
notes require lengthier pauses, and more of them.

I yearn for what the poet and memoirist May Sarton called "open
time, with no obligations except toward the inner world and what is
going on there." To maintain inner Harmony it is essential for me to
ransom at least an hour's worth of solitude out of every twenty-four
and to defend this soul-sustaining respite against all intruders and
distractions.

Deliberately seeking solitude—quality time spent away from family
and friends—may seem selfish. It is not. Solitude is as necessary for our
creative spirits to develop and flourish as are sleep and food for our bodies to survive.

"It is a difficult lesson to learn today—to leave one's friends and family and deliberately practice the art of solitude for an hour or a day or
a week," Anne Morrow Lindbergh admits. "And yet, once it is done,
I find there is a quality to being alone that is incredibly precious. Life
rushes back into the void, richer, more vivid, fuller than before."

I believe that Anne Morrow Lindbergh, who endured more than any
of us could even bear to think about (beginning with the kidnapping
and murder of her baby from his crib), demonstrated with her courageous and creative life that it is not enough for us simply to endure or
survive.

We must surmount the chaos, confusion, and cacophony of living
in the world while mastering how we play our notes. We must move
to a higher octave or a lower one, whichever is necessary to finding
the delicate balance between our deepest personal passions and our

commitment to family, friends, lovers, and work. As for me, I have discovered that the surest way to hear the soft strains of Harmony is in the
Silence.

Snatch Stolen Moments of Solitude

*She was not accustomed to taste the joys of solitude except in
company.*
—Edith Wharton (1862–1937)
American novelist, interior and landscape
designer

What is needed, then, is a plan.

Through trial and error I have tried spending quality time alone in
the early morning and late at night when the rest of the house is asleep.
Both solutions have proved impractical because I'm too tired to function at those hours, never mind be reflective or creative. I suspect I'm
not alone in my need for sleep.

If you work in an office, perhaps you can use your lunch hour for
solo excursions a few times a week. No one need be privy to this information except you. Is there a beautiful old library, museum, cathedral,
or public garden that you can visit for time alone during the middle of
the day? Why not investigate the possibilities?

Perhaps, however, your work requires you to conduct business at
lunchtime; this is the situation for several of my close friends. Block
off a half hour for yourself before and after official working hours to
close your door and collect your thoughts. One friend thought this was
impossible until she began doing it; now her snatched hour is inviolate.

If this seems impossible, then it's vitally important for you to have
some quality time alone at home, at least two nights during the week,
no matter how busy you are. Schedule "home" on your calendar and
commit to it.

Now what if you're home and you're not alone? Claim an hour in the
evening, after supper, after the kids are put to bed or while they do their
homework, even if you spend half the time soaking in the privacy of the
bathtub. Be inventive, even sneaky, if you must. Why not retire an hour
earlier than your partner during the week to read and relax in bed by
yourself?

One of my friends has a high-powered and exciting, but extremely
stressful, career as a network television executive and must burn the

midnight oil every night during the week. Her solitude solution comes on the weekend when she stays in bed all day on Saturday to recharge, joining her husband for dinner in the evening. If you're juggling family, home responsibilities, and an outside job, claim two hours on Sunday afternoon as your own. Give yourself permission to embrace the sacredness of seclusion.

Or perhaps you're home with young children who aren't yet in school. Plan your solitary pleasures when they take their naps. This is not the time for housecleaning. Use it for your own renewal. And don't be discouraged if your children have outgrown the need for naps (although I don't believe any of us ever do). Change your strategy. Call the hour immediately following lunch "Quiet Time." Take your children to their rooms gently but firmly, offering them a few special toys that they only get to play with at this time. Tell them you will see them in an hour and then retreat to your own special place.

"Being solitary is being alone well," Alice Koller explains in *The Stations of Solitude*. "[B]eing home luxuriously immersed in doings of your own choice, aware of the fullness of your own presence rather than of the absence of others."

JULY 24

Paying a High Price

[Certain] high-achieving women are imploded with demands, both external and internal, and lack the skills to filter them. These women complain that the first thing they sacrifice is their private time or private pleasures.

Harriet B. Braiker (1948–2004)
American author and psychologist

Those of us who don't spend regular time alone to rest and recoup are likely to suffer from what psychologists call "privacy deprivation syndrome." Symptoms include increasing resentment, mood swings, chronic fatigue, and depression. Sound familiar? Sound grim? It is!

Sufferers struggle through their days in a vacuum of unfulfilled exasperation, only to drop into bed too emotionally depleted to sleep well at night. The littlest thing can set them off, bringing tears and tantrums—and not only from the children in the family. Soon work and personal relationships begin to suffer. Why? Because the never refreshed are really not that much fun to be around. The cycle may continue unabated until physical illness sets in. Remember the flu you had last year for five weeks? The two weeks you were laid up with lower-back pain last summer? The sinus infection you couldn't shake last month?

We don't have to make ourselves sick before we can call a psychic time-out. Unfortunately for many women, it is only when we do get sick that we allow ourselves a dispensation for time and space alone. This may be how real life is for you right now, but it doesn't have to stay that way. If you find yourself secretly looking forward to regular rendezvous with a hot water bottle and NyQuil, then privacy deprivation syndrome is exacting a high price. Let me reassure you there is a better path.

Opening a Door That Separates Two Worlds

There are voices which we hear in solitude, but they grow faint and inaudible as we enter into the world.
—Ralph Waldo Emerson (1803–1882)
American philosopher and poet

It's impossible to experience solitude regularly for any extended length of time without personal passions and authentic longings surging to the surface of your awareness. Once you have embarked on the search for your own authentic style, followed the wisdom of your own heart, and have seen the results begin to blossom in your life, you realize that solitude cracks open the door that separates two worlds: the life we lead today and the life we yearn for so deeply.

We can all find ways to regenerate once we realize how essential solitude is to our experience of inner harmony. Tillie Olsen wrote in her story "Tell Me a Riddle" of a woman who "would not exchange her solitude for anything. *Never again be forced to move to the rhythm of others.*" While most of us probably find ourselves moving to the rhythm of others more than we would like, once we learn to respect and cherish our need for solitude, opportunities will arrive in which we can learn to nourish our imaginations and nurture our souls.

Begin slowly but resolutely. Take comfort in knowing that even stolen moments of solitude—quarter-hour increments—eventually can add up to a lifetime of serenity. Be patient. Don't expect too much too soon, especially when rearranging your schedule means dealing with your family's expectations of what you're supposed to do and when you're supposed to do it. Be patient.

And for those days—maybe even today—when you don't have a moment to yourself, take to heart the advice of photographer Minor

White, who discovered that "No matter how slow the film, Spirit always stands still long enough for the photographer It has chosen."

JULY 26

Discovering What You'd Like to Do, If You Ever Had the Time

Develop interest in life as you see it; in people, things, literature, music—the world is so rich, simply throbbing with rich treasures, beautiful souls and interesting people. Forget yourself.
—Henry Miller (1891–1980)
American writer

In the beginning spending regular time alone just to collect your thoughts will seem like indulgence enough. Spending time alone to nurture your authentic vision, to express yourself creatively, to enjoy a personal pursuit that brings you contentment and pleasure will seem— well, impossible. Incredulous. Impractical. Inconceivable. Out of the question.

"Right. In another life," is the usual response, along with audible sighs and the rolling of eyes when I broach the subject in my workshops. Then wistful looks appear. "You mean to have fun?" the women want to know.

"Yes. Have fun."

"You mean, by myself?"

"Yes, by yourself. Fun. What would you like to do if you ever had the time?"

"Fun?"

You can see where this leads. Most women I meet have a hard time holding up their end of the conversation when fun is the topic. Let the discourse be on diaper rash or Einstein's Theory of Relativity and we can hold our own. But fun for its own sake? The plain truth is that somewhere between family and careers during the last twenty years, most of us have misplaced an essential part of ourselves. Once we begin embarking on solitary sojourns to get reacquainted with our Authentic Selves, we usually discover that something is missing.

It's called zest. Exuberance. *Joie de vivre*, as the French would say, or "the love of life." The great delight that comes when the pieces of our particular puzzle finally fit. The heartfelt happiness we derive when something brings us keen pleasure. Something uniquely our own. They used to call this magical something a hobby.

But what to do? The writer Brenda Ueland tells us that our imaginations need *"moodling*—long, inefficient, happy idling, dawdling and puttering" to flourish.

Perhaps we also need a little personal sleuthing to uncover what solitary pleasures might be fun. It's been so long since we've consciously set aside time solely for rewarding reveries that many of us can't fathom what to do (except, of course, take a nap) when we have a couple of golden hours in which to answer to no one but ourselves. We lose what little leisure time we have available through attrition.

Today, give in to your need for *moodling*. And while you're dawdling and puttering, consider what rewarding reveries you've put aside that brought you pleasure in the past. "How I think about my work is indistinguishable from the way I think about my needlepoint or cooking: here is the project I'm involved in. It is play. In this sense all my life is spent in play—sewing or needlepoint, or picking flowers or writing, or buying groceries," says the American writer Diane Johnson, whose novels often feature heroines revising their lives after moving to Paris.

Once you commit to bringing more of a sense of play into your daily round with authentic personal pursuits, life will begin to take on a harmonious lilt.

JULY 27

Solitary Pleasures

Alone, alone, Oh! We have been warned about solitary vices. Have solitary pleasures ever been adequately praised? Do many people know they exist?

—Jessamyn West (1902–1984)
American Quaker author

Remember, once upon a time, when we all knew how to play? We're going to have to travel back to when we were younger to look for clues.

Did you love to play alone when you were ten? What were your favorite extracurricular activities in high school and during college? Nothing in our past lives is wasted. Nothing that once made us feel happy and fulfilled is ever lost. There's a golden thread that runs through each of our lives. We just need to rediscover this thread before the joy of living completely unravels.

Why not have a brainstorming session to excavate your buried bliss? Write out a quick list of ten solitary pleasures. Don't give this a lot of thought, but don't be dismayed if it takes you a few minutes to come up with something.

Need some help? Well, what was your favorite childhood game? Your favorite sport? Your favorite movie as a kid? Your favorite book? Comic book hero or heroine? Your favorite singer or musical group? What was the best time you ever had as a youngster? As a teenager? As an adult? Can you remember? Can you re-create the memory?

If you could instantly acquire three additional skills, what would they be? Playing the piano? Figure skating? Taking really great photographs?

What three outrageous things would you try if no one knew about it? Belly dancing? Clowning? Hot-air ballooning? What three daring things sound intriguing, even if you'd probably never attempt them? Stand-up comedy? Mountain climbing? Scuba diving?

What three all-expenses-paid vacations appeal to you? An archaeological dig in Egypt? A train trip on the Orient Express? A visit to the Paris haute couture collections? Do you like to work with your hands? Needlecraft? Bookbinding? Gardening? Or does the visual appeal to you? Framing pictures? Working in stained glass? Creating shadow boxes?

Get the idea? There's a fabulous world out there just waiting to be explored. We simply have to be willing to experiment. A hobby affords us a marvelous opportunity to awaken our natural talents. It does require a little bit of effort. First of all we have to figure out what we'd like to do to shake the doldrums. Then we have to carve out time to do it. Alice James, the sister of Henry and William James, believed that in life, "Truly nothing is to be expected but the unexpected." By seeking and finding a solitary pleasure that would make you jump out of bed each morning to pursue it, you'll discover just how right she was.

JULY 28

The Plié of Pleasure

What is your hobby? Every woman ought to have some pet interest in life, outside of the everyday routine which composes her regular occupations. What is yours?
—*The Mother's Magazine*, January 1915

There is a vitality, a life force, an energy, a quickening, that is translated through you into action and because there is only one of you in all time this expression is unique," modern dancer Martha Graham advises us. "And if you block it, it will never exist through any other medium and will be lost."

Where are you blocked? A hobby is a wonderful way to start freeing ourselves creatively. That's because no one expects us to be perfect at a hobby. Hobbies allow us to experiment, to dabble with the paint, the poem, the pot, the plié. When ballet dancers speak of doing pliés, they mean bending their knees. Doing pliés at the beginning of rehearsal warms up the leg muscles before the dance begins. Pursuing a hobby warms up our talents and illuminates our natural inclinations. We get to try on imaginary lives and see how they fit.

Now that you've done some moodling and have discovered some personal pastimes that bring you pleasure, today choose one to pursue. If you need materials such as yarn or paint, make a list of the necessary supplies. Give yourself a week to assemble what you need to get going, and one week from today plan an hour to begin. By doing this, you commit to bringing more fun into your life, and what was once inconceivable will soon become impossible to live without.

JULY 29

The Home as a Hobby

Only a very exceptionally gifted mind could cope singly with all the problems which present themselves in the perfecting of a home.
—Arnold Bennett (1867–1931)
English novelist, playwright, and essayist

One of my new hobbies is my new home. I began to think of my home as a hobby after discovering a delightful series of magazine essays written in 1924 by English novelist, essayist, and playwright Arnold Bennett. Although he is largely forgotten now, Arnold Bennett was once as famous as H. G. Wells and George Bernard Shaw. Bennett's niche was as "everyman," a middle-class neurotic who elevated his neurosis to near-genius by brooding, with wit and wisdom, on the meaning of life, its conundrums, and simple pleasures. One of his best-loved books was *How to Live on Twenty-Four Hours a Day*, an art we all should aspire to master.

In "The Home as a Hobby," Mr. Bennett writes, "The home exists. The home is accepted. Life can be, and is, lived in it. That vase does not suit that mantelpiece. That carpet will not go with that wallpaper...The foot of the bed interferes with the swinging of the bedroom door. The whole of the dining-room furniture is seen to have been a mistake. The hall has a poverty-stricken aspect. The two principal pictures in the drawing-room are too high on the wall. A hundred things are just a little wrong and a few things dreadfully wrong! But no matter. The apparatus somehow works. The desire after perfection has failed. The home has become immutable. There the home is! It will do. It must do."

But for the true artist with real life as his or her canvas, a golden opportunity awaits, says Bennett. "Nobody has the right to be bored in a half-made home. A home which is not a fair expression of us at our best, a home which lacks what it might have, a home which is in any part more ugly or in any part more uncomfortable than it absolutely need be... a home which cannot be run without waste, a home which by any detail gets on the nerves of its inhabitants and so impairs the harmony of their existence—something ought to be done about such a home... Why not make the perfecting of the home a hobby?"

An intriguing proposition. Most of us don't think of fixing up our homes as a pleasurable pursuit because we usually approach it as a feat requiring more physical, psychic, creative, and financial resources than would be necessary to scale the most formidable mountain in the world. This morning, for instance, I would rather go over Niagara Falls in a barrel than tackle the forty-foot container of my belongings that has finally arrived from England with my name on it, waiting for me at the Long Beach Pier.

"Your home may be a small one—most people's homes are—but you will never have finished perfecting it," Arnold Bennett tells us. "The subject is vast and knows no bounds." You know, he just may be right. Perhaps it's time for me to see the contents of that container as the start of a pleasurable hobby instead of a complicated chore. Our attitude is all.

JULY 30

Habits That Steal Precious Moments

I like to do weird things in the shower, like drink my coffee, brush my teeth and drink a smoothie. You don't have to spend time sitting down to eat breakfast. It's good time management.
—Michelle Williams
American actress

Nothing dies harder than a bad habit. Usually we know whenever we're doing something that's not good for us because the small voice that resides in the center of our heads can be a vigilant nag. "Please don't," it will whisper when we light up that cigarette, pour an extra glass of wine, or stand in front of the refrigerator inhaling cold spaghetti because we're nervous. The trouble is, of course, that until now, we haven't been willing to listen.

Before changing any behavior, it's helpful to know why you want to get rid of habits that don't nurture or contribute to your sense of well-being. If you change, what will be your positive payback? A healthier lifestyle, more energy and vitality, the joy and serenity of emotional sobriety, a slimmer body? Going within opens the eyes of your awareness in gentle ways. You find that you're kinder to yourself. As you become more intimate with your Authentic Self and see glimmers of the woman you truly are inside, you shore up the courage to take the first tentative steps necessary to help her evolve and emerge outwardly.

Soon we'll begin hearing whispers that encourage and comfort, not berate us. Then one thirsty evening, instead of automatically reaching for wine while we fix dinner, we'll enjoy a refreshing glass of sparkling mineral water, especially if it's served with lemon in a pretty cut-glass goblet. Instead of the unconscious snacking every time we enter the kitchen, we'll start eating only when we're sitting down and only what's on our plates, especially if we take the time to prepare delicious meals that satisfy the eye as well as our appetites. Instead of impulsively vaping or smoking an e-cigarette to calm our nerves, we'll pick up needlecraft or a crossword puzzle.

Too often we're unaware of the ways in which we rob ourselves of precious moments that could be spent nurturing our creativity. These are unconscious habits that the Surgeon General doesn't warn us about but that our Authentic Selves will. For as long as we continue to cling to bad habits that may not be life threatening but certainly aren't life enhancing, we only steal from our potential.

JULY 31

Do Try This at Home: The Home Front

The main figure in the Home Front is the woman. It is she who must make the stand, rally her family around her like a general, and plant her own feet firmly on the home ground. Everything depends on her wisdom, her enthusiasm, her vision of what home can produce, what home can be.

Harper's Bazaar, May 1942

In October 1939, a month after Germany and England were at war, Jan Struther's collection of her London *Times* essays was published as a book entitled *Mrs. Miniver.* It became an immediate best-seller. For two years English readers had adored Mrs. Miniver's musings in the newspaper. Now at war, her readers were frightened as they watched their own daily rituals disappear. There was a lot to be frightened about: As food was rationed, gas masks were distributed, blackout curtains were hung, and many families experienced evacuations to rural areas, Mrs. Miniver became more than a fictional character. She became their best friend, a sister, a mother, a wife—just like them.

One of the most important concerns for the government was keeping up morale and mobilizing women to consider themselves crucial to sustaining normalcy at the Home Front. Since Mrs. Miniver had boosted her readers' morale during peacetime, she was needed now more than ever.

In July 1940, Jan Struther's Mrs. Miniver crossed the Atlantic. An American edition of *Mrs. Miniver* was published as a Book of the Month Club selection, and it immediately topped the best-seller lists. As America teetered on the edge of joining the war, the powers behind the scenes knew Mrs. Miniver's wartime potential could serve as a similar inspiration for the American public. Those supportive powers included Sir Winston Churchill, President Franklin Roosevelt, Louis B. Mayer, the head of MGM, and the film's eventual director, William Wyler. All of them felt that a domestic drama demonstrating the importance and power of the Home Front could be more influential than a propaganda film depicting battle footage.

However, it was going to take two years before the film version would be ready for distribution. How to keep the fictional Mrs. Miniver's spirit alive to the public in the interim, they wondered? Ysenda Maxtone Graham, Jan Struther's granddaughter, recounts in her biography *The Real Mrs. Miniver:* "During the height of Mrs. Miniver's fame and success during the war, Jan Struther toured America as an unofficial ambassadress for the war effort, giving hundreds of lectures about Anglo-American relations to enchanted audiences. The public wanted to believe that she was the embodiment of her fictional creation—a sensible, calm, devoted wife and mother. She felt it was her wartime duty not to disappoint them."

When we were stocking our Caution Closet with emergency rations last month, our interest was in the easiest way to keep up our strength with protein bars and shakes once we were safely out the door. But woman is not meant to live on protein bars forever.

The good news is that we don't have to look far to find inspiration for delicious eating, because many items that belong in our well-stocked pantry are terrific choices for eating during an emergency. All pantry staples will be canned or vacuum-sealed. Using these suggestions as a guide, think of your emergency food supply as a portable pantry.

Let's concentrate on canned goods. You'll be surprised at how many kinds of foods can be found canned, including:

Canned liquids (think juices such as pineapple, apple, and vegetable)

Canned fruits

Canned vegetables, stews, and soups (this includes bone broth)

Canned beans

Consider who is with you; whom you will need to feed, the age range of your group, and what you like to eat. Pulitzer Prize–winning journalist Julia Moskin, of the *New York Times,* points out in her article "How to Stock a Modern Pantry" that we should only stock what we have the confidence to cook and what we like. As she suggests, "There's no reason to stock black beans if you only like red." If you don't like sardines, you certainly won't be comforted having to eat them during an emergency.

Think of foods that can serve double duty, like tomato paste (which comes in pouches). It can be used in stews, soups, or sauces. Your favorite hot sauce, salt, and pepper should make the list. Most grocery stores have pouches of herbs that will spice up any dish. Above all, take your time with this project, add a few items to your shopping list each week, so the "portable pantry" won't break the budget.

Joyful Simplicities for July

July was the month when summer, like bread in the oven, might change color, but it would rise no higher. It was at its height.
—Jessamyn West (1902–1984)
American Quaker author

- Make the pursuit of happiness real and personal: Hang and wave the flag; find a local parade, and then arrange to get together with friends and family for a barbeque. Watch the fireworks in the evening. Declare your personal independence: Choose to live authentically as a dreamer, not an "expecter."
- Guess what? Those pajama onesies I received from my mother many years ago have made a fashion comeback. Proof positive that if you hold out long enough, the Universe will be impressed. You can find them online at various retailers in a variety of patterns and colors!
- If you have a beach sojourn this month, try to enjoy it at different times: an early morning wander to collect shells before the crowds come, a late afternoon visit to fly kites after they've left. Save one evening for a moonlight walk. If you're not alone, hold hands.

☞ Stand at the water's edge or sit on a towel to gaze out across the water. Just let the rhythm of the waves wash over you. Experience and savor the suspension of time. If you've not yet read Anne Morrow Lindbergh's *Gift from the Sea*, this is the perfect month to do so. Every year I bring this treasured book to the beach with me, and I can tell from the different color of highlighting what I was thinking and feeling. Highlighting a cherished book over the years is like having a secret diary.

☞ Bring home a bottle of sand; place the sand on a tray. If you're in a meditative mood, do your shell searching on the shore to have as a decorative keepsake.

☞ When was the last time (if ever) that you stargazed? If you find yourself somewhere with a clear view of the night sky, take advantage of it. Lie on a blanket with a good bottle of wine or sparkling cider, cheese, crackers, and fresh fruit. Look up into the night sky. Stargazing is one of the oldest human pastimes and there's good reason for it. Gazing at the stars reminds us that there's more to this wonderful world than we'll ever fathom and that every day is another chance to follow the clues. Find a star to wish upon and then choose a wish worthy of your future happiness to make.

☞ During a summer thunderstorm, sit in the middle of your bed in the dark and watch out the window or from a screened-in porch. Experience the beauty and power of Nature unleashed. Now think about harnessing that Power in your life by asking for the Light to be switched on.

☞ While waiting for the potatoes to boil, or lying in a hammock, dip into books with culinary themes, such as the romantic and bittersweet novel *Like Water for Chocolate* by Laura Esquivel; *Crescent* by Diana Abu-Jaber; *Coming to My Senses: The Making of a Countercultural Cook* by Alice Waters; or Jacqueline Deval's *Reckless Appetite: A Culinary Romance*. Especially satisfying is Diane Mott Davidson's delicious series featuring a caterer turned sleuth in *Catering to Nobody*, *Dying for Chocolate*, and *Cereal Murders*.

☞ Arranging a dinner around a film might seem old hat, but not if you pair the cuisine with the film. Enjoy Mexican enchiladas with chocolate molé sauce while watching the sensuous *Like Water for Chocolate;* order Chinese carryout to accompany the delectable *Eat Drink Man Woman;* make French *cuisine de femme* to counterpoint the sumptuous *Babette's Feast;* try a recipe or two from Julia Child's iconic *Mastering the Art of French Cooking* to go with *Julie and Julia;* try your hand at some home sushi making and then check out *Jiro Dreams of Sushi*—or simply binge watch on the lives and inspirations of chefs with Netflix's multi-season series *Chef's Table* or my favorite, *The Great British Baking Show*, the ultimate comfort cooking show. TCM now has a wine club, which pairs movies with wines (www.tcmwineclub.com). It's a fun idea and proves that just a little flourish turns an everyday occasion (watching a movie) into an enjoyable special treat.

To make your cake-baking meditation as inspirational as possible, you might want to take a look at *The Cake Bible* by Rose Levy Birnbaum with its over two hundred suggestions for meditations you'll never forget. Remember, no matter what life throws at us, we can *always* bake a cake.

AUGUST

August is a wicked month.

> —Edna O'Brien
> Celebrated Irish novelist, playwright, and
> short story writer

Aficionados of August revel in relinquishment. When it's one hundred degrees in the shade, it's too hot to be anything but receptive and reflective. Let a seasonally sanctioned sojourn of slow joys refill the authentic reservoir of creative energy. This month on the *Simple Abundance* path we commit to discovering, acknowledging, appreciating, owning, and honoring our authentic gifts, transforming not only our own lives but the lives of those we love.

AUGUST 1

The Harmonic Convergence of an Authentic Life

You mustn't be afraid to dream bigger, darling.

—Christopher Nolan
English filmmaker

Do you remember what you were doing the weekend of August 16–17, 1987? (Were you even born yet?) I don't. However, I was probably folding clothes, thinking about what to have for dinner, changing kitty litter, and trying to make a deadline.

If you do remember, perhaps you were among the more than 144,000 people who journeyed to "power points" around the world, such as Egypt's Great Pyramids; Peru's Machu Picchu; Japan's Mount Fuji; the Temples of Delphi in Greece; Mount Shasta, California; Sedona, Arizona; the Black Hills of South Dakota; and New York's Central Park to hold hands, hum, and "resonate in harmony" in the New Age global event known as the Harmonic Convergence.

What made this weekend so significant was a rare astronomical occurrence known as "a grand trine" (when all nine planets were in their astrological fire signs and positioned exactly one hundred twenty-three degrees apart from one another). It had been 23,412 years since the last one. Now add an esoteric interpretation of ancient Mayan and Aztec calendars and a Hopi legend about a gathering of enlightened teachers meant to awaken humanity, and it's not surprising that thousands of people (at the time they were referred to as New Agers) decided that circumstances were as perfect as they'd ever be to direct the earth, through meditation, toward a peaceful spiritual awakening instead of a cataclysmic one for the next millennium.

Since then, there have been countless books published encouraging spiritual evolution as "the road less traveled" on the inspirational superhighway. With so many voices offering clues, glimmers, and insights on how to achieve harmony through the Divine grand trine of mind, body, and Spirit, how do you discern your own truth? And there are so many spiritual paths. Which one should you follow?

"In undertaking a spiritual life, what matters is simple," American Buddhist master and teacher Jack Kornfield reassures us in his wonderful book *A Path with Heart: A Guide Through the Perils and Promises of Spiritual Life*. "We must make certain that our path is connected with our heart... When we ask, 'Am I following a path with heart?' we discover that no one can define for us exactly what our path should be. Instead, we must allow the mystery and beauty of this question to resonate within our being. Then somewhere within us an answer will come, and understanding will arise. If we are still and listen deeply, even for a moment, we will know if we are following a path with heart."

For me, bearing witness to my Authentic Self is the most joyous and fulfilling spiritual path I have ever followed. It is truly "a path with heart." It began when I acknowledged that creativity is holy. Perhaps this August you might like to convene a personal harmonic convergence with me through rediscovering, recovering, and celebrating your creativity, the sacred conduit to access your Authentic Self. It's never too late to reclaim your individual gifts, resuscitate a dream, create an authentic life. Consider this: what if "original sin" is *denying* instead of *celebrating* your originality?

Each of us possesses an exquisite, extraordinary gift: the opportunity to give expression to Divinity on earth through our everyday lives. When we choose to honor this priceless gift, we participate in the re-creation of the world. When we follow our authentic path with love, embracing our creative impulses, we live truth even if what we think we're doing is just planting a flower bed, cooking a meal, nurturing a child, editing a book, producing a television show, sewing a curtain, writing a business report, painting a picture, composing a song, or closing a deal. As the Vietnamese Buddhist monk, poet, and writer Thich Nhat Hanh reminds us, "Our own life is the instrument with which we experiment with truth."

AUGUST 2

The Gentlest Lessons Teach Us the Most

What a wonderful life I've had!
I only wish I'd realized it sooner.
    —Colette (1873–1954)
     Celebrated twentieth-century French author

All of us know about learning life's lessons through pain, struggle, and loss. But few of us realize that it is often the gentlest lessons that teach us the most.

Many years ago I went to a political convention held at a resort. While my husband attended workshops, Katie—then five—and I played on the beach. One afternoon there was a surprise activity for the children: a ride on an elephant around the hotel parking lot. Katie was delirious with excitement at being able to do this. That night, as I tucked her into bed, I said, "Life is always full of wonderful surprises if we're open to them. Some mornings you wake up not knowing what will happen during the day and you get to ride an elephant!"

A couple of days later we returned home, and awaiting me was an invitation to join a group of American journalists on an all-expenses-paid, weeklong junket to Ireland to cover Dublin's celebration of its millennium.

The group was departing in ten days. Now, there are many things that I am, but spontaneous is not one of them. After I had come up with every conceivable reason to turn down a free trip to my favorite country in the world—my passport was out of date, who would look after Katie, I'd have to juggle my work schedule, I'd just *returned* from a vacation—my husband said quietly, "So you're not going to ride the elephant?" I smiled at his gentle reminder that the important lesson when following a path with heart is the ability to gratefully receive. I went to Dublin and enjoyed one of the most delightful weeks of my life.

If we are willing to learn our lessons gently, they patiently await us in countless ways. Today, try listening to the wisdom of children; accepting the loving-kindness of a friend; reaching out to those in need; asking a colleague for advice; acting on your intuition; laughing at your foibles and frailties and accepting them with love; observing how your pets live so contentedly in the present moment; rediscovering the surprising healing power of spontaneity; focusing on the good in any situation you are now encountering; expecting the best of every day; and realizing what a wonderful life you're living—sooner rather than later.

Of course, the unexpected often catches us by surprise. But if we are open to and grateful for gentle lessons, new teachers will appear in our path. Serendipity can instruct us as much as sorrow.

AUGUST 3

A Net for Catching Days

A schedule defends from chaos and whim. It is a net for catching days...A schedule is a mock-up of reason and order—willed, faked, and so brought into being.
—Annie Dillard
American Pulitzer Prize–winning author

A friend of mine has a theory that it's not so much all we *have* to do in any one week that kills us, it's *thinking* about all we must do.

Alice came to this awareness the week she forgot to attend the annual mothers' volunteering session for her daughter's Girl Scout troop. Being an extremely organized person, she assumed she'd remember it. *No need to write it down.* But she forgot because on that crucial day she experienced scheduling system failure, when all available RAM in her brain's circuitry became overloaded. The next morning, when a sinking feeling in the pit of her stomach awakened her, it was too late. All the easy jobs were gone; only one job remained. Which is how Alice became that year's Girl Scout cookie sales manager.

Here's a *Simple Abundance* strategy—even for the organizationally challenged—to bring more harmony into your life. It will free up those vital memory RAM so you don't end up tracking the sale of Samoas versus Chocolate Thin Mints. Unless, of course, you want to, in which case perhaps you'd like to get in touch with Alice.

Every Sunday take twenty minutes and sit down with your calendar to map out the next six days with a thorough to-do list, then take a preliminary look at the following three weeks.

In order to cast a net that really catches days, you need to consider all the tasks you do in one week, both professional and private. This is not for the fainthearted, but it's crucial. Be of good courage. Here's what we really do each week.

THE UNIVERSAL TO-DO LIST

Work: Meetings, prospecting, marketing/publicity, desk tasks, planning, ordering, billing, reading, researching, writing, traveling, answering phone calls and emails

Errands: Banking, cleaners, post office

Children (if applicable): School, health, lessons, sports, scouts, car pool, clubs, play dates, parties

Appointments: Health, fitness, beauty, car, animals

Shopping: Food, clothing, drugstore, home, gifts, misc.

Correspondence: Emails, bills, letters, texts, cards, and packages

Home: Cleaning, laundry, decorating, improvements, cooking, repairs, entertaining, gardening

Family: Fill in your necessary obligations

Friends: Fill in your necessary obligations

Church/Community: Fill in your necessary obligations

Personal: Inspiration, introspection, rest, recuperation, relaxation, grooming, creative excursions, education, pleasurable pursuits

After doing most of the above in any given week, it seems there'd be no time left for the last and most important category: *you.* The way to solve this real-life dilemma is to move Personal from last to first on your list, making it a top priority as you plan. Here's a radical thought: *Plan your week around you.*

Start by blocking out an hour each day on the calendar—label these windows with your initials as a subliminal code for self-nurturance. I yellow-highlight them as well, because it makes it more important: urgent, inviolate. A meeting with She Who Must Be Obeyed.

The subversive beauty of this method is that once a task is committed to a list, whether it be errands or personal, you don't have to give it another conscious thought, because the left side of your brain—the location of logic—*loves lists.* It goes on automatic pilot when making lists, sorting and shifting until a schedule appears that can accommodate everything. Sometimes it's even manageable. If you ever hope to get it done, write it down.

Scan your list morning and night. When you've completed a task, ceremoniously cross it off. It imparts a great sense of satisfaction to see the list get smaller during the week. If you feel you spend too many days accomplishing little or nothing, keep a "What I've Done" list for a week. This will be a real attention grabber. I'm betting you'll be astonished to discover that you do a lot more than you realize—or give yourself credit for—in one week. And because you do, once again, there's no time for you.

You'll probably also discover that golden moments were unconsciously squandered because there was no net to catch them. Moments to grow, to dream, to nurture your authentic vision. Writer Annie Dillard believes, "How we spend our days is, of course, how we spend our lives." And we all know truth when we hear it.

AUGUST 4

Desire, Ask, Believe, Receive

Difficult times have helped me to understand better than before how infinitely rich and beautiful life is in every way and that so many things that one goes worrying about are of no importance whatsoever.

—Isak Dinesen (1885–1962)
Pen name of Baroness Karen Blixen-Finecke

Are you a worrier? We all are to a certain extent, but some of us are more pessimistic than others, and when *we* worry, it's always the worst possible thing that comes first to mind.

Worrying is a great thief of time. I have a good friend who can soar from distress to disaster in five seconds, and it has caused her no end of sorrow. Now that she recognizes the pattern and can stop herself in midflight with a gentle reminder, she experiences much more inner harmony even under difficult circumstances.

Often when we stew, we think that we're doing something positive about the problem; at least we're thinking about it. Instead, what we're doing is setting off an escalating spiral that can ruin an entire day—for ourselves and those in our vicinity. If you find yourself fretting over an issue that literally you can't do one thing about today, instead of working yourself into a frenzy, just stop. One of the more brilliant time-management secrets shared by Jesus is "Don't worry about tomorrow, tomorrow has enough worries of its own" (Matthew 6:34). And you know what? This advice is spot on. *Mañana*, she comes with her own worries and can't wait to tell you about them.

However, if the upset is too much for you to handle today, can you have a conversation with Spirit? I love the brilliant, compassionate, and extraordinary writer Julia Cameron's suggestion that we should start to think of spiritual intervention in our lives as "Good, Orderly Direction." GOD equals a soul-directed GPS.

Many of the worries that keep us up at night are about money. Julia reminds us that God does finances. "In fact, turning over our finances… to God's care has often been a route not to poverty but to prosperity. God is an expert at husbanding resources. God is an expert at increasing the worth of what we hold. To involve God with our finances is to ask the source of all abundance to have a hand in our affairs."

Do you remember when I told you that now I've started to call anything that appears to be a crisis or is upsetting me a "blessing"? I know, it sounds so counterintuitive. However, in all the inspirational books on my bookshelves, beginning with the Bible, the one constant thread that runs through them all is the power of our *own* words to change our *own* lives.

Did you know that some cars come with an emergency reserve tank of gas that only kicks in when the regular tank is completely empty? That's how we feel in crisis mode when we can see no way out of our current dilemma. We're driving on fumes. Well, I believe that Spirit has endowed each of us with a spare tank of spiritual moxie, and when we call a crisis a blessing, our Soul automatically switches over to the emergency tank. Maybe it's not the blessing we were praying, expecting, or hoping for but there's enough gas in the moxie tank to get us safely home.

"I learned that simply to ask a blessing upon one's circumstances, whatever they are, is somehow to improve them, and to tap some mysterious source of energy and joy," the marvelous spiritual writer Marjorie Holmes confides. "I came upon one of the most ancient and universal truths—that to affirm and to claim God's help even before it is given, is to receive it." Lift up your worries and ask for grace to get through the rest of the day. There is an abundance of amazing grace available to all of us if we simply learn to ask for it.

One of the reasons we worry is because we feel powerless to control our futures. "I have spent most of my life worrying about things that have never happened," Mark Twain admitted at the end of his life. We all do this. So let's stop.

"Desire, Ask, Believe, Receive," Stella Terrill Mann, the mystic and popular spiritual writer during the thirties and forties, advised. Begin praying or rearranging your thinking in that order and you'll understand why she did.

AUGUST 5

The Gift of Sacred Idleness

Work is not always required...there is such a thing as sacred idleness, the cultivation of which is now fearfully neglected.
—George MacDonald (1824–1905)
Scottish novelist, poet, and Christian fantasy writer

It was a gorgeous summer's morning—sunny, but not too hot or humid. The kind of day that should make you feel grateful to be alive. But I was too exhausted to acknowledge the gift. All night I'd tossed and turned, drifting in and out of consciousness but not really sleep. With a work deadline looming, the end of summer camp, another month to go before school resumed, and the need to visit my sick mother, I had new appreciation for what the English poet Stevie Smith meant when she confessed that she was "not waving but drowning."

Letting the cats into the backyard, I stepped outside for a moment. A refreshing breeze rustled the green branches. Sun-dappled patterns of light and shadow created a lovely mosaic on the grass that I'd never noticed before. A natural concerto—birds singing, cicadas chirping, bees buzzing—resonated in the early morning stillness. The hush of harmony hovered around me. I didn't want to leave. Reluctantly I went inside to get a start before Katie woke up.

But the sight of my books and papers sprawled on the floor near my bed where I'd wearily flung them late the night before gave outward expression to my inner chaos and overwhelmed me. I burst into tears.

After I'd had a good cry, the gentle, reassuring voice I have come to know as Spirit suggested that I return to the backyard. Oddly enough, instead of protesting, I did. I spread an old cotton bedspread on the ground, borrowed pillows from the living room, and propped them up against a tall oak tree to create a chaise longue on the earth. Then I carried out a tea tray and my work basket, assuming I was settling outside to write. But when I sat down, all I could bring myself to do was sit quietly and breathe slowly. I didn't want to meditate, have an authentic conversation with anyone, think, create, be clever, or be a conduit. So I just sat there, sipped tea, looked up at the blue sky through the leafy canopy overhead, and observed a butterfly's graceful path through the garden. My surroundings were ordinary, but this morning, so beautiful—so familiar, yet so different.

Within a few minutes my dark mood began to lift. Soon the cats joined me, curious at this unusual detour in the day's rhythm. A little while later, Katie wandered out, still drowsy with sleep, carrying a blanket and pillow to nest and read with us. She asked what I was doing. I told her, for want of a better explanation, that I was conducting research: letting Mother Nature nurture so that I could write a meditation. I invited her to join me.

Because Mom seemed so calm and receptive, she decided to seize the day and asked me to sort through the boxes of her baby memorabilia. Who knew how long this unusual opportunity would last? Well, it lasted for eight lovely, languid, summer hours and included an alfresco lunch as well as a nap. In between laughter, family stories, confidence sharing, animal watching, and dreaming aloud, I did absolutely nothing at all except live and love.

At the end of this simply abundant day of bliss, I realized that I'd been given a restorative gift: sacred idleness. An unexpected, melodic day of undoing to balance the discordant days of doing too much. Like grace, this blessing had come out of the blue; it was completely impractical but necessary, and it was savored with thanksgiving.

AUGUST 6

The Courage to Be Happy

The only difference between an extraordinary life and an ordinary one is the extraordinary pleasures you find in ordinary things.
—Véronique Vienne
French designer, author, and artist

We know what bliss is, even if we can't define it. Because bliss is a spiritual benediction, unbound by limits of language, the best that even sublime writers, such as New Zealand writer Katherine Mansfield, can do is to describe its sensations. In her stunning short story "Bliss," we are privy to Bertha Young's unexplained sensuous seizure of ecstasy. She "wanted to run instead of walk, to take dancing steps on and off the pavement, to bowl a hoop, or throw something up in the air and catch it again, or to stand still, and laugh at—nothing—at nothing, simply."

We often think that happiness and bliss are the same because both induce smiles and laughter. But the smiley face that comes when we're happy is often contingent on external circumstances. Something *happens* outside the normal course of our dreary, repetitive daily routine, and suddenly, life's not so bleak. We get the loan, job, lucky break. We make the deal or set the date. However, if the deal eventually unravels and the wedding doesn't take place, we're not going to be so happy. In fact, because so much of what we call happiness is dependent on the choices of other people, not to mention whims and vagaries of fate, you'd think *happy* and *happened* were derived from the same root word.

They're not.

Bliss doesn't involve other people, places, or things. Bliss is bestowed upon us as a gift of Grace, the whopping, exultant generosity of Spirit carried to wild, reckless, extravagant extremes. Manifesting as visceral sensations of unspeakable joy, moments of bliss often begin with a ripple of quivering that's frankly almost unbearable, unaccustomed as we are to sustained pleasure. When Bertha is overcome with bliss, "She hardly dared to breathe...and yet she breathed deeply, deeply. She hardly dared to look into the cold mirror—but she did look, and it gave her back a woman radiant with smiling, trembling lips, with big, dark eyes and an air of listening, waiting for something...divine..."

Bertha discovers that bliss is the intense awareness of the sensuous in the ordinary, an erotic echo of the everyday. As she arranges a centerpiece for her dining room table, she notices that even the fruit has a "strange sheen" that hadn't been there the day before. Or had it?

"There were tangerines and apples stained with strawberry pink. Some yellow pears, smooth as silk, some white grapes covered with a silver bloom and a big cluster of purple ones. These she had bought to tone in with the new dining room carpet. Yes, that did sound rather far-fetched and absurd, but it was really why she had bought them. She had thought in the shop: 'I must have some purple ones to bring the carpet up to the table.'"

Although down through history, saints, seers, poets, and philosophers have waxed lyrical about the sacred imperative of embracing ecstasy on earth instead of waiting for Heaven, it was the historian, scholar, and world-renowned mythologist Joseph Campbell who popularized the concept of "bliss" in Bill Moyers's landmark television series *The Power of Myth* (1988). "If you follow your bliss, you put yourself on a kind of track that had been there the whole while, waiting for you, and the life that you ought to be living is the one you *are* living."

Campbell was referring to the hero's (or heroine's) quest for desire and fulfillment as a universal theme throughout mythology, romance, religion, and legend. One person who was so utterly influenced by Campbell's work is George Lucas and his creation of *Star Wars*. In acknowledging Campbell's impact upon his work, Lucas admitted that Campbell was "my Yoda."

After the airing of Moyers's interview with Campbell, suddenly, people everywhere were talking about following their bliss—the 1990s version of a harmonic convergence—even if they weren't quite sure what their bliss was. Support groups sprang up, coffee mugs wondered why you were doing other people's taxes if you really wanted to be a jazz singer, and bumper stickers in traffic jams jolted awake the sleeping giant of discontent: *Follow Your Bliss!*

Many people interpreted Campbell's advice as an exhortation to "answer" their calling or "life's work." "If you follow your bliss, doors will open for you," he counseled. And, of course, he's right. It's just that the doors to happiness aren't always found either in the corridors of power or at the ashram. Often the door to bliss leads to your own backyard, which is probably why we immediately disregard it. What? Ordinary bliss? Everyday happiness? That's not what I'm looking for. Precisely.

Like making love, the pursuit of happiness and the rapture of bliss involve intermingling senses. Think fantasia to the seventh degree. And while bliss sometimes calls our name, it's not necessarily our life's work; it could be palpable pleasure beckoning us to try something new, which can lead to a new interest, which then becomes our life's work. Our journey to find our bliss is never as neat as a straight line.

Thankfully, bliss doesn't discriminate against those who decide they must stay with a job they dislike, or in a relationship going through a rough patch. In fact, as Shakespeare observed, often "the contrary bringeth bliss/and is a pattern of celestial peace." I think Will S. means that moments of bliss act as spiritual salve that soothe our souls when our bodies are ravaged, and our minds are at the breaking point from the onslaught of "Breaking News" and we have no bandwidth to cope. It's been my experience that bliss isn't just a Band-Aid, but the Divine Rescue Remedy.

Although bliss, like prayer, is private, peculiar, and deeply personal, because women share the same seven senses (sight, sound, smell, taste, touch, knowing, and wonder), we have similar bliss triggers as well as bliss blockers. One woman's ecstasy might not always be another woman's euphoria (you may not, for example, share my passion for sheep, although I'm at a loss to explain why you wouldn't). Still, I'd hazard a guess that watching the sunset, walking barefoot on the sand, eating a juicy plum, showering outdoors, having an entire day to call your own, and waking up after eight hours of uninterrupted sleep might put a smile on your face as they do mine.

Please notice that these blissful triggers don't require anyone else's presence, nor do they cost money. They only cost your attention. They will, however, require your active willingness to experiment daily with idiosyncratic self-indulgence until you discover that you're smiling a little bit more this month. Tomato sandwiches and margaritas, anyone? Bliss triggers also require that we put the *pursuit* of happiness on the to-do list and make it a priority at least once a week.

How happy are you right now? Yes, the last time I asked this provocative question was seven months ago. Are we making progress? Let's try to muse upon our happiness this summer. The English novelist Fay Weldon's book *What Makes Women Happy* suggests that our bliss triggers are sex, food, friends, family, shopping, chocolate, and love. That's not a bad list to begin with, but I want us to get much more specific. I want to hear about arranging dark purple peonies and pink roses with lilacs in a creamware pitcher, rustling up some garlic parmesan baked scampi, getting out your vintage tea towels hidden away and beginning to use them.

Observe yourself for the next few days. Record fleeting moments of happiness or blissful interludes in your Gratitude Journal. Be courageous. Ask yourself, what is it I truly need to make me happy? And remember, only you know the answer.

AUGUST 7

Bliss Blockers

You look as if you lived on duty and it hadn't agreed with you.
—Ellen Glasgow (1873–1945)
American Pulitzer Prize–winning novelist

The cruelest and most cunning way that we deceive and deny ourselves the benediction of bliss is through the misconception of our duty to others. But "is devotion to others a cover for the hungers and needs of the self, of which one is ashamed?" the French memoirist Anaïs Nin confessed, surely for most of us. "I was always ashamed to take. So, I gave. It was not a virtue. It was a disguise."

We all hide behind masks, and role-playing Lady Bountiful is one of our favorites. What we don't understand is that the most important missing link between gratitude and fulfillment is when the circle of generosity is never completed. Women find it very easy to give goodness and virtually impossible to accept the return goodness with grace. And I'm talking about myself as well.

How do we block bliss? Let us count the ways. Through ignorance, often, although we call our bliss blockers by many aliases. However, the gardening writer Ruth Stout reminds us, "The bliss that comes from ignorance should seldom be encouraged for it is likely to do one out of a more satisfying bliss."

Like our peculiar patterns in making choices and giving out promises, come one, come all, our bliss blocking is highly developed, deeply personal, and very sophisticated self-sabotage. Our left hand barely knows what the right hand has agreed to. Here, I've rounded up the usual suspects; care to look at the rogue habit lineup with me? How many of these soul snatchers do you recognize?

Wanting what you can't have

Not wanting what you do have

Seeing the world as hostile

Believing life is hard

Overreliance on outside circumstances to initiate change

Believing that money is the answer for everything

Believing you're unlucky

Believing that things will never change for the better

Exhaustion

Not eating well

Not exercising

Not listening to your body

Feeling unworthy of happiness, love, success

Not knowing what you love

Not knowing who you are

Not recognizing addictive behavior patterns or dependence

Workaholism in the name of getting ahead or staying on top of things

Perfectionism

Lack of humor

Inability to laugh at oneself

Shyness in social situations

Lack of spontaneity

Thinking you're too inexperienced

Pretending that you're more experienced than you are

Believing the world will fall apart if you're not holding it together

Inability to ask or receive help

Inability to be part of a team

Inability to say no gracefully

Needing to please

Seeing everything as competitive

Confusing being argumentative with being articulate

Always needing to be right

Putting others down so you can feel superior

Not trusting your intuition

Not pursuing your dreams

Making promises you dread

Making promises you know you won't or can't keep

Making promises just to keep the peace

Thinking that worrying will make it better

Inability to relax

When I first assembled this list, I found it quite amazing to think that all these bliss blockers had become so familiar that I barely even noticed them. But as Hannah More wrote in 1811 in a little tract entitled *Self Love*: "The ingenuity of self-deception is inexhaustible." This week just pick one bliss blocker. (Start with the one that made you wince when you read it. They all made me wince when I assembled them.) See if you can't exchange these controlling habits with a little kindness toward yourself.

Eighth Day of Creation: Honoring
Our Personal Gifts

Explore daily the will of God.
—Carl Jung (1875–1961)
Swiss psychiatrist and psychoanalyst

Martin Buber, the great Jewish philosopher, told a story about a Hasidic *tzaddick*, or enlightened master, named Rabbi Zusya, who often pondered whether he was living an authentic life: "If they ask me in the next world, 'Why were you not Moses?' I will know the answer. But if they ask me, 'Why were you not Zusya?' I will have nothing to say."

How well we'll hold up our end of this revealing conversation is what begins to interest us now, as the fourth *Simple Abundance* Grace— Harmony—starts to stir within our souls. Discerning our personal gifts is essential if we are to experience Harmony in our lives. "Because our gifts carry us out into the world and make us participants in life, the uncovering of them is one of the most important tasks confronting any one of us," Elizabeth O'Connor writes in the *Eighth Day of Creation: Discovering Your Gifts*. "When we talk about being true to ourselves— being the persons we are intended to be—we are talking about gifts. We cannot be ourselves unless we are true to our gifts."

However, it's difficult to be true to our gifts if we don't know what they are. And while masters, mystics, saints, sages, poets, and philosophers have borne witness to the authentic path down through the ages, many of us have tuned out. Why? I believe it's because the lesson of authenticity is often prefaced with the four most terrifying words known to humans: *The Will of God*. Divine Will is frequently associated with suffering, so it's no wonder many of us choose—consciously or not—to slip into a spiritual abyss of unknowing. Trust God? Trust Divine Providence? Been there, done that. Thanks, but no. Prefer to go it alone.

But even in the black hole of doubt, we want to believe that a Force greater than our own power or understanding is with us. And it is. The Force is with our Authentic Self. As Obi Wan Kenobi tells Luke Skywalker in *Star Wars*, "The Force is an energy field created by all living things. It surrounds us, it penetrates us, it binds galaxies together."

The Force binds your dreams and desires with your personal gifts so they can find outward expression. "Follow your feelings, trust your feelings," the Jedi knight urges us all, because it is within the Force that we live and move and have our being.

The Force is Love.

Love wants, wishes, and wills nothing less than your *unconditional* happiness, harmony, Wholeness.

Commit this month to discovering, acknowledging, appreciating, owning, and honoring your personal gifts.

And the Force will be with you.

AUGUST 9

Calling Forth Our Gifts

Do not weep; do not wax indignant. Understand.
—Baruch Spinoza (1632–1677)
Dutch Jewish Philosopher

You long to call forth your gifts. To explore your talents. To discover and recover your creativity. But where do you begin? You begin by offering an open heart and a willingness to serve.

"The artist is a servant who is willing to be a birthgiver," writer Madeleine L'Engle tells us in *Walking on Water: Reflections on Faith and Art.* "I believe that each work of art, whether it is a work of great genius, or something very small, comes to the artist and says, 'Here I am. Enflesh me. Give birth to me.' And the artist either says, 'My soul doth magnify the Lord,' and willingly becomes the bearer of the work, or refuses."

Madeleine L'Engle certainly knew what she was talking about. Her young adult science fiction novel *A Wrinkle in Time* was rejected more than twenty-six times before it was published in 1963. It would take another half century before it became a film and was read around the world. She speaks elegantly of the despair an artist feels when their work is rejected in her memoir *The Circle of Quiet*. My personal rejection ritual that Madeleine inspired: Cry your eyes out, have an argument with the Great Creator as loud as you need, drink a tumbler of an Irish whiskey called Writer's Tears, and go to bed. In the morning, offer thanks that you're still here and can have another go with a full tank of moxie. You are a servant of the work. You are not allowed to judge it. Your task is to do it. Every day, especially on those days when your heart is broken, we have to go to work. Ask Lady Gaga, who says, "As artists, we are eternally heartbroken."

Blessed be the writer who has no publisher rather than one whose publisher doesn't get the book you're writing and, more importantly, doesn't get you. If this is happening to you, someday, many years down the road, you'll thank me for this advice. Many, many years down the road.

When we call forth our gifts, whether we serve is entirely our choice. The Great Creator's first gift to us is free will, which distinguishes mortals from the angels, who—after having seen the glory—joyfully exchanged free will for the passion of serving. Being higher than the angels, we can have the best of both worlds: free will *and* the passion of serving. Perhaps one day we'll realize it's *not* the will of God we need fear as much as being left to our own deceits and devices. We can always say no to the next *Harry Potter, Gone with the Wind,* or an idea for a historical doll series called American Girl.

"Sorry, find someone else."

And Spirit will.

To be fair, sometimes we don't literally use those words. Sometimes we say, "Sorry, I just can't get my act together right now. Come back later."

So the Great Creator moves on until a willing artist with an open heart offers to become the creative conduit.

This scenario goes a long way toward explaining why you are even more heartbroken, stunned, bewildered, and furious when, after diddling around for years, someone else takes out a patent on an infant carrier that resembles the one you made for your first baby; or the woman who cut off the feet on her irritating pantyhose and invents a new shapewear called Spanx. Didn't you do that? What ever happened to that tape of your Aunt Toby's stories about working in New York advertising during in the sixties? She was so funny! Weren't you going to try to make them into a television series?

Now, I don't mean that someone else has literally ripped off your exact book, design, name, or recipe. What I'm talking about occurs when someone else introduces into the world a creative idea so like yours it makes you dizzy. You feel crushed, but you're also freaked. How on earth could this be possible unless somebody read your mind?

Well, it wasn't *your* mind that was tapped. It was Divine Mind. Remember, before anything exists on earth, it exists fully formed in Spirit. The Great Creator does not play favorites; each of us came into being to carry on the re-creation of the world through our gifts.

And while you are offered many dazzling opportunities in a lifetime, Spirit only comes once for each Work seeking creative expression through you, then moves on. The bottom line is that the Work must be brought forth. If you don't do it, someone else will.

So when that great idea flashes across your mind surrounded by neon lights, pay attention! Once it exists in your mind, realize that other brainwaves soon will be able to pick up the creative energy pattern if they are receptive. Think of your mind as a satellite dish. Creative celestial messages are continuously being transmitted. The frequency is jammed—privy to your soul only—for an infinitesimal, proprietary moment. Just long enough for you to lift up your heart, accept the assignment, and give thanks.

Is the idea absolutely fabulous? Can you see it completely finished in your mind's eye? Does it take your breath away? Novelist Gail Godwin tells us that "Some things…arrive in their own mysterious hour, on their own terms and not yours, to be seized or relinquished forever."

So for God's sake—and your own—please just say, "Yes."

AUGUST 10

Second Thoughts

Whatever you can do or dream you can, begin it;
Boldness has genius, power and magic in it.
—Johann Wolfgang von Goethe (1749–1832)
German writer and statesman

Today you realize how blessed you are. In secret you nurture the nascent dream—the work entrusted to you for safekeeping—in the sanctuary of your soul. In quiet moments you overflow with excitement at the golden possibilities that stretch endlessly before you. Because happiness is the most difficult emotion to bear alone, you confide your dream to your partner, best friend, lover, sister, mother, children.

Their lack of enthusiasm hits you at point-blank range. Now the "for your own good" litany pours forth, a tsunami of discouragement: You're too old, too overextended to try something new right now, too broke, too inexperienced. You don't have the resources, the talent, the contacts, or one chance in a million to bring this dream to fruition.

Oh, really? Can we consider the track record of your naysayers? How many dreams have *they* successfully brought into the world?

I thought so. *Please* be careful about confiding your sacred dreams, especially in the first trimester after creative conception—the period that the nineteenth-century Danish philosopher and theologian Søren Kierkegaard called the "dreaming consciousness" prior to creation. A disgruntled dreamer is a risky mentor. Never seek somebody's advice if you even *suspect* you know what they'll say. You cannot afford to hear the negative tape again.

Second thoughts have aborted more dreams than all the difficult circumstances, overwhelming obstacles, and dangerous detours destiny ever could throw at you. Undermining your authenticity by succumbing to someone else's second thoughts is a sinister, subtle, and seductive form of self-abuse. Few of us are immune to the opinions of others. We need to learn how to dispassionately assess the advice, ponder the source, weigh the opinion. If the information is insightful and is something you hadn't considered, retain it. If it's destructive criticism, let it go. End your conversation politely but firmly. Better yet, in the future, don't even start it.

"I made a conscious decision not to tell anyone in my life," admits Sara Blakely, that savvy woman who cut the feet off her pantyhose twenty years ago and is now a self-made billionaire. "Now I tell people—don't tell anyone your idea until you have invested enough of yourself in it that you are not going to turn back. When a person has an idea at that conception moment, it is the most vulnerable—one negative comment could knock you off course."

William Hutchinson Murray, the deputy leader of the Scottish Himalayan expedition team that scaled Mount Everest in 1951, urges the dreamer in you to take a leap of faith: "Concerning all acts of initiative (and creation), there is one elementary truth, the ignorance of which kills countless ideas and splendid plans; that the moment one definitely commits oneself, then Providence moves too. All sorts of things occur to help one that would never otherwise have occurred. A whole stream of events issue from the decision, raising in one's favor all manner of unforeseen incidents and meetings and material assistance which no man could have dreamed would have come his way."

AUGUST 11

The Great Collaboration

We can't take any credit for our talents. It's how we use them that counts.

—Madeleine L'Engle (1918–2007)
American writer of young adult fiction and memoirist

Don't worry that your talent won't be adequate to the task. Spirit always assigns possible servants of work *perfectly* suited to our personal gifts, even if we beg to differ. A low opinion of our abilities is a handy cop-out when facing creative challenges, but the Great Creator is on to us by now. Feeling inadequate to the task we're asked to do seems to be a spiritual prerequisite.

Anyway, our degree of talent is a moot point, because the Work *always* knows more than we do—a fact for which we can all be eternally grateful. Agreeing to serve really means just showing up to make the calls, mix the paint, boot up the laptop, pluck the strings, shape the pot, fill the blank page, and then get out of the way.

We do not create in a vacuum. Art is a Divine collaboration, a sacred covenant between the artist and the Great Creator. Inspired artists, the ones who write the books you can't put down, pen the poems you must memorize, paint the pictures you can't walk away from, and compose the music you must listen to repeatedly are the first ones to admit it.

The great Italian composer Giacomo Puccini confessed that his opera *Madame Butterfly* "was dictated to me by God; I was merely instrumental in putting it on paper and communicating it to the public." Harriet Beecher Stowe swore that it was "Another Hand" writing through her at the kitchen table—in between caring for six children, cooking, and sewing—because she never knew what was going to come next in *Uncle Tom's Cabin*. George Frideric Handel believed he was hallucinating for twenty frenzied days as he composed *The Messiah*: "I did think I did see all Heaven before me, and the great God Himself."

Painters from Piet Mondrian to Hilma af Klint have viewed their role as channels. Robert Motherwell knew that to let the brush take over was the surest way to render the vision on canvas: "It will stumble on what one couldn't do by oneself." And one of the world's most savvy creative geniuses, Steve Jobs, confessed, "Creativity is just connecting things. When you ask creative people how they did something, they feel a little guilty because they didn't really do it, they just saw something. It seemed obvious to them after a while."

And once *you* begin to nurture Divinity's dream—with your creativity, craft, courage, discipline, devotion, discernment, energy, enthusiasm, emotion, intelligence, imagination, inventiveness, passion, perseverance, patience, skill, sweat, savvy, tenacity, tears, and tantrums—you will *grow* into your talent. What's more, you'll be astonished at what the Great Artistic Alliance accomplishes, for now you know and trust that the Force is with you.

The world needs your gift as much as you need to bestow it. May Sarton warns us that "The gift turned inward, unable to be given, becomes a heavy burden, even sometimes a kind of poison. It is as though the flow of life were backed up."

When you remember that you're not creating alone, the Flow can't be stopped.

The Artist's Way: Tuning to the Higher Harmonic

Become willing to see the hand of God and accept it as a friend's offer to help you with what you are doing.

—Julia Cameron
Author, artist, teacher

Many of us wish we were more creative. Many of us sense we *are* creative, but unable to effectively tap that creativity. Our dreams elude us. Our lives feel somehow flat. Often, we have great ideas, wonderful dreams, but are unable to actualize them for ourselves," Julia Cameron concedes in her peerless *The Artist's Way: A Spiritual Path to Higher Creativity.* "Sometimes we have specific creative longings we would love to be able to fulfill—learning to play the piano, painting, taking an acting class, or writing. Sometimes our goal is more diffuse. We hunger for what might be called creative living—an expanded sense of creativity in our business lives, in sharing with our children, our spouse, our friends."

Many of us have unconsciously erected seemingly insurmountable barriers to protect ourselves from failing or succeeding. We may think we're protecting ourselves by ignoring or denying our creative impulses, but really all we're doing is burying our Authentic Selves alive.

However, as you slowly learn to remove the rubble of opinions and judgments of others (including your own internal censor) and exchange a limiting, toxic interpretation of a miserly, mean-spirited God for what Julia calls the "good, orderly direction" of a loving and supportive Great Creator, not only will you encounter the inner artist, but you'll come to respect your art as a powerful, personal form of worship.

"Once you accept that it is natural to create, you can begin to accept a second idea—that the Creator will hand you whatever you need for the project," Julia reassures us. "The minute you are willing to accept the help of this collaborator, you will see useful bits of help everywhere in your life. Be alert: there is a higher harmonic, adding to and augmenting your inner creative voice."

Spirit speaks to you constantly throughout the day. You may experience a hunch, perk up at the suggestion of a friend, or follow an urge to try something new on a whim. Train your heart to listen. Today, adjust your spiritual satellite. Tune in to the higher harmonic frequency for help as you continue your authentic, artistic pilgrimage to Wholeness.

Artist of the Everyday: Creating a Life That Works

But if you have nothing at all to create, then perhaps you create yourself.

—Carl Jung (1875–1961)
Swiss psychiatrist and psychoanalyst

The other day a friend and I were talking about the difficulty that most of us have in grasping the concept that we are artists—that life is our canvas. She confessed that she had no domestic skills and didn't think of herself as a particularly creative person. I adamantly disagreed. I believe with all my heart that the ability to bring forth art from real life is a gift every woman possesses. Whether we choose to nurture this perfectly natural endowment is quite another matter. Admittedly, the concept is almost impossible to register when we're exhausted, overwhelmed, and frazzled. But it's certainly worth meditating on as we savor the last days of summer.

You may not draw, paint, sculpt, sew, knit, sing, dance, or act, but baking a cake *could* be as much a work of art as choreographing a ballet, if you approach it with as much dedication. So is coaxing a tired, hungry toddler (with infinite patience and persuasion) to do whatever it is you need them to do at a given moment. So is graciously entertaining unexpected company with what's on hand and turning it into a memorable feast with candlelight, wine, laughter, and lively conversation. So is helping a friend through a personal crisis, comforting an aging parent, or planning a preteen's birthday party. Whatever you're about to do today *can* be transformed into art, if your heart is open and you're willing to be the Great Creator's conduit. Women are Artists of the Everyday. The world does not acknowledge or applaud everyday art, so we must. We are the keepers of a sacred truth. We must cherish this wisdom and pass it on to those we love.

As an artist I have come to know that there are three very different layers to creation: the labor, the craft, and the elevation. St. Francis of Assisi explains the creative process this way: The woman who works with her hands only is a laborer; the woman who works with her hands and her head is a craftswoman; the woman who works with her hands, her head, and her heart is an artist.

Labor in creation is showing up to do the work. Craft is *how* you go about doing it. Are you there in mind, body, and spirit? Are you taking your time or are you rushing? Are you concentrating on whatever it is you are doing or thinking about twenty other things that need to be done?

Let's take baking a cake and its elevation to an art. Do you just throw the flour, eggs, butter, sugar, and salt into a bowl all at once, stir the lumpy mess with a flick of your wrist, stick it in the oven, and hope for the best?

Or do you sift the flour three times, beat the eggs, cream the butter and sugar together before you combine them? Do you spend fifteen minutes stirring the batter? Do you preheat the oven, grease and flour the pan? Do you hum while you're doing it, enjoying the process of creating, as well as the anticipation of the product? If you do, Love is present. Love is the spiritual energy that induces elevation—the transcendent moment in creation when craft becomes art.

It takes a lifetime to create the work of art for which we were born: an authentic life. But it only takes five minutes to center yourself before you begin each new task today. Five minutes to acknowledge in your soul that you are an Artist of the Everyday. Five minutes to give thanks for your personal gifts. Five minutes to offer your love, creative energies, and enormous talents to the person, idea, or project awaiting your attention.

So say it with me and say it aloud: *I am a brilliant, gifted Artist of the Everyday. My art is a blessing for me and mine.*

AUGUST 14

The Courage to Create

Now for some heartwork.

—Rainer Maria Rilke (1875–1926)
Twentieth-century German poet

Write the truest sentence you know," Ernest Hemingway encourages the writer in you. Paint the truest image you can render. Wait all day with camera poised to capture the five-second sliver of light. Express the rage and range of raw emotion through your dialogue. Convey passion's power with the curve of your dancer's body honed through discipline and denial. Set the angel free when you carve. Make the heavens weep when you compose.

But in order to be true to a creative work, the artist must journey to the center of the self. Past the conscious sentries in the brain, beyond the barbed wire barricades of the heart, into the trenches of "truth or dare." You can't write a true sentence or live authentically if you don't trust yourself. You can't trust yourself without courage.

Let's pause a moment to ponder about courage—our own courage—because that's what we're going to have to count upon as we take our leap into the future. The word *courage* comes from the same stem as the French word *coeur*, meaning heart. As a woman, you give from you heart in all that you do. Spirit returns to you in equal measure "courage" as needed in a continuous flow of blessings—from your heart to the hearts of others and from their hearts to yours. This is an essential life-affirming Divine exchange that transcends time and space.

You might not be aware of these blessings, but they are continuously working on your behalf, an unseen force acting in your life as gravity does on the earth. This understanding is so important as we continue our sojourn together, especially if you think you have no new ideas, opportunities, or energy with which to start over as an Artist of the Everyday. My go-to mantra when I feel like that is "Nobody can take your future away." Let's create our futures together.

I know it requires courage. Here's my take on that: Courage is the mystical alchemy of priceless experience, savvy wisdom, fortitude's savoir-faire, intrepid intelligence, and the pluck of intuitive daring. "Courage," as the American poet Karle Wilson Baker originally wrote in 1921, "is Fear that has said its prayers."

And after those prayers, we're blessed with the only kind of courage that matters, as the 1950s essayist Mignon McLaughlin confessed: "The kind that gets you from one moment to the next."

These definitions of courage work for me, every minute, every hour, every day, every page. How about you? Always remember, never forget, when it comes to talent and transformation, which are among Gratitude's blessings: *First the gesture, then the Grace.*

So how do we do that? By showing up. Day in, day out. And giving thanks. By not judging how it's going. If it's going at all, that's enough. You can't afford to think about how the Work will be received when you're finished. That's not your job. Remember, we're learning to surrender the delivery details of our dreams. Our job, then, is just to do it. It can't be published, produced, performed, or purchased if it doesn't exist.

Consider this: What if the woman who wrestles with God but doesn't live to tell the tale is the one who refuses to create a work of art. Worse yet, an authentic life? What if the fatal wound, the one from which we never recover, is regret? Today it's time for authentic "truth or dare." Dare yourself to believe in your creativity, wherever it may take you. Trust that where it leads is exactly where you're supposed to be. Your Authentic Self knows where you're headed. Don't wrestle with Spirit. Collaborate with It.

AUGUST 15

Sometimes Ignorance Is Bliss

Ignorance gives one a large range of probabilities.
—George Eliot (1819–1880)
Pen name of celebrated Victorian novelist
Mary Ann Evans

Trust me, you don't want to know. Ignorance is a protective blessing. Do you want to know that one month after your hard-won promotion your company will go belly up? Do you want to know that you won't get the grant, that it will be your third novel that gets published first, that your film acting debut will end up on the cutting-room floor, or that none of your artisanal donuts will sell at next week's farmers' market?

I don't think so. "Ever tried? Ever failed? No matter," Samuel Beckett insists. "Try again. Fail again. Fail better." Would you fight for the promotion, apply for the grant, attend the audition, rent the commercial oven, if you knew that failure always precedes success? Failure is a crucial part of the creative process. Authentic success arrives only after we have mastered failing better.

Another thing we don't need to know is just how much we took on when we accepted the artistic assignment. "I must frankly own, that if I had known, beforehand, that this book would have cost me the labour which it has, I should never have been courageous enough to commence it," Isabella Beeton confessed about her *Book of Household Management*, written in 1861—a book that has yet to go out of print.

There's a reason Isabella Beeton was kept in the dark, as we all are when creating. If we ever had an inkling of the intense labor required to bring the Work into the world, we'd be out of here.

When the visitation comes, it's the razzle-dazzle of golden possibilities that seduces us. Ignorance is part of Infinite Intelligence's inviting come-hither. Why else are heavenly encounters accompanied by brilliant, blinding Light? Because we're not supposed to see too far ahead. We're not supposed to know. Don't forget that the forbidden fruit in the Garden of Eden was from the Tree of Knowledge.

In the military and high-tech industries, there is a qualifying code assigned to information: "Need to know." If you can do your job effectively without knowing the big picture, you're kept in the dark. All we need to know is that Spirit knows what we don't. If we get out of the way, we'll be shown the next step, including how not to sell ourselves short as we gracefully grow into our gifts.

You Can't Be Original—You Can Be Authentic

Whatever your passion is, keep doing it. Don't waste time chasing after success or comparing yourself to others. Every flower blooms at a different pace. Excel at doing what your passion is and only focus on perfecting it. Eventually people will see what you are great at doing, and if you are truly great, success will come chasing after you.

—Suzy Kassem
American poet and philosopher of Egyptian heritage

One of the reasons many of us have trouble getting our Work out into the world is that unconsciously we're competing instead of creating, which always short-circuits the flow of inspiration. A friend of mine is a gifted playwright. She denies herself the pleasure of seeing anything on the stage other than revivals of classics, preferably Greek. It's too painful for her to watch contemporary work because she is addicted to comparisons.

Why do we make ourselves sick competing against strangers? I believe it's just another sophisticated, seditious form of self-sabotage. If we don't measure up, why even try? The fault line of comparison runs so deep in the lives of many of us it's heartbreaking.

Thirty years ago, when I published my first book, which updated Victorian family traditions for modern families, there were few popular books on the Victorian era available. But within two years, the late nineteenth century was the hottest thing and the market was completely saturated. Today it would be extremely difficult to find a commercial publisher for a Victorian book even if you channeled Queen Victoria as a spirit guide. This doesn't mean if you're writing one that you should stop. The cycle of creation is cyclical. There's a reason the past is prologue.

Sometimes you're ahead of your time. Mozart was known to qualify his genius by declaring he was composing for future generations. There are literally millions of aspiring and working artists writing books, publishing poems, selling scripts, directing movies, auditioning for roles, designing clothes, entering juried craft exhibitions, creating start-ups, looking for an agent, praying for a lucky break. *Don't panic.* It is impossible for you to be an original. But you *can* be authentic.

Once you accept an artistic assignment from the Great Creator, it's yours. Nobody can take it away from you, unless, of course, you relinquish it. Others can imitate, but they can't duplicate what you do, because there's no one in the world like you. Your work is born of your sensibilities, temperament, experience, emotion, passion, perseverance, attention to detail, idiosyncrasies, and eccentricities.

When you're authentic, so is your art.

AUGUST 17

Taking on Quite a Task

A record deal doesn't make you an artist; you make yourself an artist.

—Lady Gaga
American songwriter, singer, actress

I had a difficult time after my first book was published because it was impossible for me to believe that I had written a successful book, especially since I had created a character who had a life of her own.

Fictional though she was, my character, Mrs. Sharp, was the storybook mother we all longed to have, and if we have children of our own, the mother we all try to be. It was frequently pointed out that this "perfect" Victorian mother was my alter ego, but I passionately denied it. To my way of thinking, Mrs. Sharp was everything I clearly was not: serene, incurably optimistic, and deeply spiritual. Her life was harmonious because she successfully managed the delicate balance of living in the world yet remaining apart from it. She lived each day to the fullest with a deep appreciation of the past, an enriched sense of the present, and a joyous anticipation of the future. Her home was a haven of hospitality, reflecting her authentic style in its beauty, order, comfort, and good taste. She was a compassionate confidante and true friend, who empathized, encouraged, and inspired. I adored Mrs. Sharp and so did many other women.

How could I claim to be this extraordinary woman's alter ego? I came closest as her amanuensis, someone who takes down dictation. Good or bad, the book was Mrs. Sharp's. But by distancing myself I was unable to bask in the accomplishment of its creation, although it represented five years of work and struggle. I graciously accepted compliments, praise, even gratitude for having written it. But inside I was the bewildered go-between, always looking over my shoulder to see if there was another woman behind me who really deserved the compliments. Having achieved a long-sought dream, I wondered why I felt so empty, unfulfilled, and confused.

A couple of years later I was having a heart-to-heart with my sister.

Throughout our conversation, unconsciously I kept referring to Mrs. Sharp. "Stop this," Maureen said gently but firmly. "Stop referring to Mrs. Sharp as if she's a separate person. You're Mrs. Sharp, even if you don't believe it. She is who you are deep within. You have got to start owning your talent or you'll lose it."

My sister believed that my discontent came from my refusal to accept responsibility for my talent. I wouldn't "own" my talent, as in "claim it." Nor would I "own up," as in "admit to," the truth that I was an artist even if I lived in a suburban home and not a New York loft. I credited myself only with being a diligent wordsmith who worked very hard at creating viable sentences, paragraphs, pages, columns, features, finished books. By minimizing my value, I had bludgeoned my identity as an artist with the blunt instrument of disbelief, then buried my Authentic Self with denial.

But *why* didn't I own my talent? This is a question I asked myself for years. Perhaps it was because if I failed, I would have to own any failure as much as any success, and I didn't want to "fail better" anymore. I wanted to live a creative life. I believed my creativity could only be owned if the world acknowledged that I possessed it. I had many lessons to learn before acknowledging that Spirit had used my personal gifts to give outward expression to something that would not have existed if I had refused to take up my pen. And, having accepted the Great Creator's assignment and run with it, I had both the right and obligation to own—and to share—the work that resulted. So do you.

AUGUST 18

Owning Your Talent

Each time I write a book, every time I face that yellow pad, the challenge is so great. I have written eleven books, but each time I think, "Uh, oh, they're going to find out now. I've run a game on everybody and they're going to find me out."
—Maya Angelou (1928–2014)
American poet, memoirist, and civil rights
activist

Perhaps because I so often felt like a fraud, authenticity decided I'd be the perfect host. "Explore me," she whispered. "Peer behind the curtain. Look under the rock. See who's really there." Believe me, I had no inkling when I started *Simple Abundance* that I was embarking on a safari to discover my Authentic Self. I thought I was writing a lifestyle book on downshifting and getting rid of clutter.

Many artists feel they'll be "found out," sooner or later—and probably sooner. For when we create, although we know that a Higher Power works with us and through us, the Work comes into the world with our name on it. This is the artist's struggle. If we don't create, we snuff out the Divine Spark. If we do create, we feel we're showing a false face to the world because we know we didn't do it alone, even if nobody else does.

But the struggle stops once we cease denying our talent and become willing to own it—humbly, gratefully, and respectfully—and then *share* it with the world. If we're not exploiting our gifts only for our own good, we're covered.

In a New Testament parable, a rich man is about to go on a journey, so he entrusts to three of his servants "talents" of money. The first servant is given five talents, the second, two, and the last, one. The first servant immediately puts his talents to work and doubles his owner's investment, as does the servant with two talents. The servant with one talent, however, is afraid of the responsibility, so he buries his talent in the ground.

When the rich man returns, his servants are called for an accounting of their work. Both servants who have increased their talents receive praise for their efforts. They have done wonderfully, so they're invited to share in their master's happiness.

Now the third servant arrives to explain that because the rich man is such a hard taskmaster, he thought it better to play it safe by burying his talent so that nothing would happen to it. The master is so enraged that the fool didn't possess the common sense to deposit the money in the bank, where at least it could have collected interest, that he angrily seizes it back and gives it to the most successful servant. The master then says, "For everyone who has will be given more and he shall have an abundance."

The cautious servant is thrown out into the darkness where he begins weeping, wailing, and gnashing his teeth—and with good reason. It hurts like hell when the world won't invest in you. But it's excruciating, almost more than you can bear, when you don't believe and invest in yourself.

This is a parable about creative risk. We feel sorry for the servant who buried his talent because, as Elizabeth O' Connor points out, "his cautious, protective measures seem very reasonable." The master comes off as a thug, throwing the poor soul into darkness without comfort or pity just because he's played it safe. Since most of us do play it safe in life, this story makes us very nervous.

It's meant to.

Many of us squander our precious natural resources—time, creative energy, emotion—comparing the size of our talents to those of others.

Today, ask Spirit to call forth your authentic gifts, so that you might know them, acknowledge them, and own them.

Do you want to live more abundantly? Have you buried your talents? How can we live richer, deeper, and more passionately if we aren't willing to invest in ourselves? Many of us have played it safe for too long and wonder why we are miserable.

Because playing it safe is the riskiest choice we'll ever make.

AUGUST 19

Back to the Future

*The initial Mystery that attends any journey is
how did the traveler reach [her] starting
point in the first place?*

—Louise Bogan (1897–1970)
American Poet Laureate

What comes to mind when you hear the phrase "spiritual journey"? Many people immediately think of difficult lessons, painful realizations, heartbreaking sacrifices, or the frustrations and abject loneliness of unanswered prayers. I've had all of them, which I collectively call my "intimate conversations with the ceiling." But difficult lessons and unanswered prayers are part of life's required course, so it's easier for me to search for a tiny Divine hallmark in a challenge or difficulty, much as a jeweler might mark gold or silver. The Holy Grail of our seeking is our authentic destiny.

I was born into an Irish Catholic family, which means I was born into a world of black and white and veils of one kind or another. Every Sunday—religiously, as one would say—we went to mass. However, after the Latin mass and frankincense were exchanged for American English and folk music in 1965, I felt as if I had been born into the wrong side of the aisle. I found peace in the mystery, wonder, beauty, and awe of ritual; reverence in words that I might not understand but responded to in my heart and soul on the deepest level.

Of course, I attended Catholic high school during the mid-sixties, when the word *vocation*—from the Latin *vocare*—meaning "to call"— was frequently heard as synonymous with entering a religious community. I was distressed that this was suggested as the ultimate life path because I really wanted to be an actress. My future was to be found in the theater or the movies. Good gracious, I had a dozen stage names by the time I turned twelve. Then, like most teenage girls at that time,

I also *knew* that someday I would be swept off my feet by a handsome man, get married, have a big family, and live happily ever after in Great Neck, New York.

I must confess that, while dead set on becoming an actress, I found the notion of being "chosen" by God very magnetic, even hypnotic. I also thought the nuns' black-and-white habits were incredibly romantic. How much I was influenced by Audrey Hepburn in *The Nun's Story* (1959), I can't really say, except that Sister Luke pushed every emotional button I had. Hepburn was playing a young woman who enters the convent to become a missionary nursing sister in the Belgian Congo during the 1920s. She is *so certain* of her path, until she isn't, and you just know what's coming even when you don't. I love watching favorite movies every decade or so, because it's always a different film than the one my younger self remembers. I wish one didn't have to grow older to become wiser, but there you have it.

Well, as I stated emphatically to my parents and Mother Superior, my life was going to be on the stage. The way I figured it, the theater was about as far away from God as I could get. Do you want to know how to make the angels laugh? Tell Heaven *your* plans.

So I went to New York and discovered that there was the Actors' Chapel at St. Malachy's Roman Catholic Church. Hmm. Then I traveled to London seeking my fame and fortune and found the Actor's Church at St. Paul's Covent Garden (Anglican). I also discovered that the theater and church share a passion for language. I love the language of the King James Bible (1769 version, please, I'm very modern), the services of Morning Prayer (*Book of Common Prayer* 1928, thank you) and evensong. I love ending The Lord's Prayer with "For Thine is the Kingdom, the Power and the Glory, forever and ever" and never forgetting that "All things come of Thee, O Lord, and of Thine own have we given Thee." I felt safe. I also thought I stashed my spirituality into a box that I could handle. I kept the Divine Mystery at bay.

Obviously, I did not become an accomplished actress. Rejection, self-doubt, financial insecurity, and public criticism are all part of an actress's daily round. I briefly became a playwright and wrote a one-woman show about Sarah Bernhardt. Then I became a theater critic, but that didn't last very long because editors don't really want raves; flops inspire such creative turns of phrase. It's so much more colorful when you spew derision instead of encouragement. Break someone's heart with your words? The poisoned pen really is sharper than the sword. But all artists "spread their dreams under your feet" (thank you, W. B. Yeats) and I could not trample on another soul's dreams.

So I stepped away from the footlights and later was blessed with a beautiful, cherished baby girl, and I got the role of a lifetime as her mother. When she was about four, since I had never left her overnight, I asked her father if I could have a weekend away to collect my thoughts. I really had visions of a hotel, sleep, and room service, but then someone told me of an Episcopal convent that conducted weekend silent retreats. Perfect. The moment I drove into the convent grounds it seemed as if a spell came over me; by the time I walked down the hushed stone hallway to enter the chapel, I knew I was home. It was very unsettling.

After a silent weekend spent praying and working besides the cloistered, contemplative women who had answered God's call so dramatically, I felt compelled to finally try and reconcile the irreconcilable. Yes, I confessed to God that I had been called and I turned away from Heaven's request to serve. But now I had an even greater calling: I was a mother. I had been entrusted with a precious child to safeguard as best I could.

On Sunday, at the conclusion of that life-changing weekend, the guests were invited to speak to one nun in a confessor role about anything troubling our hearts. We were to unburden ourselves. A beautiful nun about my age sat with me in the convent garden bathed in the golden sunlight of an exquisite Indian summer day. I shared with her that I believed I had been blessed with a spiritual calling and I had said no to God. My sorrow was not that I had taken the path that I had, but that I did not possess the courage to even consider, never mind pray, about my true vocation. Now it was too late because my path was resolute: I was to be the best mother that I could be. Oh, yes, and I wrote a bit, too.

Sister was silent for a few moments with her eyes closed and her hands together. She sighed. And then she asked me to look at the families greeting each other and coming together after a weekend apart. Look at the smiles. The hugs. Hear the laughter. Take in the bliss of their connection and communion. She confided that there were some Sundays when she wondered if she could not have served God better in the world as a wife and a mother. Then she asked me quietly: "Why do you think that you have not already answered God's call? God needs mothers. God needs writers. There must be some special work that only you can bring forth into being. Perhaps, my dear, your convent is the world."

"The notion of vocation is interesting and rich. It suggests that there is a special form of life that one is called to; to follow this is the way to realize one's destiny," John O'Donohue reminds us. However, "the faces of the calling change" and so we must play many roles during our lifetime. "To be born is to be chosen."

And who knows? The role in life's drama that frightens us the most, may in turn lead to a gold star on the dressing room door and a dozen unexpected curtain calls, not to mention a favorite pew in the Actors' Chapel.

AUGUST 20

We'll Always Have Paris

*I always return to Paris, taking my selves along—past self, custom-
ary self, the self I never had.*
—Helen Bevington (1906–2001)
American poet

The only theater job in London I could get was as secretary to the
American producer Sam Wanamaker, whose passion project was
rebuilding Shakespeare's Globe Theater. After the summer season was
over, I decided I needed a new dream. If I was going to type, at least I
wanted to type something of my own and I didn't want it to be my personal take on George Orwell's 1933 memoir *Down and Out in Paris
and London.*

But that blistering August afternoon in 1974—down to eleven francs
in my wallet, with yesterday's breakfast the last bittersweet memory
of a meal and no place to sleep that night—it seemed certain that published works and literary accolades would come to me posthumously, if
indeed they came at all.

Desperate and sick of drowning in my unfulfilled dreams, I walked
the crowded Left Bank streets of Paris's Latin Quarter in search of
something, anything that could be an answer to my prayers. Clearly
what was needed at this point was a little Divine intervention. I was
back to basics: lighting a votive candle to pray for a miracle. Mind you,
miracles to Irish Catholic girls are daily occurrences. Wasn't I living
proof? Existing the way I had been for the previous three years, living
from hand to mouth like a nomad, in truth a little lost soul.

Of course, I kept up appearances and pretended to my family that I
was traveling throughout Europe "in order to write from experience,"
as I'd scrawl hastily on very infrequent postcards.

Avoiding the cafés along the Boulevard St. Michel, I stopped at
Notre Dame Cathedral. How very easy it is, when you live in Paris and
are lost, lonely, and scared, to sit in a café for hours or days or weeks
(if your money holds out) nursing a café crème or some aperitif with an
exotic name instead of trying to solve your problems. In French cafés
problems seem romantic; solving them is secondary. But I needed a
franc to pay for the candle, and that would leave me only a thin ten-
franc note. Believe me, life can seem extremely precarious indeed, if the
sum total of one's earthly existence is only ten francs. Still, if ever there
was a place to light a candle, it was Notre Dame Cathedral in Paris.

The dark, cool, cavernous cave set aside for Divine entreaties was
filled with more tourists than pilgrims, but I was able to make my way

to a small shrine dedicated to the Virgin Mary. I remember asking Her for whatever miracle I needed, although at that moment the main thing I thought I needed was more money. Of course, I also needed a safe place to sleep, something to eat. I needed encouragement. I needed confidence. I needed moxie. So a miracle with my name on it would have done the trick.

I sat for a long time in the protective darkness of the cathedral's side pews, having a conversation with myself and Providence. "Nobody cares if you quit. Go ahead, just pack it in." It was a tempting thought. But at the price of having to admit to my family and incredulous friends, who'd never really believed I'd accomplish anything anyway, it was way too expensive. They say that pride cometh before the fall, but sometimes in life, it's our pride that keeps us on our feet, stumbling out of the wilderness. "Oh, please, Lord and Lady, keep me at it," I prayed. "Don't let me give up or sell myself short." Making a bargain with Heaven, I remember promising that if my writing could just be published, I'd never ask for anything more.

Recalling this young girl, her future self can't help but smile and shake her head. To begin with, there have been many more prayers after I saw my words in print, and those were just as passionate. But I didn't know then, as I do now, that a writer is someone who writes—puts words down on paper, doesn't just talk about it. For the past six months I'd been cemented in inertia. Although I'd come to Paris to write my play about the French actress Sarah Bernhardt and had done a considerable amount of research into her life, which included visiting her old haunts in search of inspiration, I'd done no writing. In fact, I couldn't bring myself to lift a pen or strike a typewriter key. With no money to pay the remainder of my bill, I'd left my small hotel empty-handed, my suitcases remaining as ransom. All my earthly possessions consisted of what I was wearing and a depressing portable typewriter that now rested at my feet and screamed "fraud." And now it seemed that the management of the hotel where I'd been staying would, too.

There was nothing more to do but call home collect and ask for the airfare back to the States.

Just as I left the cathedral, I added a footnote to my prayer—requesting something that before now had never, ever occurred to me—a blessing in defeat. I wanted Heaven to help me remember that there would be other opportunities to replace the lost ones I had so foolishly thrown away or blown through naïveté, bad timing, wrong choices, stupid mistakes. And that the next time I'd be ready to act on my dreams. I learned the hard way that dreams wait for no woman. Dreams have their own timetable and their prime directive is to become real. Dreams wait for no one.

Guided by an unseen hand steering me in a sure direction, I headed across the street to a public telephone. Needing change, I stopped at No.

37, Rue de la Bucherie. From the outside, the establishment looked like a French flea market, but in reality, it was a bookstore. The yellow and red sign above the door read "Shakespeare and Company."

"Welcome," a thin and goateed Ezra Pound stand-in said to me from behind a large maple table stacked high with books. "You look like you've traveled far—as in 'travail'—and are in need of refreshment. You've come to the right spot, for we're just about to have tea."

I remember thinking at the time that this is what happens when despair gives way to hallucinations. I was handed a tall glassful of tea with lemon in the Russian style, and an outstretched hand passed me a plate of tiny butter cookies, mandarin oranges, and chocolate. The unexpected, pungent smell of the lemon floating in a sea of hot ambrosia acted on my senses like a whiff of smelling salts would for a fainting woman. And as I began to eat the cookies, I started to feel incredibly happy, despite everything. Around me were similar contented looking faces, a small group of travelers chatting amicably in different languages, amid bohemian disorder. There were books piled helter-skelter everywhere from the floor to the rafters of the ceiling. On the walls colorful posters announced upcoming Parisian literary events. A curious combination of small sunflowers and rather tired lilies arranged in a jelly jar brightened up a sale table of English paperbacks. Over the front window hung a giant lithograph of William Shakespeare. Outside the door was the Seine. I felt as if I'd just fallen behind the looking glass.

Spying my typewriter, the man spoke to me again, his hands and wrists fluttering in punctuation marks. "You're a writer, I see, who travels light—typewriter only. Certainly, more cumbersome than Hemingway's notebooks, two pencils and sharpener, but still, at the heart... the meat of the matter... You're published, no doubt?"

"Where am I?" a rather dazed voice enquired. I vaguely recognized it as my own.

"Why, the Tumbleweed Hotel for Writers, at Kilometer Zero, Paris," he said, surprised that he should be asked.

"What?"

"Shakespeare and Company. Come now, the home of Joyce, Hemingway, Neruda, Anaïs Nin, Durell, Ginsberg, and every great writer of the twentieth century. Henry Miller's favorite bookstore. George Whitman, at your service. What kind of a writer did you say you were? You're published, I assume. This is a commune for serious, published writers only. No tourists."

I still had absolutely no idea what this man was talking about, but if there was anything I wasn't, it was a tourist.

"From whence have you journeyed to join us?" Whitman asked, still talking to me as if I'd been expected all along and had simply showed up three days late.

"Washington," I answered. In August 1974 when you were an American traveling anywhere, this admission could get you into heated conversations, but I was too tired to make anything up.

"Ah, Watergate country. You've come to escape the sordidness. It's the decline of the political system in the West as we know it," he discoursed to those clustered around him. People were nodding their heads in agreement.

"Who is this man?" I whispered to a young college student reaching past me to finish off the butter cookies and the mandarin oranges. The chocolate was long gone.

"George? He's a nephew or cousin or something, son for all anybody knows... of Walt Whitman," the student said in between swallows. "The poet."

"And Shakespeare and Company?" I needed the Cliffs Notes version of this place really quickly.

"What kind of a writer doesn't know about Shakespeare and Company? Don't you know you're standing on hallowed ground?" He began eyeing me suspiciously.

Whitman graciously saved me, or at least I thought he did.

"Yes, now where were we? You're published, no doubt," he asked again.

I was beginning to get the drift of this crazy conversation. "Published, ah, well..."

"We only take in published writers at this commune. This may be the Free University of Paris, but there are standards."

"Of course, I'm published." Well, wasn't everyone?

"Where?"

"Where? Various places. Small, literary journals, and of course, the *Post*. The *Washington Post*. I mean I have had... on occasion... in the past... written for them."

I was lying very badly. "But I'm on leave, extended leave... of absence... to write a play. I don't know if I want to continue to be a journalist and I've come to Paris to sort things out."

Whitman smiled benevolently. I hadn't fooled him; he'd seen too many like me before and there would be thousands more in the next three decades to come.

"Ah, well. Yes. Rules of the house: You are allowed to stay here, free of charge, as long as you need, but no one stays longer than ten days. We've not the space for extended sojourns. Every day of your stay, you must read one book and write for a minimum of two hours. All food is shared—this is a commune—and silence is observed at all times in the study rooms upstairs, except when there are exceptions, which I'll decide. You must clean up after yourself; we've no housemother here at the moment, unless, of course, you'd like to apply for the job. In that case, you can stay as long as you like or can stand it." Then with a Cheshire grin, he added, "Housemothers don't have to be published authors when they arrive here. They only need to have the potential. That's it. With you, it makes six. Tight squeeze, but we've had tighter. Do you know how to cook? It's settled then. Enjoy yourself and remember, as Hemingway said, 'All you have to do is write one true sentence. Write the truest sentence you can.' What's the play about?"

"Sarah Bernhardt, before she was famous," I answered, somewhat stunned.

"Good, this is the perfect place for the project. Everyone here is pre-fame. But once they leave us," he leaned toward me and whispered as only a Divine co-conspirator could, "the world awaits. Remember, one true sentence. Glad to have you with us. Someday your picture will be on the wall with the rest of our friends."

I wish words could truly convey the immense sense of gratitude and relief I felt as I climbed the narrow, rickety stairs in the back of the shop, up toward Heaven, which consisted of two main rooms called the "Old Smokey Reading Room" and "Blue Oyster Tea Room" plus a tiny alcove and walk-in kitchen. The walls were lined with framed autographed pictures of now legendary writers whom Shakespeare and Company had encouraged, fostered, and protected from penury, the world's rejections, and their own doubts. Certainly, that miracle I'd invested in just a few hours earlier had paid off handsomely. I had become a writer in Paris.

AUGUST 21

Answered Prayers and Angels Unaware

Be happy. It's one way of being wise.
—Colette (1873–1954)
Celebrated twentieth-century French author

The original Shakespeare and Company was founded by Sylvia Beach, the daughter of an American Presbyterian minister, who came to Paris with the American Red Cross during World War I and stayed on afterward to open up an English bookstore at No. 8, in the Rue Dupuytren, and later at No. 12 rue de l'Odéon, which operated from 1919 until 1941. Quickly it became an oasis for American ex-pats and a group of writers known as the Lost Generation during the twenties and thirties that included James Joyce, Ernest Hemingway, Ezra Pound, Thomas Wolfe, F. Scott Fitzgerald, John Dos Passos, and Gertrude Stein.

Of Sylvia Beach, Ernest Hemingway wrote, "No one that I ever knew was nicer to me." And most likely James Joyce had said something similar, for it was Sylvia Beach who published his *Ulysses* on her own printing press after it had been rejected by every publisher in the world.

After the Germans occupied Paris, Sylvia's legendary bookshop was forced to close in 1941 and she was sent to an internment camp. When she was released in 1942, she was allowed to return to Paris. Gradually she recovered from her ordeal but never reopened her bookshop and under the Nazi occupation hid all her books in an apartment. After George Whitman arrived in Paris after World War II, he opened up an English language bookstore in 1951 to continue the literary legacy.

In one of her Paris diaries written during the fifties, Anäis Nin described the scene: "And there by the Seine was the bookshop... an Utrillo house, not too steady on its foundations, small windows, wrinkled shutters. And there was George Whitman, undernourished, bearded, a saint among his books, lending them, housing penniless friends upstairs, not eager to sell, in the back of the store, in a small overcrowded room, with a desk, a small stove. All those who come for books remain to talk, while George tried to write letters, to open his mail, order books. A tiny, unbelievable staircase, circular, leads to his bedroom, or the communal bedroom, where he expected Henry Miller and other visitors to stay."

The restorative rhythm of the days spent in the book-lined apartment overlooking the Seine nourished by reading, writing, good companionship, and Whitman's enormous respect for the "serious work" of his guests restored my self-confidence. For the first time in my life I felt that what I was attempting to do was worthwhile. This total approval and acceptance shaped a commitment, one so positive that it enabled me to rid myself of the fear of failure and bolstered my courage to write. Four weeks later, the first draft of my play about Sarah Bernhardt was finished.

At the end of my "miracle" month, I went back to Notre Dame and lit a candle of gratitude. I was no longer afraid of what the future held for me. It was time to leave. For traveling expenses, I sold my typewriter, for far more than it was worth, to a wealthy young man from California whose rich parents had underwritten his trip to the Continent before he started college. He, too, wanted to be a writer, he told me over several exotic aperitifs at Les Deux Magots, another Lost Generation literary haunt.

"A writer is someone who writes, not just talks about it," I told him, passing on Whitman's wisdom. "Remember, just write the truest sentence you know. It's the first sentence that's the hardest." After I crossed the street and glanced back, he had put the portable typewriter on the table and ordered another drink. He had just become a writer in Paris.

Spinning Straw into Gold

*Stories are medicine... They have such power; they do not require
that we do, be, act anything—we need only listen. The remedies
for repair or reclamation of any lost psychic drive are contained in
stories.*

—Clarissa Pinkola Estés, PhD
American author, Jungian psychoanalyst,
and spoken word artist

Next to knowing what to do with a few loaves and fishes, knowing
how to spin straw into gold is probably the most important talent a
woman can possess. It can make the difference between living a life of
lack and living one of *Simple Abundance*. Gratefully, this mystical gift
was bestowed upon all of us. But, like any other talent—alchemy—the
ability of transforming nothing into something—must be called forth,
treasured, owned, respected, and nurtured.

As the story goes, a poor miller who is given to bragging meets a
king who is known for his interest in accumulating riches. Wanting to
impress him, the miller tells the king that his daughter possesses a rare
talent: the ability to spin straw into gold. Skeptical but intrigued, the
king orders the maiden to his castle, where he shows her a large room
filled with straw. He then commands her to transform the straw into
gold by the morning or lose her life.

Because this is an impossible task, the young woman succumbs to
anguished weeping. What can save her? Suddenly, a strange little man
appears in the room.

"*I* can spin straw into gold. What will you give me in return?" he
says. Stunned, the miller's daughter takes off a necklace that had been
her mother's and gives it to him. At once the little man sets to work. The
last thing the maiden remembers before she falls into a deep slumber is
the soft droning of the spinning wheel. At dawn the king finds the miller's daughter still asleep, surrounded by hundreds of spools of golden
thread and not one wisp of straw.

The king is delirious with joy at what she's accomplished. And
though she wants to explain that it wasn't she who performed this
incredible feat, she cannot bring herself to admit her incompetence. If
she did, what would become of her? But her silence only increases her
dilemma, for the greedy king leads her to an even larger room filled
with straw, and again, she hears the royal command to spin it into gold
if she values her life.

The second night passes like the first. This time the maiden offers the strange little man her ring in exchange for his magic. The following morning the king is again ecstatic to find the room overflowing with golden spools. But the miller's daughter still conceals the real story. By the time the king leads her to a third straw-filled room, this one the size of a great hall, she realizes she has made a terrible mistake. Why has she not confessed her secret collaboration? But it's already too late, for the king has promised to make her his bride if she will spin the straw into gold once more.

This time, when the mysterious little man arrives during the night, he finds the miller's daughter nearly beside herself because she has nothing left to offer him. "Never mind," he says. "I will help you one more time in exchange for your firstborn child."

"How can I possibly make so terrible a promise?" she asks herself. Then she reasons that, since no one will ever know about her secret accomplice, she won't have to keep her end of the bargain. And so, with her consent, the little man spins the straw into gold for the third time. The next day, the king makes the miller's daughter his queen, and, in her happiness, she soon forgets her promise.

A year passes, and the queen gives birth to a handsome baby boy. However, soon afterward, the little magician suddenly reappears in her bedchamber and demands the baby. The queen pleads for her child, offering the little man all the wealth of the royal kingdom, but he refuses. Overcome with grief, she falls to the floor weeping. Her clandestine collaborator, moved to pity, grants the queen three days to discover his name, which he has always kept a secret. "If, by the end of that time, you can name my name, you may keep your child." Eventually, with the help of a clever, faithful servant, the queen discovers that the little magician is called Rumpelstiltskin. She can keep her child, her crown, and her contentment.

"Stories are embedded with instructions which guide us about the complexities of life," Jungian analyst and *cantadora* storyteller Clarissa Pinkola Estés reminds us in her powerful evocation of the female psyche, *Women Who Run with the Wolves*. Today, contemplate the psychic path taken in this story. When reflecting on dreams or fairy tales, it's important to remember that all the characters are inner aspects of ourselves. You are not only the miller's daughter, but the miller, the king, the faithful servant, the baby, and Rumpelstiltskin. Even more important, you are both the straw and the gold.

The Golden Storehouse of the Subconscious Mind

Infinite riches are all around you if you will open your mental eyes and behold the treasure house of infinity within you. There is a gold mine within you from which you can extract everything you need to live life gloriously, joyously, and abundantly.

—Dr. Joseph Murray (1898–1981)
Irish-American author and Divine Mind minister

Did you figure out who Rumpelstiltskin really was? He was the miller's daughter's subconscious mind. "You can bring into your life more power, more wealth, more health, more happiness and more joy by learning to contact and release the hidden power of your subconscious mind" than any wizard could ever conjure, Joseph Murphy tells us in his classic work on metaphysical principles, *The Power of Your Subconscious Mind.* Just as there are two sides of the brain, there are two spheres to our minds. The conscious mind is where reason resides, and the subconscious, or deeper mind, is where our emotions and creativity dwell.

"The main point to remember is once the subconscious mind accepts an idea, it begins to execute it," Dr. Murphy explains. "It works by association of ideas and uses every bit of knowledge that you have gathered in your lifetime to bring about its purpose. It draws on the infinite power, energy, and wisdom within you. It lines up all the laws of nature to get its way. Sometimes it seems to bring about an immediate solution to your difficulties, but at other times it may take days, weeks or longer...*Its ways are past finding out.*"

In the fable Rumpelstiltskin, the cycle of creation begins with the command given to the subconscious mind. For dreams to be called forth to the physical plane, a declaration must be made: "My daughter can spin straw into gold."

Sometimes the task we agree to take on seems virtually impossible. We think we don't have the time, talent, resources, or support to achieve it. But we are intrigued by the possibilities, just as the king is captivated by the thought of more wealth. Our authentic longings embolden us to obey the command: Spin the straw into gold or suffer the consequences. Let the dream die and with it will die the authentic life for which we long.

So we try to spin our straw, using all the skills of our rational mind— our reasoning, our experience, our craft. But when we rely solely on reason to manifest dreams, all we end up with is straw. However, we have a strange creative collaborator who knows how to spin straw into gold. It is Rumpelstiltskin, our subconscious mind. Instead of a necklace or a ring, we surrender pride and control of the dream. Instead of our firstborn child, we surrender our ego; we admit we cannot do it alone. We must give the order to our subconscious to work it out, then slip into a creative slumber so that the subconscious mind can go to work on our behalf.

When you are creating and you find yourself stuck, let go and turn it over to the Deeper Wisdom dwelling beyond your reasoning. When you are perplexed, you need to ask the subconscious to take over, preferably at night. In the morning, the answer should be forthcoming. But if it's not, continue asking questions before you go to sleep. How do I proceed? How do I spin my straw into gold? Tell your subconscious mind to awaken you with the answer. By the third morning—three is a very mystical number—the answers should start to be revealed.

Amazingly, when we harness the incredible power of the subconscious in our lives, we can accomplish whatever we set out to do, no matter what obstacles we must overcome. Hold the vision of the completed dream in your mind. See your heart's desire. Feel the thrill of accomplishment. Offer grateful thanks in advance. Don't ask how it will come to pass, just know that it will. Now go to work.

Today, prepare to evolve from a poor miller's daughter into a queen. In your heart, mind, and soul, be willing to turn it over to Infinite Intelligence. Get out of the way, name the source of your Power, and begin to spin straw into gold.

AUGUST 24

Meditation for Bad Girls

Embrace what makes you unique, even if it makes others uncomfortable. I didn't have to become perfect because I've learned throughout my journey that perfection is the enemy of greatness.
—Janelle Monáe
American songwriter and singer

Reckless, wanton, sultry, too hot to handle. August is breathing down our necks and it's not even noon. Hold it right there. When it's 100 degrees in the shade, gals turn bad, if they know what's good for them.

"Bad girls make it happen. A bad girl knows what she wants and how to get it. She makes her own rules, makes her own way and makes no apologies. She knows when to work a room, when to work the angles and when to work her curves or do all of the above," Cameron Tuttle tells us in her cheeky Bad Girl Guide series. "She's attitude in overdrive, coast-to-coast confidence and fast-forward fun. She's your boldest dreams and your inner wild. A bad girl is you at your best—whoever you are, whatever your style."

And whatever your age. "There are no good girls gone wrong," Mae West confided. "Just bad girls found out." Unfortunately, for too many of us, our Bad Girls stay in the closet in all their dazzling bodycon. That's because we often confuse bad girls with the archetypal feminine shadow—the brazen hussy. The bitch. The witch. Strumpet, wench, trollop, tart, floozy, nympho, slut, libertine.

Yes, historically that is what men have called women who rule, women they couldn't control, and the women of rock and roll. I call her my Woman with a Past. "Great women throughout history were bad girls. They were passionate about what they wanted. They were dreamers, risk-takers, and visionaries who defied the norm of their times," Tuttle points out. "They didn't conform, and they didn't take no for an answer. They weren't afraid to break the rules or scare the hell out of men to get what they wanted. You don't have to change the world to find your badness. But you'll definitely change yours."

When I think of my inner bad girl I think of "The First of Her Name" and "The Princess That Was Promised," my personal icon Khaleeshi, the Mother of Dragons: Daenerys Stormborn, as she was called, for she "had come howling into the world in the greatest storm in the memory of Westeros; a storm so fierce that it ripped gargoyles from the castle walls and smashed her father's fleet to kindling." Not a bad beginning for any woman destined to change not just the world, but worlds.

Funny story, but completely true. I was washing dishes not long ago and I was having one of those spats with Whoever might be at the listening post and I yelled at the ceiling, "No, I won't...Why do I always have to be the good one? Yadda, yadda, yadda. I'll tell you who I want to be: the Mother of Dragons!"

I immediately felt a satisfying relief from my outburst and continued to clean the kitchen. When I was done, maybe fifteen minutes later, I took out the garbage, and when I returned to my front door, there was a huge salamander right next to the door frame on the outside wall, which looked every bit like a baby dragon. "Whoa. Okay, okay," I said out loud, looking up. "Just let me ease into this. I get it. No Mother of Dragons today." And the salamander looked at me and then scurried away into the underbrush of plants.

As a "good girl" who grew up to be a well-behaved woman, I've tried to bury my passion for most of my life. But when a "good" woman snuffs out the spark of wildness she was born with, the very nature she's been endowed with as a blessing to keep her not just alive, not just surviving, but thriving, she turns her passion inward. Passion pushed down can end up dormant, eventually revealing itself through chronic depression, cringeworthy choices, debilitating illness, addiction, or in desperate measures (think Thelma and Louise driving off a cliff). A woman shouldn't need to be diagnosed with breast cancer to be motivated to take up mountain climbing or landscape design. Nor should she find it necessary to pretend she's having a root canal when she's really getting a haircut. However, speaking personally, I've known one too many women who have done just that.

Perhaps we need to reconsider our concept of exactly what makes a Bad Girl. Cameron Tuttle suggests we consider "Cleopatra cruising the Nile...Dorothy Parker at the Algonquin...Rosa Parks in the front of the bus...Miss Piggy hitting the high notes...Aretha Franklin getting some respect...Tina Turner strutting her stuff..."

How about *The Hunger Games*'s Katniss Everdeen? Or Lucy from *Peanuts*? The turn of the century rebel rouser from Nova Scotia, Anne Shirley in *Anne of Green Gables*, who confesses hopefully for all of us: "It's so easy to be wicked without knowing it, isn't it." Gee, I wish I could at least try.

Personally, my favorite Bad Girl is Tinker Bell. This gal was so bad, she'd just fall down, hold her breath, and pretend to be dead until she got her way. Jane Austen? One of the most subversive women ever to lift a pen: "I always deserve the best treatment because I never put up with any other."

What about Marilyn Monroe? Granted, she remains the greatest sex symbol there ever was, but regrettably she wasn't a Bad Girl. She just wanted to be loved. Bad Girls might wear only Chanel No. 5 to bed, but their survival instincts are powerful and admirable.

"Do you have the idea that it's unladylike to want? Snap out of it!" Cameron Tuttle urges us. "Don't be afraid to want things, to yearn, crave, or lust for anything. And don't be afraid to go after what you want. If you can't satisfy yourself, then how can you expect anyone else to satisfy you?"

Still, for a woman of any age, whose deepest, unarticulated fear is that someday she will end up alone, friendless, homeless, and on the street, the dark shadow of the fallen woman is menacing. "The word *shadow* itself suggests a dark, secretive, possibly malevolent countenance that looms in the background of our nature, ready to do harm to others as well as to ourselves," the brilliant writer and pioneer in spiritual energy medicine Carolyn Myss explains in her book *Sacred Contracts: Awakening Your Divine Potential*. However, "a much more appropriate understanding of the shadow aspects" of our personalities is "that they represent the part of our being that is the least familiar part of ourselves."

And for too many women the least familiar part of ourselves is the girl who just wants to have fun. It's quite illuminating to discover that often what a woman calls the search for true love isn't a hankering for another person. It really turns out to be the suppressed desire to do something that she loves, something that makes her feel alive and joyful. I've rarely had as much joy in my life as the weekend I spent learning on the job how to midwife rare-breed pregnant ewes by doing it, rubber gloves up to my shoulders. A weekend and eighty newborn lambs later, I could barely move and spent two days sleeping. But it was the best sleep I'd had since the night my own beautiful lamb, my daughter, was born. There's a soulful connection there, and I'll find it. After all, I'm the Mother of Salamanders.

AUGUST 25

The Smell of the Greasepaint, the Roar of the Crowd

I seem to wish to have some importance in the play of time... What is deep, as love is deep, I'll have Deeply. What is good, as love is good, I'll have well. Then if time and space have any purpose, I shall belong to it.

> —Jennet Jourdemayne in *The Lady's Not for Burning*
> Christopher Fry (1907–2005), English playwright
> and poet

Although I adored acting—the art, the craft, the lifestyle—I reached the point where I could no longer handle the pain of rejection when I didn't get a part, which happened most of the time. Casting has absolutely nothing to do with how talented an actress you are and everything to do with how you look. If your physical appearance doesn't match the director's interior preconception of what the character looks like, you may not even be able to read for the part.

Holly Hunter virtually stalked Australian film director Jane Campion for more than a year while Jane was searching the world for an actress to play Ada, her mute, mid-nineteenth-century Scottish heroine in *The Piano* (1993). Campion didn't initially believe that Holly was right for the part, probably because she couldn't get the indelible image of Holly's previous incarnations as a southern floozy out of her mind. But Holly possessed soul knowledge; she knew this part had been the reason for all those piano lessons as a child and that this part was the role she was born to bring to life. The tremendous obstacles she'd overcome to get the role must have made winning an Oscar for her soul-stirring performance all the sweeter. All I know is that it did for me, as I watched her accept it.

Rejection, self-doubt, financial insecurity, and public criticism are all part of an actress's daily round. We forget this when we watch these women all dressed up for the Academy Awards. Another actress in *The Piano*, and many years before she would fall for a vampire on the long-running series *True Blood*, was then eleven-year-old Anna Paquin. Anna won an Oscar for her role as Ada's obstinate daughter; her only previous acting experience had been as a skunk in a school ballet. She beat out five thousand other little girls in an open audition. Now this is the stuff that dreams are made of: sagas on which entire lives can turn. Why, then, was I surprised when Katie, then in high school, informed me one year that she would not be returning to the art school she had attended for the past three summers, but would be signing up for a young actors' workshop run by a professional theater company? Oh, God, the twig is bent early.

The moment we walked into the darkened theater and I saw the bare stage and spotlights, it all rushed back: the smell of the greasepaint, the roar of the crowd, the chills, thrills, magic, mystery, and wonder. An empty theater pulsates with palpable creative energy. Katie's face was flushed with excitement, her eyes were ablaze, and she radiated joy. I wondered if I'd ever seen her like that before; surely I would have remembered, wouldn't I? Wistfully, I exited the stage door that had just opened for her.

Over the summer we worked together on her monologue, as character motivation, line reads, rehearsals, and costumes became part of my everyday life again in a recycled sort of way. I shared memorization and makeup tricks, the power of pacing and pausing, and stories from my "illustrious" stage past. When she got anxious, nervous, and hysterical, I reassured her that tension is an important part of the creative process and tried to show her how to work with it, instead of fighting it.

Being a traditionalist, I wanted her first opening night to be unforgettable, rich in stage lore and luck. Her aunt Dona (her godmother, director, author, and professor of screenwriting) sent her a telegram from Hollywood (which certainly created a buzz backstage), her dad bought her a beautiful bouquet of flowers, and I told her to "break a leg," the stage invocation for success.

Katie's theatrical debut was terrific—her intensity, energy, and passion caught me completely off guard. I was very surprised and so proud I thought I'd burst. The next day, when I excitedly shared all the details with Dona, she laughed. "Well, what were you expecting? She's *your* daughter." Then my old friend gave me a memory gift. She vividly recalled another passionate young actress wearing a red wool vest, matching gauchos, and black riding boots who confidently walked into an open audition for Christopher Fry's play *The Lady's Not for Burning* as if she knew something the director did not. "She had fire in her eyes and possessed more theatricality just walking to the stage than most people have on it. At that moment I knew I'd found my Jennet Jourdemayne." Jennet, Fry's high-spirited heroine, was my first leading role.

No matter how brilliant at it we are, a life in the performing arts is not always possible. But a life enhanced by the performing arts is. We don't have to join Actors' Equity to explore the world of theater, dance, or opera as a passionate, personal pursuit. Either side of the footlights can illuminate your path toward authenticity. As the seventeenth-century English poet Francis Bacon reminds us, in life's theater only God and the angels are permitted to be onlookers.

AUGUST 26

Reel Life Lessons

For so many people, television and movies may be the only way they understand people who aren't like them.
—Michelle Obama
American lawyer, author, and first lady of the United States

Instead of meditating today, let's just watch a movie. Sneak away in the middle of the day, hunker down in the dark, with popcorn, to ponder the meaning of life. It doesn't matter whether we choose to watch it at home or venture out to the movie theater, truth can pleasurably be discerned one frame at a time.

"Studying movies for their mystical message empowers us. We gain insight and greater self-awareness," Marsha Sinetar suggests in her fascinating book *Reel Power: Spiritual Growth Through Film*. "So much of life today is centered on problems, recovery, and the painful struggles of *trying* to meet the unrelenting demands of twenty-first century living. Unfortunately, by dwelling only on problems, and thus failing to see ourselves and our dilemmas in a heroic, promising light, we limit ourselves. Movies elevate our sights, enlarge imagination. Film, like poetry, is one of our heart's most subtle agents. It reminds us of what we know, helps us stretch and change, provides us with a sensory catalyst for creative, cutting-edge change." Reel power is "the ability to dig out, and use, whatever is spiritually valuable in a movie."

Films are celluloid fairy tales for a culture that no longer sits around the campfire listening to the wisdom of its elders. I use movies to replenish my creative well. I crave period films with lush sets and costumes for my visual fix, rely on comedies for relief from stress, and seek out black-and-white mysteries and romantic classics from the 1930s and 1940s for sheer escape. I collect movies about angels, reincarnation, the afterlife, and everlasting love.

Meditatively matching your mood to a movie is very restorative and rewarding. Put a list together of films that sound good to you. Refer back to it or save it to your streaming platform of choice. And don't forget to go to the theater sometimes. While we live in an age of anything on demand in our living room, it is still great fun—and an occasional treat—to experience films the old-fashioned way.

AUGUST 27

Becoming Your Own Heroine

Don't just write a strong female protagonist. Be one.
—A. D. Posey
Author and screenwriter

I once had an interesting conversation with a professional screenwriting coach, and she told me that you can tell if a student is developing a truly authentic voice by "who's the central character of their stories."

This made me curious. One of the most common problems of novice screenwriters is that they write heroes by default; characters whose names are on almost every page but who are only the leads due to their frequency of appearance. They're victims of circumstance or malice, and they don't drive the story through their choices. They only react, so they're constantly focusing their creative energies on the bad guys and the continuing escalation of crises.

Wow. I think the same is true in our personal stories. All of us have had bad actors in our personal plays, but like George Bernard Shaw's heroines, from now on it will be our choices that shape our emotionally satisfying ending. "The real moment of success is not the moment apparent to the crowd," G. B. S. tells us. Becoming our own heroine doesn't occur until we triumph in our own eyes.

Because if we didn't make the choices that got us where we are, then it can't be our fault, right? And if it's not our fault, then we shouldn't bear the blame or the shame? Am I creating enough weasel room for us? I'm trying my best.

So as of today, there's no one else to blame. No more mitigating circumstances. No more copping a plea or copping out. For when we choose to react instead of acting for ourselves, not only do we give up our chance to be the heroine, we surrender every ounce of our creative energy, our vitality, our passion. We become a wind-up doll in our minds, sitting in the closet waiting for someone to come in and take us out to play.

Perhaps the mistake that novice screenwriters as well as younger selves make is thinking that heroines must be perfect. They aren't. We don't want heroines to be perfect, we just need them to get themselves out of the snafu they didn't anticipate. It's the attempt that makes their story riveting and becomes our inspiration, whether they ultimately succeed or not. In fact, if a person doesn't have real challenges to face, they can't possibly be heroic. Who sees triumph in an Olympic long distance runner crossing the street at noon? But someone with a champion's heart is running laps in the dark and damp at four a.m. Years of such grueling training make us take notice and earn our admiration.

When you're embroiled in a perplexing situation that pushes all your emotional buttons, realize that you can't cut through the thicket of fear, benign neglect, and confusion all at once. But you can make a gigantic spiritual leap by simply acknowledging that you don't want to live any longer crippled by fear. At the very moment that you choose the forest path to find your way home, rather than being chased into the thickets by the villain, you become the lead character—the heroine—of a whopping good yarn. A legend, shall we say, in your own mind, which is the best place for legends to practice their winning moves.

It can't be your life until it's your story. By claiming one, you begin to own the other.

AUGUST 28

Perfect Pleasures: The Bliss of Period Films

Only connect! That was the whole of her sermon.
Only connect the prose and the passion, and both will
Be exalted...Live in fragments no longer...
—E. M. Forster (1879–1970)
English novelist

I close my eyes and hear the clip-clop of the horses' hooves upon the road in the opening of *Sherlock Holmes*, the click-clack of Miss Marple's knitting needles, or the beginning of the symphonic suite from the stunning television series *Victoria,* about a young girl who becomes a great queen. There are only two words in the suite composed by Martin Phipps. The two words are "Gloriana/Alleluia." But I can't get these words out of my head and neither will you. I've been singing them for weeks and I've never felt better. Maybe it's because those two words contain all the Power and the Glory. In a few beats of the music, Phipps chose notes to mimic the beating of the human heart—how it sounds when we're in love, happy, or frightened.

Gloriana/Alleluia: I'm carried aloft with a haunting Divine swoosh, transported in a finely tuned personal time machine, and probably as close to the Rapture as I'll ever get.

Today let us praise the simply abundant bliss of the period film. Let me pull you back from the brink, far, far away from the world of atomic blondes, girls with dragons, or even with dragon tattoos. Fabulous role models but not the serene and soothing reprieve I'm searching for right now.

Instead, let us rejoice and riff upon the parallel reality of historical films rather than the raucous, rowdy, rude here and now. Let us turn a page back to the twilight elegance of a Paradise that became lost; a change of mise-en-scène. Let's celebrate another time, another place: a costumed life at the pace of grace.

Lavish sets, hushed hallways, fringed drapes, secret passageways. French doors, Parisian drawers. Perfect manners. Forbidden love. Veiled hats, kid gloves, pearl buttons, hat pins, haberdashery worth a queen's ransom. Flushed cheeks, silk corsets, voluminous petticoats. Beguiling parasols, ostrich fans, ruffled necklines, cascading curls, sherry and chintz, paisley shawls, burgundy tufted leather fire fenders. Scheming plots and cheeky bon mots, roaring fires and decanted Cockburns 1947 port—a legendary year—so glad we made it.

Drawing room, morning room, conservatory, mud room, butler pantries; no servants at breakfast, help yourself from the sideboard, and aren't you glad you know this coded behavior and won't be embarrassed at your next Saturday to Monday invitation to the Great House.

Shooting parties, riding to hounds, hunt balls, galloping glorious women in black riding habits on sidesaddle, men in white flannels swinging bats and bowlers, billiards and badminton.

Pimm's and punts, tennis anyone, we need a fourth? Meet you on the lawn. Strawberries, clotted cream, cucumber sandwiches, and champagne. Sophisticated conversations in cut-glass accents, clipped phrases, lengthened vowels and crisp consonants, punctuated by wicked irony, endearing eccentricity, subtle nuance, the arched eyebrow, and tea, not at three, but at 4:20 in the afternoon to be as precise as Her Majesty, the Queen. No matter what today's conundrum or shock, sweet tea in paper-thin porcelain cups is the rescue remedy.

Personally, I think we all need the uplift provided by films that inspire, encourage, affirm, and celebrate the human spirit—and if we ever needed home-grown serenity and heaping portions of comfort it's now.

"Movies mirror us and invite us to go beyond the obvious," Marsha Sinetar tells us. "Their themes and images can powerfully equip us to see ourselves as we are at our worst, and our best, or help us invent new scripts about who we hope to be."

And with period films, we can be back home before they even notice we're gone.

AUGUST 29

Creature Comforts

Our perfect companions never have fewer than four feet.
—Colette (1873–1954)
French writer famous for *Gigi*

One of the most important life lessons I have ever learned—the transformative power of unconditional love—was taught to me by a four-legged mystical master. Jack was a feral cat who showed up in my Maryland backyard many summers ago. Even though he was obviously starving, he kept his distance; for the first week he simply watched, sizing me up as he cased the joint. Every day I set food and water for him outside the kitchen door, but it was at least a month before he would eat in my presence.

Gradually, I was permitted to pet him, and he would reward me with a deep, resonant purr of contentment. One chilly morning, as autumn turned to winter, he decided to finalize my adoption and came indoors to live with me and be my love.

Soon after our passionate affair began, Jack developed an eye infection; I took him to our vet and discovered that he had feline leukemia. The diagnosis was devastating. But my Belgian veterinarian practiced holistic as well as conventional medicine and suggested, along with antibiotics, a course of homeopathic remedies, particularly massage and meditation (rhythmically stroking him for ten minutes to induce deep relaxation), which bolstered both our immune systems.

Eight comforting years of constant companionship passed. Jack would sit in the window next to my word processor and keep me company as I wrote *Simple Abundance,* and we had many marvelous conversations. I particularly loved our afternoon meditation/purring sessions, which lowered my heart rate as well as his.

At the vet's clinic, Jack became known as the "miracle cat" because he lived longer after having been diagnosed with feline leukemia than any other cat the clinic had treated. In fact, Jack appeared so healthy that occasionally his doctor would test him to see if he'd not had a spontaneous remission.

But eventually our time together became finite and Jack began to fail rapidly. Every cutting-edge veterinary procedure was attempted in order to buy us just a little more time. Finally, the moment of profound loss that no prayer could put off arrived. "Only his love for you is keeping him alive," my vet said softly. "Your love for him must now let him go." Gently I wrapped my soul mate in my old bathrobe and cradled him in my arms. As I kissed Jack farewell, he licked away my tears and purred until his last heartbeat. After bringing my daughter into the world, it was one of the holiest moments I've ever known.

Jack was buried in the same backyard where he once played, and where our paths first crossed so many years before. A little brass marker offers the Scottish poet Robert Burns's remembrance to the "Harried orphan who found tender refuge in our hungry hearts." It's a sentiment that applies not only to the pets we have loved, lost, and mourned, but to those we share our dreams with today.

What long-lost dream is seeking tender refuge in your hungry heart today?

Physicians and psychologists say that loving, caring for, and spending time with animals enhances our well-being. Anyone who has ever been adored by a dog or adopted by a cat probably can't convey in words the emotional bond that grows between them. That's because dogs love us unconditionally and cats are big on redemption. Our sins and shortcomings don't bother them if we delight in their presence and make sure they're fed.

If you don't have animals living with you, this doesn't mean you can't make a connection: visit the zoo at different seasons, offer to pet-sit for a friend, walk a neighbor's dog, put out dried corn and nuts for the squirrels in your backyard, or toss bread to the ducks on a pond, the pigeons in the park, the seagulls at the beach. I hope to begin volunteering at a sanctuary for abused horses.

If you do have pets, don't just feed, walk, and ignore them. You invited them into your life, so open your heart. Pets need to be stroked, cuddled, caressed, indulged, pampered, and played with; dote on them and they'll return the kind of devotion most of us can only dream about receiving from human beings. Talk to them and you'll discover a trusted confidante who'll never betray your secrets. Laugh at their silly antics—a sure stressbuster—and learn how to live by observing them. Dogs make friends easily, are loyal, and aren't moody. Cats are spontaneous, content to live in the present moment. They're small, shedding, scratching, inscrutable Zen masters sent to teach us the paradox of undoing in a hectic world where things always must be done. As the ball of fur presently curled up on my desk clearly demonstrates, the more naps you take, the more awakenings you experience.

Today, be grateful for the gift of sharing your earthly span with creatures who comfort. Animals are our spiritual companions, living proof of a simply abundant source of Love. None of us need feel alone. And if there is a gift, then surely, there must be a Giver.

AUGUST 30

This, Too, Is God

One must also accept that one has "uncreative" moments. The more honestly one can accept that, the quicker these moments will pass. One must have the courage to call a halt, to feel empty and discouraged.

—Etty Hillesum (1914–1943)
Dutch mystic and writer

Whether you're a professional, poet, parent, or performance artist, one morning you'll wake up, begin to prime the well to continue in the re-creation of your authentic life, only to discover that the well has run dry. It might seem disconcerting to end this month of meditations on a downbeat, but accepting uncreative days as part of the creative cycle is crucial to your serenity. Uncreative days are real life. Every artist knows them, although few of us care to acknowledge this except in confidential whispers. But as you make authenticity your art you will know them, too. Uncreative days are the part of the yin/yang of artistic yearning.

Once in the middle of a creative drought I sat in a New York coffee shop with my agent and confessed softly, as if I was admitting a great personal failing or the discovery of a terminal illness, that for months I had been unable to dream. I couldn't fantasize, visualize, or even make a wish. Since I'm Irish, the inability to dream is the emotional equivalent of a chemical imbalance in the soul. I needed her advice because Chris has a knack for knowing how to finesse things. We'd just come from a meeting with an advertising agency where she'd made a deal for my creative consulting services that astounded me, especially since at that moment I was convinced there was nothing going on inside worth more than two nickels.

"What do I do?"

"You don't do anything," she told me. Zilch. Nada. Zip. Wait it out.

Accept the fallow period as graciously as you can and get ready for a quantum leap in creativity or consciousness.

However, it's so difficult to come to a halt, especially when we want to get on with our careers, relationships, health, creativity. But when you're too parched to pray, beyond tears, or too drained to give a damn, it's time to cease and desist. Not all our hours are billable.

No, this does not mean you can quit. You still must go through the motions, keep showing up for work: on the page, at the drawing board, stove, sewing machine, computer. Continue to prepare the canvas, moisten the clay. Pretend you're a creative temp, here to fill in until your Authentic Self arrives.

In the meantime, defer making any life-altering creative decisions until you receive operating instructions. Your only assignment is to replenish the well. Search for the underground spring through creative excursions. Keep in touch with your Authentic Self with the Gratitude Journal and the little things that bring you pleasure. Resurrect any old creative projects that might have fallen into the sinkhole of second thoughts or back of the closet. Give them another glance. When I'm deeply discouraged, I retreat to my *Illustrated Discovery Journal* searching for visual clues to indicate the next turn in the path.

Often the derailment of too many dreams can bring on a drought, but whenever there's a dry period, there's still plenty of Light. We're just blinded by dark dust storms. Arid despair can often result from nurturance deprivation: not eating well, not sleeping enough, working too hard and too long without anything to look forward to. If you're creatively barren, give yourself a break. Dona Cooper, one of the most creative and productive women I know, frequently reminds me, especially when my plans don't proceed at the speed of light, that "This, too, is God."

And it is. Four months after I stopped trying so hard, the creative incarnation of *Simple Abundance* occurred. The hardest thing we'll ever do as Artists of the Everyday is learn to call an occasional halt. Today, if you're feeling uncreative, don't despair. Start getting excited and save your strength. You're being prepared for a quantum leap in authenticity.

In the natural world, droughts depart as suddenly and as mysteriously as they arrive. This, too, is God.

AUGUST 31

Do Try This at Home: The Victory Garden

Tomato and oregano make it Italian; wine and tarragon make it French. Sour cream makes it Russian; lemon and cinnamon make it Greek. Soy sauce makes Chinese; garlic makes it good.
—Alice May Brock
Alice's Restaurant Cookbook

For Mrs. Miniver, having a fully stocked pantry would have been a miracle, not just a luxury. That's because in January 1940, just four months into the war, the British Ministry of Food was established, and the serious rationing of food began. It would continue another fourteen years, until 1954. The Home Front was also responsible for victory gardens for the armed services as well as civilians. Cookbooks from that time show recipes for eggless, butterless, dairyless baked goods accompanied by as many leafy greens as you could grow.

We're blessed to be able to stock up on whatever we fancy.

For our canned provisions, now we're going to add another canned type: meat and fish. Many of the emergency prepper advice lists include canned meats. All these brands are available at your local supermarket, big box store, or via online merchants such as Amazon:

Yoder's Canned Bacon

Armour Potted Meat

Smoked Salmon Pate

Yoder's Variety Pack

Pack of 3 Dak Ham

Roast Beef with Gravy (Kirkland brand)

Vienna Sausages

SPAM Classic

Think of canned tuna, clams, mackerel, and salmon in olive oil. And don't forget that sardine lover in your crowd. Remember how food was preserved long ago. Add some dried organic grass-fed beef sticks to the mix. Or how about some paleo chipotle chicken jerky? Look for minimally processed and natural food protein and fats that will keep you satisfied and your blood sugar stable. There are several providers online that offer sustainably fished products that are safe and delicious. Canned smoked mussels and linguine is the start of the sur-vivalist version of linguine in clam sauce.

While we're thinking of camping pasta, add your favorite pasta, noo-dles and rice, quinoa, and other grains, but don't forget the pot you'll need to cook them in. In fact, if the pot is large enough, you can pack your dried ingredients in it.

Now remember, we're grateful to have this choice, because it's an emergency, but we can also add some sauces, mustard, and other con-diments to it. Amazon, for example, sells individual packets of Heinz condiments.

While we're putting together our "rations," I also suggest you get an old-fashioned can opener that needs no batteries, a pair of kitchen scissors, a bottle opener, a corkscrew, one serrated knife, one set of plastic utensils—large spoon, soup ladle, spatula. Place them all in a clear bag and then into the storage bin where you're storing your canned foods.

Hard cheese wrapped in wax can be included, as can crackers in large tins and cans of beer, boxed wine, and long-life milk. And if you have nothing to do for Labor Day weekend, why not have a prepper's potluck to see which of all these choices suits your tastes best!

Joyful Simplicities for August

How softly summer shuts, without the creaking of the door.
—Emily Dickinson

- Rediscover the books you loved as a child. Head off to a library (there are still some around!) and wander into the children's sec-tion with or without your own little ones. Sit in the child-sized chairs and recall moments of contentment curled up with a good book. What was it? *Little Women? Black Beauty? Anne of Green Gables?* The Little House books of Laura Ingalls Wilder? Any-thing by Judy Blume or Beverly Cleary? The Babysitters Club? *The Giver? Goosebumps?* Harry Potter? The vintage adventures of the ace girl detective Nancy Drew? (Remember Nancy's little blue roadster, twinsets, Bess, George, and Ned, and such baffling cases as *The Secret in the Old Attic* and *The Mystery at the Moss-Covered Mansion?* Solve them once more with feeling.)
- Gloria Steinem tells us it's never too late to have a happy child-hood, and I believe her. The childhood I would have chosen is captured in Maud Hart Lovelace's wonderful Betsy-Tacy series. If you want pure and simple escapism run away to Deep Valley, Minnesota, at the turn of the century to enjoy escapades with Betsy Ray and her friends, Tacy Kelly and Tib Muller. There are

ten books in the series, beginning when Betsy and Tacy are five in 1892, and ending with Betsy's wedding after World War I. What I like most about reading children's books from the past (now that I'm old enough to appreciate their subtle nuances) are the charming domestic details of these cozy worlds—the kinds of cooking, decorating, entertainments, and pastimes that filled their lives.

- Consider joining or starting a book club. Sharing a good book is as rewarding as reading one. Explore plot twists and character development over food and drink with a congenial group of people once a month. A wonderful resource is the free online directory for reading groups, www.readerscircle.org. Please check out www.sarahbanbreathnach.com, www.SimpleAbundance.com, or Grand Central Publishing for a new *Simple Abundance Reader's Guide* and info about any upcoming book club webinars we might be doing.

- Artists need to support one another in their sacred endeavors. I cannot praise Julia Cameron's compassionate and compelling *The Artist's Way* highly enough. It's the first book I recommend to my workshop participants and the one I packed in my daughter's suitcase when she left for California to pursue a film career. Julia's twelve-week course in discovering and recovering your creative self is an intimate tutorial with a gifted and generous mentor. Her many other books are equally inspiring and encouraging. Visit her website www.juliacameronlive.com for her blog and online classes.

- Visit (in person or virtually) Shakespeare and Company, one of the world's most iconic bookstores, and browse tempting reading possibilities at www.shakespeareandcompany.com. It's now run by George's daughter, Sylvia Beach Whitman, and there's a café next door just as George wanted there to be so long ago. So many happy and grateful memories of mine come from there. We'll always have Paris. For a wonderful book that captures sixty-five years of literary memories and photographs, there's *Shakespeare and Company, Paris: A History of the Rag & Bone Shop of the Heart* edited by Krista Halverson, which will entice you to plan a literary adventure of your own.

- Attics are great August destinations. Even if you, unlike the rest of womankind, have everything neatly packed away in labeled boxes, "the past is never where you think you left it," the novelist Katherine Anne Porter tells us. When we depart on sentimental journeys, we discover how right she is.

- Where is your past? Is it in your attic or basement, or at your mother's or sister's? Was it accidentally left behind at your former spouse's house? If remnants of your childhood or your private selves aren't physically located in places where they can be easily retrieved, you might want to have a gentle conversation about recovering them. This is especially important if you, like a woman in Carrie Fisher's novel *Delusions of Grandma*, have become "a chronicler of absence," devoted to recalling what is missing from your life. So drag a box outside under something shady and take along a pitcher of iced tea with mint. Give yourself the gift of a couple of idle hours revisiting your past and sorting through your memorabilia.

↪ The scent of love enveloped in a folded handkerchief; the feel of plush bears, flannel shirts, an old beach blanket (still with sand after all these years!); a pair of white go-go boots or a pressed flower found in a book of poems reunites us once again with what we never were meant to lose. We may never have left the house, but as the Victorian novelist Sarah Orne Jewett says, "The road was new to me, as roads always are, going back."

↪ Pretend that you're a tourist and you've selected your hometown as the perfect spot to visit for an unpretentious, relaxing, and delightful exploration. Or, is it possible for you to take a road trip to where it all began? When I went back to visit my first home, I was so shocked to find out how tiny it was! In my memory it was a mansion. And the three-block walk to my grammar school was one of the most satisfying trips I've ever taken. You can't imagine how wondrous it was to tell that little girl, still walking and dawdling slowly by herself, that she had, in fact, moved on.

↪ What does summer taste like for you? Lobster roll, blueberry pie, chocolate egg cream, root beer float? Potato salad? Make sure you revisit your taste sensations again!

SEPTEMBER

Autumn...asks that we prepare for the future—that we be wise in the ways of garnering and keeping. But it also asks that we learn to let go—to acknowledge the beauty of sparseness.
—Bonaro W. Overstreet (1902–1985)
American poet and writer

September's song is a two-part harmony, as summer's light-hearted serenade ends and a deeper melody begins. For eight months we've plowed and sowed the soulful seeds of Gratitude, Simplicity, Order, and Harmony into our lives. Now an authentic harvest of contentment waits to be gathered in, as the fifth *Simple Abundance* Grace—Beauty—beckons us to partake in her bounty. Begin to reap the rich harvest that Love hath sown.

Turning Over a New Leaf

Autumn to winter, winter to spring,
Spring into summer, summer into fall—
So rolls the changing year, and so we change;
Motion so swift, we know not that we move.

—Dinah Maria Mulock Craik (1826–1887)
Victorian English novelist and poet

Since ancient times, September has been viewed as the beginning of the new year, a time for reflection and resolution. Jews observe the high holiday of Yom Kippur, the day of public and private atonement, a sacred withdrawal from the world for twenty-four hours in order to become right with God and others, so that real life might be renewed with passion and purpose.

Change in the natural world is subtle but relentless; seasons seem to give way gently to one another, even if the monthly motion is so swift, we don't realize we're moving. But when the leaves start turning colors, it's time for turning over a personal new leaf so that our lives might be restored.

"What we need in autumn is an emotional or spiritual shot in the arm," Katharine Elizabeth Fite wrote in *Good Housekeeping* in 1949, urging the beginning of a new tradition for women: personal and positive resolutions in September. "Why do you suppose so many of us waste the autumn? Why don't we make the effort that would provide something new in our lives?" January's negative resolutions "are made when we are worn out in spirit, body, and pocketbook, and have no real urge to do anything but rest."

It seems to me that January resolutions are about will; September aspirations are about authentic wants. What do you want more or less of in your life, so that you can love the life you're leading? It could be as simple as seeing friends more often, setting aside time to have adventures with your children while they still want your companionship, rekindling romance, calling a solitary hour a day your own, introducing more order into your daily round, or just taking more walks in the dazzling sunshine.

The beauty of autumnal inspirations fueled by imagination, pluck, and purpose is that they're private; no one else knows we're making them. Autumnal resolutions don't require horns, confetti, and champagne. September asks only that we be open to positive change. I can try to do that. So can you.

The Work of Understanding

Somewhere there is an ancient enmity between our daily life and
the Great work. Help me in saying it, to understand it.
—Rainer Maria Rilke (1875–1926)
Twentieth-century German poet

Many of us believe that if Adam and Eve hadn't blown it in Paradise, we wouldn't have had to work for a living, and we'd be on easy street in Eden.

Unfortunately, that biblical interpretation is fanciful. For if you read Adam and Eve's story more carefully, you'll discover that God always intended for human beings to work and for work to be a joy. Consider Adam's soulful occupations: to name all living things after studying them and to tend a beautiful garden. In the beginning, work was meant as a gift.

But then came the fall, and our work became labor. All kinds.

There are private works: nurturing children, taking care of the home, preparing meals, chauffeuring, financial management, horticulture, tending animals, and *husbandry* (which is a fabulous old word referring not to a spouse, but to managing resources or the thrill of thrift).

Then there are public works: employment, school and church activities, youth groups, community and charitable volunteering. In real life we must take care of reality, so that we can afford to take care of what's real.

If you're employed outside of your home, you're paid money for your efforts. But the greatest portion of a woman's work is gratis and largely unsung. Because we spend so much of our earthly span working, one way or another, this deserves profound contemplation, and I'm not just referring to coping with the hassles of adulting: commutes, day care, sick children (or partners), snow days, teacher conferences, cooking and cleaning and laundry. Juggling swords, flaming torches, and conflicting commitments deserves its own meditation. But so does the numinous nature of work. Each of us was created to give outward expression to Divinity through our personal gifts. Sharing our gifts with the world is our great work, no matter what our job description might be or how our resume reads.

I don't think many women today can honestly say that their work life—private and public—is in balance with their personal life. Matthew Fox, the radical philosopher and former Catholic priest, believes "to live well is to work well." I wholeheartedly agree. But just how do women today accomplish that? I wish I could serve up a quick and easy solution to such a complicated, emotionally charged dilemma. For we can't work well or live well if we don't live authentically. Like Rilke, we need to acknowledge aloud the ancient enmity between real life and work. It exists. It tears us to pieces every day. We need to help each other understand it, because we will never understand it on our own. We can start by holding one another's hands, by listening to one another's concerns, by reassuring one another, today, that everything will be all right.

Somehow, together, we will figure it out. We always do, together.

SEPTEMBER 3

Scrambled or Fried?

At work, you think of the children you have left at home. At home, you think of the work you've left unfinished. Such a struggle is unleashed within yourself. Your heart is rent.
—Golda Meir (1898–1978)
Former Israeli prime minister

More women than you realize have a secret fantasy that has absolutely nothing to do with erotica. But in its own way, it focuses on the forbidden. I call this fantasy, "Scrambled or fried?"

One more perfectly normal day of incessant demands, neglected children, needy partners, family, or friends, unfinished work, and everyday money worries, and you feel you can't cope anymore. An overwhelming impulse to disappear without a trace comes over you. Methodically, you withdraw all the cash you can from your bank account (credit cards can be traced), pack a small suitcase, head for the bus terminal or the airport, and begin life all over again as a waitress in a diner somewhere out West or a bartender at a beach shack in a tropical locale.

Of course, you're not going to do it, but contemplating a plan of escape is an imaginary mechanism to let off steam from life's pressure cooker. No more overdue bills, arguments over cooking, cleaning, carrying out the garbage, spending, or custody; no more clashes between children and career, no more exhausting caretaking of an elderly parent, no more emails from bosses at all hours of the night. No more responsibility than what you can serenely handle in any twenty-four-hour period. When you think you can't take it anymore, a life that revolves around asking customers if they want their eggs scrambled or fried holds a certain allure.

When I lived in Maryland, many years ago, a thirty-nine-year-old woman, the mother of five children between the ages of eight and sixteen, vanished off the face of the earth not far from where I lived. Earlier in the day she had been a chaperone on an elementary school field trip. After the class returned to school, she put her daughter on a bus for a basketball game and told her that she would walk the short distance home since it was such a beautiful day. She never arrived. Around dinnertime, her frantic family called the police and a massive search began, complete with prayer vigils.

Of course, everyone feared the worst, because for this particular woman to disappear without a trace was completely out of character. She had everything: a Wellesley education, a beautiful family, a lovely home, an extremely comfortable lifestyle, and a perfect marriage to a diplomat. Three days later the woman who had everything, but obviously not enough of what she truly needed, turned up unharmed (thank Heaven), confused by her own conduct, and dazed by all the commotion.

Here's what happened. As she started for home, she sought a solitary spot to sort some things out. On the spur of the moment she walked a few miles to her favorite place, Washington's National Cathedral, an exquisite sanctuary. In the silence she could hear herself think. After a few hours of quiet and serenity, she could not bring herself to leave its peace to return to the chaos engulfing her at home, so she slept for two days on a pew in a small chapel.

When I heard that she hadn't been abducted but had voluntarily vanished, I felt a tremendous sense of relief and said as much to my then husband. His response was that this woman was obviously mentally unstable. Unbalanced. There was no other explanation for her bizarre behavior. I disagreed—it seemed like the weight of her life had become too heavy to carry alone—but as I had a meditation to write (on coping with stress), I chose not to challenge his interpretation. A long conversational detour would have been necessary to point out that under her particular circumstances, which, of course, we did not know, her disappearing act might have been extremely sane. Desperate, no doubt. Heartrending, no question. But not necessarily unrelatable or unhinged.

This much we did know: For whatever reason, her heart was rent. Her center could not hold. Her life was not, after all, as perfect as it appeared. Real lives seldom are, even if the surface has a pretty sheen. I only wish I'd been able to say to her, "Darling, disappear if you must, but phone home and let the children know that you're okay."

When our waitress or bartender fantasy surfaces, we're physically, emotionally, psychologically, and spiritually exhausted by the struggle within. We're seriously wounded by the ancient enmity between daily life and the Great Work. Band-Aids don't work anymore.

Actually, the fantasy of running away can be very therapeutic because it waves a psychic and spiritual red flag warning us that our real life has become unmanageable, we're at a dangerous crossing, and the barrier arms are coming down. Changes need to occur, creative choices need to be made, conversations need to be started and *finished*. If the fantasy persists to the point of action, asking for help is much better than buying a one-way bus ticket.

"If you knew how often I say to myself: to hell with everything, to hell with everybody, I've done my share, let the others do theirs now, enough, enough, enough," Golda Meir, the only woman prime minister of Israel, once confessed candidly.

You won't have to run away if you can learn to just say: *Enough. Enough. Enough!*

And mean it.

SEPTEMBER 4

What Women Do When They Are Alone

"I wish I knew when I was going to die," ninety-six-year-old Dame Frances Anne often said. "I wish I knew."
"Why, Dame?"
"Then I should know what to read next."

—Rumer Godden (1907–1998)
In This House of Brede

Have you read a good book lately? I hope so. Reading is one of my passions, and what to read next is like finding something fabulous in a Cracker Jack box, where there has been a prize in every box for a hundred years. But is it a decoder ring or a fairy girl with wings charm we fancy?

Let's ponder the glorious, extravagant blessing of reading and choosing the perfect book for bibliotherapy, as carefully as an Artist of the Everyday (or Bob Ross) chooses the colors for her palette—burnt sienna, yellow ochre, cerulean blue, scarlet lake, titanium white.

When I was young enough to still be impressionable, we were visiting my Granny at her home in Kentucky. One hot, sticky, summer day I was bored, restless, and roaming in rooms, in that stir-crazy way that drives grown-ups stark raving mad. Then I chanced upon a pile of *National Geographic*s in a small back room, sat down, and started looking through them. Obviously, I was too quiet, because the next thing I heard was Granny wondering where I was.

"I'm okay Granny, just reading a book."

"Book? What book? What book in the back room?" she boomed in a loud voice, suddenly standing over me and pulling it from my hands.

"Are you calling this magazine a book?"

Looking up, saying nothing.

"This, child, is *not* a book. This is a *ma-ga-zine*, Missy. *Magazine*."

Saying nothing, looking up.

"Only krogers call magazines 'books.' I do not *ever* want to hear you call a magazine a book, for the rest of your natural born life." Then, to make her point, she reached for a *Reader's Digest* anthology volume of four abridged novels, and said, "Now this is a 'book,' but you're not old enough to read it."

"Yes, Ma'am."

Having successfully learned the lesson of how to identify reading material in their different species at a very young age, I can now distinguish between two different types that are used interchangeably in the modern world: books and ebooks.

They are not the same.

There are books, which you hold in your hands as you lovingly or excitedly turn the printed, paper pages; and there are reading devices that display information, sometimes, if you can get your finger to slide across the damn abomination's screen. An ebook might be handy, I suppose, if you are racing around the world in a hot air balloon for eighty days. But ever since the first printed book, the Gutenberg Bible, appeared in 1454, books are chosen precisely so that you can cease all outward movement to retire within and regain your balance.

"Only one hour in the normal day is more pleasant than the hour spent in bed with a book before going to sleep," the English novelist, poet, historian, and literary critic Dame Rose Macaulay wrote in 1926, "and that is the hour spent in bed with a book after being called in the morning."

I hope you have your hour today.

SEPTEMBER 5

Back to the Future

She would read anything from a dictionary to a treatise on turnips. Print fascinated her, dazed her, made her good for nothing.
—Kylie Tennant (1912–1988)
Australian novelist, playwright,
and historian

Probably because I've always felt that I was born out of time and place, not meant to be here, now, but stranded somewhere in between the lines of an old life cut short or someone else's life, I always have gravitated toward the world of books, knowing that my lifelong search was hidden in between two covers. I will find my destiny by reading and writing.

I once consulted a highly esteemed astrologer who specialized in past lives. This was after *Simple Abundance* was first published and pre-internet. I didn't reveal any personal information and went incognito because I was very interested to hear her opinion without her knowing any peripheral information that might influence her.

What she found was fascinating. She said she saw one very strong karmic connection. In this previous life, I had once been a monastic scribe during the Middle Ages, at the time of the Crusades. I created beautiful illuminated manuscripts of secret sacred texts. But I was very conflicted because I believed that this forbidden spiritual knowledge should be shared with everyone, not just the king or church, so that we all could experience the Divine in our everyday life. At the end of my session, she asked if I was a writer now, and I told her I was. We laughed. She smiled and said, "I think you've honored your sacred contract very well."

We all experienced a sense of déjà vu, the feeling that a situation or person is familiar to us from a past life if we are open to receiving unexpected knowledge. That's the key—being open to receiving information or insight that we weren't anticipating, especially if the source or the flash seems weird or random but opens our eyes. We call this synchronicity—when two or more events occur that are meaningful to us.

Have you ever heard of the television show *Ghost inside My Child*? It's a "reality" program where small children talk about their previous lives in such detail that their current and curious parents can't ignore it as nonsense anymore.

One story was especially affecting, in which a three-year-old says: "Mommy, why don't you watch *my* movie?" And so secretly his parents investigate on the internet, and guess what? They follow the clues and discover that their toddler *could have been* Sidney Coe Howard, the screenwriter of *Gone with the Wind,* who died in a 1939 farming accident before the most famous movie ever made was released. He's miffed he missed that golden moment in his life, and who could blame him? The Academy Awards bestowed the first posthumous Oscar in 1940, but that's not quite the same, especially if you must head off to an after party thrown by Casper the Friendly Ghost instead of *Vanity Fair.*

I've experienced shivery goose bump moments when I pick up a used book—and I always find these encounters fascinating, especially when I follow up on an author I've never heard of before.

There are so many ways to enjoy books as a personal pursuit: belonging to a book club, rediscovering the old favorites you loved as a child, and searching for that next irresistible volume in which to lose yourself. Unfortunately, the good books that provide comfort, consolation, chuckles, and the companionship we all crave cannot be conjured up without a little curation. Since the choice of what we curl up with is often crucial for our solace and sanity, we need to learn how to nurture the talent of selection.

"The wonderful thing about books is that they allow us to enter imaginatively into someone else's life. And when we do that, we learn to sympathize with other people," the gifted writer Katherine Paterson reminds us. "But the real surprise is that we also learn truths about ourselves, about our own lives, that somehow we hadn't been able to see before."

Or as the great Yankees Hall of Famer Yogi Berra so succinctly put it: "It's déjà vu all over again."

SEPTEMBER 6

The Comfort of Good Old Books

I do love secondhand books that open to the page some previous owner read oftenest.
—Helene Hanff (1916–1997)
American author of *84, Charing Cross Road*

Book browsing is a meditative art and a sleuthing escapade. Every woman should have three well-paved avenues for page-turning adventures: a proper bookstore stocked by bibliophiles, a choice secondhand haunt, and an online specialty bookseller. This last category is a treasure because what you're looking for is probably the bookseller's passion project and you've tapped into their knowledge and expertise. What subject fascinates you? The Irish Famine, the Duchess of Windsor, the creation of NASA, political memoirs, the French designer Maggy Rouff, the evolution of *Homo sapiens*. Trust me, whatever you are interested in today, there is a specialty bookseller somewhere in the world who would love to help you find the perfect volume. I've found some marvelous books from Australia and New Zealand, when the bookseller said "Leave it with me and I'll see what I can find for you." Seek and you will find.

Books are as essential as breathing. In my experience, when going down for the third time, it was often word-to-word resuscitation that saved the day.

We have much to be grateful for: the proper brick-and-mortar bookstores that have survived after the culling of their breed need to be applauded and supported by our buying books there at least twice a year, even though we can get the book delivered overnight by an online retailer.

Visiting a special secondhand bookstore can trigger a religious experience for me. Here I glimpse eternity as time stands still: hours become minutes and I am suspended in the hereafter. The dog-eared, gilded-paged, embossed, and foxed with age receive me with the knowing embrace of an old flame. But instead of arms, I am enveloped by the fragrance of leather mingled with a slight, sweet, musty scent.

Occasionally, stumbling down a dusky corridor, I will be embraced by the Light, as a sunbeam sliver or an angel's wing leads me to exactly the book I need but wasn't consciously aware of. Frankly, this has happened so many times it's no longer paranormal but standard operating procedure. If you'd like to become more aware of hidden helpers as you begin to call forth your talents, a visit to a great secondhand book shop is a fabulous way to begin. My favorite book exploration invocation is: "Divine Guidance is my only reality and Divine Guidance richly manifests for me in the perfect book at the perfect price. As I seek, I shall find, and I give thanks."

Some secondhand stores are ramshackle affairs with vague subject categories, but others can be very prim, especially if they deal in rare books or particular obscure subjects. But the choice available is astonishing and it's akin to having a tutor; secondhand stores can have entire rooms devoted to subject categories. You'll find these volumes alphabetized according to author or book series, and occasionally still in their original jackets. Here's where I find my treasures—and for me it's the lost domestic tomes from the turn of the century to the 1950s, the ghosts of all things once bright and beautiful. I also find old magazines and booklets that were given away as free bonuses from manufacturers, which are a wealth of inspiration and information.

I call this true self-help treatment "bibliotherapy," seeking Divine guidance through books, which is an ancient form of prayer.

It is also referred to as Divination. "Divination is the means by which you engage in dialogue with the Divine. Communicating with the deity provides proof that you are not alone, that the Universe is alive, and that it is aware of your presence, your longings, fears, wounds, gifts, and truest self," the English spiritual writer Phyllis Curott tells us. One of her favorite sources of Divination is consulting her "library angel" by going to a row of books in her home, or a friend's house, as well as to libraries and bookshops all over the world. In each place she would ask to be led to the right book to give her the guidance and comfort she sought at a particular time. This is her prayer: "I invite the numinous spirit that resides within these volumes to guide my hand, and my inquiry. Please help me find wisdom." She then closes her eyes, moves her hand back and forth and up and down over the bookshelf and, when the moment is right, honors the gentle pull toward a particular volume. She waits to see if there's a feeling of certainty and then takes it from the shelf, saying, "I acknowledge you as my guide."

Phyllis suggests, "Allow the book to open in your hands. Open your eyes and let them light upon the page. Read what is before you. It may take time to meditate upon the answer you have received, or the message may be absolutely clear immediately...Write down the passage you received and, even if it does not seem immediately meaningful, let it evoke feelings. And end the divination by giving thanks to the book, the library angel, and the Divine for their assistance."

I've been exploring a similar prayer ritual for decades and have never failed to be nudged toward the next step or given the knowledge that I needed. When I'm searching for new women friends on the page to guide me through rough or daunting life passages, I start meditating on the type of advice I need even before I leave for the bookshop. And the swiftness of the Divine Librarian's help makes me smile with thanks through my fears.

Virginia Woolf believed that "a perfect treat must include a visit to the second-hand bookshop." Put finding a fabulous one on your list of personal priorities.

SEPTEMBER 7

The House Was Quiet and the World Was Calm

The house was quiet and the world was calm.
The reader became the book; and summer night
Was like the conscious being of the book.
The house was quiet, and the world was calm.
—Wallace Stevens (1879–1955)
American twentieth century poet

All I've ever needed in life has been found in between the lines, paragraphs, pages, chapters, and covers of a book. The ones I've read, of course, but even more mysteriously, the books I write.

After all this time, it's been quite a revelation to discover that the books I write are the very books that I need to live or propel me safely into the next stage of my life.

My books become personally prophetic, for unbeknownst to my conscious mind, my Authentic Self has sent a soul scout to the territory up ahead, ready to stake a new claim in my heart and name. Then like a gold rusher, I work my vein, panning for spiritual moxie: nuggets of truth, wisdom, grit, gumption, and grace to sustain me through the changes, choices, and circumstances ahead, but have not yet been revealed. Gratefully, however, by now I've learned to distinguish between the real thing and fool's gold.

I sort my books by categories: writing books (on the craft of writing), art, interior design, cookbooks, women's memoirs, my cherished canon of forgotten women writers, women explorers, biographies, cinema (which includes film history, costume design, and art decoration), sleuth mysteries, Irish history, Celtic mysticism, gardening, natural studies, literary domesticity, philosophy, spiritual, fashion and style, poetry and literature. I keep all the books written by one author together.

Then there is the reference bookcase filled with Oxford dictionaries and quotation tomes, and books on words themselves, literary quips, forgotten phrases. When I feel dry, I peruse the shelves.

When I moved recently, I drove everyone crazy with the packing and sorting of the books.

It was the perusing, I tell you. The perusing of the pages and the euphoric discovery that I possessed this unread book, and then, the deciding to leave this one out of the box marked "Women's Lives" because I might want to read it before I move (ridiculous notion) until what ended up happening was a huge wardrobe box labeled "Miscellaneous" was loaded onto the moving van. Last one in, first box out. As I write, its enormous edifice of brown cardboard sits patiently, waiting to be opened. That might happen soon, as the cats are using the cardboard as a shedding post. However, I do pray it's not a complete karmic cycle before it's unpacked. I miss my books.

To be completely candid, when I'm writing a new book, I only read nonfiction for information and don't read contemporary novels because I don't want to have the slightest influence of anyone else's voice in my head. A writer's voice is a mirror of her soul and as indelible as fingerprints, and it must be guarded like the treasure it is. After twenty years of journalism, I finally found my voice during the five years of writing *Simple Abundance;* and at forty-five years old it was a thrilling adventure and accomplishment. Every writer will confess, if they're honest, that it takes a lifetime trying to "find your voice," and that can happen only when you allow your mind and creative life to become quiet enough to hear the end of a thought. Your own. And then, like a singer whose voice is insured by Lloyd's of London, you protect it.

My prime directive as a go-between is that there should be no separation between the words I write and the words the woman I write for reads. That would be you, lovely one.

"The words were spoken as if there was no book, except that the reader leaned above the page ... The quiet was part of the meaning, part of the mind: The access of perfection to the page," the American poet Wallace Stevens tells us in his exquisite poetic meditation on reading "The House Was Quiet and the World Was Calm." Just repeat slowly and aloud that glorious sentence: *The house was quiet, and the world was calm.* Isn't that very thought a prayer? Nine words only, but if it had taken Wallace a lifetime to craft and convey them, there wouldn't have been a moment wasted.

When we are going through turmoil and challenge, sorrow and difficulty, I find it very reassuring to view my present from the vantage point of my future. Then, with our backward glance at our past lives in this one, we discover that whatever tries our soul and breaks our hearts now will be remembered as a "period" that we courageously sailed through, past shoals to safe harbor.

But here's the very thing that wears us down—the constant contradiction between needing space and the desire to hold on, even if we don't know what to hold on to or why. *It might come in handy someday ... Or I loved that time so much ...* If you are feeling overwhelmed in the sifting and sorting process of your life or home, then know you're not alone. We all need a homeopathic rescue remedy. This morning I let my thoughts drift back to a safe, cozy childhood reverie and how all my favorite rooms were illustrated in comics and books. Before *House and Garden,* there were Archie, Betty, and Veronica comics. Prior to *Architectural Digest,* there were *Anne of Green Gables* and *Calling All Girls,* the compact magazine for pre-teens in the forties, fifties, and sixties.

My favorite childhood books were the Little Golden Books illustrated by Eloise Wilkin (1904–1987). Eloise was a successful children's book illustrator who accepted a contract from Simon & Schuster in 1943 to illustrate four Little Golden Books. She ended up illustrating more than a hundred books, even into her eighties.

What a timeless exquisite gift she left women of all ages and how grateful I am that she shared her heart and home with the world. I so loved Eloise Wilkin's world as a child, that I wanted her cozy, safe world for my baby. Now we've both grown up, but the power of Eloise Wilkin's magic is still potent. To sip a cup of tea and slowly turn the pages of her books *We Help Mommy, We Help Daddy, The New Baby, Prayers for Children, Baby's Christmas* is to take a brief sojourn in serenity—a tour of a happy childhood.

Our constantly changing circumstances ask us to think again about what our absolutes are—those things we cannot bear to be without— no matter where we live. For me it's a big, comfortable bed where I can stretch out with my books, pads, pen, cats; a great reading light; good English tea; a cozy chair and ottoman; a scented linen closet; a fireplace; bookshelves; the ticking of the grandfather clock; and my beautiful collection of still-life paintings. Still, while I've not yet been reunited with all my absolutes, I know it won't be long, because I can see the vision so clearly.

But today, once again, I return to my Little Golden Books. My finger traces the picture on the page of a colonial rag rug, a stenciled border, blue-and-white china, a maple rope bed, a blue hutch with its walls of cherry pink, a small world all cozy and contained. I realize that the feelings inspired by the treasures I have found for myself in books by and for women of all ages are beyond measure. Yes, I have decorated the homes of my life in different ways, yet all were inspired by Eloise Wilkin's loving energy and influence. And here is where wonderment accompanies me as I begin to live again through my books, both written and read.

It looks like I'll need to create a new category and space to display them! Back go my strays into the special box labeled "Happy Books."

Today, dearest friend, I wish for you a quiet house and a calm world, beginning in your heart. And wonderful words to read and hold close to enwrap you in a hug and a hush. And more Amazing Grace than you can imagine or ask for, in full measure, pressed down and overflowing.

SEPTEMBER 8

Howards End Is on the Landing

I only really love a book when I have read it at least four times.
—Nancy Brooker Spain (1917–1964)
Prominent English broadcaster and journalist

I've described the *Simple Abundance* journey as a safari of the Self and Spirit. In *Something More: Excavating Your Authentic Self,* we embarked together on an archaeological dig. But even though there have been eleven other books in my body of work, to some extent I always feel like an archivist/archaeologist when I begin a new one. This is because I can carbon date distinct periods of my life by the books on my shelves. Or rather the books I *remember* as being on my shelves during a particular time and place.

The sublime English writer Susan Hill describes such an adventure in her delightful memoir *Howards End Is on the Landing,* based on a year of reading all the books she had crowded on her bookcases. It's always so mysterious how minor happenstance can morph into a new trajectory of one's sense of belonging. "It began like this. I went to the shelves on the landing to look for a book I knew was there. It was not. But plenty of others were and among them I noticed at least a dozen I realized I had never read." So, forsaking any new purchases, she embarked on a pilgrimage of her own heart, mind, and opinions—both past and present.

What books are crowded on your bookshelves? Do you even know? Now here's a crisp September pastime for you. Sometimes we find ourselves completely at loose ends trying to figure out how to inspire change in our lives and we don't have a clue where to begin. I say begin with your bookshelf. As Susan Hill explains: "I wanted to repossess my books, to explore what I had accumulated over a lifetime of reading, and to map this house of many volumes. There are enough here to divert, instruct, entertain, amaze, amuse, edify, improve, enrich me for far longer than a year and every one of them deserves to be taken down and dusted off, opened and read. A book which is left on a shelf is a dead thing, but it is also a chrysalis, an inanimate object packed with the potential to burst into new life. Wandering through the house that day, looking for one elusive book, my eyes were opened to how much of that life was stored here."

Because I love both film and books equally ("...two lovers and I ain't ashamed, two lovers and I love them both the same..." Thank you, Mary Wells, the first queen of Motown...), I created my own cinema/bibliotherapy ritual that's a fusion of film, food, reading, and fun.

Let's take *Howards End* by the Edwardian English novelist E. M. Forster (1879–1970), who was very interested in social classes during the height of the British Empire and its decline, and in the restraints on women's lives and independence. By layering simultaneous stories of the haves and the have-nots throughout his novels, we can examine both sides without looking away from what is uncomfortable. That's possible because he reveals the truth so gently, through happenstance, such as when Helen Schlegel absentmindedly picks up the umbrella belonging to a stranger, Leonard Bast, at a concert, setting in motion a series of circumstances that changes the lives of three families forever.

We're familiar with Forster's work because of the cinematic versions of his novels, including *A Room with a View* and *A Passage to India*, the stunning movies made by the Anglo-Indian collaboration of filmmakers called Merchant-Ivory (the late producer Ismail Merchant, the director James Ivory, and their screenwriting partner Ruth Prawer Jhabvala were a team that defines harmonic convergence!) during the eighties, nineties, and early 2000s. Strangely wonderful is the alchemy of Merchant-Ivory films, part of a genre known as "heritage cinema," in which houses always play a supporting role and a difficult love affair is featured. History, heritage, houses, and throbbing hearts. Forster had me at hello. Merchant-Ivory never let me go.

And as the Mary Wells song explains about the one man she loves who embodies two distinct aspects, both representations of Howards End—the book and the movie—equally delight me. The Merchant-Ivory film (1992) of *Howards End* starred Emma Thompson and Anthony Hopkins and won three Academy Awards. It is the epitome of a period film, and while watching, we feel that we are voyeurs held at bay, looking through gauze made of golden threads. The lighting and the rich colors are so luxurious, the period touches so authentic, the dialogue so ironically precise that soon "Merchant-Ivory-esque" became a generic description, used when attributing the special look and feel of their work to other things.

Recently a new version of *Howards End* was made into a four-part series for Starz, by the American film director and screenwriter Kenneth Lonergan (who gave us *Gangs of New York* and *Manchester by the Sea*) which was a very unexpected choice for that screenwriter. Contemporary, fresh, energetic, golden gauze removed and no spoilers—you'll just have to have a contrast-and-compare cinematherapy weekend. Invite as many friends as you like or just revel by yourself: Take one book, two films, a flagon of wine, olives, Genoa salami, provolone cheese, a crusty baguette, dark chocolate with sea salt, and have a blast.

E. M. Forster has been described as a novelist who can be read over and over because you learn something new every time you do, which is exactly why we love certain movies. Sometimes I read the novel before watching a film or watch a movie and then find the book—do whatever gives you pleasure on a certain day.

"The only books that influence us are those for which we are ready," E. M. Forster reminds us, "and which have gone a little farther down our particular path than we have yet got ourselves."

SEPTEMBER 9

On Becoming a Woman of Letters

People read everything nowadays, except books.
—Madame Anne Sophie Swetchine (1782–1857)
Russian mystic and nineteenth-century
woman of letters

Imagine with me that tonight we're traveling back in time to 1836. We've been invited to a lively French literary party at the apartment of the esteemed salonnière, Madame Sophie Swetchine, at 71, Rue Saint-Dominique in Paris.

And what is a salonnière? So glad you asked.

"A salonnière is a party host," entertaining expert Carla McDonald explains, an influential contemporary salonnière in her own right. "The term (pronounced 'sal-on-yair') was first used to describe the clever women in seventeenth and eighteenth century France who hosted parties—called *salons*—in their homes to celebrate and promote the most important writers, philosophers, and artists of the day. Highly influential, the salonnières would select the topics to be discussed at their parties, determine the list of thinkers, politicians, aristocrats, and other influencers who would be invited to attend, and artfully lead the discussion. Conversation was the principal activity of the salon, and the goal of the salonnières, these feminine power brokers of the day, was to keep the discourse civil enough to encourage enlightenment for all in attendance."

And who doesn't love a swell party? Polite, witty, intelligent banter, an exchange of views, and a respect for the other guests (especially if one was meeting for the first time), these parties brought together the most important thinkers and creators of their day to meet and exchange opinions. Their hostesses were the original social and power influencers.

Madame de Pompadour, who was the royal mistress of French King Louis XV, is probably the most famous salonnière, but the extraordinary, intelligent, and savvy women whose names or stories we might not be familiar with (but can now learn about) knew that a suggestive whisper in the right ear and a smile behind her fan was far more persuasive than a boisterous shout in a crowd, especially since intelligent, animated, and witty conversation was the purpose of the evenings.

So, whose party are we crashing? Madame Sophie Swetchine. Here's her backstory. As the daughter of the Russian secretary of state, Sophie was a member of the imperial Russian Court of Catherine the Great. She was well-educated and spoke several languages. But there were many lessons the young Sophie learned through watching, and above all, by *listening* to the candid conversations she was privy to because she happened to be a young girl and practically invisible to her seniors.

At seventeen, Sophie married a man much older than herself, but it was a good match. Unfortunately, she was childless, and found comfort in spirituality, converting to Catholicism when she was thirty-three. However, any member of the Russian nobility who left the Russian Orthodox Church was exiled from Russia. Sophie chose Paris as her new home and, using her sophisticated background and connections, set up a salon "that soon became the talk of the town," Kristen O'Brien tells us. "Some of the most distinguished thinkers in literature, politics, and ecclesiastical high society, including the Archbishop of Paris, came through her doors, as did a number of other Russian exiles."

From 1826 to 1856, Madame Swetchine was the grande dame of

Paris, so let's imagine that we are there with her. Who is on her guest list tonight? Victor Hugo (*Les Misérables*), Alexandre Dumas (*The Three Musketeers*), Gustave Flaubert (*Madame Bovary*), and the French romantic novelist George Sand (one the most successful female writers of the nineteenth century). Did she bring Frédéric Chopin? Is that *Nocturne op. 9* we hear in the background?

As the other guests have taken seats to listen, Madame Sophie glides serenely toward us and asks if we will do a favor for her. Of course, with pleasure, anything. She asks us to travel ahead into the twenty-first century with an urgent message, and she slips a small piece of paper into my hand before closing it with her own. Softly she says, "*Que Dieu bénisse l'assemblée et recompense ses efforts* . . . May God bless you and reward you for your efforts."

It's time for us to return to our day jobs. Why don't you stash some of those beautiful Ladurée macarons in your pocket for our trip home.

But Monsieur Ladurée will not open his Paris bakery until 1862.

Then we'll just stop there on our way back to the future. Reading collapses time.

SEPTEMBER 10

The Great Acceleration

One glance at a book and you hear the voice of another person, perhaps someone dead for 1,000 years. To read is to voyage through time.
—Carl Sagan (1934–1996)
American astronomer, cosmologist, astrophysicist, and author

In the beginning was the Word. And frankly, the Word was all that was needed to separate the heavens and earth. Still is, still can.

As the Word spread, its importance to the act of creation increased in myriad ways, whether it was chiseled onto clay tablets, pressed into wax, drawn on papyrus, painted in illuminated gold leaf on vellum, or printed by rolling ink over iron type on parchment. For thousands of years, the progression from darkness to light, not to mention from the hammer to fonts, has always required that words be written down for someone else to read, speak, interpret, inspire, inform, act, visualize, direct, educate, and entertain.

Still is, still can, as long as the word remains sacred, saved, savored, and shared. Remember the note Madame Sophie asked us to bring back from Paris, 1836? Did you guess what it said? "People read everything nowadays, except books." Nearly two centuries after her astute observation, time isn't just collapsing, it's accelerating, faster than ever; now a blink of an eye is considered lollygagging. We're speeding so fast we don't even notice we're moving. In fact, environmental scientists now refer to the rapid speed of the earth's climate change crisis as "The Great Acceleration." And the Great Acceleration has spread like a contagious rogue virus to technology and society as well.

How can this be even remotely good for our psyches or our souls? Well, it's not and we know it. But that doesn't mean today I won't be on my computer working, then distracted by a diversion like a $699 blush-colored Nuit Ephemere off-the-shoulder, short-sleeve, sheer lace one- piece bodysuit. It's very pretty, the color is scrumptious, and why is it luring me away from my tasks today, such as writing this meditation? Because I made the mistake last week of clicking to get more information. That's when I noticed its price, which was all the information I needed. However, guess what? Bergdorf Goodman now knows that I didn't resist clickbait and they have been trolling me ever since. Oh, no kidding, it's on sale today for $349.

"The Internet and social media have trained my brain to read a paragraph or two, and then start looking around. When I read an online article from the *Atlantic* or the *New Yorker*, after a few paragraphs I glance over at the sidebar to judge the article's length. My mind strays and I find myself clicking on the sidebars and the underlined links," writer Philip Yancey shares, surely for all of us. Yancey is the author of thirty books, exploring provocative and contemporary spiritual issues in the age of social media, and he's experiencing a personal crisis he calls the death of reading, which is threatening our souls.

Yancey writes surrounded by twenty-seven tall bookshelves which contain the 5,000 books he's read over a three-decade career. "Books help define who I am. They have ushered me on a journey of faith, have introduced me to the wonders of science and the natural world... More importantly, they have been a source of delight and adventure and beauty, opening windows to a reality I would not otherwise know." But Yancey admits that what is happening to us all is our increasing inability to focus and concentrate.

Just as our health and well-being—mental and physical—are nourished, preserved, and expanded by what we eat, so are our brains nurtured by what feeds our imagination, emotions, and creativity. These soul sources need preservation. In the last twenty years, we have become activists in trying to save not only our planet but rare-breed animals and plant species from extinction. Even so, how can we save the world, if we can't save the Word? One of the blessings of the internet is that we have so much information and knowledge now available to all of us. It's not that important and life-changing books aren't being written. But what's being read?

I've shared my belief that the Authentic Self is the soul made visible. But only you can make sure that She's a soul survivor.

SEPTEMBER 11

A Lesson from Loss

Loss as muse. Loss as character. Loss as life.
—Anna Quindlen
American author, Pulitzer Prize–winning journalist

It was just another manic Monday for Nancy, Cheryl, Valerie, Kathleen, Gilda, Elizabeth, and Patricia. Just another business trip, another swing on the flying trapeze. Children were kissed and sent off to school; babies were left with sitters; spouses were reminded about soccer practice, the casserole in the freezer, the laundry that needed to be picked up. Their day was frazzled or pleasant, successful or disappointing. Does it really matter? At the end of it, perhaps there was an opportunity to grab some small treat in the gift shop before boarding American Eagle commuter Flight 4148 to Chicago's O'Hare Airport. Waiting for them were loved ones eager to report on the day's happenings, cabs to catch, connections to make.

Instead, there were news bulletins, phone calls, disbelief, devastation, shock, pain, grief, hearts broken, dreams dashed as Nancy (forty-eight), Cheryl (forty-four), Valerie (forty-four), Kathleen (forty-seven), Gilda (forty-three), Elizabeth (thirty-seven), and Patricia (forty-two) never made it home. For, as the plane was descending, the inconceivable occurred. All the women perished in a fiery crash, along with sixty-one other souls. In their final moments, did they realize they weren't going to make it? What were their last thoughts?

It certainly wasn't the deal made or lost or how hassled their day had been. Surely their last thoughts were real. Maybe the faces of those they loved pushed away the fear. Maybe there was no time for regrets. I hope so. I pray so.

If we are alive, we cannot escape loss. The litany of loss is a part of real life. The World Trade Center. We all know where we were when we heard the news. Sandy Hook. First graders. After Sandy Hook we said never again. But then Again paid us a visit before Never arrived.

"Have you ever thought, when something dreadful happens, a

moment ago things were not like this; let it be *then* not *now*, anything but *now*?" the English novelist Mary Stewart asks. "And you try and try to remake *then*, but you know you can't. So, you try to hold the moment quite still and not let it move on and show itself."

Today might be tough for you. You might not want the next moment to show itself, to reveal the twists and turns of life's mystery. But at least you have it. You still have life. A choice as to how you will live this precious day.

Don't wish it away. Don't waste it. For the love of all that's holy, redeem one hour. Hold it close. Cherish it. Above all, be grateful for it. Let your thanksgiving rise above the din of disappointment—opportunities lost, mistakes made, the clamor of all that has not yet come.

And if today is so horrendous that the gift doesn't seem worth acknowledging; if you can't find one moment to enjoy, one simple pleasure to savor, one friend to call, one person to love, one thing to share, one smile to offer; if life is so difficult you don't want to bother living it to the fullest, then don't live today for yourself.

Live it for those who cannot.

Live it for Nancy, Cheryl, Valerie, Kathleen, Gilda, Elizabeth, and Patricia.

SEPTEMBER 12

You Now Have a Shorter Attention Span Than a Goldfish

Storytelling—that's not the future. The future, I'm afraid, is flashes and impulses. It's made up of moments and fragments, and stories won't survive.

—Dexter Palmer
American novelist

According to *Time* magazine, a Microsoft study determined that people now lose their concentration or ability to focus after eight seconds, down from twelve seconds in 2000 when the study began, demonstrating the physical effects of an increasingly digitalized lifestyle on our brains.

A goldfish's attention span is nine seconds.

Hold that thought.

Whether it's smartphones, tablet computers, video games, the Cloud, free wi-fi and hot spots—as the number of digital devices grows, so too are new ways created to catch our attention. As Satya Nadella, the chief executive officer of Microsoft, concluded, in the future "the true scarce commodity" will be "human attention."

After reading this, I tried to source how many content varieties we all deal with every day without realizing it as we scroll and click. There are 101 categories of digital content popping up on our screens in little boxes and in our discombobulated brains. And the number of digital media companies who will provide these digital traps is growing as well.

"There are no new stories in the world anymore, and no more storytellers. There is nothing left but fragments of phrases that signaled their telling; once upon a time; why, and then, the end. But these fragments of phrases have lost their meanings through endless repetition, like everything else in this modern, mechanical age," Dexter Palmer writes in his beautifully rendered novel *The Dream of Perpetual Motion.* "And this machine age has no room for stories. These days we seek our pleasures out in single moments cast in amber, as if we have no desire to connect the future to the past. Stories? We have no time for them; we have no patience."

A world without stories. We can't let that happen.

On the brighter side, we've dramatically increased our multitasking skills! Gratitude, find it where you can.

SEPTEMBER 13

The Poetry Prescription

Instructions for living a life. Pay attention.
Be astonished.
Tell about it.
 —Mary Oliver (1935–2019)
  Pulitzer Prize and National Book Award–winning poet
  Best-selling poet in America

One of the gems I unearthed in a choice secondhand book haunt was the October 1925 issue of *Good Housekeeping.* In it was a surprising remedy for weariness called "The Poetry Cure." It suggested that when we are frazzled, ruminating on a line or a stanza of poetry can induce a sense of serenity. This suggestion led me to a marvelous form of meditation, especially if I think I don't have twenty minutes to sit down or take a walk—a situation that happens more often than I care to admit.

Many of us resist the power of poetry to illuminate our path because we have such bad memories of dissecting stanzas in high school English.

Some of us also have an inferiority complex about poetry, viewing it as an esoteric art that only the well-educated, literate, and erudite can appreciate. But poets are the first to disagree; they know poetry is real and personal. Rita Dove, America's youngest and first African American poet laureate, tells us, "Poetry connects you to yourself, to the self that doesn't know how to talk or negotiate."

When we allow poetry to slip slowly beneath the sinews of our conscious mind, connection to our Authentic Selves becomes simpler; an emotion or an experience is captured in evocative word melodies that bestow harmony and balance on everyday encounters. Rita Dove believes that poetry has the ability to restore "a sense of mystery, a sense of wonder" to our daily round. Once I heard her read a poem she had written about waiting to board a flight to go home. I was cooking as I listened, but in that instant I was waiting to board my own flight. It was an exquisite reminder that our specific lives can mirror the universal experience. Nowhere is this more passionately expressed than in poetry.

To begin exploring this simply abundant art there are several voices I suggest you listen to and in turn help you to find your own: Warsan Shire, Rupi Kaur, Tracy K. Smith, Morgan Parker, Yrsa Daley-Ward, Rita Dove, Anne Sexton, Louise Bogan, Diane Wakoski, Emily Dickinson, Maya Angelou, Adrienne Rich, Audre Lorde, Muriel Rukeyser, Judith Viorst, Elizabeth Barrett Browning, Maxine Kumin, Diane Ackerman, Shirley Kaufman, May Sarton, Cherrie Moraga, Marianne Moore, and the glorious Mary Oliver.

Read one poem a day. Write a favorite verse from it on a card and commit it to memory. Follow your favorite contemporary poets on Instagram and Facebook, too. Discover the marvelous Maya Stein, who teaches ten-line poems on her website www.mayastein.com. Poetry possesses many secrets just waiting to be revealed to patient seekers of truth. I love to meditate on a line just before drifting off to sleep.

Explore writing your own poems. Don't tell me you're too old or that none of us are interested in what you have to say. Few literary debuts were as stunning as the publication of Amy Clampitt's first full-length book of poetry, *The Kingfisher*, in 1983, when she was sixty-three. Although she had been a poet all her life, she didn't find her authentic voice until she was in her fifties. If you have lived all your life hearing another voice in your heart, maybe it's time to take inspiration from her life's path?

And consider the advice of Yrsa Daley-Ward, who said, "If you are afraid to write it, that's a good sign. I suppose you know when you're writing the truth when you're terrified." So start with the truth, write a poem with your Authentic Self, as if you're both collaborating on a country and western song.

Trust that you will discover, as did the Russian-born writer Anzia Yezierska, that "The real thing creates its own poet."

Job, Career, or Calling?

The pitcher cries for water to carry
and a person for work that is Real.
                —Marge Piercy
                American novelist, poet, and social activist

There are significant differences among a job, a career, and a calling. Jobs are what we do to keep bodies, souls, and families together. But as the Pulitzer Prize–winning historian Studs Terkel wisely pointed out in his oral history *Working: People Talk About What They Do All Day and How They Feel About It*, the search for daily meaning is as important as daily bread, and recognition as necessary as cash. For when we work, we are searching "for a sort of life rather than a Monday through Friday sort of dying."

One of the people Studs Terkel interviewed was Nora Watson, who then worked as a staff writer for a health-care magazine: "I think most of us are looking for a calling, not a job. Most of us, like the assembly line worker, have jobs that are too small for our spirit. Jobs are not big enough for people." But jobs are crucial; we need to "earn a living," we need to pay our bills and take care of ourselves and our loved ones.

A career can be a calling, but not necessarily. Usually a career occurs when we stick to an occupational path—accounting, advertising, nursing, publishing—because we do what we do quite well and get paid for doing it. Sometimes careers resemble long-standing marriages in which passion is exchanged for comfort, security, and predictability in an uncertain world. Of course, there is nothing wrong with this choice; for many it is absolutely the right one—although some may wonder what psychic price is being exacted for playing it safe. It is certainly true that every day we don't strive to live authentically we do pay a price, with compounded interest.

Many of us eventually move from jobs to careers, but often we hesitate to answer an authentic calling, especially in midlife, because we're torn—between the financial realities of a mortgage and debt, between raising children and caring for aging parents, between a proven track record and the unknown, between a regular paycheck and uncertainty, between circumstance and creative choice.

But the Game of Life has changed. We're living and working into our eighties and nineties. Authenticity is ageless. Consider the glorious Carmen Dell'Orefice, the world's oldest working model. She began when she was only thirteen and was discovered on a New York crosstown bus, six decades ago!

She's now eighty-seven. Two years ago, she closed out the haute couture runway show of Chinese designer Guo Pei, resplendent in red as she slayed the audience and media. When asked how long she was going to continue working, she said: "I'm going for 105, then I'll see if I want to change professions." No matter what your age as you read this, you have several decades ahead of you. Shouldn't you be doing a few things that you absolutely love?

It's a mistake to accept as our reality the illusion that many are called to fulfillment, but few are chosen. What Spirit has done for other women can be done for you—when you're ready. The truth is, we're all chosen; most of us just forget to RSVP.

Novelist Mary Morris tells us that "Pursuing what you want to do and achieving your goal is not like finding the burning bush or discovering a gold mine. There are usually no epiphanies, no sudden reversals of fortune. Fulfillment comes in fits and starts...Fulfillment comes in many guises, and it can come to us in our lives at any time...But only *we* can make sure we will be fulfilled. If we feel empty, no amount of water can fill our well. It has to come from within, from the underground springs and streams."

SEPTEMBER 15

Working from the Heart

Work is love made visible.

—Khalil Gibran (1883–1931)
Lebanese-American poet

Most of us do not consider our work a personal form of worship. Work is worldly. Worship is withdrawing from the world to honor Spirit. But could there be a more beautiful way to honor the Great Creator than by contributing to the re-creation of the world through our gifts? This is what we're called to do each day through our work. Yet it is very difficult to get even a glimmer of the holy when we are harassed, unappreciated, overwhelmed, frazzled, and burned out.

Marianne Williamson believes that the workplace is "but a front for a temple, a healing place where people [can] be lifted above the insanity of a frightened world." Once, when she was working as a cocktail waitress—years before she answered her calling to become a spiritual guide and writer—she realized that people only thought they were coming to a bar for a drink. Really the bar was a church in disguise, and she could minister to people with warmth, conversation, and compassion.

"No matter what we do, we can make it our ministry," she writes in her illuminating *A Return to Love: Reflections on the Principles of a Course in Miracles.* "No matter what form our job or activity takes, the content is the same as everyone else's; we are here to minister to human hearts. If we talk to anyone, or see anyone, or even think of anyone, then we have the opportunity to bring more love into the universe. From a waitress to the head of a movie studio, from a dog trainer to the president of a nation, there is no one whose job is unimportant to God."

It's easier to imagine that our work could be our worship if we could perceive the sacred in how we spend at least eight hours of the day. Perhaps the secret to coming to this awareness, no matter what our present circumstances, is to discover the work we would *love* to do. But until we do, we need to learn to love the work we're presently doing.

Today you can begin to transform your workplace and your working style by considering how much you have to be grateful for. If you have a job, even one you dislike, it's a safety net as you take a leap of faith toward your authenticity; if you're out of work, the path already has been cleared for you to answer your authentic calling. Invoke Spirit as your personal career counselor. The mystical poet Khalil Gibran tells us, "When you work, you fulfill a part of earth's fondest dream assigned to you when that dream is born."

Fulfilling your part of the earth's fondest dream occurs when you work from the heart.

SEPTEMBER 16

On Keeping a Notebook

It is a good idea to keep in touch, and I supposed that keeping in touch is what notebooks are all about... I think we are well advised to keep on nodding terms with the people we used to be, whether we find them attractive company or not... Remember what it was to be me; that is always the point.

—Joan Didion
American literary journalist, novelist, and
memoirist

Recently my daughter surprised me with a box of my old notebooks, which had been stored for decades in the attic of her childhood home. I was gobsmacked to discover an enormous number of diaries, yellow pads, journals, calendars, artist's sketchbooks, and single pages dating back to years before I married her father or she was born. But here was the body of proof: *prima facie* ("on first look") evidence of the girl I left behind. At that time I was working as a legal secretary by day (which explains why there are so many Latin legal terms jotted in the margins of my memories) and aspiring writer by night, burning the candle at both ends because I was in my twenties and could.

For all the experiences I was convinced I wouldn't survive (survival is a theme writ large during one's twenties), here I still am, and gratefully so. As for all those heartbreaking leaps in the dark, romantic obsessions, and daring misalliances, the majority of them have faded in their passionate intensity, leaving only such literary references to their many charms as "a git lower than whale-shite on the bottom of the ocean" and "His knuckles scraped upon the sidewalk as he tried to walk upright…" Wisdom honed, no doubt, after a few evenings of fish and chips and lager or Pimm's cup and cucumber tea sandwiches with sympathetic girlfriends. Other life experiences left behind reluctant ragged-edged lessons or losses so deep they've scarred over and I'm not going back there again.

Nevertheless, those scribbled passages I did manage to lasso and rope to the page bring me curious wonder. One declaration, in particular, from Saturday, March 29, 1976, could be fluky coincidence, ornery stubbornness, or mysterious clairvoyance, an art I had not yet realized was in my personal bag of tricks:

*"I have decided to take radical complete control of my life and go after what it is I want. This year I want to **write**."*

I was at the hand-wringing-but-hopeful beginning stage of living my calling, a phase that every burgeoning creator experiences. My determination was to become a writer, but the process is familiar to all creators: Close your eyes, hold your nose, feel the adrenaline, and jump in.

And that was all I did, from that day forward. Write.

But I didn't become a writer on that day, because declaring to the Universe your intention and wishing to be a writer is not the same as becoming one. A writer is someone who *completes* the act of writing: a poem, play, short story, novella, novel, nonfiction narrative, biography, essay, script, feature article, a blog post. One really bad page. Or a terrible paragraph. Even a sentence. Heaven knows, I've spent entire days on one sentence: putting a comma in during the morning, then taking it out in the afternoon. (Thank you, Oscar Wilde.)

Those examples may be mine, but they're familiar to anyone who yearns to follow a dream. It doesn't matter whether you get paid or not—paid, of course, is preferable—but that's not likely to happen for a long time. So, in my case, it was the legal secretary's gig that kept body, if not soul, together. In the beginning you do a lot of work "on spec." For me that meant an editor showing a bit of interest in an idea, leaving me to write it on my own dime in hope she'd commit to it later. What matters is that you do it. Bake the artisanal donuts. Go for the audition. Build beautiful birdhouses. For me it was to write. Show up on the page and keep a disciplined schedule so the Muse knows where to find you. Then, finish the damn thing, whatever it is. Turn it in and begin another.

The dreamer I was, who kept this notebook years ago, tells me: "I have the following goals. To finish my play on Bernhardt, to write 'Mock Memoirs,' to write at least the first draft of the Irish novel and to earn at least a living wage from writing." I love her moxie, although she hasn't a clue yet about the discrepancy between *chronos* and *kairos*, earth's time and Divine dispatch. God knows I wish I'd understood this spiritual truth earlier, because it would have made things easier. Or I think it would, at any rate. However, a retrospective look tells us that she will learn her way, the hard way, the long way, the only way she knows how, falling asleep over the pink typewriter, which explains the black carbon crease on her forehead in the morning.

Still, when she does finally take a backward glance, all the hard-scrabble years of naïveté, disappointments, detours, wrong choices, bad timing, bungled efforts; all the threadbare years of struggle, loneliness, failure, second-guessing, and despair it took to get her to the right moment at the right time (a publisher's "yes" after thirty rejections, five years' work, and a whopping advance of $22,500), it will only seem like a blink of an eye.

However, years later, I can report the results:

I did finish and have produced my one-woman show on Sarah Bernhardt. The play ran for a month.

The first draft of the Irish novel on yellowing, curled foolscap from the Dark Ages, with its one carbon paper copy, is in a file cabinet just arrived from England. I vaguely recall abandoning that one when I ran out of rent money and had to pawn that gorgeous pink typewriter. But you can bet that I'll be rereading it when I have some time, to see if there's even a kernel of an idea there.

Regretfully, I haven't a clue what "Mock Memoirs" is or was, but it sounds like a delicious romp, so let's dwell in grateful possibility.

Finally, the most difficult and harrowing lesson of them all: it would take twenty years to achieve the last goal of 1976, to be able to earn a living as a writer.

I'm grateful that Heaven operates on a "need to know" basis. It's one of life's most overlooked blessings.

SEPTEMBER 17

Upon Reading Her Books

Like most—maybe all—writers, I learned to write by writing and,
by example, by reading books.

—Francine Prose
American novelist, short story writer, essayist,
and critic

Joan Didion burst on the scene in 1968 when her first book of essays written for magazines was collected into an anthology called *Slouching Towards Bethlehem*. This was during the heady days of "New Journalism"—the American literary movement that pushed the boundaries between what journalism had been and what nonfiction could be. It combined the research of journalism with literary technique and narrative storytelling.

Tom Wolfe (author of *The Right Stuff* and *The Bonfire of the Vanities*) coined the phrase, Truman Capote (*In Cold Blood*) copied it, and Gay Talese's elegant prose cemented the genre in his blockbuster *The Kingdom and the Power* about the *New York Times*, where he'd worked for twelve years as a journalist.

But Joan Didion. Joan Didion was revelatory. Joan Didion was unlike anyone I had ever read before or since; she was more a composer creating arias or an illusionist performing sleight-of-hand magic than a mere journalist using words. The emotional tension inherent in her sentences suspends the reader on a tightrope of tenacity, intrigue, and innuendo. If any writer has ever lived between the lines of her work, it's Didion, who creates a cozy, confidential, even conspiratorial sojourn with her reader, hinting at self-revelation without the slightest intention of disclosure. Yet what she does reveal is breath-gasping, a piercing honesty that stops you in your tracks. As you shake your head and read that paragraph again to make sure this isn't some mystical incantation, suddenly, like a phantom, she's vanished, leaving behind an intoxicating aura in her wake; disappearing in a fragrant fog of unforgettable poetry-like prose.

And therein lies the magic. The alchemy. You read Joan Didion and somehow you believe you are reading about yourself.

Just the memory of reading her for the first time while sitting at the bar in a Capitol Hill hangout, the Jenkins Hill Saloon, and the flush of excitement she triggered all floods back. My usual Sunday ritual in those days was reading the Sunday *New York Times* at the bar with two Bloody Marys and eggs Benedict and then home to a nap. (I really knew how to treat my girl good back then.) But that Sunday, at the bookstore where I picked up my papers, I glimpsed a book called *Slouching Towards Bethlehem*. The cover was rather psychedelic, and I was most definitely not a flower child. Still, I wanted to know any writer who borrowed lines from W. B. Yeats for her book's title. And then I read:

"Once, in a dry season I wrote in large letters across two pages of a notebook that innocence ends when one is stripped of the delusion that one likes oneself... The dismal fact is that self-respect has nothing to do with the approval of others—who are, after all, deceived easily enough; has nothing to do with reputation, which, as Rhett Butler told Scarlett O'Hara, is something people with courage can do without... That kind of self-respect is a discipline, a habit of mind that can never be faked but can be developed, trained, coaxed forth."

Joan Didion taught me the meaning of the Latin verb *vocare*—to answer a call or another Voice. This Voice is distinct and like no other. It invites you to follow it. To peek around the corner of your life or open an old notebook with a stain on its cover or to start taking notes. Reading her was effortless, which means, of course, that she worked harder than any other writer in the world. Writing is not supposed to show. You're not supposed to see the brushstrokes on the canvas. Like Sherlock Holmes's admiration for the beautiful, mysterious adventuress Iréne Adler, always and simply known as *the* Woman as revealed in *A Scandal in Bohemia*, Joan Didion became *the* Writer to me. I wanted to learn how to write, not like Joan Didion, but like Sarah Ban Breathnach.

After winning *Vogue*'s famed and prestigious Prix de Paris essay contest in 1956 (which promised college seniors a shot at winning a week in Paris and an entry-level job at *Vogue*), Joan Didion began her writing career on the bottom rung, at twenty-one, writing fashion promotional copy.

In the marvelous Netflix documentary *Joan Didion: The Center Will Not Hold*, directed by her nephew Griffin Dunne, we get to see the woman behind her half century's work. The entire film is such a wondrous experience, but I'll just recount Joan's anecdote about working with her *Vogue* editor, Allene Talmey. Talmey would go through her copy with violent slashes, a huge aquamarine knuckle ring sparking like flint against a rock as her pencil raced across the page, crossing out and calling for "Action verbs! Action verbs!" She spoke of Talmey's trick of asking for a 350-word paragraph on something, only to tell the young writer when she turned it in to now cut it down to fifty words. I couldn't stop laughing because I've had some harsh editorial episodes like that in my career, and it all comes back to you—but you really do learn how to write. A few years later, the understudy will get her big break, when a cover story article commissioned by *Vogue* from another writer isn't turned in but the cover is already set. Joan has forty-eight hours to write a replacement essay called "Self-Respect: Its Source, Its Power" and down to the character count allotted she pulls off this enormous feat like the stunning star she truly is with panache, verve, style, and piercing insight.

Even though in the documentary the self-respect essay (August 1961) is cited as Didion's first *Vogue* break, it's really her second. My favorite part of writing is research, and I heard a whisper on the internet that Didion had written a cover story on "Jealousy: Is It a Curable Illness" (June 1961), so I searched and finally found a copy on eBay. Life often makes one feel like the poor oyster with a piece of irritating grit instead of grace, but discovering Joan Didion's lost pearl is worth the price.

So here's how Joan Didion helped me learn to write. I recognized in her a distinct voice, which was music to my ears. I realized that music is the mathematics of the spheres. So I would write down a paragraph and then copy it as if I were learning to write for the first time. Joan Didion confesses that Ernest Hemingway taught her how to write a true sentence. We all learn from someone else. We're all taught. We are never alone as long as we can find beauty and truth in the amazing, astonishing combinations of only twenty-six letters. Think of that for a moment: only twenty-six letters and what we can do with them. The wonder of it all. The magic and the majesty. We are our own code-breakers. We are our own ciphers seeking our Authentic Selves.

Copy book after copy book, I wrote out her words in my hand, hearing the cadence, the melody, the harmonies. Feeling the rhythm. The intake of breath, the exhalation. I read her out loud. I heard her music. And then I began writing/composing my own words/musical notes. Gradually, I discovered my own beat. I fell in love with the words; I read dictionaries for pleasure. And by the time I began writing *Simple Abundance* a decade later, I had found my own voice. No longer a copy or an imitation but now an adagio of solace, one singular sensation, a solo for soul and pen.

Why do I write? To find out what I think and feel and know. To lay it all on the line, all of the time. Because the Great Creator loves a pageturner. And when I do that, read it aloud, I notice that a chord might be missing, so then the rewrites begin, over and over again until it brings me tears of joy, surrender, acknowledgment, gratitude. Sheer delight. For at long last, I'd finally found the woman I've been searching for my entire life. My Authentic Self is sharing stories of where we've been and where we're going—the Territory Up Ahead. I am not alone. She promises she'll always be with me on the page and to keep us company, Joan Didion will be in my pocket.

The Courage to Answer the Call

You gain strength, courage and confidence by every experience in which you really stop to look fear in the face.... You must do the thing you cannot do.
— Eleanor Roosevelt (1884–1962)
American first lady, political figure, diplomat, and activist

Just before her death in 1848, Emily Brontë wrote that she did not possess a coward's soul. She was only thirty. At her end, at an age that is really only the beginning for many of us, came the inner awareness that she had lived courageously. She had lived authentically.

Of course, she had known dark moments, but in the darkness, she'd come to trust that a Power greater than her own would never leave nor forsake her. This Love was so transformative she wrote to her sister, Charlotte, that It "Changes, sustains, dissolves, creates and rears" as It leads. This steadfast Love endowed her with courage and confidence as her great novel *Wuthering Heights* was rejected by one publisher after another.

Make no mistake, when you start on the path to authenticity, Love will change you, transforming your life in countless ways. Your family and friends might not notice the changes in the beginning because they're so small. But you will, and you'll know that miracles are taking place. Love will sustain you when passion's path takes unexpected twists and turns. Love will dissolve your fears by creating opportunities you couldn't have imagined before you began the search to discover and recover your Authentic Self. And when doubt, despair, and denial threaten to dismantle your dreams, Love will rear up in your defense. The next time you feel frightened and fragile, stand very still. If you do, you might feel the tip of an angel's wing brush against your shoulder.

No coward's soul is yours. I know this, even if today you don't. I know this because you wouldn't have come this far on the *Simple Abundance* journey if you were a coward. Reluctantly (literally kicking and screaming), I have come to the realization that feeling afraid is Spirit's signal to ask for grace and Power. So take a deep breath, seek your quiet center, and push on. As Alex Honnold, an American rock climber who is the first and only person to free solo Yosemite National Park's El Capitan—a feat chronicled in the riveting, Oscar-winning documentary *Free Solo*—says: "I've done a lot of thinking about fear. For me the crucial question is not how to climb without fear—that's impossible—but how to deal with it when it creeps into your nerve endings."

One of the hardest lessons we ever must master is accepting that experiencing fear is out of our hands, but how we deal with the fear is not. The closer we get to giving our dream to the world, the fiercer the struggle becomes to bring it forth. Why should this be so? Because we will be inexorably changed, and life can never return to the way it once was. Of course, we're scared; we wouldn't be sane if we weren't. But how many exquisite, glorious dreams sent to heal the world has Heaven mourned because the dreamer, weary and discouraged, relied only on her own strength and could do no more?

Today if you feel afraid, take comfort in remembering once more that courage is fear that has said her prayers. "I've dreamt in my life dreams that have stayed with me ever after, and changed my ideas," Emily Brontë confessed. "They've gone through and through me, like wine through water, and altered the color of my mind." Dreams are gifts of Spirit meant to alter us. Trust that the same Power that gifted you with your dream knows how to help you make it come true.

SEPTEMBER 19

Setting Your Own Pace

One sad thing about this world is that the acts that take the most out of you are usually the ones that other people will never know about.

—Anne Tyler
American novelist, short story writer, and literary critic

Novelist Anne Tyler tells a wonderful cautionary tale about pursuing your authentic calling. Arriving to pick up her children at school one afternoon, she was met by another mother who casually asked, "Have you found work yet? Or are you still just writing?" Ouch.

Just because you do something doesn't mean the rest of the world will think it's wonderful or even worthwhile. The sooner you realize that other people won't necessarily bless or appreciate your efforts to follow your calling, the happier you'll be. A lot of people—including your partner and close friends—might wonder aloud for years if you're ever going to become sensible again.

No, you're not. Shrug off their skepticism with a smile and go back to mining your acre of diamonds. Eventually they'll come around, either as cheerleaders or as astonished spectators. In the meantime, do your best to pay as little attention as possible to doom, doubt, and derision. You've only got so much psychic energy. If it's squandered on converting the heathens, you won't have any left to do the work waiting for you. Remember, the prophetess is rarely recognized in her own household.

Next, if you're trying to bring forth a dream while caring for a family and holding down a job, you must set your own pace. You know your commitments better than anyone else. We've all got to live with them as well as work around them.

Authentic fulfillment through your work is a marathon, not a sprint. Long-distance runners prepare for marathons with a lot of shorter runs, increasing their length and speed as they become stronger. In order to hear your calling and answer it, you must generously give yourself the gift of time. Certainly, no one else in the world will do it. If you have children living with you or are employed full-time during the day, you should have a five-year plan to secure that dream job, publish that book, organize a one-woman show, win that grant, fund your start-up. It took me three years and so many rejections to launch a nationally syndicated newspaper column, I lost count. The bottom line is not how fast you make your dream come true, but how steadily you pursue it.

Anne Tyler reveals in a collection of essays, *The Writer on Her Work*, how difficult it is to create around family life. Writing is her frame of reference, as it is mine, but the same principle applies to any passion. One March a character arrived in her consciousness as she was painting the downstairs hall. She knew if she "sat down and organized this character on paper, a novel would grow up around him. But it was March and the children's spring vacation began the next day, so I waited." By July she was finally able to start. Even with the inevitable creative delays that daily life brings, there is tremendous gain in the struggle to answer your calling with children growing up all around you. "It seems to me that since I've had children, I've grown richer and deeper," Anne Tyler confesses. "They may have slowed down my writing for a while, but when I did write, I had more of a self to speak from."

A Psalm for Life

Let us, then, be up and doing
With a heart for any fate;
Still achieving, still pursuing,
Learn to labor and to wait.

—Henry Wadsworth Longfellow (1807–1882)
American poet

Here, in four lines, is the essence of mystical moxie: the secret to achieving what you want out of your life. Written more than a hundred years ago, this wisdom is as relevant today as when it was penned. This psalm to life is one of my favorite poetry meditations, especially when I'm discouraged because I'm not seeing results as quickly as I'd like to. I know that if you mull over Longfellow's advice, you'll receive an emotional and spiritual boost today.

"Let us, then, be up and doing..." Dreams are not enough. They must be backed up with effort. Success is as simple and as profound as that. Always remember that *striving* and *struggle* precede success, even in the dictionary. We must be doing something about bringing our dreams into the world *every day*, even if we only have fifteen minutes out of every twenty-four hours to concentrate on our calling. Is there a phone call you can make? An email you can send? An inspirational Ted Talk segment you can watch? Five pages of a book you can read? Some quick research on a local organization in your dream field you can do? You'll be amazed at the power of fifteen focused minutes.

"With a heart for any fate..." Opening our hearts to the possibility of failing is easier said than done. That's why we must surrender expectations, delivery details, and the world's reception to Spirit. Become open to Divine fine-tuning or finishing touches. Birthing a dream is a collaborative effort "Still achieving, still pursuing..." If you're actively pursuing your dream with a practical plan, you're still achieving, even if it feels as though you're going nowhere fast. It's been my experience that the very moment I feel like giving up, I'm only one step from a breakthrough. Hang on long enough and circumstances will change, too. Trust in yourself, your dream and Spirit.

"Learn to labor and to wait." This is the most difficult of Longfellow's suggestions. Most of the time we wait much longer for a dream to manifest itself in our lives than we ever imagined we'd have to at its conception. That's because *our* concept of time and Spirit's are not the same. Be extra kind to yourself while waiting, making it as pleasurable as possible. Remember, the longer it takes for a dream to make itself manifest, the more comfortable you'll feel owning your talent.

SEPTEMBER 21

Uncommon Women and Others

Self-doubt is so insidious that it not only renders us stuck in our lives, but it also actually weakens our ability to dream about what living unleashed would look like first.

—Danielle LaPorte
Canadian author, speaker, and publisher

When we're twenty-five," Rita declares, "we'll be *pretty* incredible." Rita is one of seven Mount Holyoke seniors featured in Wendy Wasserstein's play *Uncommon Women and Others*. The young women are about to leave their privileged and sheltered college existence to seek fame and fortune in the real world. They will discover that fulfillment is a lifelong process, even for uncommon women. At the end of the play, six years later, their lives have changed in unexpected ways, but Rita still has high hopes: "When we're forty-five, we can be *pretty* amazing."

Uncommon Women and Others's first professional reading was during the summer of 1977 at the Eugene O'Neill Theater Center in Waterford, Connecticut—an elite, idyllic, three-week summer camp for the country's most promising young playwrights and theater critics. Each year ten new plays are selected from the thousands submitted in hope of receiving a high-gloss polishing by the professional actors, actresses, directors, and script doctors who are assigned to each young playwright.

After two weeks of preparation, showcase evenings are performed in the handsome white wooden barn and attended by representatives of regional theaters around the country and off-Broadway. Everyone who visits the beautiful farm overlooking the Long Island Sound is searching for the next season's hit. Of course, they're supposed to be focusing on promise, but it's the next sure thing that always has the famous and near-famous buzzing in the O'Neill Center's cafeteria line.

Although it didn't receive the most attention during the session, Wasserstein's play turned out to be the jewel in the O'Neill's crown that summer, launching a major career for her as well as for some of the actresses who appeared in the New York production: Glenn Close, Swoosie Kurtz, and Jill Eikenberry. In 1988, Wasserstein's promise was confirmed when she won both the Tony Award and the Pulitzer Prize for her play *The Heidi Chronicles*.

Like the self-absorbed *Uncommon* characters, most of the playwrights, actors, directors, and critics at the O'Neill Center were very full of themselves—puffed up with their reputations or potential. However, I remember Wendy Wasserstein as a rather shy, funny, and self-deprecating young woman who stood apart from the glitterati. She seemed much more focused on the work at hand—which was getting her play into shape for a professional production—than on making contacts. Of course, it was precisely because she concentrated on calling forth her authentic gifts that the play was eventually such a success and the theater world began lining up to contact her.

One of the most wonderful truths you will discover on the path to authenticity is that your aspirations *are* your possibilities. "Each year I resolve to believe there will be possibilities," said Wendy Wasserstein. "Every year I resolve to be a little less the me I know and leave a little room for the me I could be. Every year I make a note not to feel left behind by my friends and family who have managed to change far more than I." This passion for authenticity is what made Wendy Wasserstein not only an uncommon woman but an extraordinary one. She gave birth to her daughter, Lucy, at forty-eight and, sadly, died in 2006. But the legacy she left all of us is extraordinary—trust yourself, and begin believing that you are "Uncommon."

SEPTEMBER 22

Thoughts on Success

When you are young, you are surprised if everything isn't a success, and when you get older, you're mildly surprised if something is.
—Kathleen Norris (1880–1966)
American journalist and author of
ninety-three novels

Few women *believe* they are successful because they don't *feel* successful. In the deepest recesses of our hearts, we feel like failures—counterfeits, frauds. But even if we know we are successful, we rarely admit it. The world does not like braggarts. And we want the world—every last person in it—to like us. We suffer from a potent combination of public and private conditioning over a lifetime.

Webster's Dictionary defines success as "the attaining of a desired end," as well as "the attainment of wealth, favor or eminence." When we succeed, we "prosper, thrive, flourish." When we don't, we want to sink to the center of the earth until the shame subsides. Success and failure are a black-and-white issue. It's good or bad. It's a lucky break or tough luck. Actually, it's none of these things. Failure and success are the yin and yang of achievement, the two forces in the Universe over which we have absolutely no control. We keep forgetting that all we can control is our *response* to failure and success.

During the Victorian era, success, power, and wealth were considered physical manifestations of Providence's Divine approval. They still are. William James regarded the pursuit of success as "our national disease" and cautioned that the "exclusive worship of the bitch goddess" could kill you if you weren't careful. A century later, even though we can see the bodies dropping all around us, we still don't believe him. We must *never* forget that what the world giveth, the world taketh away— and frequently does.

Most of us were not taught that there are two kinds of success: worldly and authentic. But in order to live happy and fulfilled lives, we need to know the difference between what's real and what's not, because success is part of Life University's required curriculum. There is absolutely nothing wrong with the pursuit of worldly success and financial independence; I'm pursuing it as I write this meditation. But *Simple Abundance* has taught me, as I know it will teach you, that authentic success is living by your own lights, not the glare of popping flashbulbs.

And they can't take *that* away from us.

SEPTEMBER 23

Giving Yourself Credit

It was the first operatic mountain I climbed, and the view from it was astounding, exhilarating, stupefying.
—Leontyne Price
First African-American prima donna at the
Metropolitan Opera

One of the reasons women often don't feel successful is we never give ourselves credit. Should we slip for a moment and bask in the glow of accomplishment, we immediately feel the need to downplay our achievement, especially in front of our family and friends. Before we know it, we're practically denying we ever attained anything. But many successful people do revel in their achievements, covering the walls of their offices and homes with their photographs, and magazine covers, displaying golden statuettes and awards on their mantels or in specially built cabinets. They've succeeded, and not only does the world applaud them, they congratulate themselves.

Do you remember the song we used to sing as children on lengthy family car trips? "The bear went over the mountain, the bear went over the mountain, the bear went over the mountain, and what do you think he saw? He saw another mountain, he saw another mountain, he saw another mountain, and what do you think he did? He climbed that other mountain; he climbed that other mountain..." until our parents were smart enough to stop for gas, the toilets, and something to eat in the car.

Many women suffer from the climbing-bear syndrome. We scale one mountain after another, overcome every obstacle, smash the glass ceiling. But is the promotion savored? Do we celebrate graduating from night school, closing the deal, delivering the goods? No! We shrug off our personal triumphs as if they were flukes, then wonder why we feel so unfulfilled.

If we trace this un-nurturing behavior back to its source, many of us will find ourselves standing quietly, waiting patiently for the parental approval that never came, no matter what we achieved. Decades later, because we have been conditioned to believe that *nothing* we do is ever good enough, we continue this destructive cycle of withholding approval from ourselves.

Once, over a five-year period, I wrote and narrated a twelve-part series for public radio, launched a nationally syndicated newspaper column, wrote and published two books, and gave numerous lectures and workshops. On the surface I looked successful. Looking back, I now recognize this frenzy to "succeed" was the climbing-bear syndrome. But I had also succumbed to the self-destructive illusion of believing that the next creative project would be *the one* that would bring me the recognition I'd been hungering for all my life. My breakthrough. The big break would finally arrive, the brass ring would at last be within my reach, or my ship would come in. Since I hadn't received recognition or approval from my parents and certainly didn't give it to myself, the only possible source was the outside world. Surely the world would notice, in a meaningful way, my next project.

I experienced this awakening one day when I was rewriting my résumé for a new venture. As I listed my accomplishments, I wondered, "Who is this woman? Do I know her? Do I have multiple personalities?" If CSI detectives arrived at my door to search for her, they wouldn't have found a shred of physical evidence. So I started searching for clues in cardboard boxes buried in the basement, rescuing proof that mountains had been climbed. I took some of my favorite memorabilia—my book covers, the announcement of my column—to the framers. When

I hung them up in our living room, I stood back and looked at them the way a stranger might. Wow! It was astounding, exhilarating, stupefying. Then I began to congratulate myself out loud for jobs well done. Now I seize moments of achievement by making them concrete. Having the physical evidence of accomplishment has gone a long way toward making me feel successful.

Although it may crown you queen for a day, the world cannot confer the recognition that will make you feel fulfilled. Only *you* can. So chill a bottle of champagne and toast yourself upon the *completion* of a creative project, personal accomplishment, professional achievement—no matter how small. Can we really afford to wait for the world's approval? "I am doomed to an eternity of compulsive work," Bette Davis confessed in her memoir, *The Lonely Life*. "No set goal achieved satisfies. Success only breeds a new goal. The golden apple devoured has seeds. It is endless."

SEPTEMBER 24

Authentic Success

We must all pay with the current coin of life
For the honey that we taste.

—Rachel Blumstein
American poet

Authentic success is different for each of us. No single definition fits all, because we come in all sizes. One autumn afternoon years ago, while wandering through an abandoned cemetery, I discovered a wonderful definition of authentic success inscribed on the headstone of a woman who died in 1820: "The only pain she ever caused was when she left us."

Authentic success is having time enough to pursue personal pursuits that bring you pleasure, time enough to make the loving gestures for your family you long to, time enough to care for your home, tend your garden, nurture your soul. Authentic success is never having to tell yourself or those you love, "maybe next year." Authentic success is knowing that if today were your last day on earth, you could leave without regret. Authentic success is feeling focused and serene when you work, not fragmented. It's knowing that you've done the best that you possibly could, no matter what circumstances you faced; it's knowing in your soul that the best you can do is *all* you can do, and that the best you can do is always enough.

Authentic success is accepting your limitations, making peace with your past, and reveling in your passions so that your future may unfold according to a Divine Plan. It's discovering and calling forth your gifts and offering them to the world to help heal its ravaged heart. It's making a difference in other lives and believing that if you can do that for just one person each day, through a smile, a shared laugh, a caress, a kind word, or a helping hand, blessed are you among women.

Authentic success is not just money in the bank but a contented heart and peace of mind. It's earning what you feel you deserve for the work you do and knowing that you're worth it. Authentic success is not about accumulating but letting go, because all you have is all you truly need.

Authentic success is feeling good about who you are, appreciating where you've been, celebrating your achievements, and honoring the distance you've already come. Authentic success is reaching the point where *being* is as important as *doing*. It's the steady pursuit of a dream. It's realizing that no matter how much time it takes for a dream to come true in the physical world, no day is ever wasted. It's valuing inner, as well as outer, labor—both your own and others'. It's elevating labor to a craft and craft to an art by bestowing Love on every task you undertake.

Authentic success is knowing how simply abundant your life is *exactly as it is today*. Authentic success is being so grateful for the many blessings bestowed on you and yours that you can share your portion with others.

Authentic success is living each day with a heart overflowing with gratitude.

SEPTEMBER 25

Shepheard's Hotel

She had been forced into prudence in her youth. She learned romance as she grew older—the natural sequence of an unnatural beginning.

—Jane Austen (1775–1817)
English novelist

Christmas, Dublin, 1878. I'm hiding a handsome Irish patriot on the run from the British police in a room beneath Neary's pub. No thought of the risk.

But that's just one of my many lives. Other nights it's 1915 and I'm on the veranda of the Muthaiga Club, the "Moulin Rouge of Africa." Or I may be watching for the guanacos in the mist of the Andes, running with the bulls with Hemingway in Pamplona, sailing down the Nile, trekking through Karakoram, whizzing across the frozen Neva River in a sleigh, descending the steps at the Paris Opera House with a suave Guy de Maupassant (or is it the fiery young Toscanini?).

And I can do all these things because of one gentleman, J. Peterman, the last romantic man on the earth. Peterman believes I'm mysterious, powerful, irresistible, smart, sharp, sassy, funny, and sexy. And beautiful, it goes without saying, but he tells me that all the time.

Not too surprisingly, when I'm with him, I become that woman. My Authentic Self. Sentimental. Incurably romantic. Emotional. Impulsive. Passionate.

If you're reading this and still wondering who this mysterious J. Peterman is, then that tells us both a lot about our ages, and where you were in the 1990s when the J. Peterman clothing company was at its peak. This was the period where Peterman (and in this case a fictionalized Peterman) was so popular he was regularly spoofed on *Seinfeld* where Julia Louis-Dreyfus's Elaine Benes worked for the eccentric catalog owner/businessman/world traveler for three seasons. This was also the same period when the company struck gold (no icebergs on this trip) in a deal to sell both original and authorized replica costumes and props from that small arthouse flick *Titanic*, including the only authorized replica of the famous blue diamond necklace (one million's worth, to be precise).

And although popularity for J. Peterman may have waned, my love for him never will. Like Peterman, I lament the passing of a period of time when romance was a part of the daily round. With Peterman's help, the days of ocean liners, crepe de chine, train cases with secret compartments, and Morris Minor roadsters can be summoned back at will. When he finds a little piece of it, he has it reproduced and tells me all about it in his mail order catalog (yes, a real one) known as "Owner's Manuals." No glossy pictures, no hard sell. Just beautiful clothes and accessories with literary copy–style descriptions that tell me where I was when I last wore this stunning outfit and evocative watercolor sketches in lieu of photos.

My trysts with Peterman are nocturnal, and always take place in bed. There, my soul mate and I reminisce, retrace roads not taken, and recall risks not ventured, until there is no longer a trace of regret, only fond remembrance. I knew J. Peterman was my soul mate when he poured out his regrets for not spending a night in Shepheard's Hotel in Cairo. It burned to the ground before he could afford to check in. "That night it became my code word for everything unobtained, undone." I thought there was not another soul on the face of the earth, who mourned missing out on a romantic sojourn at Shepheard's Hotel in Cairo.

Peterman knows the woman I truly am, even if I forget. He knows that I was created in a burst of passion, for romance. So were you.

Plumb the female psyche and you will find an elegy of romantic remorse—the unattained, the undone. Melancholy fragments of unrequited loves that stretch from our cradles to our graves. Regrets not necessarily caused by lovers who chose to live without us, so much as by the recollections of the things we loved once but learned to live without.

It could be the opera master class you never took, the art fellowship in Paris you never pursued, the black velvet cape that finally found you at an antique stall but you passed up because, where would you wear it? (Everywhere.) The love you couldn't return, the love that frightened you, the love that you were afraid to express. The loving gesture that died in hesitation. The romance of living that we let slip away every day because real life forces us into prudence.

When you acknowledge your romantic impulses, no matter how implausible or impractical, you strengthen the intimate connections with your Authentic Self. Connection with those who cherish and love you unconditionally. Connection with those things that fuel your passions, nourish your soul, keep you alive.

Care to check in with me? They have a weekend special for two. I'm sure you're going to love it. It's my favorite place in the world.

Bogart and Bergman will always have Paris. Peterman and I will always have Cairo. I have the bathrobe to prove it.

SEPTEMBER 26

On Becoming Ravishing Renegades

It's never too late to be what you might have been.
—George Eliot (1819–1880)
Pen name of celebrated Victorian writer
Mary Ann Evans

For more than a century, the Victorian golden age of travel was a mesmerizing mélange of exotic locales, steamer trunks, gangplanks, mosquito netting, and pith helmets with the globetrotting smart set all heading toward one destination: Cairo and Shepheard's Hotel, the most glamorous, luxurious, and sensational watering hole in all the world.

Shepheard's Hotel's heyday stretched beyond a century. Built in 1841 by Samuel Shepheard, it soon became an international setting for intrigue and romance. Travelers of the Overland Route, riding camels across the desert to Africa, India, and the Far East, flocked to its legendary two-tiered terrace, high-backed wicker chairs, whirling ceiling fans, exotic plants, and long-fringed palms.

"One gets another view of exotic life from the orchestra seats on the terrace of Shepheard's Hotel overlooking the only original streets of Cairo," Miss Blanche McManus wrote in 1911 in her spine-tingling travelogue, *The American Woman Abroad*. The mind boggles with the history lessons we could have absorbed—before they occurred—over a refreshing sip of chilled hibiscus juice with an ear cocked underneath our wide-brimmed straw millinery marvel, held down with a ten-inch hat pin: a proper lady's formidable defense weapon.

From Shepheard's Hotel adventurers, fortune hunters, artists, writers, archaeologists, diplomats, foreign correspondents, stars of the stage and screen, playboys, heiresses, spies, scoundrels, rogues, royalty, European aristocracy, and the upper echelons of society gathered to reconnoiter and recuperate. Back from discovering the source of the Nile, building the Suez Canal, establishing the Raj, strategizing over the Crimean War, the Boer War, the Great War, excavating the boy King Tutankhamun, and fighting World War II, they marched into the Long Bar to quench their thirst.

Then there were the clandestine romantic rendezvous that would have scandalized nations—not to mention the hoi-polloi—that took place beneath its mosquito-netted beds. Or the literary inspiration enjoyed by both Sir Arthur Conan Doyle and Agatha Christie, who plotted coups in Khartoum and murders in Mesopotamia during their annual sojourns at Shepheard's.

Unfortunately, Shepheard's Hotel burned down in 1952. I was five years old at the time and not yet permitted to travel on my own, but as my incurable romantic nature grew, I succumbed to vicarious wanderlust during my twenties. Should you ask me today what the greatest motivating influence of my life was, my answer would be missing out on one impossibly perfect stay at Shepheard's Hotel. And so "Shepheard's Hotel" and the tittle-tattle about what went on there became my secret passion, its very name a secret code for the unattempted and untried, particularly those misalliances sure to be tinged with sighs and smoky singed regrets.

What must you do before you die? Where must you go? What worlds must you conquer? Perhaps they only exist in your imagination, but the ability to traverse time has never stopped a clever woman with a romantic temperament before and it certainly won't now. So one day a week we're going on location to check in at Shepheard's Hotel. Aliases are optional. I'm going to work on a screenplay that's lived too long tucked away in my heart, and you'll begin a secret project for your new fabulous, splendid life.

Let's sustain each other's hope and nourish each other's dreams. Now remember, if you undertake this with me, we can't share our secret with anyone else, not until my script or your new project is completed. This is because our dreams are extremely fragile, and just as we would protect our unborn child, the creativity stored within us must be guarded as it grows in strength, and until it births/bursts into expression on the outside and can breathe on its own. Nothing kills our dreams faster than other people's opinions of them, particularly people who think they know us intimately, such as family and friends. No one had a clue what I was writing when I wrote *Simple Abundance* until it suddenly appeared in the world.

So how about a little reconnoitering with our cherished reveries and perusing soulful memories, especially the ones we haven't yet created. *Et quelle coincidence!* For once in our lives, we'll be right on time. But let's not keep our glorious futures waiting a moment longer than we must.

SEPTEMBER 27

Passion and the Plate

We tell ourselves stories in order to live.
—Joan Didion
American literary journalist, novelist, and memoirist

What have you been craving, I'd guess for a while now? You might be a ceramicist and long to throw pots but haven't managed to do more than a couple of pieces over the last decade.

Your passion might be restoring antique textiles or collecting vintage notions. You know more about hat making and the history of millinery than anyone you know but you've surrendered your hat designing days to the more practical pursuit of teaching. We all have.

Read it here first: your days devoted only to practicality are almost finished.

I still remember the crackling, creative energy on the day I went to what I swore would be my last secretarial job. I made myself a soul promise that if I was going to type, it would be my own words. I kept that promise, too. It's time for you to make a similar promise. You might not be in your dream life at this very moment, but I'm coordinating your calendar for the next year, and guess what? You're booked two days a week. I've got plans for us. Details will be provided.

Why? Because you still adore making your own clothing from 1950s Vogue patterns; your knees go weak when you hear the rustle of taffeta, glimpse ruffles of silk tulle, or find a bolt of Hawaiian bark cloth from the 1930s. There isn't a tapestry to be found that you can't turn into the most irresistible ottoman. They're all over your house, and every woman who sees them tries to figure how to get you to do one for her.

Or, *ma chèrie*, perhaps you mysteriously inherited an enormous Goyard trunk filled with Parisian costumes. Now it's clear why your Great Aunt Mary Frances never was mentioned without someone in the family making the sign of the cross. It turns out she was the notorious "Fifi de la Folle," a Lido showgirl famous for playing Salome! Who knew? And you thought she'd become a French nun! Wouldn't you love to know her real story and what to do with these fabulous egret plumes and ostrich fans? It's going to be thrilling! *Please* let me go through the trunk with you.

You might dream of starting a retail lifestyle website, or have friends ask you to do flowers for their special events, or calligraphy or framing. I feel a little happy percolating going on right now. When the reveries come, there's no figment of your imagination that's too much of a good thing.

Don't stop dreaming, sweetie. Start.

Let's say your first summer job was at a small department store where you learned and loved to do window displays. You've never told a living soul about those happy hours, but you remember them, and they still make you smile. Your windows were amazing, and they helped pay for your law degree. Then you spent the last three decades writing briefs with nary a smile on your face.

Now we're getting somewhere.

You dwell in a high-rise apartment and work in a city but secretly live for the rare times you visit rural towns on the way to your coastal beach condominium. It's not just the ocean that's singing the siren's song, but the sheep, cows, horses, pigs, and roadside stands groaning under homemade jars of fruit preserves, green tomato chutney, and curried marmalade. Your lemon curd won first prize at the church fair and still you didn't take it as a serendipitous sign!

Clues, clues, clues to the cosmic mystery of you and your passion project abound. Any and all of these examples can become your new calling. This may not have been true twenty years ago, but now with the explosion of e-commerce and the fact that we're not ready for the rocking chair (unless woodworking is your passion and you design them) there's nothing stopping us. Except, of course, the opinions of others. This is why *we're not telling anyone what we're doing for the next year. There is no one on the face of this earth about to tell us what we can or cannot do or that our still passionate dreams aren't practical.*

You might want to read that again and then take the pledge. By the time they put together our increasing good mood, vitality, optimism, and the vintage silver Airstream you've been restoring in the driveway, we'll be long gone down Route 66.

The only words you won't hear from me in the next few months are "impractical" or "unrealistic." Quixotic or screwball, maybe, but look how far "screwball comedy" got Lucille Ball, Tina Fey, Kate McKinnon, Carole Lombard, Tiffany Haddish, Jean Arthur, and Kristen Wiig. So here's looking at you, kid.

When we acknowledge our romantic impulses, no matter how implausible or improbable, the soul-craft of Divine restoration kicks in. It's imperative for us to discover or reconnect with what we cherish and love unconditionally. This is why we were created by Divine Love. In turn, Divine Love cherishes and loves us unconditionally. If you do not jump out of bed every morning, grateful to the point of glee that you have another day on earth, then these words are specifically being written for you. In a year's time when you *do* have a smile on your face before opening your eyes and a "thank you" on your lips as you go to sleep, my work on these pages will be complete, and I'm getting on my filly, heading out yonder to find my ranch and work on my screenplay. I've got a few of my own overdue dreams, too.

Everything you've ever loved is part of the riddle of your incandescent mystery, inimitable style, and inevitable good; the life you should be living now, the life that's been waiting in the wings. It whispers the next line in the one woman show of your dreams. "Go for it."

SEPTEMBER 28

Becoming Real in a World Not of Our Choosing

Again. Another start.
—Dorothea Lange (1895–1965)
American documentary photographer

You can almost hear the bone-weary sigh—the searing truth in these words: "Again. Another start."

Yes, dammit. Again.

I adore and admire Dorothea Lange. She has taught me how to honor my intuitive sense of "knowing" more than any other person in history. Throughout this acclaimed photographer's life, Lange was forced to begin again, and again, *and again*; so many times, in fact, that she ended up transforming the medium of photojournalism. Lange's most iconic photograph is "Migrant Mother," a black-and-white portrait of despair—an exhausted mother holding an infant. Published in 1936, this harrowing image gave the world a human face to the Great Depression and did far more than any unemployment statistics and newspaper headlines could. Suddenly, Americans understood the trauma beyond the urban bread lines: the barren, staggering, starving Dust Bowl—from the Midwest to California.

But what makes Dorothea's personal struggle so inspirational for me is the amazing backstory of that remarkable photo. As she tells it:

It was raining, the camera bags were packed, and I had on the seat beside me in the car the results of my long trip, the box containing all those rolls and packs of exposed film ready to mail back to Washington. It was a time of relief. Sixty-five miles an hour for seven hours would get me home to my family that night and my eyes were glued to the wet and gleaming highway that stretched out ahead. I felt freed, for I could lift my mind off my job and think of home.

I was on my way and barely saw a crude sign with a pointing arrow which flashed by at the side of the road, saying PEA-PICKERS CAMP. But out of the corner of my eye I *did* see it.

I didn't want to stop and didn't. I didn't want to remember that I had seen it. I drove on and ignored the summons. Then, accompanied by the rhythmic hum of the windshield wipers, arose an inner argument [with herself]:

[Inner Voice:]
Dorothea, how about that camp back there?
What is the situation back there?
Are you going back?
Nobody could ask this of you now could they?
To turn back certainly is not necessary . . .
Having well convinced myself for twenty miles that I continue on, I did the opposite. Almost without realizing what I was doing, I made a U-turn on the empty highway. I went back those twenty miles and turned off the highway at that sign, PEA-PICKERS CAMP.

I was following instinct, not reason; I drove into that wet and soggy camp and parked my car like a homing pigeon.

I saw and approached the hungry and desperate mother, as if drawn by a magnet. I do not remember how I explained my presence or my camera to her, but I do remember she asked me no questions. I made five exposures, working closer and closer from the same direction. I did not ask her name or her history. She told me her age, that she was thirty-two. She said that they had been living on frozen vegetables from the surrounding fields, and birds that the children killed. She had just sold the tires from her car to buy food. There she sat in that lean-to tent with her children huddled around her and seemed to know that my pictures might help her, and so she helped me. There was a sort of equality about it.

The pea crop at Nipomo had frozen and there was no work for anybody. But I did not approach the tents and shelter of other stranded pea-pickers. It was not necessary; I knew I had recorded the essence of my assignment.

And indeed, she had. But who gave Dorothea that assignment: Heaven or the Farm Security Administration? After the photograph was published, the federal government rushed a shipment of 20,000 pounds of food to the camp. Later the writer John Steinbeck would recall that his 1939 Pulitzer Prize–winning novel *The Grapes of Wrath*, which was cited in Steinbeck's Nobel Prize for Literature, had been inspired by Lange's "Migrant Mother."

We have no idea the ripple of blessings *we* will set in motion as we begin our lives again or the how and why that might change others' lives for the better. But I've come to a point where I don't need to know anymore. I only need to follow orders, and there is such an amazing freedom in this. These instructions are given to us through our sacred, creative, intuitive prompts and when you're edging out further and further on that swaying limb for the fruit dangling at its end, don't look down. Keep looking for the next inch and trust that there is a net or wingspan underneath. Because there will be. Just recall the soul assignment Dorothea Lange was on, even though she didn't know it. Her willingness to follow her soul's direction, however reluctant at first, is one of the most inspirational stories I've ever heard, and it always moves me forward. Ponder it in your heart as you travel on the dark, wet, and gleaming highway toward your dream.

Little Steps + Tiny Choices = Big Change. Our yearnings are our blessings. We're going to honor and respect our creative urges. Most importantly, we're going to ease our way into this new world. We will be brave, and we will be real. Once we acknowledge that from this moment on, our soul assignment is the sacred work of beginning our lives over, we are not alone. You have me. I have you. And we both have the loving support, guidance, and resources of our Authentic Selves. We have Gratitude. Thank Heavens.

Remember, Dorothea Lange thought her photograph was going to be "just one more of the same" that cold, rainy night. She didn't want to turn back. We, too, will have nights when we don't want to turn back, and days when we don't want to begin. So hold this thought: When you're willing to go in over your head, your life isn't the only one that's changed for the better. As your agent provocateur, your secret mission is safe with me.

The Fear of Success

The conflict between what one is and who one is expected to be touches all of us. And sometimes, rather than reach for what one could be, we choose the comfort of the failed role, preferring to be the victim of circumstance, the person who didn't have a chance.
—Merle Shain (1935–1989)
Canadian author and journalist

Many women fear success much more than failure. Failure we can handle, failure feels familiar. But success means we must leave our comfort zone, the well-padded perimeter of predictability. Whether or not we like to admit it, a woman's success is secondary to her relationships. We fear success because we fear the impact it will have (and it most assuredly will), not only on our own lives but on the lives of those we love.

Even the financial rewards of success don't entirely belong to us, unless we're single and without children or elderly parents to care for. If we're not, the checks may have our name on them, but they go to pay for groceries, tuition, winter coats, braces, summer camp, vacations, medical bills. Not to mention mortgages or rent, utilities, food, health insurance, and much, much more. Why should it come as a surprise that personal indulgences become figments of feminine imagination?

So we fear success with good reason. We've got a lot at stake. Success brings change, and change is uncomfortable. But by attempting to achieve one challenge at a time, we redefine success for ourselves and those we love. As we become more comfortable with our accomplishments, we learn that success doesn't have to pull, tug, or chafe if we wear our real size.

Do Try This at Home: Mother Courage's Curriculum

I've been through it all, baby, I'm mother courage.
—Dame Elizabeth Taylor (1932–2011)
British-American actress, businesswoman,
and humanitarian

As we have been preparing our Caution Closets over the past few months, you may not have noticed a subtle shift in your attitude and growing confidence. While Mrs. Miniver helped us prepare for the unexpected, our next coach, Mother Courage, will now take over our final months of training. The most important item in your closet is not an item at all. It's your ability to stay calm and carry on in the face of any situation.

When it comes to being mentally prepared for whatever happens, Megan Hine, the internationally renowned survival consultant, knows that we are our own best ally when we understand and control fear. She should know, as she has worked as a survival consultant behind the scenes for Bear Grylls's television shows (the *Running Wild* series), as well as celebrities and international clients. Whether in the wilderness or conference room, her book *Mind of a Survivor: What the Wild Has Taught Me about Survival and Success* is a salve for our adrenaline-stoked, stress-filled lives. Megan puts it succinctly: "In survival people often talk about three minutes without air, three days without water, three weeks without food. I'd like to add another: three seconds without thinking." Now, we're going to add some training to build our confidence and increase our skills—beginning with CPR for adults, children, and pets.

CPR

"Walk on By" is more than a fantastic song by Dionne Warwick, it's an alarming situation when it comes to a stranger not helping the victim of a heart attack. According to research conducted by the University of Pennsylvania, bystander CPR in a public setting is considered rare, with only 37 percent of the public stepping up. In physical matters of the heart, women need to take charge of an even more alarming gender disparity. Men are more likely to receive CPR from a stranger (45 percent) compared to women (39 percent). The dilemma only increases for women of color.

The American Heart Association encourages best friends to share more than a meal out. The video "Shared Moments" reminds us that doing hands-only CPR until emergency medical responders arrive is a lifesaving act worthy of Mother Courage. Hands-only CPR is easy to learn and keeps the heart pumping in a crisis. So the next time we see a red dress for Women's Heart Awareness Month, let's remind ourselves and our friends and family to take that CPR class. Is a friend having a new baby? Are you in a toddler play group? Let's all take child and infant CPR classes together. Women are the ports in life's storms, since it is more likely that the man on the street will walk on by. Recently, I heard a story of a policeman who was called to the scene of an accident and he performed infant CPR, saving the baby's life. In an interview he admitted that in twenty years he'd never needed it, but thank God he knew what to do instinctively.

First Aid on the Go

While nothing can replace taking a CPR class, the American Red Cross has two apps that you might find helpful in a pinch: First Aid by the American Red Cross and Pet First Aid. Each app provides step-by-step instructions for handling the A to Z of unexpected situations. Following our preparation motto, it is best to download the free apps before you need them (www.redcross.org).

For the Pet First Aid app, the American Red Cross has teamed up with veterinarians to provide step-by-step instructions for immediate care. Our four-legged friends, be they dogs or cats, are family, and if Miss Kitty gets a thorn in her paw, knowing how to remove it properly is a blessing. You'll be so relieved to have the first aid kit with tweezers in your Caution Closet. Although there are many first aid kits for pets on the market, the family's kit can do double duty here. Just add a spare harness or leash, a muzzle, and a portable water dish.

Bach Flower Essences offers a line of Rescue Remedies for our pets to ease stress, anxiety, and more. Now that we're thinking of it, we would be well served to add a bottle for ourselves in the first aid kit as well.

For while it is a good thing to check with the experts, most often, you will have to think for yourself. Megan Hine reminds us, "When things go wrong, it happens so fast. Thinking—whether it's thinking through your actions or being alert to the environment around you— could potentially save your life."

Joyful Simplicities for September

September is the time to begin again. In the country, when I could smell the wood-smoke in the forest, and the curtains could be drawn when the tea came in, on the first autumn evening, I always felt that my season of good luck had come.
—Eleanor Perenyi (1918–2009)
American author and gardener

Most of us have been conditioned to believe Labor Day weekend marks the end of summer, but the season of autumn or fall actually starts when the sun crosses the Earth's equator from north to south. This is called the autumnal equinox.

    ▸ *L'été c'est fini*, as the French say, so end summer on a high note. Make a really big deal out of the last cookout of the summer. Serve your favorite summer recipes with a final flourish. Sit outside if you can. Linger in the twilight, watch the sun go down, and bid summer a fond *adieu*.

On Labor Day weekend take fifteen minutes to write down all the things you wanted to do over the summer but never got around to. Put your list in an envelope. Put a note on your calendar for June first next year reminding you to look at your list. Try to block in some time on your calendar to make postponed pleasures a priority when summer returns.

Stock up on your own school supplies. They're on sale this month. Get your pads, notebooks, scissors, tape, and crayons—just for you. Get pencils that make you smile. It's inexpensive and fun. Take a creative excursion to find exactly the kind of pen you prefer writing with. Once you've identified your brand, stock up on them at discount office supply stores.

Did you know that there are 7,000 varieties of apples worldwide? In the United States there are approximately 2,500 different apple varieties with only 100 types of apples grown commercially. Go apple picking (it can actually be quite fun, I promise) and bring your bounty home to experiment with in the kitchen. This is a wonderful activity to do with single friends and friends who have children. Everyone will love this new soon-to-be tradition. Make taffy or caramel apples, apple pie, apple fritters, apple butter (just to name a few). There are so many things you can do with apples, just a quick look online or through your recipe book or app and you're sure to find something to inspire you.

Enjoy fresh apple cider and pear nectar.

Experiment with different types of popcorn.

Bring out your woolens. Do you have a favorite sweater that you absolutely adore? If not, why not?

Celebrate the autumn equinox with a festive dinner of home-style cooking. Do this especially if you live alone and rarely cook a decent meal for yourself. Bring home a small pot of mums for your dining table. Draw hearthside and light the candles, pour wine or cider, and enjoy the simple pleasures of comfort food.

Have you ever tried an English fidget pie, a traditional harvest meal? It's composed of potatoes, onions, apples, and ham pieces in a vegetable stock seasoned with a little brown sugar, salt, and pepper. Pour into a pastry shell, cover with a top crust (a frozen one works beautifully), and bake as you would any filled pie.

Observe the autumnal festival of Michaelmas on September 29, which is the feast day of St. Michael the Archangel. This ancient English harvest festival dates back to the sixth century. Legend has it that on this day the devil was driven out of Heaven by St. Michael and landed in a patch of blackberry brambles. It's traditional to have blackberry treats—pies, tarts, or jam on scones—for tea on this day.

🖎 Start making your Christmas list this month so that you won't be frantic in December.

🖎 If you have children, this is the time to have them decide on their Halloween costumes. Don't despair. They don't divide the children into two groups at school: those wearing store-bought costumes and those wearing homemade ones! Order the costumes sooner rather than later (if going this route) or assemble all your supplies if you're being crafty. If you do construct homemade costumes, always keep in mind exactly whose costume it is you're making. Some of us get carried away and end up creating costumes designed more to impress other women than to please our children.

🖎 Look at farmers' markets for dried flowers to create your own bouquet. Prepared bouquets can be wonderful, but they're expensive. Creating your own bouquet on a September Sunday afternoon is a relaxing restorative that reminds you all winter long that beauty is simply abundant if you look for it.

🖎 J. Peterman is happy to contact you by email, but ask for his new catalog at www.jpeterman.com, and there will be lots of adventures you might be inspired to dream about.

OCTOBER

The fields are harvested and bare,
And Winter whistles through the square.
October dresses in flame and gold
Like a woman afraid of growing old.

—Anne Mary Lawler (1908–1980)
Irish-American poet and novelist

Now autumn arrives, a change of season that's more a sense memory than a date on the calendar. Finally, the heat is passing. Gradually familiar surroundings don a rustic palette of jewel tones that dazzle with their beauty. Let October seduce you with her charms. "Beguile us in the way you know," poet Robert Frost entreated this season of abundance. "Release one leaf at the break of day."

OCTOBER 1

Recognizing Burnout Before You're Charred

My candle burns at both ends;
it will not last the night; but ah, my foes,
and oh, my friends—it gives a lovely light!
—Edna St. Vincent Millay (1892–1950)
American Pulitzer Prize–winning poet

Burnt offerings.

Burned to a crisp.

Burned beyond recognition.

Burned alive.

Burned out.

Setting the world on fire comes with risks. Unfortunately, we usually don't realize this until smoke gets in our eyes.

Burnout is a condition caused by unbalance: too much work or responsibility, too little time to do it, over too long a period. We've been cruising in the fast lane, but we've been running on fumes rather than on fuel. Often, we think that burnout is something that just happens to other women—to workaholics and perfectionists.

But careaholics are also at risk—women who care deeply about their children, work, relationships, parents, siblings, friends, communities, issues. This sounds like every woman I know. Perhaps we would pay more attention to burnout if it were as dramatic as a heart attack. But a smoldering flame can be just as deadly as a flash fire.

Sometimes burnout manifests itself as a sense of complete exhaustion at the end of a project that has taken months of challenging and intense work. Taking a week off to rest, then resuming work at a slower pace is usually enough to bring about a speedy recovery. But first-degree burnout—the soul snuffer—comes from living unbalanced for years; when what was supposed to be a temporary situation becomes a lifestyle.

Burnout often begins with illness—anything from a bout of flu you can't shake to chronic fatigue syndrome—and is usually accompanied by depression. Sometimes burnout is hard to distinguish from a creative dry spell, especially if you're good at denial, which most women are.

It's burnout when you go to bed exhausted every night and wake up tired every morning—when no amount of sleep refreshes you, month after weary month. It's burnout when everything becomes too much effort: combing your hair, going out to dinner, visiting friends for the weekend, even going on vacation. It's burnout when you can't believe, under any circumstances, that you'll ever want to have sex again. It's burnout when you find yourself cranky all the time, bursting into tears or going into fits of rage at the slightest provocation. When a glass of spilled milk becomes an avalanche, it's burnout. When you're frightening the animals, it's burnout. It's burnout when you dread the next phone call. It's burnout when you feel trapped and hopeless, unable to dream, experience pleasure, or find contentment.

It's burnout when neither big thrills nor little moments have the power to move you—when nothing satisfies you because you haven't a clue what's wrong or how to fix it. Because everything's wrong. Because something is terribly out of whack: you. It's burnout when you feel there is not one other person on the face of the earth who can help you.

And you're right.

When you're suffering from burnout, *you* are the only person on earth who can help because you're the only one who can make the lifestyle changes that need to be made: to call a halt, to take a slower path, to make a detour. When you have no strength left, you have no choice but to rely on the strength of a saner Power to restore you to Wholeness.

OCTOBER 2

The Ultimate Seduction

It is your work in life that is the ultimate seduction.
—Pablo Picasso (1881–1973)
Spanish painter, sculpture, ceramist

Like a phantom lover, work charms, cajoles, comforts, and caresses. Our work—especially if it's our grand passion—can be so seductive that we can find ourselves completely caught up in its rapture, unable to resist.

However, work doesn't have to be a grand passion for us to be swept away; an infatuation can just as conveniently distract us from whatever is disappointing, disagreeable, or disturbing elsewhere in our lives. When you simply can't deal with real life, an email or phone call that needs to be answered immediately can be a fine friend.

The ultimate seduction is often accompanied by the ultimate addictions: workaholism and perfectionism. What makes these two reckless behavior patterns so dangerous is that they're sanctioned, supported, and sustained by a society still shackled to the Puritan work ethic. The

Puritans frowned on anything enjoyable, believing that God's favor could be achieved only by grueling struggle, stringent self-discipline, and backbreaking work. But Spirit can't use us to heal the world if we can't heal ourselves.

I and many of my friends are workaholics. Even kryptonite can't stop us. For years, we've all vehemently denied it. Now, in conversations, we're able to admit "tendencies toward," much the way an alcoholic admits being a social drinker. These tendencies include working long hours during the week; bringing work home with you on weekends and vacations; turning on the computer after the kids are in bed; sneaking in work, one way or another, seven days a week; referring to the perusal of contracts as "reading"; canceling dates with friends and family to finish up "one more thing"; postponing pleasure until a deadline is met; setting your phone notifications to tell you of every text and email at every hour of the day and night; and then responding to said communications in social settings; beginning one project before finishing another; letting work interrupt precious private or family time; squeezing the only "vacations" you take into business trips.

Tendencies?

If you hear yourself frequently muttering under your breath, "This is insane," the time has come to quietly scrutinize your working style. Authentic success doesn't come wrapped in a shroud.

Start small. Be sneaky. Think baby steps. The same savvy that got you into this mess can help you escape. Take the work home but don't open the computer—or at least your email app. Put the phone on silent and leave it in the other room during dinner. Take a day off every two weeks. A woman I know has reached the point of taking one Sunday off a month, whether she needs it or not. Secretly she believes it's her most astonishing accomplishment.

When we succumb to workaholism, what's really happening is that we've lost faith in Spirit's willingness to help us achieve success. We've separated the secular from the spiritual. Asking for Grace doesn't seem as practical as working round the clock.

When was the last time Spirit accompanied you to work?

When was the last time you asked It to?

OCTOBER 3

Little Miss Perfect

Perfectionism is the voice of the oppressor, the enemy of the people. It will keep you cramped and insane your whole life.

—Anne Lamott
American author

The road to hell is paved by perfectionists working with grains of sand. Uh-oh...missed a spot...

Like workaholism, aspiring to be Little Miss Perfect is an addiction of low self-worth. When we were young, nothing we did was ever good enough, so we just kept on doing until doing was all we could do. When doing more and more didn't make a difference, we thought if we did our work perfectly, we'd hit the mark.

When we did, suddenly voices other than our own sang our praises. It sounded like the Heavenly hosts. Champagne or chocolate couldn't begin to compare with the ecstasy of genuine compliments. We're creatures who live by our senses, and since the response we got for perfection felt wonderful—even if for only ten seconds—we wanted to repeat the experience. So we committed to doing everything perfectly, setting in motion a cycle of self-destruction that frequently felt as comfortable as a straitjacket. Still, the pursuit of perfection is the opiate of choice for millions of women.

I could tell you to stop going on social media, don't read any news articles, don't watch TV or watch any movies that continuously reinforce our belief that perfection is possible, but you're not going to listen to me. Instead, next time you see a gorgeous woman on the cover of a magazine, or floating through your Instagram feed, a room to die for, or a meal that would take a professional chef a week to prepare, begin to chant, "You're not real. You're not real. You're not real. I refuse to grant you the power to make me miserable." The woman, the room, and the meals that are depicted to inspire (but which really diminish us) are illusions conjured up by professionals paid handsomely to manipulate our reality.

Once a close friend gave me a priceless gift. She convinced me that my sanity is much more important than the subtle nuances that I adore. The subtle nuances are the essence of perfection. The subtle nuances trigger the "ah" response. But a life spent seeking the subtle nuances leaves little time to enjoy the big picture. Now, as a recovering perfectionist, I try to leave the subtle nuances to Spirit, who shows off better than I do.

Today, I would like to give you that gift: *Your sanity is much more important than the subtle nuances.*

Get yourself a small hourglass filled with sand. Place it prominently where you can see it—in the kitchen or on your desk. Turn it over once a day. Watch how fast the grains of sand flow. Those are the minutes of your life. Live them. Or pave with them. Everyday it's your call.

A point worth pondering: Upon completing the Universe, the Great Creator pronounced it "very good." *Not "perfect."*

OCTOBER 4

Homework

There are some things you learn best in calm, and some in storm.
—Willa Cather (1873–1947)
American Pulitzer Prize–winning novelist

Working from home is as popular as ever these days as both men and women try to bring more balance into their daily round. Working from home, at least part of the week, is more productive than working at the office because, with fewer interruptions, it provides a more serene environment in which to concentrate, and therefore "remote work" is common now.

Working from home is great, but it's not exactly as you might imagine it to be, especially if your main workplace is still at another location. Yes, it's fabulous to be able to work in pajamas or sweats, handy to throw a load of laundry into the washing machine on a quick work break; convenient to start spaghetti sauce simmering in the early afternoon while conducting conference calls. But if you're not careful, it's *very easy* to blur the distinction between the two spheres—home and work—until you have only "homework," which is horrendous. Homework is rolling out of bed and immediately looking at your work emails, only to fall asleep at night with your laptop on your chest. Homework is a soulless, repetitive cycle of brutality brought on by the ease and convenience of technology.

Does the hamster's wheel mean anything to you?

I've been working from home for nearly my entire adult life, and now I can't imagine another working style. But like any life choice, you must be suited to it. A dear friend fantasized about working from home for years; after a couple of months she resumed working at her office most of the time because, for her, the isolation was numbing.

You also must be extremely focused to work from home, because *you must work.* When the family heads out the door in the mornings, you must head into your office and not give your home, whatever its state, another thought until your business for the day is complete. This response is not automatic; it requires rigorous discipline not to pick up the house before settling down to work. I recommend blinders when walking through the house during the day.

Once you realize how comfortable, even pleasurable, it can be to work at home, it's easy to become reckless, taking on more than you can handle reasonably. That's because your work week is no longer structured around five days and eight to ten hours; the office is always open. Since you don't have a commute, you start working an hour earlier and continue an hour later than if you were working in an office. Since the office is right down the hall, it's easy to just pop in there after the kids are settled for the night to "finish up." Weekends are all too perfect for "catching up" on last week's leftovers or for "getting a head start" on next week's load. Eventually the days have no distinction and your working style is a sinkhole. But even if you're earning more money than before, if you no longer have a life at home you must learn to set limits.

Working from home can be a genuine step toward self-determination, once we honor the sense of balance we originally sought away from the office.

"If people are highly successful in their profession, they lose their senses," Virginia Woolf, who worked at home, cautions us. "Sight goes. They have no time to look at pictures. Sound goes. They have no time to listen to music. Speech goes. They have no time for conversation. They lose their sense of proportion—the relations between one thing and another. Humanity goes."

Heed her wise words.

OCTOBER 5

The Glad Game Reconsidered

Be Glad. Be Good. Be Brave.
—Eleanor Hodgman Porter (1868–1920)
American novelist

Remember Pollyanna? "The Glad Girl"? Now don't snicker at the thought of her name. Pollyanna's cloying determination to find the good in any situation might seem too saccharine to swallow for our sophisticated palates, but I think the instructions to her Glad Game deserve another look.

Sneer if you must, but the Glad Game is the perfect antidote when our daily rounds suddenly implode because of unexpected circumstances.

"Pollyanna did not pretend that everything was good," her creator, Eleanor Hodgman Porter, insists. "Instead she represented a cheery, courageous acceptance of the facts. She understood that unpleasant things are always with us, but she believed in mitigating them by looking for whatever good there is in what is."

When *Pollyanna* was originally published in 1913, no one was more shocked than Mrs. Porter at the sudden and widespread appeal of her eleven-year-old orphan heroine's ability to find the silver lining in any black cloud. Although the book was published without any publicity, word-of-mouth recommendation made it a best-seller, eventually selling more than a million copies. *Pollyanna* was translated into a dozen languages and was so popular that the character's name entered the English vernacular to describe irrepressible optimism.

In the novel, Pollyanna Whittier is the daughter of an impoverished missionary who continuously preaches the sermon of gladness to anyone who'll listen. The path of optimism. The Reverend Whittier points out that the Bible records *eight hundred* instances of God instructing his children to be glad and rejoice. Obviously, the Reverend concludes, Spirit must have wanted us to live that way, at least some of the time.

One Christmas these beliefs are put to a severe test when the annual holiday hamper arrives from the Missionary Ladies Aid Society. Pollyanna has asked for a real china doll for Christmas. But when she opens the hamper on Christmas morning, she finds that the good ladies have mistakenly sent her a pair of children's crutches instead. Naturally, she feels devastated. To comfort her, the Reverend makes up a game to see if they can find one good thing about receiving a pair of crutches as a Christmas gift. Of course, they do. Pollyanna doesn't need them! Thus, the Glad Game is created.

After Pollyanna's father dies, she's sent to live with her Aunt Polly Harrington, a wealthy but lonely spinster. No one doubts that the reason Miss Polly never married is her very stern and unpleasant personality.

When Pollyanna arrives in the little Vermont town, she soon transforms the community with her spunk and good cheer. The sick become well; the lonely find friends and sweethearts; unhappy marriages are saved. Everyone except Aunt Polly succumbs to looking for life's bright side. But Aunt Polly remains a hard nut to crack. At one point she explodes: "*Will* you stop using that everlasting word 'glad.' It's 'glad'—'glad'—'glad' from morning till night until I think I shall go wild." (A response we could imagine sharing occasionally!) However, even Aunt Polly comes under the Glad spell after Pollyanna has a serious accident and only pulls through because of her own pluck and the goodwill of the community.

Pollyanna may be hopelessly sentimental, old-fashioned, and outdated as a novel, but this business about eight hundred reassurances to "Cheer up, it's not so bad!" deserves reconsideration.

Try it for one day. Hey, remember we are our own research and development team. Skeptics make the best seekers.

OCTOBER 6

Attention Must Be Paid

Her work, I really think her work
Is finding what her real work is
And doing it
Her work, her own work
Her being human
Her being in the world.

—Ursula K. Le Guin (1929–2018)
American science fiction/fantasy author

One morning your predictable conscious self surprises you. The alarm rings. She shuts it off and rolls over. Doesn't get out of bed. Shows no intention of getting dressed. She's on strike. Grievances have been ignored for years, maybe a lifetime. Working conditions are intolerable.

The incomparable Annie Dillard tells us what happens next: "[Y]our worker—your one and only, your prized, coddled, and driven worker—is not going out on that job. Will not budge, not even for you, boss. Has been at it long enough to know when the air smells wrong; can sense a tremor through boot soles. Nonsense, you say; it is perfectly safe. But the worker will not go. Will not even look at the site. Just developed heart trouble. Would rather starve."

Maybe you haven't burned or bummed out, run away, landed in the hospital, or had a complete nervous breakdown. Yet. Maybe your family is still intact. At least they were still all accounted for at dinner last night. Maybe your friends are still speaking to you. Who knows? It's been six months since any of them saw you.

Today you're a very lucky woman. Don't push it. Life with you has been as much fun as getting a bikini wax. You were a walkout waiting to happen. Management—the ego—can fend for herself until a new contract is agreed on. There are labor laws but none to protect against self-exploitation. The picket line will not be crossed until there are.

The time has come for you to pay attention. Get a soothing cup of comfort and think about your ideal working day. If you could work in any style or setting, what would it be? What are your ideal working hours? Imagine your ideal workplace surroundings. What do you see? Now compare the ideal with the real. Is there any common ground?

Can you introduce one ideal element into your present working environment? Few women can wave their hands and start an authentic life over from scratch. But all of us can begin working with what we've got. Working with our real-life circumstances is *how* we render reality perfected. Perfection is unattainable. "Perfected" is possible.

Today, begin a little creative collective bargaining between choice and circumstances. Artists of the Everyday excel in elevating the simple to the level of sacred. Use whatever you have on hand—a meal, a conversation, humor, affection, a new filing system, a relatively clean desk to create comfort and content at work. Ask your soul, "What is it that would make this encounter with my work more pleasurable?" Then do it.

OCTOBER 7

Learning to Create Boundaries

Before I built a wall I'd ask to know
What I was walling in or walling out.
—Robert Frost (1874–1963)
Only American poet to win four Pulitzer
Prizes for his work

Limits are the barbed wire of real life. Boundaries are split-rail fences. When you push past limits, personal or professional, there's a good chance of being pricked as you hurtle up and over. But boundaries set apart the Sacred with simple grace. There's always enough room to maneuver between the rails if you're willing to bend.

We want our lives to feel limitless, so we must learn the art of creating boundaries that protect, nurture, and sustain all we cherish. For most women, creating boundaries is excruciating, so we don't do it until we're pushed to the outer edge of tolerance. To create boundaries, we must learn to say, *this far and no further.* This means speaking up. Expressing our needs. Indicating our preferences. These moments are tense and can easily escalate into confrontations complete with tears, misunderstandings, and hurt feelings. This is why many women stay quiet, rendered virtually mute by unexpressed rage and unable to articulate any needs at all.

But even if we are mute, we're not powerless to draw a line in the sand. A talented friend of mine who has several books to her credit has long been married to an intelligent, charming, but critical man. Because her husband is more formally educated than she, she's always asked him to read her work and make suggestions about it. Unfortunately, he's often been rather harsh in his efforts to help and didn't realize how much of a sting his words inflicted. Sometimes he would even leave her work lying around before looking at it—long enough to convey, if not disdain, then certainly disrespect. After each such episode, it would take his wife days to pick up her pen again. Finally, she stopped showing her work to him, creating an unspoken boundary to protect her dreams. When she finally published her breakthrough novel, her husband was astonished at all the praise she was receiving and seemed embarrassed that he didn't understand what people were raving about. One night, she told me, she discovered him reading her best-seller. "This is good. This is very good," he told her in a surprised voice. "But why didn't you ask me to read it first?"

"Because you had no idea I was capable of this," she replied, with relish, finding her authentic voice at last.

Speaking the language of "no" is a good place to start creating boundaries. "'No' can be a beautiful word, every bit as beautiful as 'yes,'" writers John Robbins and Ann Mortifee declare. "Whenever we deny our need to say 'no,' our self-respect diminishes," they tell us in *In Search of Balance: Discovering Harmony in a Changing World*. "It is not only our right at certain times to say 'no'; it is our deepest responsibility. For it is a gift to ourselves when we say 'no' to those old habits that dissipate our energy, 'no' to what robs us of our inner joy, 'no' to what distracts us from our purpose. And it is a gift to others to say 'no' when their expectations do not ring true for us, for in so doing we free them to discover more fully the truth of their own path. Saying 'no' can be liberating when it expresses our commitment to take a stand for what we believe we truly need."

OCTOBER 8

A Passion for Beauty

Beauty is an ecstasy; it is as simple as hunger.
—W. Somerset Maugham (1874–1965)
British playwright, novelist, and short story
writer

One baby step forward. Three giant steps back. I'd been experimenting with the first four *Simple Abundance* Graces—Gratitude, Simplicity, Order, and Harmony—for almost a year and thought I had overcome the "buy me" syndrome. I enjoyed browsing and did not feel diminished because I couldn't purchase something that captured my eye. Then I discovered a lifestyle blog full of posts with things I love. I scrolled through visions I wanted to live in. Angrily, I closed my browser—fed up that I was not living the lifestyle I thought I wanted. All I had may very well have been all I needed, but it certainly wasn't all I wanted at that moment.

After several hours of churning, I stopped. Something was going on within; this emotional response was occurring for a reason. I meditated on what had pushed my buttons. Was it that I had been living too stringently on a budget? Was I depressed about my lack of money for decorating trifles that I could once have purchased without a thought? Or was something deeper happening?

The more I thought about it, the more I realized that I hadn't been paying enough attention to my passion for beauty. My deprivation was caused by not appreciating, savoring, or celebrating the beauty that already existed in my life—so much so that my soul had erupted into a volcano of protest. When something calls to us on a deep enough level to engage our emotions, our conscious attention is sought. Beauty was calling to me, not objects. After I realized this, I headed for a farmers' market for flowers. But instead of one bouquet, I treated myself to two. When I set my lush arrangement of flowers in the living room, my authentic craving for beauty was satisfied very inexpensively and the wants immediately quieted down.

Don't feel you have to deny or ignore your feelings when you want something beautiful but can't afford it. The desire offers clues to satisfy this holy hunger. Explore why you behold something as beautiful; use your impressions to jump-start your imagination. Beauty surrounds us. It is everywhere if we search for it, if we're open to having more of it in our lives. "Here we are, sitting in a shower of gold," the Australian novelist Christina Stead wrote in 1938, with "nothing to hold up but a pitchfork."

OCTOBER 9

Coping with Stress

In this world without quiet corners, there can be no easy escapes... from hullabaloo, from terrible, unquiet fuss.
—Sir Salman Rushdie
British-Indian novelist and essayist

Is there a woman alive who doesn't suffer from stress? If there is, seek her out, ask her to share her wisdom. When you find her, I'd be willing to bet she'll offer the following suggestions:

Cultivate gratitude.

Turn your phone off.

Carve out an hour a day for solitude.

Begin and end the day with prayer, reflection, or silence.

Keep it simple.

Keep your house picked up.

Don't overschedule.

Strive for realistic deadlines.

Never make a promise you can't keep.

Allow an extra half hour for everything you do.

Create quiet surroundings at home and at work.

Go to bed at nine o'clock twice a week.

Always carry something interesting to read.

Breathe—deeply and often.

Move—walk, dance, run, find a sport you enjoy.

Drink pure spring water. Lots of it.

Eat only when hungry.

If it's not delicious, don't eat it.

Be instead of *do*.

Set aside one day a week for rest and renewal.

Laugh more often.

Luxuriate in your senses.

Always opt for comfort.

If you don't love it, live without it.

Let Mother Nature nurture.

No phones allowed at the dinner table.

Stop trying to please everybody.

Start pleasing yourself.

Stay away from negative people.

Don't squander precious resources: time, creative energy, emotion.

Nurture friendships.

Don't be afraid of your passion.

Approach problems as challenges.

Honor your aspirations.

Set achievable goals.

Surrender expectations.

Savor beauty.

Create boundaries.

For every yes, let there be a no.

Don't worry; be happy.

Remember, happiness is a *living* emotion.

Exchange security for serenity.

Care for your soul.

Cherish your dreams.

Express love every day.

Search for your Authentic Self until you find her.

Don't tweet in bed. (Thank you, Michelle Obama.)

OCTOBER 10

Poise Wreckers

The most alluring thing a woman can have is confidence.
—Beyoncé
American singer, songwriter, actress,
director, dancer

One of the most miserable days in my life graciously bestowed on me a priceless gift: the awareness that everyday poise is acquired or lost before we leave our homes.

Early in my writing career I was summoned to New York for an important meeting with a woman who, it was whispered, made Medusa (who had snakes instead of hair) seem beatific. I decided I should prepare for this encounter by appearing just as formidable. Since deep within I was paralyzed with fear, I attempted to overcompensate for it with outward trappings. In a frenzy, I bought an expensive outfit that screamed "woman of substance," although it most assuredly didn't look like me. I also dramatically changed my hairstyle and makeup.

Because I felt so strange with my sophisticated new getup, I stayed up far too late the night before my trip fussing with everything instead of relaxing, packing leisurely, and getting some much-needed sleep. I was exhausted when I finally dropped into bed, so I just left my makeup, personal care necessities, and accessories strewn on top of the dresser.

In order to arrive in New York in time for the meeting, I had to get up at four-thirty a.m. It had never occurred to me that I would be virtually dressing in the dark, so as not to wake up my family. It was difficult and frustrating feeling my way to find what I needed. I ended up rushing out in a state of utter panic to catch my train.

The meeting had not even begun before I became hot and sweaty. This was right after I felt the left sleeve of my blouse rip beneath my suit jacket. Since I'd never worn this outfit before, I didn't realize how tight the arms were or how much the skirt rode up on my hips when I sat down. The deep red nail polish that had looked so elegant in the salon the day before had chipped en route; naturally, I had no way of touching up my nails, so I tried to hide my hands. Several cups of coffee on the train, combined with raw nerves, had made my mouth dry, but I hadn't thought to carry breath freshener in my purse or ask for a glass of water before the meeting started.

I was so self-conscious during the meeting that I had difficulty focusing and certainly didn't have the confidence to offer my opinion, even though I felt very strongly about some of the decisions being made on my publishing project. Two excruciating hours later, the conference from hell was over. As the elevator doors closed, I swore I would never again leave another business meeting hot and sweaty and frazzled, much the way Scarlett O'Hara swore with raised fist that she'd never again go hungry.

Of course, I realize I'm probably not the only woman in the world to endure such humiliation at her own hands. Into each of our lives come important meetings, public appearances, and special occasions. Here are some practical antidotes for public awkwardness:

- Never dress to impress others: Dress to express your authentic sense of style. The only way we become truly at ease with ourselves is by knowing who we are.
- Never wear an outfit that you've never worn before to an important event; if your clothes need constant adjustment—pulling

down a too-short skirt, hitching up a shoulder strap—you'll be unable to relax, focus, and function. If you buy something new, give it a trial run.

↜ *Never* drastically change your hair and makeup just before meeting new people for the first time. If you want a new look, put it together thoughtfully and gradually, so that you'll be at ease with the final effect.

If your dressing table is cluttered and your closet jumbled, you're bound to feel less than confident and serene when you're trying to put together a look that presents you at your best. To achieve order within, begin with outward order.

If your hair needs washing, your breath isn't fresh, or your makeup is stale, if your nails are rough or chipped or your antiperspirant is fading, you'll self-consciously avoid close encounters, giving others the wrong impression. Poise and personal grooming are soul mates. Women known for their sense of style and poise are impeccably groomed.

Poise is often overlooked when we think of putting together our authentic look. Why is developing poise so important? Because when we're not obsessively focusing on ourselves or our shortcomings, our smiles become warmer, our laughter more spontaneous, and our thoughtfulness blossoms. Outer poise mirrors inner poise. Moments spent in quiet contemplation to nurture our inner poise should be an essential part of every woman's daily beauty ritual. Self-possession costs us only time and self-nurturance. When we feel at ease with ourselves, we feel at ease in the world.

OCTOBER 11

It's Always Something

It's always something.
—Roseanne Roseannadanna (Gilda Radner, 1946–1989)
Comedian, actress, the first performer hired for *Saturday Night Live*

And of course, it is. Sometimes it's a damn nuisance. Sometimes it's soul shattering. But it's always something. It's real life.

After Gilda Radner left *Saturday Night Live,* where she created some unforgettable, funny women characters—Roseanne Roseannadanna, Emily Litella, and Baba Wawa—she set out to create a life for herself.

For a decade she had been a successful workaholic as life whizzed by. Falling in love with Gene Wilder helped her realize the pleasure of lowering gears. By the time they married in 1984, she wanted to pursue her dream of becoming a writer. Always observant and knowing rich material when she found it, she began a book called *Portrait of the Artist as a Housewife*, a collection of stories, poems, and vignettes celebrating domesticity and the humor inherent in toaster ovens and plumbers. It would have been hilarious.

But real life grabbed her attention with a diagnosis of ovarian cancer, and a grittier book emerged, *It's Always Something*, a defiantly irreverent, moving memoir. Like other women who struggle with life-threatening illness, Gilda mourned "my lost joy, my happiness, my exhilaration with life." The day before her diagnosis, life stretched before her, luminous in its limitless possibilities. The moment after being told she had cancer, life's dimensions shrank to twenty-four-hour stretches.

In a moving essay contained in *Minding the Body: Women Writers on Body and Soul*, Judith Hooper rightly admonishes us: "We go around thinking that real life is about adding a rec room to the basement, but this is not about real life. Cancer is real life. When you accept cancer, it is as if new systems within the organism automatically open—like the oxygen masks and flotation systems that automatically drop in your lap on a 747 in an emergency. When you walk this earth on borrowed time, each day on the calendar is a beloved friend you know for only a short time."

You begin to *live*.

Why must we find a lump in our breast before this occurs? Do you know? Because I certainly don't. But I do know a wonderful woman who was very active at her children's school for many years, largely because after she had volunteered a generous amount of personal time, everyone took for granted that she'd always be there. The hours she put into her PTA work were the equivalent of a full-time but unpaid second job. When she made the terrible discovery that she had breast cancer, she admitted to close friends that in a strange way, she was relieved. Cancer meant she could start saying no, create boundaries, and finally put down the school committee burden without guilt. Now she could ransom back her life. After all, no one expects a woman fighting breast cancer to do anything but take care of herself. Of course, she was right.

When I heard this story, I wanted to scream and cry. Yes, it's always something. *But it doesn't always have to have your name on it.* I pray we never find a lump, but I pray just as fervently that we never squander or surrender another precious day for whatever reason, and that we never wait until something dire occurs to feel justified in setting boundaries.

And if you've already found a lump, I pray that you'll grow whole and old in joy, peace, and grace, gifting us for many years with your wisdom.

Heaven knows, we need it.

OCTOBER 12

A Tale of Two Times

It was the best of times, it was the worst of times.
—Charles Dickens (1812–1870)
British novelist

Once upon a time.

Up until this time.

For the time being.

Time and time again.

All in good time.

Time's up!

Since the dawn of time, we've tried to understand her nature. Why? In order to control her. But time is a holy mystery, an extravagant gift meant to be experienced, not understood. Certainly not controlled. Why do you think we're crazed half the time?

Time's mystery is difficult for most women to appreciate because we've so little of it. Although we've all been allotted twenty-four hours each day, it doesn't seem to go very far. So if we experience anything at all, it's dread, because we keep running out of time. Again, and again. And it doesn't matter what *kind* of time it is—Greenwich, daylight saving, standard, eastern, mountain, central, or pacific. All that matters is we never seem to have enough of it. Which is why all the women I know constantly feel time-worn.

For centuries those with time on their hands—saints, poets, mystics, masters, sages, and philosophers—have pondered time's enigma. They've discovered her duality. As the sculptor and poet Henry Van Dyke explains: "Time is/Too slow for those who Wait/Too swift for those who Fear/Too long for those who grieve/Too short for those who

Rejoice…" Slow and swift are time's parallel realities, the yin and yang of existence.

In order to know a semblance of serenity during the days of our lives, we also need to discover time's twin nature, which the ancient Greeks called *chronos* and *kairos*.

Chronos is clocks, deadlines, watches, calendars, agendas, schedules. Chronos is time at her worst. Chronos keeps track. Chronos is a delusion of grandeur. Chronos is always running for the subway and having the doors shut before you can get on. In chronos we think only of ourselves. Chronos is the world's time.

Kairos is transcendence, infinity, reverence, joy, passion, love, the Sacred. Kairos is intimacy with the Real. Kairos is time at her best. Kairos lets go. In kairos we escape the dungeon of self. Kairos is a Schubert waltz in nineteenth-century Vienna with your soul mate. Kairos is Spirit's time.

We exist in chronos. We long for kairos. That's *our* duality. Chronos requires speed so that it won't be wasted. Kairos requires space so that it might be savored. We *do* in chronos. In kairos we're allowed *to be*.

We think we've never known kairos, but we have: when making love, when meditating or praying, when lost in music's rapture or literature's reverie, when planting bulbs or pulling weeds, when watching over a sleeping child, when snuggling together in bed, laughing at the antics of our pets, when delighting in a sunset, when exulting in our passions. We know joy in kairos, glimpse beauty in kairos, remember what it means to be alive in kairos, reconnect with our Divinity in kairos.

So how do we exchange chronos for kairos?

By slowing down.

By concentrating on one thing at a time.

By going about whatever we are doing as if it were the only thing worth doing at that moment.

By pretending we have all the time in the world, so that our subconscious will kick in and make it so.

By making time.

By taking time.

It only takes a moment to cross over from chronos into kairos, but it does take *a moment*. All that kairos asks is our willingness to stop running long enough to hear the music of the spheres.

Today, be willing to join in the dance.

Now you're in kairos.

OCTOBER 13

Absolutely Fabulous

If you don't have any shadows you're not in the light.
—Lady Gaga
American songwriter, singer, actress

For many years I've had difficulty identifying, imagining, and personalizing my "shadow," Carl Jung's name for the darker self lurking deep within. Jung believed that our shadows are the composite of all the shameful emotions, nasty impulses, and negative aspects of our personalities that we attempt to bury in order to show an acceptable face to the world. Think of the raving lunatic the family keeps locked in a tower in gothic novels, or Robert Louis Stevenson's Dr. Jekyll and Mr. Hyde, and you get the idea.

Unfortunately, not knowing *is* what hurts us, especially when sublimating our shadow. In *Guilt Is the Teacher, Love Is the Lesson*, the stress and mind/body specialist Joan Borysenko describes the fermentation of our "ghostly double" as "getting up a head of steam, getting wilder and wilder inside us, informing our behaviors without our consciously knowing they are there" until they express themselves "quite suddenly and explosively in accidents, impulsive behavior, illness, lapses of judgment...In other words, an unexplored shadow leaves us stuck without understanding why, assaulted by strange impulses, and powerless to change."

To be honest, even though I understood Jung's concept of the shadow, I had no real desire to get to know her better. Then another of life's lessons opened my eyes. What I discovered shocked me but didn't send me shrieking in terror. It made me laugh.

Have you ever seen the wicked nineties British sitcom *Absolutely Fabulous?* Think *30 Rock* in the fashion world. The series revolves around two forty-something debauchees—Edina and Patsy—whose only redeeming social value is their loyalty to each other. Edina—known as "Edie" by her intimates—is a dizzy, pudgy fashion publicist, whose greatest ambition is to "look completely happening." She has two ex-husbands, one long-suffering, sensible, and disapproving teenage daughter, and a mother who can't figure out where she went wrong. There isn't a New Age fad Edie hasn't embraced in a futile effort to find enlightenment, including chanting, colonic irrigation, and isolation chambers.

Patsy is an anorexic, alcoholic, nymphomaniac fashion editor with an outrageous blond beehive. Edie's never seen in anything but designer hallucinations; Patsy's never seen without a cigarette dangling from her red lips or a glass of champagne in her hand. To Edie and Patsy, everyone is either "sweetie," "darling," or "sweetie darling"; anything pleasurable is "absolutely fabulous," including their opinions of each other.

They're vile, vain, vapid, vacuous. Shallow, selfish. Dumb and dumber. Hilarious. They're certainly not role models, but most assuredly, they're the stuff of our shadows.

The first time I watched Edie and Patsy cavorting around London, I fell off the couch in tears, hooting, howling, and holding my sides. Edie was my evil twin, my shadow. I recognized her instantly. Edie gives new meaning to the awareness of "there but for the grace of God." But I love her despite all her flaws, or maybe because of them.

I suspect there are many women who identify with some part of Edie and Patsy. Or Thelma and Louise. Or Romy and Michele. Or Ilana and Abbi. Iconic friend duos who get into all sorts of trouble. If we could shed every responsibility and inhibition for a half a day, perhaps we'd resemble one of these gals. And while that's amusing, it's not pretty. Still, whenever I am stressed to the max, I'll relax with a glass of wine and watch *Ab Fab*. I always come back to real life chuckling and, in a strange way, renewed.

Our shadows are only to be feared if we repress them, if we refuse to give them the recognition they need. In her book *Women Who Run with the Wolves*, Clarissa Pinkola Estés suggests "opening the door to the shadow realm a little and letting out various elements a few at a time, relating to them, finding use for them..." so that we can "reduce [the risk of] being surprised by shadow sneak attacks and unexpected explosions" like a "Roman candle gone berserk." But also, without darkness there is no light. Shadows are also what make us human.

Edie, self-medicating with booze, cigarettes, drugs, shopping, and sex to mask her pain, blindly embraces self-awareness trends because she's afraid to follow the wisdom of her heart. She's consumed with her appearance to avoid recognizing deeper concerns; she's a slave to fashion because she doesn't trust her instincts. But as Dr. Estés reassures us, the shadow "can contain the divine, the luscious, beautiful and powerful aspects of personhood" such as "the woman who can speak well of herself without denigration, who can face herself without cringing, who works to perfect her craft."

Edie's craft, like our own, is discovering her authenticity. But in our search, we must not ignore what Dr. Estés calls "these discarded, devalued, and unacceptable aspects of soul and self," even if they make us feel uncomfortable. Especially—sweetie darling—if we long for our lives to be rich, deep, and absolutely fabulous.

Kiss, kiss.

The Ultimate Result of All Ambition

To be happy at home is the ultimate result of all ambition.
—Dr. Samuel Johnson (1709–1784)
English poet, playwright, critic, creator of
the *Dictionary of the English Language*

The wisdom contained in this one sentence is worth meditating on for the rest of our lives; it's probably the reason Dr. Johnson earned his final resting place with the "Immortals" in Westminster Abbey.

Why are you working so hard? To be happy at home. But you're never *at* home—in mind, body, or spirit—because you're always working. So why are you working so hard? To be happy at home.

This is not a Zen koan. Life *is* a paradox, but we don't have to make it any harder than it is already. We've been on this path for ten months, but if you're on the cusp of grasping this insight, you're miles ahead of most of us.

Hold this thought: *The ultimate result of all ambition is to be happy at home.* Engrave this truth on your consciousness. Lay the track deeply, so that even when you're on your own version of automatic pilot, you'll be homeward bound. Write it on the palm of your hand; sneak a peek at it three times a day. Mutter it under your breath before attending a budget review that starts a half hour before the children need to be picked up; before agreeing to entertain out-of-town clients on your anniversary; before answering emails on Sunday or leaving voice mails at midnight.

What is the ultimate result of all ambition?

You know.

Inscribe it on your heart. Print it on a TV shirt or a poster you hang in your house. Say it out loud when you get up and just before retiring. Make it your mantra—that personal phrase that brings all things into focus. Doing so will help remind you that the greatest adventure of our lives is finding our way back home.

OCTOBER 15

The Quality of the Day

To affect the quality of the day, that is the highest of arts.
—Henry David Thoreau (1817–1862)
American philosopher and author

We know now that there are many aspects to real life in which our opinion is neither sought nor required. Sometimes, despite our best efforts and positive thinking, health, fortune, and/or peace elude us. But the one thing we do have absolute control over is the quality of our days. Even when we're grief stricken, racked with pain, sick from worry, deeply depressed, squeezed by circumstances—how we greet, meet, and complete each day is our choosing.

We hate to hear this.

Of course, when we're sick, worried, grieving, depressed, or frantic, we're not very interested in the day's quality; we just want the misery to end. But wishing the day away is also a creative choice, even if it's not a deliberate one.

Artists of the Everyday excel in elevating the simple to the level of the Sacred. You can use whatever you have on hand—a meal, a conversation, humor, affection—to create comfort and contentment—to put a positive spin, if not on the overall quality of the day, then on critical moments of it. For some time now I have been conducting a top-secret experiment with life, as Thoreau suggests we do. I wanted to see just how much influence I really had on the day's character. So the first words I speak in the morning are: "Thank you for the gift of this wonderful day in this body and this life."

Here are the initial findings, but you will not like them. Nor did I.

- All days are wonderful in direct proportion to the creative energy invested in them. No investment, no return.
- Even lousy days possess hidden wonder. Sometimes all you need is a moment of attitude adjustment to shift your perception of an entire afternoon and move forward into a pleasant evening.
- Weather does not seem to affect the experiment. Gray, cold, and rainy days spent in an office are just as susceptible to the warming influence of enthusiasm as are sunny days spent lying in a hammock sipping sangria.
- Days that are expected to be wonderful before they begin turn out to be so much more frequently than days greeted with grumbling.

♨ The results of this experiment suggest that it doesn't matter whether a day is good or bad. What matters is what we do with it. *But we knew that.*

OCTOBER 16

Ceremonials for Common Days

How but in custom and ceremony,
Are innocence and beauty born?
—William Butler Yeats (1865–1939)
Irish poet and recipient of the Nobel Prize for
Literature in 1923

Ceremony and custom give birth to beauty, restoring a sense of wonder to our daily round. Most of us are far too jaded for our own good. We've seen it all. Nothing surprises us anymore.

Which is precisely our problem. We only *think* we've seen it all. What we haven't begun to see is the abundance that surrounds us, the beauty that gift wraps the extravagance of each day.

The best way to renew our sense of the Sacred is through personal rituals. I treasure a little book called *Ceremonials of Common Days* written in 1923 by Abbie Graham. I found it languishing on a dark, dusty secondhand bookshelf and ransomed it for a dollar. Now my hand-printed oracle, with its blackboard cover of yellow and green woodcut flowers, sits on my desk. The gold lettering on its spine reminds me that perception comes only when we pace ourselves. Nothing is too insignificant in the eyes of the Authentic Self. Nothing is beneath notice.

There are numerous holidays (from the Old English "holy day") throughout the year, falling just when we need cheering up. We respond to them as if company's come to call, bringing out our special dishes, linens, crystal, flowers, and candles.

However, we actually do most of our living among the common days, taking them for granted just the way we do the people we love. Yet myriad occasions during the course of each day cry out for consecration.

A liturgy of commonplace moments ripe for personal ritual might include sipping the first cup of coffee; putting on one's public face; eating at one's desk; window shopping; crossing the threshold at night; changing into comfortable clothes; hearing the sound of a loved one's homecoming footsteps; sitting down to a simple meal; being paid; traveling; sharing a laugh, or a confidence, or both; indulging in rainy-day reveries; curling up to watch something at home; sleeping late and having breakfast in bed; starting a good book; losing five pounds; having a good cry; and so to bed. There is no shortage of common day ceremonies waiting to be enjoyed, only weary imaginations in need of inspirational transfusions.

"To make a day, it took an Evening and a Morning—at least to make the first day. But that was when the world was new and there was in it only light and darkness, day and night, and God," Abbie Graham calls to our remembrance. "The world has grown more complicated since that creative era." To make a day now it takes bells and whistles and clocks and desks and committees and meetings and money, and hungry people, and people who are too tired, and Twitter and news feeds and telephones, emails and noise and shouting and much hurrying. All these things and many others it takes now, in addition to an evening and a morning.

"Perhaps these ingredients are necessary for the concoction of a day; but when I come to observe the Ceremonial of Evenings and Mornings, they do not seem to be the reason why light and darkness were separated, and day and night created. Whatever be my philosophy, I, too, must work to make enough money to pay my share toward the bells and whistles and the gas and the personal engagements and the privilege of hurrying," Abbie Graham admits, pointing out some things that time only increases, like our proper use of it.

"But as I watch the stars of evening, and in the morning open my window toward the east, I shall observe the Ceremonial of quietness of heart, of simplicity, and poise of spirit, that I may keep my soul and the souls of others free from entanglements in the machinery of a day."

OCTOBER 17

The Habit of Being

So many worlds, so much to do
So little done, such things to be.

—Alfred, Lord Tennyson (1809–1892)
British and Irish Poet Laureate

During her lifetime (1925–1964), neither the camera nor the critics were very kind to Flannery O'Connor. She was as unphotogenic as she was unapologetic. The camera's harsh lens couldn't capture the intelligence, passion, imagination, exuberance, wit, and grace her family and friends knew and loved. For much of her adult life, the camera only recorded a body and face ravaged by illness. Her critics didn't appreciate her finely honed sense of the grotesque—that Southern specialty—with all its satire, black humor, and pathos, nor her obsession with religion. She was a cartographer of the human soul, and her searing words gave expression to the yearning of misfits. The characters in her novels and short stories were forlorn and flawed, searching for redemption whether they knew it or not.

Redemption was a major theme in Flannery's work as well as the thread that held her life together. "There are some of us who have to pay for our faith every step of the way and who have to work out dramatically what it would be like without it," she wrote, "and if being without it would ultimately be possible or not." Her rural Georgia surroundings, coupled with her affliction with lupus at twenty-five (the disease that killed her father when she was a child), contributed to a deep sense of isolation, for she was unable to care for herself and lived with her mother until her death at thirty-nine.

What her close friends remember best about Flannery was her determination to revere and savor the gift of every day. Her close friend (and editor of her letters), Sally Fitzgerald, calls it "the habit of being," a deep *joie de vivre* that animated her daily round. Flannery's passion for life, Sally Fitzgerald tells us, was "rooted in her talent and the possibilities of her work, which she correctly saw as compensating her fully for any deprivations she had to accept, and as offering a scope for living that most of us never dream of encompassing." Her mornings were sacred, reserved for her writing, but the rest of the day was devoted to being Flannery.

The habit of being—the exultation in the present moment—is an exquisite concept, one that could enrich our lives beyond measure. We're all habitual creatures, but usually we practice the *habits of doing*: getting up, making breakfast, walking the dog, exercising (if we're so inclined), getting children off to school, and getting ourselves to work.

Then there are our *habits of brooding*: projecting into the future, dwelling on the past, nursing old wounds, holding imaginary conversations, indulging in comparisons, conducting endless mental calculations about money, gnawing on regrets, second-guessing inspiration, ruminating on problems at work, anticipating the worst. The habits of brooding are rooted in the past or the future, and they can rob the present moment of all harmony, beauty, and joy.

But what if, as curators of our own contentment, we deliberately cultivated the *habit of being*: a heightened awareness of real life's abundance? The habit of being is a grateful appreciation for the good surrounding us, no matter what our circumstances might be today. What if you knew there was always going to be a simple pleasure to look forward to every few hours? What if you made sure there was? How do you think you would greet the day?

Flannery O'Connor generously offered struggling writers advice. To one she wrote: "Wouldn't it be better for you to discover a meaning in what you write than to impose one? Nothing you write will lack meaning because the meaning is in you." I believe this passion for discovering meaning extends to the Art of the Everyday as well. Once you commit to cultivating the habit of being, nothing in your daily round will lack meaning, because you'll discover that the meaning is within you.

OCTOBER 18

Choice

Authenticity is a collection of choices that we have to make every day. It's about the choice to show up and be real. The choice to be honest. The choice to let our true selves be seen.

Dr. Brené Brown
Research professor and author

Many of us don't think of choice as a spiritual gift. We believe choices are burdens to be endured, not embraced. And so they become burdens. But after breath, is there a more precious gift than free will?

Consider for a moment that there are only three ways to change the trajectory of our lives for better or worse: crisis, chance, and choice.

You may not realize it, but your life at this exact moment—it doesn't matter who you are, where you are, or who's getting ready to jerk your chain—is a direct result of choices you made once upon a time. Thirty minutes or thirty years ago.

Our choices can be conscious or unconscious. Conscious choice is creative, the heart of authenticity. Unconscious choice is destructive, the heel of self-harming. Unconscious choice is how we end up living other people's lives. "The most common despair is...not choosing, or willing to be oneself," the nineteenth-century Danish philosopher Søren Kierkegaard warns us, "[but] the deepest form of despair is to choose to be another than oneself." This is how we always hurt the one we love. The one we shouldn't hurt at all. Our Self.

We live in a world defined by duality—light or dark, up or down, success or failure, right or wrong, pain or joy. This duality keeps us in perpetual motion. Like a pendulum in an old clock, we swing back and forth through our emotions. But creative, conscious choice gives us the power to stop swinging and remain in balance, at peace. Be still, woman, and know who you are. Many women are petrified of making choices. This is because we don't trust our instincts. It's been so long, we've forgotten how. We'd opt to clean the kitty litter or work for our passage to the Congo if it meant we never had to make another choice more complex than deciding what's for dinner, which is hard enough. (How many times have you had chicken this week?) Having to decide what to wear to a cocktail party or which of forty-seven different shades of white to paint the dining room trim have been known to trigger the kind of emotional response that puts women behind bars—or on the floor of one.

The reason we're terrified of making choices, even little ones, is that we're convinced we'll make a wrong one. *Again*. Maybe you're too tired tonight to have that conversation, although you know it's long overdue. Maybe you can choose to put it off until tomorrow night. *Again*. If you're anything like me, a lot of wrong choices got you where you are today and continue to keep you there.

But a wrong choice isn't necessarily a *bad* choice.

You married the wrong man. Became a teacher instead of a country and western singer. You didn't finish college, join the Peace Corps, or move to New York. If you had, your life would have been different. But *not necessarily better*. That's because *we*, not our outer circumstances, are the catalysts for the quality of our lives. Not then. Not now. Not ever.

We don't know if a choice is wise or wrong until we've lived it. We can't ever really know where a choice will take us, although we may sense its direction. We're torn between the agonizing shoulds and shouldn'ts. An inner debate begins to rage. The English writer Jeanette Winterson describes our dilemma beautifully: "I have a theory that every time you make an important choice, the part of you left behind continues the other life you could have had."

Wow. That's a lot to mull over. So why don't we do that for the rest of the day. Or just sleep on it.

OCTOBER 19

Designing Women

It's when we're given choice that we sit with the gods and design ourselves.

—Dorothy Gilman (1923–2012)
American author of mysteries and spy novels

Good morning. You look well rested. What's your secret? Making more choices while you're awake rather than asleep? It suits you!

So you gather as much information as you can before making a choice.

You weigh the options. You ponder the possibilities. You brood. You probe the probabilities with your best friend. You ask your heart. You pray for guidance. Then you take a leap in the dark and hope you land on your feet. You live your choice. You don't look back for a long time. Eventually, with hindsight, you'll glance back and see which it was, wise or wrong. But at least it's a calculated risk, and you did the best that you could. Spirit asks nothing more. Neither should you.

But wrong choices should never be confused with bad choices. Bad choices—and we all have made them—often happen when we embark on sinuous stretches of self-destruction, usually with a smile. You don't ask your heart or a pal for advice. You don't ponder, and you certainly don't pray. Why? Because on the deepest intuitive level you know you shouldn't even be entertaining the thought of this choice. But you want to do it so badly that even its badness doesn't daunt you. In fact, it eggs you on.

Quite frankly, my dear, we don't give a damn what *anyone* thinks at times like that, do we?

If we close our eyes, we can honestly say that we never saw disaster coming. How could we? Bad choices are made while we're sleepwalking. From now on, let's call them *coma choices*. Before we even make them, we know that when we wake up, we'll ask, "How could I have been so stupid?"

But our lives are not entirely shaped by wrong or bad choices, thank God. There have been wise choices, good choices, strong choices, courageous choices, happy choices. Brilliant decisions. We just don't remember many of them. That's because we shrug off any good thing that arrives in our lives as if it were a fluke, a lucky break, a misdelivery. Certainly, we don't give ourselves credit. Only when things don't work out, only when we make mistakes, or stumble on missteps, do we feel we're responsible. Then we claim all the blame.

So it should hardly be surprising if our primary reaction to any choice is to avoid it. Put it off as long as possible. Postpone the inevitable. But by not choosing, we allow others to decide for us. It doesn't matter how well-meaning or wonderful they are. It doesn't matter *who* they are. Just remember, if you didn't make the choice, you can't blame someone else if you're unhappy.

Today, as you start to retrace your journey, be willing to reflect on the choices you made in the past, as well as on your style of choosing. Are you deliberate? Impulsive? Comatose? Do you make choices with your heart, your mind, or your gut? Are you comfortable with your style of decision-making, or do you cringe? What about trying a different approach? Whatever your style, I'll bet that your life, like mine, is choices you never even considered.

Scary, isn't it?

Choice is destiny's soul mate. In her novel *The Avenue of the Dead,* Evelyn Anthony exquisitely evokes the moment of recognition: "Long afterwards, she was to remember that moment when her life changed its direction. It was not predestined: she had a choice. Or it seemed that she had. To accept or refuse. To take one turning down the crossroads to the future or another."

OCTOBER 20

Compliments

Nowadays we are all of us so hard up that the only pleasant things to pay are compliments.

—Oscar Wilde (1854–1900)
Anglo-Irish poet, playwright, and legendary
raconteur

All women need more compliments in their lives. We need to give more of them to our families, friends, and strangers. We need to hear more of them, even if we must give them to ourselves. But most of all, we need to bask in them.

In our heart of hearts, most of us feel that we deserve more compliments than we receive. But maybe one of the reasons we don't hear as many compliments as we'd like is because whenever one has our name on it, we return it to the sender.

"Oh, this old thing?"

"I got it on sale."

"I've had this forever."

"Do you really think so?"

"It was nothing."

Remember, if we send good things away or aren't open to receiving them, at some point the Universe may no longer bother with us. And who would blame it? No one enjoys hanging around an ingrate, and that's exactly what we are when we discount the marvelous about ourselves.

It's interesting that the first dictionary definition of a compliment is "an expression of esteem." Perhaps we have a difficult time accepting compliments because deep down we don't believe we deserve them. When we aren't willing to receive praise, it's because our self-esteem is flagging.

Today, be receptive. Start with the assumption that you're beautiful, dazzling, bootylicious, absolutely fabulous. You're slaying it. Ask Spirit to reveal how gorgeous and brilliant you really are. Every time someone pays you a compliment, accept it as if an angel had just whispered Spirit's appreciation. Smile and say, "Thank you. How nice of you to notice."

Become abundant with your compliments to others. We're all so fragile, especially when we put on a brave face. A sincere compliment can penetrate beneath even the most sophisticated masks to soothe troubled souls. The woman you think needs compliments the least is probably the one who needs them most.

Cultivate the habit of giving at least one compliment a day to another human being, as well as to yourself. You'll feel good when you do, and soon it will become one of your habits of being. Just as words can hurt, words can heal.

OCTOBER 21

Complaints

I personally believe we developed language because of our deep inner need to complain.

—Jane Wagner
American writer, director, and producer

Complaints we know. Complaints we're good at. Most of us have already mastered the art of the complaint in all its many variations: gripe, groan, moan, kvetch, bitch, whine. Probably the only woman on the face of the earth who has never carried on the way we do was Mother Teresa, but I hear that she gave a withering look if someone needed to be kept in line.

One of the reasons we love our close friends so dearly is that they allow us to complain knowing that we'll return the favor. But if we really love them, don't you think it's about time we started sparing them? Some of us spend half our lives griping. It's time to get a grip. When we bitch and moan we're not much fun to listen to; just because you can't see the eyes at the other end of the receiver doesn't mean they're not rolling or shut.

Try new outlets to channel hostility: Shout in the shower, blow off steam as you walk, or scream in your car as you wait in traffic. Spirit's big enough to take it. Besides, it's all been heard before. There's nothing new under the sun.

I'm not suggesting that we suppress our negative feelings. But the petty stuff we're often foaming at the mouth about isn't worth the breath it steals. Our words are powerful, so powerful that they can change our reality—the quality of our days and nights. Moaning rarely makes either us or those around us feel better. In fact, it often makes everyone feel worse. Learning to shrug is the beginning of wisdom.

Alternatively, learn to be creative about your complaining. Barbara Sher, the inspirational author and coach, believes "in the efficacy of complaining the way some people believe in the efficacy of prayer." In fact, she encourages "hard time sessions." In her book *Wishcraft*, Sher suggests that the next time you feel as though you'll explode, announce beforehand that you need a hard time session. Tell anyone in close range that you're mad, nervous, fed up, and not going to take it anymore. Tell them for the next five minutes you're going to lose it. Tell them not to pay any attention and not to take it personally. Then run amok. You'll probably end up feeling much better without having to offer apologies or wipe away tears. You may even end up laughing.

Today, if you must complain, sweetie, at least be creative about it. I hear you.

OCTOBER 22

Comparisons

We're only envious of those already doing what we were made to do. Envy is a giant, flashing arrow pointing us towards our destiny.
—Glennon Doyle
American author, activist, philanthropist

Comparisons are irresistible but insidious, odious, and very often our self-torture of choice.

Today, let's meditate on not coveting our neighbor's figure, home, clothes, income, or career. Not to mention her accomplishments, achievements, awards, recognition, and fame. Usually it's only one woman whose bounteous blessings push our buttons of raging insecurity; we really don't care if most of the world has more than we have, we only care that she has, and we have not. Often the subject of our hostility is not personally known to us, though the life she leads on our social media feeds is. Secretly we stalk for evidence of *her* good fortune. Or she could be one of your friends (deepest sympathy), which is horrendous, because you must hear firsthand accounts of all you're missing now. Whoever she is, she's the devil in disguise, because you insist on measuring your life, success, bank account, and self-worth against hers.

Obviously, I couldn't ruminate on coveting, jealousy, envy, and making oneself utterly miserable with comparisons unless I was vaguely familiar with this sin against authenticity. (All right, intimately familiar.) Would you believe one of my favorite poems (and probably that of every other writer in the world) is Clive James's funny, spiteful ode, "The Book of My Enemy Has Been Remaindered"? You cringe as you laugh. My bad.

This is not good. This is not enlightenment. We're grown women. We're bigger than this. *Aren't we?*

Well, even if we aren't, comparisons hurt us in profound ways. They undermine our confidence. Shut down our flow of creative energy. Short-circuit our access to Power. Deplete our self-esteem. Suck the life force from our marrow. Coveting destroys what is Sacred within. Instead of comparing yourself to another woman, why not just take out a billboard at Hollywood and Vine and remind the world how fantastic you are? Or make up a smaller one and put it where you can see it every day.

The next time you're tempted to compare your life to another's, pause for a moment. Remind yourself, over and over, that *there is no competition on the spiritual plane*. The blessings your nemesis has received also can be yours as soon as you are *really* ready to receive with an open heart all the good fortune created just for you.

And when will that be? As soon as you can bless the woman you secretly curse; as soon as you can give thanks for her happiness and success as much as your own because it demonstrates the abundance of real life.

OCTOBER 23

Compromises

Compromise, if not the spice of life, is its solidity.
—Phyllis McGinley (1905–1978)
Pulitzer Prize–winning poet and essayist

Whether you're single, married, with children or without, it's not possible to get through the day without agreeing to at least one compromise. There are little compromises and there are bigger ones. Tolerable compromises are those we enter into fully—with complete knowledge in advance of exactly what we're surrendering. The other kind of compromises—the ones many of us make day in, day out—are the strong, silent type. They're strong because we're stuck with them and silent because they're unconscious or unspoken.

Compromises are the art of the bottom line. We can bend only so far, and then we break. Knowing just how far you can bend is the first step in making sane agreements, but this isn't as easy as it sounds.

The more complicated life becomes, the simpler your bottom line must be. How about this: What *must* you have from this situation? What do you absolutely *need*? If you need it, you must have it. It's non-negotiable. If you didn't *need* it to survive, it—whatever "it" is— wouldn't be a need. Then it would be a want. Unfortunately, "wants" are the currency of compromise. I want, you want, we all want, which is why we bargain. Keep in mind that your want might be another's legitimate need. The best compromises, like a workable lifestyle, cover all your needs while satisfying a few of your wants.

However, if you dread it, don't agree to it. If you do end up doing it despite your dread, you'll despise the whole deal, including the woman who agreed to it: you.

Be affable. Try to see the other person's point of view. Be flexible. Be as generous as you can without gagging. Ask that the highest good for all parties be achieved. Trust your instincts. Pay attention to physical clues, especially your gut; it's there not only to aid in digestion, but to serve as a reliable aid in discerning what's best for you.

Above all, follow Janis Joplin's advice: "Don't compromise yourself. You are all you've got."

OCTOBER 24

The Ladies' Man: George Bernard Shaw

You can be as romantic as you please about love,
But you mustn't be romantic about money.
—George Bernard Shaw (1856–1950)
Irish playwright, critic, and political activist

From the desk of Virginia Woolf:

May 15, 1940

Dear Mr. Shaw,

Your letter reduced me to two days silence from sheer pleasure. You won't be surprised to learn that I promptly lifted some paragraphs and inserted them into my proofs. You may take what action you like...

When imagining the quintessential ladies' man, one doesn't immediately think of the Irish dramatist George Bernard Shaw. Indeed, the public persona he projected over eight decades as scathing curmudgeon, showman, intellectual, critic, pundit, Socialist, playwright, and Nobel laureate seems to have been carefully constructed to leave the impression that he hated women. He was also a strange-looking man—likely not a bundle of cuddles. The English novelist Edith Nesbit described him as "very plain, like a long corpse with a dead, white face—sandy sleek hair, and a loathsome straggly beard, and yet is one of the most fascinating men I ever met!"

For all his aloofness, which was really acute shyness, Bernard Shaw adored ladies, believing them to be the world's saving grace, and, in turn, it was impossible for women to resist his charm. And why would they? Here was a thinking woman's crumpet, especially if you were a woman who believed that the sexiest part of a man is his brains. (Don't you wish men knew that?) Women fell under his spell and delighted in every minute of it, from famous actresses such as Stella Tennant (Mrs. Patrick Campbell) to feminist authors such as Virginia Woolf, who confessed a lifelong passion to him in a rapturous letter:

"As for the falling in love, it was not, let me confess, one-sided. When I first met you at the Webb's, I was set against all great men, having liberally been fed on them at my father's house. I had only wanted to meet business men and say, racing experts. But in a jiffy you made me re-consider all that and had me at your feet. Indeed, you have acted a lover's part in my life for the past thirty years, and I should have been a worse woman without Bernard Shaw..."

Of course, women love those who love us, believe in us, urge us to strive for our personal best and help us do so. G. B. S. was a staunch supporter of woman's rights, including equality of income as well as the vote and the right to serve in public office. He marched for the suffragettes in 1908, supported them financially, and seems to have endowed all of his women characters—from Eliza Doolittle to St. Joan—with the extraordinary qualities he found in Everywoman, championing the women's issue in popular culture and great art. ("The only difference between a Duchess and a flower girl is how she is treated.") More prolific than Shakespeare, Bernard Shaw wrote fifty plays and was the only writer to win both the Oscar (in 1938 for the film script of *Pygmalion,* which years later became the basis for *My Fair Lady*) and the Nobel Prize for Literature in 1925 (for his play *Saint Joan*). In a true cantankerous streak, he accepted the honor but refused the money.

Ironically, it's George Bernard Shaw's attitudes on money and women that have me inspired today, and I think they'll bring a smile to your face as well.

In a little book I cherish, *George Bernard Shaw on Women*, G. B. S. takes on the economics of marriage in a correspondence with his cousin Georgina, who writes to her aged relation to ask him for money for a trousseau. She's pretty but rather clueless, and he takes her to task for not being precise about her request. How much money does she want? What will she be using it for exactly? (He recommends spending it on undergarments, which last longer than fashion.) What does her fiancé do for a living? Is he a millionaire or a pauper? "You are not taking this seriously enough," G. B. S. writes. "Nobody is going to throw a £100 note to a young woman who has never had to handle such sums..."

Finally after getting his cousin to create a budget (sixty-five pounds for clothes, five pounds for a trunk, ten pounds for odds and ends and pocket money, ten pounds for the wedding breakfast), he offers to give her a hundred pounds as a wedding present with the proviso that she is to open up a bank account and "to keep it open for the rest of your life—a separate account in your own name." Can you imagine how every woman's life would be different and how the trajectory of our journey would have altered if we had been given this advice instead of having to learn it the hard way?

Perhaps it was because Shaw grew up in poor circumstances (his father was a "drunkard," which prompted G. B. S. to be a lifelong tee-totaler) that from an early age he was distressed about the lot of his mother and sisters. The themes of women, money, and self-reliance run as a vein of gold throughout his work. From *Pygmalion*'s heroine, Eliza Doolittle, accepting Professor Higgins's efforts to transform her from urchin to lady when all she really wants is to own her own flower shop to *Mrs. Warren's Profession*, written in 1894, the importance of a woman handling her own money is a dominant theme.

In *Mrs. Warren's Profession*, we meet a Cambridge University–educated young woman, Vivie Warren, who is eager to begin her career in finance. Full of storm and thunder and strong opinions, Vivie has been raised in boarding schools and has an awkward relationship with her mother; she really doesn't know her nor the source of her wealth or even the name of her own father. What *is* the profession of Mrs. Warren that has financed her daughter's position in "good society," thus enabling her to marry into the upper class?

Well, you don't have to take a very big leap to guess that Vivie's mother doesn't want her to find out that she's a madam. "I was a good mother," declares Mrs. Kitty Warren, "and because I made my daughter a good woman she turns me out as if I were a leper."

When Mrs. Warren defends her choice to become a high-class prostitute to give her daughter a good life and proper education instead of a life of poverty and drudgery, Vivie accepts her mother's history and even begrudgingly begins to appreciate the sacrifices her mother has made for her. But after the shock of this revelation, mother and daughter are tested to extremes when Vivie discovers that Kitty, now a woman of substance, runs successful brothels from Brussels to Vienna. Vivie recoils in horror and wants nothing more to do with her. If ever there was an iconic play for its time and ours, it's *Mrs. Warren's Profession*, but a century ago just the whiff of its subject matter caused a scandal on both sides of the Atlantic. It took Shaw eight years to get it produced, and when it was finally performed in New York in 1902, the actors were arrested for indecency.

In these uncertain financial times, it's instructive to reacquaint ourselves with the juncture in our own personal history when our family's attitudes toward money and the meaning of life became our own—where the twig was bent—and if these attitudes are not serving us, learn to discard them. I've always found dramatic literary heroines to be my first line of defense, and the women of George Bernard Shaw, as he knew, "all-together are a superior species." Indulge yourself and stream some of Shaw's plays, and then read the plays and you'll enjoy the witty banter. If you don't know Eliza, Kitty, Joan, Major Barbara, or Candida, you are in for a treat.

Shaw's fabulous Epifania Ognisanti di Parerga in *The Millionairess* is absolutely a personal female mentor for me. She's the richest woman in the world, who gives each potential suitor six months to transform £150 into £50,000 before she'll consider having a glass of champagne with him. Let the tutoring begin! Some of the best financial advice I've ever received is from literary mentors.

One last thought (or the beginning of many more!): George Bernard Shaw took great delight in the fact that he married in 1898 a "green-eyed millionairess" named Charlotte Payne-Townsend and once commented to an Inland Revenue tax official in 1910 that he could only guess at his wife's wealth. "Her property is a separate property. She keeps it at a separate banking account at a separate bank. Her solicitor is not my solicitor... I have no more knowledge of her income than I do of yours." They were happily married for nearly forty-five years, and at his own death in 1950, G. B. S. requested that their ashes be mingled and scattered together.

One last bit of inspiring truth Shaw always seems to bestow upon his heroines until they discover it for themselves: "Life isn't about finding yourself," Shaw tells us. "Life is about creating yourself."

Improbable Happy Endings

*If you want a happy ending, that depends, of course, on where you
stop your story.*

—Orson Welles (1915–1985)
American actor, director, writer, and
producer

When we begin searching for what we'd like to be doing with the rest
of our life (and remember, Carmen Dell'Olio already eliminated the
first excuse, which is age), we really don't have to look very far. The
clues are usually hiding in plain sight on bookshelves, bulletin boards,
or a few parcels from the past that you can't bring yourself to part with,
stored in your attic, basement, utility room, garage, or the universal
catch-all underneath the stairs. You may have even hidden your secret
desires in attractive display boxes. You've probably moved these boxes
for decades and never bothered to open them because you know the
longings that are buried in them.

Here's what I save and have held on to my entire life. Clips, cartoons,
photographs, theater programs, newspaper headlines, and memorabilia
from my bulletin boards that trace, as surely as Egyptian hieroglyphics,
my longings in this lifetime on earth. Not the actual achievements of
my life, mind you, but my unfilled yearnings. I know you have a similar cache somewhere, so this week might be the perfect opportunity to
retrieve the traces of some of those discarded dreams. Those dreams
still believe in us, even if we've lost track of them.

My dream of becoming a screenwriter is at least as old as the June
1980 issue of *Esquire* magazine, which features a chimp in a red polo
shirt at an electric typewriter with the headline: "Is Anyone in America
Not Writing a Screenplay? How to Hustle, Pitch, and Sell Your Story
to Hollywood." Like carbon dating my bookshelves and an archaeological artifact, I can pinpoint the moment I abandoned all hope of ever
actually writing a screenplay, because I pinned the cover on my bulletin
board. There was some insurmountable challenge I was facing—or I
thought there was, which is the same thing and meant I couldn't follow
this dream. If you think you can't do something, you're right, you can't.
Press on, and you'll discover you are doing it.

In the movies, an "insurmountable challenge" is called "transformation."

Transformation has three acts, which include spiritual, physical, and
psychological change, and this is called "The Story." The emotional arc

between what an ordinary woman was and what outside circumstances force her to become—a heroine—isn't for the faint of heart, but who doesn't adore cheering her on as she activates her improbable happy ending?

I love Steven Spielberg's observation that "In the best stories, someone loses control of his/her life and must regain it." Doesn't that sound familiar?

Right at this moment we couldn't be better positioned for success. We've lost control of our lives if we're not living the life we've dreamed of, but as Heaven is our witness, we're going to regain that better life just waiting over the horizon. When I imagine the future that I want, it's so exciting it sends shivers down my spine. But then, a split second later, when I think about how much I have to do between the dreaming and its coming true, the future morphs into Alfred Hitchcock heroine scary.

In fact, my dream feels a bit like Eva Marie Saint scaling Mount Rushmore in high heels in the film *North by Northwest*. We're in the middle of the ascent and the future seems so far away. If we look down, we'll get dizzy because we've had to climb so far from our past. If we look up to see how far it is to the top, we'll start hyperventilating.

But experienced rock climbers as well as stunt performers don't climb alone. A knowledgeable climber is above you with a top rope harnessed around you. Falling is expected and planned for in rock climbing, so you prepare for all contingencies. Your partner feeds you rope, lowers you down, helps you lift yourself up, and catches those falls. I always ask for Divine Grace to send me the right spiritual help, because, frankly, I don't know what I need, I just know I need bolstering. Prayer has become my primary practical skill because it's the only way I know how to do "life."

Each time you experience the new, you become receptive to inspiration. Each time you try something different, you send the Universe a message that you are awake, alive, and listening. We're going to have to slowly learn how to trust our instincts again. The truth is that we *all* have ignored those flashing intuitive red flags at the railroad crossings in our life. The regret and remorse that truly keep us up at night are because we received plenty of warning signals and didn't slow down. At some point we *didn't follow our intuition, did we?* So naturally now we're afraid of making any more mistakes. But we need to remember that the misjudgment came from *not* following our intuition. Next, we need to learn to forgive ourselves if we're ever going to begin again, and then we need to learn once more to trust our creative nudges. Now's there's a list for the essential transformation of our heroine.

So let's recap. In the new "Story" of our renaissance there will also be three acts:

Act 1: Our Heroine swears never to go against her intuition again.

Act 2: Our Heroine forgives herself for the past.

Act 3: Our Heroine trusts her new creative nudges, which lead her to the happiness she truly deserves.

Little steps + tiny choices = Big changes. We are going to believe once again that our yearnings are blessings. We're going to honor and respect our creative urges. More important, if we're going to ease, edge, or elbow our way into this brave new world with vision, vitality, and verve, we need recurring moments of success and episodes of encouragement in our daily round and throughout the rhythm of the year.

"You can have anything you want if you want it desperately enough," the British writer Sheilah Graham, the last lover of F. Scott Fitzgerald before his death, wrote in *The Rest of the Story* in 1964. "You must want it with an inner exuberance that erupts through the skin and joins the energy that created the world."

OCTOBER 26

Mount Rushmore Moments

There's something more important than logic: imagination.
—Sir Alfred Hitchcock (1899–1980)
British film director and producer

Although the great film director Alfred Hitchcock had his heart, mind, and ego set on filming his masterpiece *North by Northwest* (1959) at Mount Rushmore, in real life those scenes were never filmed there because the National Park Service wasn't about to let Hitchcock climb and film on a national monument. This decision incensed Hitchcock, a man who knew how to throw his considerable weight around.

That didn't matter, because when a movie's director is upset, everybody else below inherits the problem. It was up to the real-life movie "stars" of the special effects, production design, and stunt departments to perform magic on an MGM soundstage. And the glorious Eva Marie Saint climbed as if her very life depended upon it, with a pile of mattresses below her.

I adore this story because it just goes to prove that it doesn't matter how successful you are, how much power you think you have, or how right you are, there's always going to be someone in life's National Park

Service who's going to put the kibosh on your filming the chase scene across Lincoln's nose.

So what do you say we keep making a little magic of our own by discovering not only what we loved in the past but what we love now. I know there are a lot of things you'd like to have figured out right this minute. You want answers right now. But we don't have answers, because we haven't even figured out the questions.

There are going to be days where every time you turn around there's another stumbling block to your dreams, when the perfect scenario turns out to be not as perfect as you originally hoped or as doable as you planned. We're going to learn to think of these days as our "Mount Rushmore moments." Down for a day but pulling a pile of mattresses behind us the next. Making it work.

"Do you remember the fun we had when we started out all those years ago? We didn't have any money then, did we? We didn't have any time, either. But we took risks...we experimented," Alfred Hitchcock recalled wistfully about his movie-making Mount Rushmore moments. "We invented new ways of making pictures because we had to."

We will, too. Because when they tell us we can't use Mount Rushmore, that's when the magic really begins.

OCTOBER 27

By Love Possessed

Your possessions express your personality. Few things, including clothes, are more personal than your cherished ornaments. The pioneer women, who crossed a wild continent clutching their treasures to them, knew that a clock, a picture, a pair of candlesticks, meant home, even in the wilderness.
—Good Housekeeping, August 1952

In July 1846, Margaret Reed reluctantly left her beloved home in Springfield, Illinois, with her husband, James, their four children, and her ailing mother and set off for California. Margaret had stubbornly resisted her husband's entreaties to move for months, begging him not to abandon the charmed life of comfort and culture they enjoyed. But her Victorian husband, who was a wealthy furniture manufacturer, sought even more wealth, as well as adventure, and in the end, his will prevailed.

Much of James Reed's success in persuading Margaret lay in his promise that she would travel in unsurpassed luxury and style, with all her prized personal possessions. He kept his word.

Never before had a covered wagon been built like the Reeds' and never would one be built like it again. Two stories high, with a sleeping loft, it was outfitted with spring seats just like the best stagecoaches, an iron stove, velvet curtains, and her cherished organ. It was stocked with six months' supply of the best food and wine money could buy. As the wagon pulled into formation with the rest of the Donner party to head west, it was difficult not to stare and gasp.

The tragic saga of the Donner party is the most indelible tale of triumph and despair ever written in the history of the American West. Twenty-five hundred miles away from home and only two days from safety, thirty-one men, women, and children were stranded for an entire winter in the Sierra Nevada mountains by a succession of the worst blizzards on record. Out of provisions and starving, some members resorted to cannibalism in order to survive. Margaret and her children were not among them. She kept them all alive on snow, bark, and leather broth until James, who had left the group to ride on ahead to California seeking a rescue party, returned. The fact that her family did not perish—physically or spiritually—had absolutely nothing to do with the worldly goods she had counted on, for the wagon and all it carried had to be abandoned along the way because it was too heavy and cumbersome to travel through the mountains. The possessions that saved Margaret and those she loved were of Spirit—her wits, her faith, and her courage.

While I've been on the *Simple Abundance* path, I've consulted a century's worth of decorating books and women's magazines, searching for simple pleasures to share. They all express the commonly held belief (at the time they were written) that possessions define a person. During the Victorian period, worldly goods were viewed as evidence of God's favor, and I think that attitude is still very much part of the American consciousness. Certainly, I believed it until I began the journey to authenticity. But as I meditated, ruminated, mulled over, and tried to write about how our possessions define us, the Spirit within balked. Reared up and refused to cooperate. Shut down so that I would shut up and stop perpetuating such nonsense. If a writer has a block, it's usually because she doesn't believe in what she's writing.

Here's what I believe. I believe our possessions can be very revealing, offering insights into our personalities in intimate and illuminating ways. I believe surrounding ourselves with objects that speak to our souls can bring us authentic moments of pleasure. *But I do not believe our possessions define us.*

Instead, I believe it's what you *love* that expresses the authentic woman you are, not what you own. When Jacqueline Kennedy Onassis died, much was written about her style and strength, her grace and beauty. If ever there was a woman who lived by her own lights it was Jackie. Yet here was a woman who could have had virtually anything she wanted in the world, and yet her most prized possession was her privacy, a gift you and I probably don't think about very much.

But what struck even a deeper chord in me was her son's recollection of what meant the most to her: "The love of words, the bonds of home and family, and her spirit of adventure." Her passions defined this extraordinary woman.

Today I wish for you, as I wish for myself, that when our authentic adventure comes to a close, we can also be remembered as being by Love possessed.

OCTOBER 28

The Spiral Path

I don't believe that life is linear. I think of it as circles—concentric circles that connect.

—Michelle Williams
American actress

I am often asked if I am now living authentically after following the *Simple Abundance* path for the last twenty-five years. Some moments, some hours, some days feel wholly right, completely authentic. And more frequently than not, I can attest that my conversations with family, friends, colleagues, acquaintances, and even strangers are authentic encounters. So are my choices, even the difficult ones, and my joys, my griefs, my hopes, my loves. But every minute of every day is not yet authentic. I think it takes an entire lifetime to live authentically. It is the *striving* to be authentic that makes you so, not the end result. When you think you've arrived, you realize you've come all this way just to prepare yourself to begin again.

The biggest surprise on the soulful journey to authenticity, whether as a philosophy or a spiritual path, is that the path is a spiral. We go up, but we go in circles. Each time around, the view gets a little bit wider. Somehow the circle has length and width to it. The psychologist Carl Jung believed that our spiritual experience of "the Self," which I call the Authentic Self, could only be truly realized by "circumambulating."

The ancients revered the power of the circle. In the African tradition, as well as in Disney movies, our earthly span is called "the circle of life." Black Elk, the leader of the Oglala Sioux, taught that "The power of the world always works in circles." Buddhist and Hindu pilgrims circle the base of Tibet's Mount Kailash as an act of worship. Muslims circle the Kaaba in Mecca. For thousands of years the creation of mandalas—circular geometric designs—has been part of both Eastern and Western spiritual traditions. Seekers create personal mandalas in order to invoke the sacred through the visual. Circles are found at sacred sites throughout the world. There is a circular maze at the base of Chartres Cathedral in France. The gigantic prehistoric sculptures at Stonehenge, England, form a circle. The communion host offered at Catholic mass is a round wafer. If we search for circles, we will find them everywhere. Plato believed the soul was a circle. If it is, and the Authentic Self is the Soul made visible, how could our awakening to authenticity be straight and not circular?

I am reminded of just how much of a spiral the authentic journey is when I get stuck in a set of circumstances from which escape seems impossible. When this occurs, I ask myself, "What's the lesson here, so that I can move on?" I usually discover that I've stopped using the *Simple Abundance* Graces as my stepping-stones to Wholeness. I've been too busy to write in my Gratitude Journal; I've begun dropping in my tracks because I've been unable to say no; I'm cranky because my house is cluttered and I can't find anything; I'm frazzled because I've let myself forget that moments of solitude and meditation are necessary to center myself. I've been down this route many times. I *know* that if I'm not experiencing Harmony in my daily round, I'm not participating in the process.

So I start again. Begin at the beginning. Make Gratitude an active rather than a passive prayer, consciously bring Simplicity and Order to my daily round, honor moments of *being* rather than of doing. It's not enough to know or write about *Simple Abundance*; it must be *lived* to realize its beauty and joy. When I do resume living by my own lights, I usually discover that I'm able to move on. But even if I can't change my outside circumstances, *Simple Abundance* enables me to change how I react to them.

"The life we want is not merely the one we have chosen and made," poet Wendell Berry tells us. "It is the one we must be choosing and making."

OCTOBER 29

A Bounty of Goodness

Autumn, season of earth's maturing... asks that we prepare for the future—that we be wise in the ways of garnering and letting go.
—Bonaro W. Overstreet (1902–1985)
American author, poet, and psychologist

As the daylight hours decrease and the air turns crisp, we're reminded that it will soon be too cool to take leisurely strolls through our ordinary

Edens. "Nature has been for me, for as long as I can remember, a source of solace, inspiration, adventure and delight: a home, a teacher, a companion," Lorraine Anderson writes in *Sisters of the Earth*. Finally, so it is for me, which is funny considering that I spent my teenage years trying to run away from a small rural New England town, then settled in a small English hamlet over a decade for love of a stone cottage, an apple tree, and the turning of the year. Now I live half a world away in a strange, different landscape in California and prepare to begin again.

As the year winds toward its end, the sixth *Simple Abundance* saving Grace called Joy joins her sisters—Gratitude, Simplicity, Order, Harmony, and Beauty. On the *Simple Abundance* path, we are urged to be willing to let go of struggle so we might learn some of our life lessons through Joy.

One of my joys is collecting out-of-print country journals, especially from the twenties through fifties, that track the seasons through observing Mother Nature's and Mother Plenty's journey through the year. Today when the natural rhythm of life has been completely obscured by technology (although people have been complaining about that since before the nineteenth century's Industrial Revolution), I was so blessed to have lived in the back of the beyond where work began when the sun rose and ended toward the end of the afternoon, bookended by a pot of tea and other women's thoughts on paper. There was no more comforting ritual than coming in the kitchen door at day's end, drawing the curtains, and turning on the soft, small lights to settle down before a "cheery" in the fireplace and a fragrant aroma of something wonderful baking in the Aga.

You quickly learn Heaven's laws when living close to the earth. "If the workings of cause and effect were everywhere as visible as in the world of seed and harvest, much human folly might reach a happy ending in wisdom," Bonaro Overstreet observed in a little book of comfort and joy for me, *Meditations for Women: For Every Day in the Year*, published in 1947. "A grocer, unlocking his store, exchanges a word with a passer-by, 'Feels like winter's coming and it's going to be a tough one for a lot of folks—all over the world.'" And this could have been written this morning. Nothing is new under the sun.

This time of the year is known in the old country books as the season of gleaning, gathering in, and letting go. I love the Old Testament's story of Ruth, a young widow living with her mother-in-law, Naomi, who was also a widow, which meant not just being poor, but destitute and homeless. But spiritual law instructed that any harvest that fell to the ground, as well as the four corners of each field, had to be left for the poor and hungry to "glean" or pick up. Ruth would follow the harvests to gather up the bounty of goodness left behind as she worked for them both. It's a wonderful meditation (Ruth 1 and 2).

The subject of gleaning was an especially fertile inspiration for Victorian artists coming after the land was abandoned and families moved to the city to find work, and it can be for us as well.

Gleaning is a blessing whether you visit a food bank, thrift shops, or hunt for berries in an English bramble. Now I glean in private moments of wistfulness through the golden fields of acceptance, grace, and gratitude. For it is up to us to distinguish between the bitter and the sweet among our memories as we glean, gather in, and let go. Weeping may endure for many seasons of our lives, but we can also ask to be surprised by joy.

OCTOBER 30

Do Try This at Home: Personal Safety

You are stronger than you believe. You have greater powers than you know.

—Antiope to Diana,
Wonder Woman (2017)

Did you see the movie version of *Wonder Woman*? While I was watching, it became a mythical heroine experience for me. Not just the marvelous Gal Gadot as Diana, but the lineage of her women ancestors, including her mother and aunt. I kept thinking, now that's how you raise a girl today.

Diana is an Amazonian princess, raised on an island of only women warriors. Her destiny is to leave her home and embark on a journey during World War I to save the world. No small feat there. I remember being transfixed by Wonder Woman's garb, including her weapons, which included her body, a shield, arm cuffs, her crown, and the Golden Lasso of Truth. Of all her weapons, it was her martial arts skill that impressed me the most. The fierceness of her ability to fight and defend herself while saving others resonated deeply for me.

Perhaps this movie made such an impression because I couldn't be more physically different from the Amazonian women if I tried, fictional though they may be. I couldn't have saved anyone, including myself. And that truthful acknowledgment was both sharp and galvanizing.

I've been wanting to increase my physical strength for several years to be able to resume my two favorite activities: horseback riding and fencing. However, while writing is not the most physically active endeavor, try to convince my exhausted brain and body after eight intense hours of work to "work out."

Still, even as I have been physically sidetracked for the last couple of years, the desire to become as strong as I can be has only increased. It always amazes me how the most profound positive choices and changes we can make in our lives start out as small as a mustard seed. All that's required for a plant to grow in the natural world or an idea to bloom in our inner world is for it to take root.

A related, but perhaps more difficult, topic to embrace emotionally is how to feel safe in our day-to-day lives. Wouldn't we all feel more comfortable if we exuded an invisible force field of confidence when we're out and about in the world? Think Wonder Woman.

Dr. Jocelyn Hollander, an academic expert from the University of Oregon, is an advocate for empowerment self-defense (ESD). Dr. Hollander believes that the "mindset in ESD may be more important than physical techniques." ESD teaches boundaries; how to create, preserve, and protect our boundaries is an essential skill we need to develop.

In an article for *The Economist*'s 1843 magazine called "Fight Club for Feminists," journalist Emma Goldberg describes a self-defense class she took from the founder of Feminist Self-Defense, Rachel Piazza. Piazza believes that "it is an intuitive skill-set." What is important to note here is there is a *difference* between traditional self-defense classes and empowerment self-defense. Women may experience less vulnerability in an all-female class; however, the effectiveness of defense techniques varies between genders, and shared experiences are often the catalysts for new communities.

As Emma points out in her article, "Even for the non-athletically inclined woman, a workshop in self-defense can do wonders for self-confidence. It gives you that surge of assurance you might otherwise get from a compliment, pep talk or a shot of tequila."

Personal Safety Gadgets

There may be some occasions where you will feel more comfortable walking to your car with a personal safety alarm on your key chain. So why don't we just get one now? Most models have an LED light to illuminate your steps and emit a loud, high-pitched sound on activation. Small step, big payoff. Never underestimate the power of the small.

If you have a home security system, like ADT, check and see if they have a panic button key fob. While this type of button would work great at home should an intruder visit, you may also want a Bluetooth device that works with GPS. Look for a police-approved personal safety key fob that connects with your cell phone app. If you have an older relative, a medical alert system that works both at home and away might deliver peace of mind wherever you are. There is a monthly service fee for some of these systems.

Video doorbells, like Ring, keep you connected with home. They have thwarted package thieves and unwanted solicitors through their video and audio communication system. There are a number of home security systems on the market, and if you are a fan of Google Home or Amazon's Alexa, look for systems that integrate with them to build a smart home safety grid.

Since we're talking about safety, here's an item I've gifted to friends and family. It is a car emergency escape tool. This inexpensive item will safely break a window or cut a seat belt should the need arise. Flash floods, pets in cars, and accidents make this a must-have for the First Responders in all of us.

Learning how to implement Mother Courage's curriculum into our daily round increases our capacity for becoming the women who keep calm as we carry on protecting those entrusted to our care. The safety poster at the Twitter office in New York City says it all: "In case of fire, exit the building before tweeting about it."

OCTOBER 31

Make Room for Mystery, Awaken to the Magic

To work magic is to weave the unseen forces into form; to soar beyond sight; to explore the uncharted dream realm of the hidden reality.

—Starhawk
American writer, teacher, and ecofeminism activist

At last the bewitching hour hath come upon us: All Hallow's Eve. Tonight, some of us will be accompanying little goblins on their appointed rounds; our love, care, and concern providing their protection during the dark of night. Many other women will be greeting high spirits at the front door with sweet bribes, choosing to treat rather than be tricked. Wise choice.

Halloween comes down to us from the pre-Christian Celtic festival of Samhain (pronounced *saw-wind*), held October 31, the last autumn night before the cold and bleakness of winter. On this night—considered the Celtic New Year—the Druids believed that the supernatural world drew closer to the physical world, so human beings were more susceptible to the power and influence of the unseen. Magic spells could be cast more easily, divination (predicting fortunes) was more revealing, and dreams held special significance.

Being Celtic, I still believe this. Being human, I believe Halloween is the perfect reminder that magic flows through us, mystery infuses every encounter of every day. We conjure up the shoe that cannot be found anywhere in the house, transform leftovers into a feast, coax bounty from barren earth, banish fear, heal hurts, make money stretch until the end of the month. We carry, cradle, nurture, and sustain life. We do all this and much more. But most women are not aware of their tremendous power for good. We are asleep to our Divinity. We've not consciously awakened to the realization that we are descendants of an ancient, sacred lineage: the She.

Isn't magic what you're performing when you're creating an authentic lifestyle for yourself and those you love? Aren't you shaping unseen forces with your creativity and soul-crafts, bringing into the physical world through passion what has only existed in the spiritual realm? If you can do this unconsciously, how much more could you accomplish if you were fully aware of your powers?

O blessed daughter of the She, much power has been gifted you. It is the power of Love. Tonight, by candlelight or by the light of the full moon in your backyard, commit to use your power wisely for the Highest Good of all. *You have no idea of the countless souls you will touch in the course of your lifetime.* Souls searching for Wholeness that could be healed with the magic at your command. Go directly to the Source. Acknowledge your lineage and your authentic gifts with a grateful heart.

"I am sure there is Magic in everything," Frances Hodgson Burnett observed, "only we have not sense enough to get hold of it and make it do things for us."

Now we do.

Joyful Simplicities for October

Mrs. Miniver suddenly understood why she was enjoying the forties so much better than she enjoyed the thirties; it was the difference between August and October, between the heaviness of late summer and the sparkle of early autumn, between the ending of an old phase and the beginning of a fresh one.

—Jan Struther
Mrs. Miniver

✍ Plan an outing to a pumpkin patch or farmers' market. Select the perfect jack-o'-lantern, but get an assortment of smaller pumpkins on which to carve different designs, like checkerboards, hearts, or the moon and stars. Pie pumpkins are the perfect size for creating luminarias for steps or driveways, and the midget pumpkins make charming votive candle holders for dinner tables.

- Save the seeds from your pumpkins and roast them with salt. If you feel experimental you can even add seasoning (sweet or savory) for an extra kick.

- Put your house in a festive mood with autumnal details: wheat sheaves, pumpkins, gourds, Indian corn, or bittersweet. Instead of fresh flowers mix it up with bouquets of dried flowers and preserved autumn leaves.

- Pumpkins make very attractive natural vases for autumn bouquets. Scoop out the center as you would for a lantern and fill with a damp oasis (the floral sponge) cut to size. Arrange jewel-tone flowers, preserved leaves, and vines in the oasis for a long-lasting arrangement. Occasionally test the oasis to see if you need to add more water.

- Halloween is traditionally the night for fortune-telling. A delicious and fun way to do this is with a fate cake. Make a spice cake and insert specially made silver charms into the batter after it is poured into the pan. When the cake is cut, the charms will reveal the future: the bell is a wedding; the thimble blesses the owner; the wishbone grants one wish; the coin promises prosperity; the horseshoe ensures good luck; and the button, domestic bliss. Remember how many charms you insert in your batter and count them afterward! A safe alternative for kids (under twelve) is a charm pull, where the charms are attached to ribbons and stuck into a ready-made cake. For a great selection, visit the website www.jewelrybyrhonda.com. I also use the charms for the Christmas plum pudding.

- Dress up for Halloween, or at least find yourself a wonderful mask to wear when opening the front door.

- This is the month to plant crocus, daffodils, and tulips outdoors for next spring's season of showing off.

- If you live in a four-season climate, take a Sunday drive in the country to revel in Mother Nature's flamboyant fancy dress. Pack a picnic. Linger as long as you can.

- Mull cider and/or wine on the weekends for an autumn cup of cheer, especially delightful after raking leaves! The best mulling spices I've ever found are the Williams-Sonoma brand, available from their shops and online.

NOVEMBER

She stands
In tattered gold
Tossing bits of amber
And jade, jewels of a year grown old:
November

—Zephyr Ware Tarver (1886–1974)
American poet

November loves the pilgrim soul in you. But with the holidays fast approaching, it's all too easy to grumble away the month's gifts of grace. Take heart! Family, feasting, and fussing might be en route, but November knows how to take care of you. So let her, with cold comfort charms, a winter's tale or two, sumptuous pajama suppers, splendor in the glass, and the stunning Ordinary in the simply overlooked. Let thy cup runneth over with sensuous self-preservation.

NOVEMBER 1

Embracing the Ebb

Everything in life that we really accept undergoes a change.
—Katherine Mansfield (1886–1974)
New Zealand short story writer

There once was a mighty queen with a short fuse. One autumn, as the year was beginning to ebb, the queen fell into a deep melancholy. She could neither eat nor slumber, and tears of an unknown origin fell frequently, which infuriated her, triggering angry fits that made those around her quake in fear.

Each day the queen summoned a new adviser from her esteemed circle of sages to explain the cause of her baffling condition. In they came and out they went: the court physician, the stargazer, the psychic, the alchemist, the herbalist, the philosopher. All were dismissed as charlatans for their inability to unravel the mystery of the royal black spell. They counted themselves lucky to have only their illustrious careers shortened.

"Surely there must be one among you who knows the source of my suffering," the queen cried in despair. But her pathetic wail was greeted only with awkward silence, for all were wary of her wrath. Finally, the royal gardener was moved by compassion for the poor woman and slowly approached her throne.

"Come into the garden, Majesty, beyond the walls of your self-imprisonment, and I will disclose your dilemma." The queen was so desperate, she did as she was bid. When she went out to the garden for the first time in many weeks, she noticed that the bright, vivid colors of summer had faded. But it was not, she saw, wholly bereft of beauty, for it was regal in autumn's brilliant hues of crimson and gold. The air was refreshingly cool and crisp, and the sky pure blue. "Speak, gardener," the queen ordered, "but choose your words carefully, for I seek the truth."

"Majesty, it is not your body or your mind that is ailing. It is your soul that needs healing. For while you are a mighty and powerful queen, you are not Divine. You are suffering from a human condition that afflicts us all. Earthly souls ebb and flow in sorrow and joy according to the seasons of emotion, just as the seasons of the natural world move through the cycle of life, death, and rebirth. These are the days to be grateful for the harvest of the heart, however humble it might be, and to prepare for the coming of the year's closure. Even now, the season of daylight diminishes, and the time of darkness increases. But the true Light is never extinguished in the natural world, and it is the same in your soul. Embrace the ebb, my beloved queen, and do not fear the darkness. For as night follows day, the Light will return, and you will know contented hours once again. Of this I am sure."

The unhappy queen considered this wisdom thoughtfully and asked the gardener how he possessed the secret knowledge of inner peace during the seasons of emotion. The gardener led her to a brass sundial. It read:

This, too, shall pass.

NOVEMBER 2

Caring for Your Soul

Let us imagine care of the soul, then, as an application of poetics to everyday life.
—Thomas Moore
American psychotherapist, former monk, and author

Soul. Created on the sixth day. After the cherubim and seraphim. After the dominions, virtues, powers, principalities, archangels, and angels. After Light was called forth from the void of darkness. After morning and evening were delineated. After space and time. After air, fire, water, earth. After the sun, moon, and stars were hung in the heavens. After the Universe began spinning. After its Power was switched on and its Energy was charged. After the music of the spheres began the celestial concerto. After the beasts ran upon the fields and birds soared. After the garden was in full bloom.

Only after *all* was made ready—and the Great Creator pronounced it very good—only then, was it the Beloved's moment. For the Beloved—to be known through all eternity as Soul—was sent into the world on Divine breath as Spirit laughed and cried. Soul was born in both joy and pain. Blown into a handful of dust. Divinity was to live and move and have its being in a creature made of mud.

There you have it. Go figure. Which is precisely what men and women have tried to do down through the ages. But even reason, intellect, imagination, passion, poetry, prayer, art, sex, song, and saxophone cannot unravel or fully reveal the mystical nature of our souls, let alone understand it.

Obviously, after twenty-five thousand years of trying, we're not meant to understand the essence of Soul. But we can come to know her. For we were created *for no other reason* than to love, nurture, nourish, sustain, protect, uplift, inspire, delight, charm, and comfort the beloved presence within each of us. Psychotherapist and spiritual writer Thomas Moore calls this profound attention to the authentic needs that stir deep within "caring for our souls."

Today is All Souls' Day, a solemn day set aside since the Middle Ages for remembrance of the beloveds who no longer laugh and cry with us on earth. But All Souls' Day is a beautiful occasion for contemplating how we care for our own souls, the degree of hospitality we extend to these guests in our daily round, and the quality of their visit so far. In order to approach "the depth that is the domain of the soul," Moore urges us to become "artists and theologians of our own lives."

It is through "the small details of everyday life" that we make our souls feel welcome. "Tending the things around us and becoming sensitive to the importance of home, daily schedule, and maybe even the clothes we wear are ways of caring for the soul," Moore tells us in his deeply moving meditation, *Care of the Soul: A Guide for Cultivating Depth and Sacredness in Everyday Life.*

Today, be willing to ask your guest what she requires to make her stay more pleasurable. Ask often: "What do you need at this moment? What would bring you peace, contentment, joy?" It may be to slow down, take a walk, hug a child, caress a cat. Go to the farmers' market. Call your sister. Send a funny GIF to a friend. Take a nap. Order Chinese delivery. Watch a favorite movie. Have a good cry. Find an old-fashioned diner and have a root beer float. Turn in early. Dream. Fantasize. Pray. Whatever it might be, she will tell you. Ask.

" 'Stay' is a charming word in a friend's vocabulary," Louisa May Alcott reminds us. Stay, my Beloved. Stay. Say it now. Say it often. Come live with me and be my love.

Stay.

NOVEMBER 3

For Thine Is the Kingdom, and the Power, and the Glory

When I look into the future, it's so bright it burns my eyes.
—Oprah Winfrey
American media executive, actress, talk show
host, producer, and philanthropist

Many years ago, I read a profile of Oprah Winfrey in *The New York Times* magazine. This was just when she was beginning what would become *The Oprah Winfrey Show* and she started her own production company, HARPO, to do it her way. Nobody in television was doing anything like it.

In the interview Oprah expressed her belief that the concept of God never giving us more than we can handle refers to much more than just the stoic bearing of pain and suffering. God's giving also includes the goodies—wealth, worldly success, power. If you think you're not strong enough to bear the Glory, rest assured, it *will* be withheld until you believe you can and ask for it.

Today, meditate on this possibility. I know I've been thinking about it for decades, and it's just beginning to register.

We know that Power is available to each of us, every moment of every day, but we must ask that the spiritual electricity switch be turned on. Next, we've got to be ready to bear the Glory. We prepare ourselves by gradually growing into our talents, one creative challenge at a time. With each accomplishment that is personally acknowledged and celebrated, our self-confidence increases, and we begin to trust our abilities. Furthermore, we realize we weren't intended to do this alone. That takes care of the Power and the Glory. Now what about the Kingdom?

Spiritual seekers are told to search for the Kingdom of Heaven before anything else. Could the Kingdom of Heaven be an authentic life? I believe so. Because once you find your authentic path and follow it, all the other puzzle pieces start to fall into place: the money, the job, the relationship.

Remember Joseph Campbell's intoxicating inspiration tells us to "follow our bliss" if we want life to be rich, deep, and meaningful. "Follow your bliss and doors will open. Follow your bliss, and you'll get on the track created especially for you at the beginning of time."

Could your bliss and an authentic life be one and the same? What if whatever it is that makes you ecstatic, brings you joy, sends you soaring, satisfies your hunger, fulfills your yearning, ignites your passion, makes you reach out to others, and gives you peace—in other words, your bliss—*is* also the Kingdom of Heaven?

Thy kingdom come, thy will be done, on earth
as it is in heaven...

"Your life is not static. Every decision, setback, or triumph is an opportunity to identify the seeds of truth that make you the wondrous human being that you are," Oprah tells us in her marvelous book *The Path Made Clear: Discovering Your Life's Direction and Purpose.* "When you pay attention to what feeds your energy, you move in the direction of the life for which you were intended. Trust that the Universe has a bigger, wider, deeper dream for you than you could ever imagine for yourself."

NOVEMBER 4

Return of the Goddess

And write about it, Goddess, and about it.
—Alexander Pope (1688–1744)
Eighteenth-century English poet

She's ba-aa-aack! The goddess has returned with another book to lead us from desire to fulfillment. Which one? Doesn't really matter! The goddesses of gracious living, entertaining, decorating, fitness, fashion, beauty, and relationships regularly appear this time of year, keeping in motion the cycle of worship and words. It used to be that goddesses performed miracles. Now they write books or blogs or posts on social media telling us how to perform our own. And the biggest bookselling season is now before the holidays, which is why you see so many new titles competing for your attention.

It was four o'clock on a cold November afternoon, and it was already dark. Disciples from all over the Washington area had left their jobs, homes, and families to await the Appearance, Signing, and Rapture at the ceremony of the book signing. The goddess would not arrive for another hour, but already the faithful number two hundred. The first in line have camped out here all day. My daughter, then twelve, and I have only been here for half an hour conducting field research on the contemporary goddess scene, but already there are two dozen women behind me.

Every now and then a bookstore employee comes out to remind the flock that the goddess is signing *only* her latest offering and *only* two books per customer. This particularly irks one woman who just minutes ago bought ten copies of the latest tome to give to family and friends as Christmas presents; no one ringing up the $250 sale told her she couldn't get eight of them signed. Now there is much grumbling about nerve, fame, wealth, business empires, and goddesses who forget who elevated them from divas to divinities. But we are resourceful. Not all of us have more than one book for signing; up and down the line her books are distributed, and the problem is solved. Women acting together are a force to be reckoned with.

Instead of loaves and fishes there will be canapés. Occasionally, Katie comes back to give my aisle the latest reconnaissance on the goddess's estimated time of arrival. Katie is starving; it never occurred to me to pack provisions. I snatch two cranberry tartlets the size of postage stamps from a passing tray, wrapping them in a tissue for safekeeping in my pocket until her next report.

After another hour, fearing that I won't get to the front before the great one must leave, I sneak behind the barricades up to the front. I haven't waited this long not to get at least a glimpse of the goddess in the flesh.

But I get much more than I imagined. For behind her is an altar: a gorgeous French country table of washed pine covered in checked homespun. Upon it are mountains of fruits, vegetables, loaves of bread, copper cooking utensils, and candles. In front of the altar, she sits in a tapestry chair behind a desk bearing an arrangement of exquisite flowers. Nearby, tokens of devotion from the disciples have created a shrine; individual bouquets of flowers and a large pile of presents, many of them wrapped in homemade wrapping paper, variations on a theme of potato stencils.

Frankly, I've seen more than enough. The goddess is as lovely as her images; the altar is beyond belief, except that I saw it with my own eyes. It gives me the shivers. I want to leave, but my sweet girl is horrified at the thought of going without getting our book signed. We stay.

By now, it's much too late to cook dinner, so we stop off for burgers and fries. A few minutes later, I'm fishing for my house keys and pull out the crushed tissue containing the cranberry tartlets. The house is dark, cold, and forlorn. No fire, no candlelight, no animation, no inviting aromas to welcome us. "A house is no home unless it contains food and fire for the mind as well as for the body," Margaret Fuller wrote in *Woman in the Nineteenth Century* in 1845. Alas, the crust is delicious, but the cranberry tartlet is not as filling as I imagined it would be.

NOVEMBER 5

The Goddess Within

Come, Vesta, to live in this Beautiful Home.
Come with warm feelings of friendship.
Bring your intelligence,
Your energy and your passion
To join with your Good Work.
Burn always in my Soul.
You are welcome here.
I remember you.

—Homeric hymn
(Translation by Frances Bernstein)

Ever since civilization began, women have turned to goddesses for intercession and inspiration. For Roman women, the most beloved goddess was Vesta. She, like her Greek counterpart, Hestia, was the goddess of the hearth. Vesta is the one who urges women to be quiet, to sit, to gaze, to listen, to prepare delicious meals, to bring beauty into our daily round, to live through our seven senses, to create a sacred haven of security and serenity set apart from the world in order to protect all we cherish. Vesta is the ancient goddess who calls on us to focus our creative energies on the real.

In her book on ancient women's spirituality, *Classical Living: A Month to Month Guide to Ancient Rituals for Heart and Home*, Frances Bernstein notes that the Latin word for *hearth* is *focus*. Focusing is the sacred art of Vesta. Focusing is also a crucial need today for women who spend much of their time rushing to fulfill the inexhaustible demands of family and work, or both. The faster we run, the more conflicted we become. As we get nowhere fast, we lose focus and clarity, existing in a perpetual state of confusion.

Have you ever noticed how many times during the day we'll speak of feeling "off," "out of it," or "off the wall"? These expressions are quite apt because they accurately describe a lack of centering within. When the center isn't holding, it's because we've lost touch with the tremendous healing power of our Vesta aspect. We have wandered far away from the sacred hearth and don't know how to find our way back to heat, light, and warmth.

In order to regain focus, women need to restore a sense of "at homeness" to their lives, which is what we are really attempting to do when we create domestic goddesses. We glorify women whose public personas cleverly exploit our private yearnings. It's far easier to live vicariously through their books, social media, magazines, blogs, and television shows than it is to nurture our own gifts. It is much more comfortable to create goddesses we worship than honor our own Divinity.

Don't misunderstand me. I love the goddesses. They are clever, savvy, and possess marvelous creative talents. They have much good to offer us; certainly. I've done my share to make them all wealthy women. I want an impeccably organized and joy-filled home just as much as you do. What parent wouldn't want to send their kids off to school with lunch works of art in bento sized boxes? But there is a significant difference between being an avid fan and a rabid follower. You don't have to belong to a cult to become brainwashed.

When admiration leads to adoration, we unconsciously create graven images that diminish rather than enrich our lives. We deny our own authenticity. Disown our passion. Siphon off our own power by endowing women who clearly have enough with our portion. Is this what "the rich get richer and the poor get poorer" really means? Being poor in self-confidence and creative energy keeps us in lack much more than a lean purse.

By worshipping false goddesses, we make another woman the Creatrix, instead of honoring the Creatrix within. If you're really seeking an authentic goddess, you know where to find her.

Rising to the Occasion

*To be really great in little things, to be truly noble and heroic in the
insipid details of everyday life, is a virtue so rare as to be worthy of
canonization.*

—Harriet Beecher Stowe (1811–1896)
American abolitionist and author

In real life, serenity depends on coping and coping well. Rising to the
occasion.

Consider the following scenarios. You have a flat tire on the way
to an important business meeting. You find yourself locked out of the
house. You discover that your spouse's college roommate is coming for
dinner in two hours. The pipes freeze. The roof leaks. The dog swallows
an earring. Someone's sick or snowed in. You're asked to lend money,
switch car pool trips, show up for jury duty. One minute you're called
out of town, the next you're taking someone to urgent care.

Real life is the collision—day in, day out—of the improbable with
the impossible. Henry Wadsworth Longfellow believed that situations
that call forth our coping abilities are "celestial benedictions" in dark
disguises, sent not to try our souls but to enlarge them. Just as dough
rises in a bowl, expanding before it becomes bread, we become larger
than we ever thought possible when we rise to occasions, performing
miracles with good humor and grace. Coping well enables you to see
beyond the circumference of circumstance, so that the real in the center
of your daily round is not hidden by happenstance.

Most women are geniuses at rising to the occasion. But we've never
realized how extraordinary this talent really is, because it's second
nature by now. We've never given credit where credit is due, because
we've never given coping much thought. But if women who cope well
ran everything, Nirvana wouldn't only be the name of a Seattle band.

We become more adept at rising to the occasion each time we see
ourselves doing it. Every time we cope well with whatever real life
throws our way, it's another deposit of confidence, creativity, and courage in our self-esteem account. So congratulate yourself each night for
handling the unexpected with finesse. Well done.

Today, when you need to rise to the occasion, do it with style. Do it
with a knowing smile. Confound them. Astound yourself. Make it look
easy, and it will become so.

How to Start Over

*She saw now that the strong impulses that had once wrecked her
happiness were the forces that had enabled her to rebuild her life
out of the ruins.*

—Ellen Glasgow (1873–1945)
American Pulitzer Prize–winning novelist

The day that I finally put my beloved English home on the market, my
first copy of *The Hollywood Reporter* arrived in the post.

I took it as a sign: my brand-new, big adventure as a screenwriter in
sun-drenched California was about to begin. Finally, I was letting go of
my dream of English rural life, which had begun with so much promise
and excitement. But to my great astonishment and dismay, the life I had
created in England was not willing to let me transition to my new life as
easily as I'd hoped.

So let's get right to it. Who or what did you want to be or become
when you grew up? After trying to be her for the last ten or twenty years,
do you feel you just don't have the energy anymore? That's because you
were forcing yourself into a role everyone thought you'd be perfect at,
except you. We've all done it.

Have you wandered through Shepheard's Hotel yet? When you close
your eyes to imagine a different way of living, what does your dream
day look like? Or do you find your thoughts are still pulled into a thousand different directions? Can you conjure up happy images? This isn't
a trick question, because I've had a bit of difficulty with this dream-
scape, and I want you to know there's a good reason. Sometimes on our
way out of the past, for all the progress we think we've made, suddenly
we feel as if we've been sucked back, perpetually detoured in the "waiting place" by the centrifugal force of circumstances that short-circuits
our ability to cope, not to mention dream.

Perhaps you find yourself in the "waiting place" as well. For a house
to sell, for a new job, to decide about where you'll live or how you'll
occupy all the time that's been freed up by a pink slip or early retirement
(which would be any time before ninety).

On the sly, washing the dishes, when you think no one's watching,
perhaps you wander as I do, like a ghost that doesn't know she needs
to head toward the Light. You find yourself somewhere in your past
wandering through the mud room to a walled kitchen garden, out to
the stables, and there you are in your riding habit again, meandering
through the green meadows where the baby lambs are gamboling. Or
maybe you're at the wheel of a shiny red vintage convertible, top down,

vintage flea market finds tied in the back seat. Or are you in a pretty cardigan twin set and pearls, gazing out the library windows down to the sea when a lavish tray is brought in and set before the fire? And now it's time for tea.

Brought back with a bump to the here and now when the dishes are finished, your imaginary travelogue is done for the night. However, you do realize that if you continue to use your time, creative energy, and emotion to revisit faded tea-stained floral dreams, fanning the embers of what was and can't be again, you just might not be sparked to envision your own red carpet of possibilities.

They say that when you hear your name called at the Academy Awards, time stops and you're suddenly floating in slow motion. I adore slow motion, because usually we're all running pell-mell over the minuscule. Still, I'm now at a stage in my life where I'd better get a move on. There's an urgency building beneath my skin, waiting to burst through. I know that if I don't seriously start writing that secret screenplay I've been "researching" for years, somebody else is going to float toward the stage and claim my Oscar.

Why don't we limber up with a little creative brainstorming about the things you dream about doing? You now know that my private dream is screenwriting. What's yours?

You've always loved the notion of spiritual gardening. You even created a labyrinth in your backyard. It's so beautiful, and I know about a thousand women who would love to have one as well, starting with me. Wouldn't it be marvelous if women could create their own sacred circular path with flowers and plants for a restorative and inspirational time out, using a gardening design stencil?

Is knitting your passion? Julia Roberts and Ryan Gosling love it, too. You've mastered the particular stiches of Aran fisherman sweaters and everyone who knows and loves you has one. But what if you rendered these sublime designs in another medium, say, in plaster of paris decorative molds or woodworking? Feeling those goose-bump shivers of possibility?

You might dream of opening a baby shop featuring adorable smocked frocks and rompers created by local seamstresses. You've always loved to bake and your cheesecakes are sublime; everyone tells you it's time you sold them. But where and how? What you'd really like is to go on an international cooking school jaunt—six weeks in Paris, a month in Tuscany, and then the twelve-week "Forgotten Cooking Skills" certificate at Ballymaloe Cookery School in Ireland. Where there's a passion, there can be a plan.

You'd love to grow medicinal herbs and create organic remedies from that "Herb Simple" scrapbook you bought decades ago at London's Portobello Road antique market. You carried it through five countries to get it home, because it meant more to you than having an extra change of clothes. It spoke to you then about mystical plants, sacred trees, and nature's alchemy, and it speaks to you now, but you still can't make out what grabbed you in its message. Now you have the time to figure it out, but even more importantly, there's an urgency to your quest. I'll do my best to help you honor this. It sounds like a soul-directed urge.

When creative brainstorming, think of your ideas as popcorn kernels popping open one at a time. That's what ideas do. We're getting deeply up close and personal in pursuing your riveting story of self-discovery.

Loving the idea of finally doing something different with your life, accomplishing some long-held desire, something that is simultaneously thrilling and terrifying, is why we're still alive. It's the reason you can still feel a pulse. It's why we're meeting on the page. But holding a finished screenplay, book, painting, play, photograph, sculpture, or libretto, debuting a stand-up routine, or launching a new website and wishing that you could are *not* the same thing. I love Eleanor Roosevelt's wry observation that "It takes as much time to wish as it does to plan."

Let's hold that thought today.

In between the dreaming and its coming true are sweat equity and magnificent obsession: the tunnel focus that keeps you glued to your seat or at the barre when your back hurts, the words won't come, or the design is faulty. You need to tap into the determination of a hungry bloodhound with a steak bone; the persistence and perseverance that has you studying when the rest of the world slumbers; the true grit of grace and faith greater than yourself.

Faith might very well be "the substance of things hoped for, the evidence of things not seen," but faith without work isn't just dead, it's fantasizing. And it will break your heart, not to mention the hearts of incalculable others who could be healed through your work. Most of all, it will break the heart of the Great Creator, the One who first entrusted the assignment to you.

There are spiritual laws at work in the Universe, and once you know how the cosmos operates, you can't play dumb. I know that the Great Creator does not play favorites; that each of us came into being to carry on the re-creation of the world through our gifts. But what matters is the Work. When you feel a dream hovering over your head just waiting to be pulled down onto the paper, canvas, new web page, or the stage, keep calm and type on.

Even though I know better, I seem to have been waiting for something outside my personal velocity to trigger forward movement toward my goal. I have forgotten the truth of Sir Isaac Newton's laws that a body at rest stays at rest. And a body in motion will stay in motion.

It doesn't matter how slight that motion is, just keep at it and it will get you there. For where we've been is a place we never expected to be, stuck in a life we don't recognize. In a life stage we've never encountered before. At a loss, at a standstill, stumped.

Good gracious—could it possibly have been for this long? Astonishingly, yes, and yet it feels, sometimes, as if it just happened last week. Whatever your "It" is, starting your life over after it's stalled requires grace, grit, and guts. So what do you say to meeting back here tomorrow and making another move, taking another step toward the future? Passion becomes you.

NOVEMBER 8

Everyday Life Is the Prayer

More things are wrought by prayer than this world dreams of.
—Alfred, Lord Tennyson (1809–1892)
British and Irish Poet Laureate

Some women know they pray. Other women think they don't because they aren't down on their knees morning and night. But they're up in the dark with sick children, visiting an elderly parent on their lunch hour, supporting the dreams of those they love with their work, helping a friend bear grief or rejoice, nourishing bodies and souls. This, too, is prayer.

For whether we realize it or not, with every breath, with every heartbeat, women pray. We pray with desire, longing, hunger, thirst, sighs, remorse, regret. We pray with disappointment, discouragement, despair, disbelief. We pray with anger, rage, jealousy, envy. We pray with pleasure, contentment, happiness, exultation, joy. We pray with gratefulness, acknowledgment, appreciation, acceptance, relief. We pray when we comfort, cheer, console. We pray when we laugh. We pray when we cry. We pray when we work and play. We pray when we make love or make a meal. We pray when we create and admire creation. One way or another, we pray. Everyday life *is* the prayer. How we conduct it, celebrate it, consecrate it. It's just that some prayers are better than others. Conscious prayers are the best.

In its purest form, prayer is conversation. Communion. Connection. Intimacy. Prayer is the dialect of Divinity. Prayer is the Authentic Conversation because you don't have to hold back; you can say whatever needs to be said, exactly the way you want to express it, when you want to express it. You won't be judged. You won't risk losing love; instead, by praying you will increase your awareness of it. You won't have to phrase your words carefully lest there be misunderstandings, because you can't be misunderstood. Even if you don't know what you want or need, Spirit knows what you're about to say, ask, beg, scream, or praise before you utter a syllable.

Then why do we need to lift up our voice in prayer?

Because it's not good for women to be silent. We need to get real life off our chests, get whatever's bedeviling us out into the open, so that we can get on with it. We can't do that when we're stuck, and women do get stuck, in a kind of self-destructive holding pattern, when they're silent. "Every person's life is lived as a series of conversations," Deborah Tannen, a professor of linguistics, tells us. Women pray because we need to talk to Someone who's really listening.

NOVEMBER 9

The Sacrament of the Present Moment

There is nothing so secular that it cannot be sacred, and that is one of the deepest messages of the Incarnation.
—Madeleine L'Engle (1918–2007)
American prize-winning novelist for young
adults and spiritual memoirist

If everyday life is our prayer, the moments we offer up to create an authentic life are our sacraments. *The Book of Common Prayer* defines a sacrament as "an outward and visible sign of an inward and spiritual grace." The outward and visible way in which we move through our daily round—the time, creative energy, emotion, attitude, and attention with which we endow our tasks—is how we elevate the mundane to the transcendent. Moments of illumination aren't just experienced by saints, mystics, and poets.

There are seven traditional Christian sacraments: baptism, penance, eucharist, confirmation, marriage, ordination, and healing the sick. But we don't have to think of the sacraments only in religious terms, as Matthew Fox notes, for "the Sacred is everywhere."

When we welcome the new day, we baptize it with our gratitude and enthusiasm; when we reconcile with another or ourselves and make amends, we experience penance. Confirmation bestows wisdom. Marriage is the sacrament of relationships. Eucharist is the sacrament of nourishment. Holy orders or ordination is the sacrament of authority, and healing the sick is the sacrament of Wholeness. It *does* matter how we braid her hair, pack his lunch, send them on their way, greet their return, make suggestions, change the contract, analyze the data, lead the group, return the telephone call, pass the pasta, pour the wine, listen to a friend, lift a burden, share a secret, visit him in a nursing home, check for monsters under the bed.

"For the wonderful thing about saints is that they were *human*," Phyllis McGinley reassures us in *Saint-Watching*. "They lost their tempers, got hungry, scolded God, were egotistical, or testy or impatient in their turns, made mistakes and regretted them. Still they went on doggedly blundering toward heaven."

NOVEMBER 10

The Gaps

Where so many hours have been spent in convincing myself that I am right, is there not some reason to fear I may be wrong?
—Jane Austen (1775–1817)
English novelist

It's difficult for me to write about faith without also writing about doubt.

I'd love to write a meditation on the comfort of absolute faith, the faith of Abraham walking in the desert with his beautiful little boy, Isaac, on their way to make a burnt offering to God. They have the fire; they have the wood. "But where is the lamb?" Isaac asks his father. "God will provide the lamb for the burnt offering," Abraham tells the son he prayed seven decades for. Of course, this being a story about absolute faith, God does provide. After an altar is built, the wood is arranged, the child is bound, and the knife is unsheathed, an angel intervenes. God provides. Faith breaks a heart in order to make it whole. But I can't write about the comfort of an absolute faith like Abraham's because you'd never have found me walking in the desert with fire, wood, my child, and no lamb.

For Abraham, there were no gaping black holes of doubt. Or were there? Not even as he held the knife aloft? Once, a friend told me of a conversation she'd had with another mutual friend on God, faith, and doubt. In passing, she mentioned that they both wished that they possessed my faith. I have no recollection of the rest of the conversation. I do recall, however, my need to hang up the phone, shocked that anyone should believe my fragile faith worth emulating.

Annie Dillard tells us that the Old Testament prophet Ezekiel was wary of those who hadn't floundered in the gaps before finding their way back across deserts of the heart. "The gaps are the thing," she points out. "The gaps are the spirit's one home, the altitudes and latitudes so dazzlingly spare and clean that the spirit can discover itself for the first time like a once-blind man unbound." I hope to God she's right.

For perhaps the gaps are what make faith possible, especially when the pain is unbearable. If there were no doubt, why would we need faith? Perhaps the doubts must be acknowledged, accepted, embraced, and pushed past before our faith is strong enough, not just to talk about, but to sustain.

It's okay if you hold your breath when you leap. Just don't look down.

"Faith is not *being sure*. It is *not being sure*, but betting with your last cent," Mary Jean Irion reassures us in *Yes, World*. "Faith is not making religious-sounding noises in the daytime. It is asking your inmost self questions at night—and then getting up and going to work."

NOVEMBER 11

Amazing Grace

Grace fills empty spaces, but it can only enter where there is a void to receive it, and it is grace itself which makes this void.
—Simone Weil (1909–1943)
French philosopher and mystic

Grace is direct Divine intervention on our behalf that circumvents the laws of nature—time, space, cause and effect, the availability of parking—for our Highest Good. Theologians tell us that grace is an unmerited demonstration of God's love, proof that we're not in this alone.

Considering that most of us operate under the assumption that daily life is a battleground, it's no wonder we're amazed when out of the blue, the Force suddenly seems to be with us. Grace is the Force—a spiritual energy field that protects and assists. Grace is Spirit's test flight; we seem to glide through the moment, the encounter, the day, without friction. We experience Real Life.

We access Grace like every other spiritual tool, by asking for it specifically and regularly. Every morning gratefully and expectantly ask for one day's portion of Grace. The kids eat their breakfast, get dressed without fuss, and are out the door on time. The bus driver waits for you. The day unfolds in blissful uneventfulness. Someone says: you look great, something seems different, what have you been doing? You realize you're smiling at four o'clock in the afternoon. You think, maybe there's something to this. The next day you ask for Grace. Eventually you get to the point where asking for Grace is as natural and as necessary as breathing.

NOVEMBER 12

Answered Prayers

God answers sharp and sudden on some prayers,
And thrusts the thing we have prayed for in our face,
A gauntlet with a gift in "it."
— Elizabeth Barrett Browning (1806–1861)
Victorian English poet

Oscar Wilde believed that there were only two tragedies in life: not getting what you pray for and getting it.

"Answered prayers are scary," Julia Cameron admits in *The Artist's Way*. "They imply responsibility. You asked for it. Now that you've got it, what are you going to do? Why else the cautionary phrase 'Watch out for what you pray for; you just might get it'? Answered prayers deliver us back to our own hand. This is not comfortable."

Very often the reason we're uncomfortable is because we've not been praying for the right thing, and on some deep level we know it. We pray to meet our soul mate, instead of praying for the grace to become the woman our soul mate would be attracted to; we pray for worldly success when what we really long for is a sense of authentic accomplishment; we pray for more money, when what we need is a change in our relationship to money. We pray for a certain outcome in any given situation, when what we should be praying for is peace of mind, no matter which outcome occurs.

Actually, our prayers are always being answered. We just don't like to think that "No" is a reasonable response to our very reasonable requests. Writer Madeleine L'Engle admits in *The Irrational Season*, surely speaking for us all: "We don't like Noes; and sometimes we like the Noes of God less than any other No."

The Noes of Spirit are more of a Holy Mystery than the Yeses; more meaningful to meditate upon, after the tears, the fury, and the cursing subside. The Noes of God don't make sense to our conscious, rational mind, especially since we're convinced we know what's best. But do we? Really?

We want the Yes, but sometimes we need the No. Consider the disaster that would ensue if we answered a child's every request with a Yes. That's too frightening even to contemplate. But we're children of Divinity. We can't begin to envision the big picture; nor do we weigh our requests against the prayers of others. Spirit hears both the hopeful entreaties for a sunny family reunion picnic and the farmer's plea for rain.

You would be astounded at the relief that comes once you stop assuming you have *all* the answers.

When your prayers seem delayed or denied, you need to ask Spirit if you're praying for the right thing. If you're not, ask that the right prayer might be revealed to you. Very often when we're told No, it's really, "No, not yet," to allow us more time, space, wisdom, and experience to prepare for the glorious moment when, because you're finally ready, willing, and able, Spirit answers you with a sharp, sudden, and resounding "Yes!"

NOVEMBER 13

Miracles

There are only two ways to live your life. One is as though nothing is a miracle. The other is as though everything is a miracle.
—Albert Einstein (1879–1955)
German Nobel Prize–winning theoretical physicist

We think of a miracle, such as a sudden physical healing, as an event. Actually, the real miracle is not the event, but how we perceive the event in our lives. Ask yourself which is the *real* miracle: when the check finally arrives, the deadline is extended, the lawsuit is settled, the exception is made? Or when you cope, serene and smiling, in the face of unbearable circumstances, triumphantly blowing everybody's mind— including your own—with your poise and courage?

Marianne Williamson describes a miracle as "a parting of the mists, a shift in perception, a return to love." The sacred continuum of Love is what makes miracles possible: Spirit's love for us, our love for each other, our love for Spirit. In her book *A Return to Love: Reflections on the Principles of a Course in Miracles*, she tells us that once miracles were all we knew, because we existed in Love. Then we woke up on earth and "were taught thoughts like competition, struggle, sickness, finite resources, limitation, guilt, bad, death, scarcity, and loss. We began to think these things, and so we began to know them." Love was replaced by fear.

When we exist in fear—which for many of us is real life—miracles become the exception, not the daily round. But it doesn't have to stay that way. What we need to do is find our way back home, back to our Authentic Self.

There are many paths to Wholeness. The one Marianne Williamson began taking in 1977 was *A Course in Miracles*, which she explains is a "self-study program of spiritual psychotherapy" based on universal spiritual truths transcribed by a Jewish psychologist in mystical dictation sessions during the mid-1960s. Through a daily meditation and workbook exercise, seekers learn to surrender all the ego's preconceptions— what we want, need, and think will make us happy—exchanging it only for the practical daily application of Love in our lives. "Whether our psychic pain is in the area of relationships, health, career, or elsewhere, love is a potent force, the cure, the Answer," she reassures us.

The introduction to *A Course in Miracles* states that the crux of the three-volume, 1,188-page course is very simple:

Nothing real can be threatened.
Nothing unreal exists.
Herein lies the peace of God.

In becoming aware of this, we experience the miracle of Real Life. "In asking for miracles, we are seeking a practical goal," Marianne Williamson reminds us, "a return to inner peace. We're not asking for something outside us to change, but for something inside us to change."

NOVEMBER 14

Heaven Watching Over

I was talking to angels long before they got fashionable…So maybe you don't believe in angels, that's all right, they don't care. They're not like Tinkerbell, you know, they don't depend on your faith to exist. A lot of people didn't believe the earth was round either, but that didn't make it any flatter.

—Nancy Pickard
American crime novelist

Do you remember the comfort and joy of an imaginary playmate when you were a child? Just because the rest of the world couldn't see your constant companion didn't mean he or she wasn't real. What's more, your reassuring companion spirit is still an immediate presence in your daily round—guarding, protecting, guiding, inspiring, and loving you—even if it's been a long time since you made mud pies together in the backyard.

Angels are our proof of Spirit's love for us, continuous reminders that we're not alone. Many people have had an experience of being pulled back from danger by an invisible force, when we're on the sidewalk about to cross the street. At that moment we felt that Heaven was truly watching over us. And we were right. Recently there was a story about a young child who was lost in a wooded area for two days in inclement weather. When he was rescued unharmed, he told his parents that a nice bear took care of him. His parents were told there were no bears in their geographical area. Sounds like an angel visitation to me.

While over two-thirds of us believe in the existence of angels, and every major faith in the world since antiquity acknowledges the angelic realms—Christianity, Roman Catholicism, Eastern Orthodoxy, Judaism, Islam, and Baha'i faith—not everyone is ready for an intimate earthly relationship with a Heavenly superior being.

Throughout my life I've enjoyed an intimate relationship with my guardian angel, whom I call Annie. As I committed to my spiritual growth, I consciously sought a mystical friendship, and it has brought me great joy, comfort, security, and peace. Much as I'd like to, I've never seen her. Angels cannot be conjured up on demand; they're not genies in magic lamps. However, we can call on these constant companions to guide, help, and inspire us.

"Our angels know us more intimately than our parents or our spouses. They care passionately about our well-being, and about our physical health, too," Eileen Elias Freeman tells us. "They know what we do, what we pray, what we see and say. They watch over the life and death of every single cell, and they love us, because they are beings who come from God, and God is love."

Although there are more books on angels today than ever danced on the head of a pin, Freeman's books *Touched by Angels* and *Angelic Healing* are my favorites. She argues convincingly that deep and abiding angelic encounters are only possible when we become aware that the special relationship we really seek is with Spirit.

As with every spiritual gift, we must ask our angels to help us. We must ask Spirit to deepen our relationship with our Heavenly guardians, offering thanks that the lines of celestial communication are continuously open.

NOVEMBER 15

The Tao of Success

Nothing in the world can take the place of Persistence.
Talent will not; nothing is more commonplace than unsuccessful men with talent.
Genius will not; unrewarded genius is almost a proverb.
Education alone will not; the world is full of educated derelicts.
Persistence and Determination alone are omnipotent.
—Calvin Coolidge (1872–1933)
Thirtieth president of the United States

This is the Tao of success—the Way—and like every other truth, it's at once very simple and very difficult. Not the understanding as much as the doing, because the Tao of success is patience and persistence.

Patience is the art of waiting. Like all high arts, it takes time to master, which shouldn't be surprising, since patience is the knowledge of time and cycles. How to use time to your advantage, how to be at the right place at the right time, how to pick your moments, how to bite your tongue. Patience is discovering the mysterious pattern of cycles that cradle the Universe and ensure that everything that has happened once will recur because few of us learn the lessons first time around.

Perseverance in life is being steadfast; persistence is being stubborn. Persistence is grittier than perseverance. Perseverance is achievement's perspiration; persistence is its sweat. Persistence is knocking on Heaven's doors so often and so loudly on behalf of your dreams that your knuckles are bloody and eventually you'll be given what you want, just to shut you up.

For example, think of an eleven-year-old child who wants to get her ears pierced sooner than her fourteenth birthday, the age her old-fashioned mother thinks is appropriate. The first request, even if it comes in a burst of emotion, doesn't succeed. Nor does the second, the third, or even the fourth. But the child who goes at you, morning, afternoon, and night, week after week, month after month; this child's voice is water to the rock of your reason. This stubborn and persisting child wears you down, which is why on her twelfth birthday, you end up shaking your head as you pay to adorn her earlobes with tiny gold balls.

The potent alchemy of patience and persistence, which together become endurance, must have been what the Lebanese poet Hoda al-Namai was meditating on when she wrote:

I have not withdrawn into despair,
I did not go mad in gathering honey,
I did not go mad,
I did not go mad,
I did not go mad.

If you are determined to gather life's honey, to stick your hand into the hive again and again and again, to be stung so many times that you become numb to the pain, to persevere and persist until those who know and love you can no longer think of you as *a fairly normal woman*, you will not be called mad.

You will be called authentic.

Affinities

*Oh, it's delightful to have ambitions.... And there never seems to
be any end to them—that's the best of it. Just as soon as you attain
one ambition you see another one glittering higher up still.
It does make life so interesting.*

—Anne Shirley
Anne of Green Gables by Lucy Maud
Montgomery

Ambition is achievement's soul mate. Action is the matchmaker that
brings these affinities together so that sparks can begin to fly, and we
can set the world on fire.

We think highly of achievement. He's a fine fellow—honorable,
desirable, the perfect gentleman. But ambition is considered more of a
tramp than a lady, a vixen rather than a virtue. If her passion and power
aren't creatively and constructively channeled, she could turn on the
one who invoked her presence. Just as electricity can be life enhancing
or destructive, so can ambition. What ambition really needs is a new
press agent. The only time we ever hear about her is when she's blamed
for somebody's downfall.

But ambition only becomes dangerous when, blinded by her charms,
we become easy marks for greed. When the soul is impoverished, the
ego is easily seduced. Greed is a very effective pimp for the dark side.

It's no wonder that many women flee from authenticity. It's too dangerous to admit, even to ourselves, that we possess not only aspirations
but ambitions.

What if ambition is a gift of Spirit? What if ambition is part of the
authentic package, generously bestowed on us all when we were given
our personal gifts? If sex can be both sacred and profane, if power
blesses as well as destroys, why should the nature of ambition be any
different?

What if we are *supposed* to be ambitious? What if our refusal to
channel our ambitions for our highest good, the highest good of those
we love and the rest of the world, is the real corruption of power? Think
of all that could be accomplished if women cherished their ambitions
and brought them into the Light where they belong. Think of how our
lives could be transformed if we respected ambition and gave grateful
thanks for being entrusted with such a miraculous gift.

One thing is certain. We cannot achieve without ambition. Action—
ambition in motion—is what produces achievement. "All serious daring starts from within," Eudora Welty, the Southern writer, reminds

us. Today the most serious daring you might engage in is an unusual creative brainstorming session. Invite ambition to sit down with your Authentic Self. Tell her what you'd like to achieve. Listen to her suggestions. Then take a closer look. Those horns you think you see might be a slightly off-center halo.

NOVEMBER 17

Only the Heart Knows

Only the heart knows how to find what is precious.
—Fyodor Dostoyevsky (1821–1881)
Russian novelist and philosopher

When Anna Quindlen, the Pulitzer Prize–winning columnist for *The New York Times*, stepped off journalism's fast track to devote her time, emotion, and creative energy to writing novels and raising her three children full-time, her peers were aghast, and her female readers were astonished. Half her readers—women who had decided to put family before career—applauded her choice. The other half—women who were trying desperately to raise happy kids and work full-time—felt betrayed. Anna Quindlen was not just Supermom, but the archetype for women who wanted to have it all. Her personal decision resurrected the old debate between mothers with careers versus mothers who work at home. If she couldn't take the juggling any longer, what hope was there for the rest of us?

But Anna Quindlen's creative choice wasn't about career versus family. It was about worldly success versus authentic success. She dreamed of writing novels instead of newspaper columns. She wanted to be there when her children came home from school. She wanted to live by her own lights. She wanted to listen to her heart. And she had the financial means to do so.

Only the heart knows what's working in our lives. The heart is our authentic compass. If we consult her, the heart can tell us if we're headed in the right direction. But the heart also tells us when we've made a wrong turn or when it's time for a U-turn. For a lot of us, this is information we don't want to know. Knowing might mean choice, and choice often means change.

I don't doubt that there are ten million women who would love to make the choice that Anna Quindlen did, but they're not in the financial position to do so. But just because you can't do it today or tomorrow doesn't mean you can't ever do it. Dreams deferred come true every day. Delay doesn't mean denial.

The heart does not charge for consultations, conversations, creative brainstorming sessions, or carrying a dream from conception to delivery, no matter how long it takes. "Dreams pass into the reality of action," Anaïs Nin reassures us. "From the action stems the dream again; and this interdependence produces the highest form of living."

NOVEMBER 18

A Time for Everything

There is a time for everything,
And a season for every activity under heaven.

—Ecclesiastes 3:1

Yes, but they are not the same time.

You cannot raise happy, secure, emotionally well-adjusted children, revel in a fabulous marriage, and work a sixty-hour week.

You want to, I know. So did I. But we can't. It is physically, emotionally, psychologically, and spiritually impossible. We have tried. We have failed.

We cannot circumvent the laws of Heaven and Earth just because it would be convenient. Just because it would fit nicely into our plans. We have tried. We have failed.

When we cannot do it all at the same time, we are meant to do only some of it. In order to find out what that "some" is to be, we need to ask: What is it I truly want right now? What is it I truly need? How do I get it? How much does it cost in life's currency?

This might be the season for you to wipe a runny nose. That doesn't mean the season of running your own business won't occur. This might be the season of living out of a suitcase. That doesn't mean the season of restoring a colonial farmhouse will never come. Making deals doesn't mean that someday you won't be making school lunches. The seasons of life are not meant to be frenetic, just full.

"You probably can have it all," Anna Quindlen muses. "Just not all at the same time. And...you might have to make certain compromises when your children are small. But your children are going to be small for a very short period of time...it will go by in a blink of an eye, and you will only be 40, 50, or 60 with another 15 or 25 years ahead of you." A quarter of a century to do what you want to do, the way you want to do it.

Blessed is the woman who knows her own limits.

NOVEMBER 19

The Enemy Within

We have met the enemy and he is us.
—Pogo
America cartoon character by Walt Kelly

It's hard to accept that you can be your own worst enemy. In fact, this realization is so painful that we go to great lengths to prove otherwise. It's always fate, circumstances, or lousy luck that messes up our best-laid plans.

When all you encounter is disappointment after disappointment as you pursue your dreams, it's natural to start feeling sorry for yourself. But if you constantly think the chips are stacked against you or that the cards are marked, pray today for the courage to check out the dealer at your game of chance. Does she seem a bit familiar? She should, because she's your Authentic Self's evil twin: the ego.

The ego has everything to lose once your Authentic Self grows strong enough to act consciously on your behalf, guiding your creative choices, decisions, ambitions, and actions for your Highest Good. What was standard operating procedure before—denial, sublimation, repression—is recognized for what it is: subtle self-abuse. When you become authentic, you become greater than you ever thought you could be, and this greatness allows you to heal yourself, your family, and your world.

Your Authentic Self is your ego's worst nightmare, and the ego will do everything in its power to eliminate her rival's influence from your daily round. The ego's heavy guns: fear and intimidation.

Fear has derailed more dreams than we can ever know. Physical distress—a racing heart, pounding head, nervous stomach—is the first assault when we edge to the perimeter of our comfort zone. It's a natural, primordial instinct, a remnant of the fight-or-flight syndrome. But although it may feel excruciating, making a telephone call, speaking up during a business meeting, or dropping off your portfolio with a prospective employer is not the same as fighting off the charge of a woolly mammoth.

We don't have to run scared. We *do* have to learn to recognize the physical manifestations of fear and acknowledge them. The next time you're physically sick at the thought of leaving your comfort zone, calmly reassure your conscious self that the feeling of fear is passing *through* you and will dissipate if you keep on moving forward. Many actresses are so scared that they feel nauseated just before walking on stage, but they've learned how to transform fear into the creative energy of forward motion. They burst through to the other side of stage fright to applause.

Intimidation works differently from naked fear. She's a shape-changer, capable of adopting different guises to control you. The moment you step bravely out from the bounds of your comfort zone, she's likely to rise up inside you like a lion tamer, complete with whip and chair. "Get back!" she'll scream. "Who do you think you are? You'll make a fool of yourself! You're risking your livelihood! You're neglecting your children! Get back to your cage immediately!"

When these scare tactics are no longer effective, intimidation often takes another shape, as the voice of reason: "Look, I don't want to alarm you but... You know you've taken on quite a lot... I wouldn't if I were you..."

The worst thing about intimidation is that she knows all our buttons and just when to push them. But if she doesn't succeed with scare tactics, she'll kill your dreams with kindness. She's your best friend: She'll enable you to dig your own creative grave by handing you the shovel. She's the only one who knows how tired you really are, so she'll encourage you to take a nap instead of making cold calls. She understands that you just don't have much time for relaxation, so what's the harm of catching a soap opera in the early afternoon instead of working on your résumé before the kids come home from school? Relax, she tells you, "You've got plenty of time... If it doesn't get taken care of today, there's always tomorrow..."

If none of the above works because now you're older, wiser, and more experienced, she'll begin a whispering campaign, sounding very similar to your intuitive voice. How will you know the difference? If the suggestion you hear doesn't bring you a sense of peace, *it is not the voice of your Authentic Self*. It's the ego in one of her many guises. Tell her to shut up. Then turn on some beautiful music that uplifts, inspires, and drowns her out.

Today, just begin observing your behavior pattern. Every woman— even the megastar whose life seems so glamorous—experiences ambivalence about success. One significant quality found in the women we admire is that they have identified their personal patterns of self-sabotage and learned to let their own best friend—their Authentic Self—outsmart the enemy within. And so can you.

How to Become a Social Media Influencer

Sometimes it's the smallest decisions that can change your life forever.

—Keri Russell
American actress and dancer

Just walk away, Renee. Just walk away.

How long have you been performing your agility calisthenics—scrolling, swiping, screening, teetering, tottering, clicking, posing, preening, and pushing to squeeze yourself into whatever size or flavor today's "likes" or "following" might be?

The escape door awaits your arrival. I put your name on the list. The muscle at this chic, private club gives a smiling nod, as he parts the velvet rope and you leave the sheer bedlam of performing on multiple media platforms.

And what awaits? Digital detox camps, which are the new growth industry in personal development. Disconnect so you can reconnect. At these self-empowerment getaways, you surrender all your digital paraphernalia and sign up for hands-on workshops in archery, spoon carving, stilt walking, rock climbing, acapella, theatrics, tango, crochet, macramé, comic book drawing, analog photography, tie-dye, mask making, embroidery, furniture design. A wealth of creativity at your fingertips once the smartphone is out of your hands.

The early days of Facebook two decades ago made it fun to share updates on what you were up to, and it was a great way to keep in touch with family and friends at a distance. But then you started hearing the opinions of people you didn't know and, what's more, didn't want to know. What about those angry political rants? And the shaming posts? The constant criticism? The tripe and the drivel among the rabble and riffraff? Or the styles of the rich and famous, who actually weren't rich or famous until they got a lot of people, like us, to follow them so they could be sponsored. "Influence which is given on the side of money is usually against the truth," Harriet Martineau wrote in 1836, proving that there is nothing new under the sun.

There are four separate reasons we use the internet: to educate or entertain, and to persuade or convert.

I adore the fact that so much information, knowledge, history, science, economics, and the arts is available to us to learn. That we can finish our degree or get another one via online universities, workshops, and master classes. It's intoxicating to think that I can see virtually any film in the world.

I'm grateful that in times of crisis and disaster we can find out what's happening and send help; that medical information can be conveyed quickly in an emergency; that by being connected online we can have a greater understanding of what's happening in the world outside of what's happening on your street. But I also believe that we're weary and wary now, too, as the educating and entertaining purposes of the internet have been trampled on by those who want to persuade, convert, and subvert.

It's time to re-examine our relationship to digital connection. Let's start by separating the wheat from the chaff, which is a marvelous old farming expression that we can use for dealing with the amount of information we are bombarded with 24/7. When a grain farmer separates the wheat from the chaff, she's pulling off the husk that surrounds the wheat seeds and getting rid of it. Do the same with your social media accounts. Consider how you use them, why you use them, and how they affect you emotionally. Do they serve you, or do they diminish you? When you use Instagram do you find yourself comparing yourself to others? Do you feel depressed or disheartened after looking at perfectly composed images and glimpses into lives that are not your own? Do you go on Twitter to gain and exchange information? To connect with others? Or do you use it to let off some steam? Could your quick and unconsidered words potentially impact another in a hurtful way?

Subconsciously we think that because these digital exchanges transpire through an inanimate object in our hand, they aren't serious. You aren't saying the hurtful comment to someone's face; you're just looking at a pretty picture; it's fine, it's not real. But consider this—if we consume content again and again and again, on one endless loop, there's a "brainwashing" effect, and those "not real" things start to feel very real in our minds.

So how do you stop? Can you stop?

I am, of course, aware that many businesses and interesting people are using the most popular social media platforms as calling cards for their work, and letting people politely know what's going on is acceptable, as is staying informed yourself. Did you know that you can turn notifications off and on your phone and computer? No more pinging every time someone comments on your comment. You can also choose when to see posts in your feed from accounts you follow. No unfriending and subsequent social awkwardness required, simply choose to unfollow them, and the political rants of your second cousin will no longer take up brain space. You can also limit yourself to only checking your accounts once a day or removing Facebook from your phone and only interacting with it on your computer. It's really that simple. We think we don't have a choice but to engage because everyone else is doing it, but the fact is we *do* have a choice, and we can choose how much and what we want to consume.

Recently I discovered a company by their announcement that they were pulling out of social media, which immediately piqued my interest. Lush UK, a bath and personal care purveyor, posted this farewell: "We are tired of fighting with algorithms, and we do not want to pay to appear in your newsfeed...So we've decided it's time to bid farewell to some of our social channels and open up the conversation between you and us...from our founders to our friends."

Nothing is stronger than the power of choice, especially when that choice is to walk away. This is how, Renee, you become the mistress of all you survey.

NOVEMBER 21

Riding the Big Kahuna

Chance is the first step you take. Luck is what comes afterwards.
—Amy Tan
American Chinese novelist

Go with the flow. Catch the wave. Ride the big Kahuna. Wouldn't I just love to! How about you? But real life rarely includes a stop at Surf City unless you live in Malibu.

Whenever we experience the flow, we experience a luminous liftoff: we're alert, soaring, unself-conscious, authentic, moving at the peak of our abilities. We forget food, drink, sex, sleep. Why? We're fueled by high-octane Love. Calling forth our gifts at the top of our lungs to a celestial "Bravo!" Reveling in our passion. We don't need positive-thinking mantras to motivate us; happiness propels us at warp nine toward our aspirations. Obstacles dissolve in the flow. Toxic emotions, anxieties, and depression disappear. We're in this world, but certainly not of it. Here we experience a profound pleasure not found in the erogenous or erroneous zones, a peace that surpasses our puny understanding. Exhilaration. Joy. Transformative transcendence. We took that first step by chance and we're riding this wave of luck all the way.

The bad news is that we don't ride the big Kahuna often enough. The good news is that the flow can be invoked and induced. For decades, Mihaly Csikszentmihalyi has been pioneering the scientific study of joy, scrutinizing altered states of "optimal experience," those moments when we feel deeply connected with real life, which he labels "flow." He believes that exhilaration can be part of everyday life, and I'm a believer. Reading his incredible book *Flow: The Psychology of Optimal Experience* might make a believer out of you.

What's more, going with the flow is most often attained with simple pleasures, even work, when we bring the right attitude and attention to our tasks. Complete consciousness—focusing our psychic energy on what we're doing—induces the flow. As we learn to shut out chaos, concentrating our creative energies within, our attention fuels our ability to accelerate beyond our normal capacities.

When working, playing, or creating, ritual plays an important role in preparing our minds, bodies, and souls to tap into the mother lode. The particular way you arrange your desk at the beginning of the day, the soft pencil you prefer, the music you listen to when you work with your *Illustrated Discovery Journal* is an invocation to the flow. Small moments—reading, gardening, cooking, arts, and crafts—take on new meaning when we honor them as waves on which to catch the flow. Exploring your family's heritage, commemorating special moments or people in your life by collecting and displaying talismans, can invite the flow by linking the past with the present.

Varying the routines of your daily round can induce the flow because novelty increases the frequency of the waves; thinking of lovemaking in new ways can fan waves of desire previously doused with familiarity. Memorizing favorite quotes, poetry, songs, and facts and enlivening our conversation with them evokes the flow. Mastering a game, sport, or new skill activates the flow process. But so do solitude and daydreaming. Indulging your imagination brings the big Kahuna within reach, because your imagination is your soul's way of communicating with your conscious mind.

Two tricks I use in order to catch the wave are listening to the same music for different long-term projects. I use movie soundtracks because they impose a rhythm without distracting vocals; I found this gold nugget through Amy Tan, and I've shared it with many people. The other discipline I follow is saying No to any appointments during the writing of the book: such as no dinner plans a week from next Thursday. If I'm writing, that is all I'm doing: writing, editing, sleeping, rewriting. The dinner invitation might be ten days in the future, but how do I know when the Muse will drop in? Good heavens, she might appear at two p.m. in the afternoon. If you've ever caught the wave once, you know how magnificent it is, and I am trying to woo her to pay me a return visit.

"How we feel about ourselves, the joy we get from living, ultimately depends directly on how the mind filters and interprets everyday experiences," Mihaly Csikszentmihalyi reminds us. "Whether we are happy depends on inner harmony, not on the controls we are able to exert over the great forces of the universe."

Weather Report

Better to be without logic, than without feeling.
—Charlotte Brontë (1816–1855)
English novelist and poet, eldest of the three
Brontë sisters

Today, variably cloudy. Moody. Didn't sleep well last night; up twice with the baby. Much tossing, turning, churning. Could be time of month, bills due. Heavy water retention. Alternating gray punctuated by streaks of light, some levity but not quite sunny. Most likely at lunchtime, if with friends. Foreboding, if lunching at desk. During the afternoon, expect thunderstorms due to deadline approaching, boss's frustrations, the results/feedback/figures coming in. Tonight, turning colder. Didn't resolve argument with husband over upcoming holidays. Possible frost late tonight, which will make for another unsettling day tomorrow.

Many women struggle with addictions in some form—drink, drugs, smoking, food, sex, shopping, or exercise—and to varying degrees. Most of these forms of self-abuse are frequently discussed on online forums, in books, and articles. But there's another habit that affects many of us but gets little airplay, and that's addiction to the highs and lows of emotions.

There was once a period in my life when I could literally cry or rage for hours—and did so frequently. I was an emotional drunk, bingeing on self-abuse with tears and tantrums until I was exhausted, unable to be a loving partner or a productive writer. Emotional binges aren't just a matter of temperament; they can spell termination for relationships, careers, and dreams. The only way I got sober was by acknowledging my dependence on personal drama to a Source stronger than my instinct for self-sabotage and finally surrendering the theatrics. I prayed every day for emotional sobriety. One day at a time. I got therapy. I got better. I started taking meditation. I became well. But I know that as far as emotions are concerned, I'll always be in recovery.

Sometimes emotional bingeing is precipitated by a physical disorder—PMS, depression—or by stress and fatigue. But significant changes in our emotional climate, such as manic behaviors that disrupt and destroy our daily round, aren't to be ignored. They are to be treated.

Becoming aware of our emotional weather patterns is essential if we want to remain sane, functioning, and well-loved members of the human race. Every woman has a pattern, and everyone's pattern is different. If you don't recognize yours, start paying attention. When an outburst of anger or tears erupts, step back. Breathe deeply. Center yourself. Count to one hundred before issuing an ultimatum. When you're calm, replay the circumstances surrounding your emotional surge. You're frustrated. Why? How much sleep did you have last night? What did you eat for lunch? How many glasses of wine did you drink? When was your last period? Your last physical exercise? How much sugar did you consume throughout the day?

You're enraged. Why? You're grief-stricken. Why? You're resentful. Why? Deal with it. Talk to a friend. Find images of how you feel to make a collage in your *Illustrated Discovery Journal*. Write a letter you don't send. Update your résumé. Clean a closet or your in box. Now that you're calmer, what one practical step could you take to make the situation, if not better, then at least tolerable? Yes, there must be one thing you can do. Do it.

Unfortunately, emotional drunks do not overindulge with the *positive* emotions: gratitude, forgiveness, empathy, admiration, wonder. But we do recover our authenticity and our equilibrium with joy.

Cultivate happiness. Hone your sense of humor; it's the most irresistible asset any of us can possess. Smile, especially if you don't feel like it. The physical workout of the muscles around your mouth increases the positive enzymes in your brain chemistry.

"The truth is that we can overhaul our surroundings, renovate our environment, talk a new game, join a new club, far more easily than we can change the way we behave emotionally," the Pulitzer Prize–winning journalist Ellen Goodman observes. "It's easier to change behavior than feelings about that behavior."

But no behavior can be changed before it's acknowledged. And no addiction is beyond the reach of Love.

NOVEMBER 23

The Gift of Failure

Flops are part of life's menu and I'm never a girl to miss out on a course.

—Rosalind Russell (1907–1976)
American actress, comedian, screenwriter, and singer

In the eyes of the world, Clare Booth Luce was one of the most successful women in the twentieth century. She was a playwright and author, a two-term congresswoman, and ambassador to Italy. She was also a mother and the wife of publishing magnate Henry Luce, cofounder of

Life and *Time* magazines. But this extraordinary woman confessed that she often thought, "If I were to write my autobiography, my title would be *The Autobiography of a Failure.*"

Now I ask you, if Clare Booth Luce felt this way about herself and her brilliant career, what hope is there for the rest of us?

Gratefully, there is a great deal of hope if we stay on the path to authenticity. Clare Booth Luce felt like a failure because she believed she had lived inauthentically, having not followed her true calling. "I would say my worst failure, paradoxically, was a rather long-drawn-out series of relative successes, none of which were in theater. In other words, my failure was not to return to the real vocation I had, which was writing. I don't remember from childhood ever wanting to do or be anything except a writer."

To begin with, she *never* wanted to run for Congress; it was entirely her husband's idea; Henry Luce was a powerful man because he knew how to wield power for his own benefit. Clare Booth's theatrical career was thriving (she had written five plays) when she married Luce in 1935, and her play *The Women* became a smash hit on Broadway the following year. But her husband believed that theater was an avocation, nothing more than "night work." So when Clare Booth added Luce to her name, she reluctantly sublimated her passion. After two terms in Congress, she tried to resign from political life to resume her writing. Then, in rapid succession, came a series of staggering losses: the deaths of her mother, brother, and of her only child, a daughter, in an accident. For Clare Booth Luce, life came to an abrupt halt, and it was a long time before she felt able to continue as an active participant.

After a while, she began to tell herself, "Maybe you're not a writer. Maybe you'll never be a writer again." And although she did eventually write articles and books, she never went back to her first love, the theater. She mourned the path she had abandoned for the rest of her life.

Clare Booth Luce's loss was a hidden one, Carole Hyatt and Linda Gottlieb tell us in their inspirational and practical primer on surmounting failure, *When Smart People Fail: Rebuilding Yourself for Success.* "Hidden failures suffer less from a sharp sense of loss than a chronic sense of disappointment. But they suffer nonetheless, longing somehow to change, often as scared and ashamed as those who have been fired. How many people, laid off jobs through no fault of their own, nevertheless feel they have somehow failed? How many of us feel stuck in jobs we hate, are terrified to risk change, and despise ourselves for doing less than our best? Often at the very moment the world is praising us, we know in some corner of our minds that we have failed our own best hopes."

Each one of us is terrified of failing. But whether we risk it all or play it safe, we cannot avoid failure—public or hidden—all our lives.

"It is impossible to live without failing at something, unless you live so cautiously that you might as well not have lived at all, in which case you have failed by default," J. K. Rowling tells us.

This is failure's generous gift. In life the worst thing that can happen isn't failing. It's never having tried.

NOVEMBER 24

The Blessing of Friends

Each friend represents a world in us, a world possibly not born until they arrive, and it is only by this meeting that a new world is born.

—Anaïs Nin (1903–1977)
French-American novelist, poet, and diarist

Our friends are the jewels in our crown of contentment. We need to treat them as preciously as we truly hold them in our hearts.

There are many ways to do this. Rituals of friendship are especially meaningful. Take each other out for festive birthday dinners. Share your favorite books. Read one simultaneously, then get together once a month for afternoon tea or coffee just to discuss it. Be on the lookout for articles, recipes, and memes to share back and forth. Remember friends with the lost art of cards and thank-you notes. Brief, encouraging notes when tough times hit will be treasured, even more than phone calls. Share resolutions or aspirations with a friend on New Year's Eve.

Go on walks together. Make annual outings a tradition: thrifting together in the summer; holiday shopping together in the winter. When a friend is sick, deliver a get-well "indulgence basket" filled with bedside comforts: something irresistible to read, cough drops, tissues, assorted fruit teas, homemade soup, a small flowering plant. Send or give friends flowers: spur-of-the-moment bouquets from the grocery store before you meet for lunch or to bring a smile during dark days. When there's a death in a friend's family, instead of making a contribution in the deceased's name or sending flowers to the funeral (others will do that), wait a couple of days and send her a beautiful plant or bouquet. It will comfort her more than you can imagine.

During tough times, put her name on a prayer list. I believe the prayers of another woman are the most thoughtful, personal, and powerful gifts there are. I have a dear friend who keeps me on convent prayer lists throughout the year, and I always feel there's backup if I need it, and probably do. Sometimes our prayers for our friends are the greatest gifts we can give them.

Start or continue collections for a friend, adding a new collectible each birthday or at holiday time. When giving a cherished pal a gift, always give her something she'd never give herself, an indulgence. Cook for your friends. During trying times—while a friend is sick or under tremendous stress—double a recipe and deliver a casserole to her home.

Above all, let your friends know how much you love them. Tell them frequently how much you treasure the gift of their friendship. Sadly, significant others come and go. Children grow up. Parents die. Siblings are separated by distance. But our friends are the continuous threads that help hold our lives together. Cherish your friends, not only in thought but in action. "Friends are people who help you be more yourself," Merle Shain reminds us, "more the person you are intended to be."

NOVEMBER 25

O Pioneer! Willa Cather's Kitchen

These coppers, big and little, these brooms...and brushes, were tools; and with them one made not shoes or cabinet work, but life itself. One made a climate within a climate; one made the days— the complexion, the special flavor, the special happiness of each day as it passed; one made life.
—Willa Cather (1873–1947)
American Pulitzer Prize–winning novelist

Many writers have been in exile when they wrote of a certain time, a certain place. Nothing soothes the broken heart holding the pen more than ritual, reverence, and remembrance.

Edith Wharton archly channeled the frantic yearnings of a poor girl dying to be rich on the fringes of New York society while Wharton was in residence on the French Riviera in 1905. James Joyce captured the dank, dreary despair of turn of the century Dublin from Paris in 1914. Ernest Hemingway portrayed the tempestuous bravado of the Spanish Civil War and bullfighting matadors in a mojito-fueled decade writing five novels, a play, and two collections of short stories while in Key West, Florida, between 1929 and 1938.

But, arguably, few writers have ever come as close to brilliantly conjuring up the soul's sacred sense of place as Willa Cather, writing about America's amber-waved prairies from the last place you'd ever expect to find her: New York's Greenwich Village. Twenty years before Gertrude Stein was lamenting "the Lost Generation," meaning the self-exiled expatriates on the Left Bank in Paris, Willa Cather went where no woman and no writer had gone before, becoming a pioneer of American fiction writing about holy hunger—food and love, home and away, the sacred in the ordinary, the secret altars where women pray in their kitchens.

Here is what is so astonishing to me: Reading between the lines of Cather's prairie fiction, the in-between is so deftly disguised and cleverly concealed, hiding in plain sight with flour finger stains still on the apron.

Now imagine with me. In the very early morning Willa goes marketing; she loved to treat herself to fresh raspberries, brioche, French Camembert cheese, and chickens sold by a particular Italian vendor. Then after returning home to a second-floor apartment at 5 Bank Street, Greenwich Village, with the superb groceries for her cook, she'd seize her solitude and in the space of two to three hours every day, while also working as the managing editor at the muckraking tabloid *McClure's Magazine* (think *National Enquirer*), she wrote three novels in five years—*O Pioneer!* (1913), *The Song of the Lark* (1915) and *My Ántonia* (1918)—which captured forever the true grit and gumption of the Nebraska Territory frontier immigrants, largely Scandinavian, Czech, and Polish homesteaders. The harsh and acerbic critic H. L. Mencken declared, "No romantic novel ever written in America, by man or woman, is one half so beautiful as *My Ántonia*."

And while Cather's pioneer novels could teach how prairie dogs build their underground society or how to kill rattlesnakes in the back garden with a club, what touched readers was her uncanny ability to blend the siren song of wanderlust and courage in the face of unimaginable hardships with the salvation of food, home, and family, and in prose as sparse as the treeless desert of dust, sky, and sun she'd left behind. Willa Cather believed that homemaking and homesteading "are activities which build a space where souls can thrive and dream—secure, protected, related, nourished and whole," and she made believers out of even the most jaded sophisticate.

Born into a prosperous Virginia family on December 7, 1873, and the oldest of seven children, when she was just nine Willa was plucked from a genteel upbringing by her father's decision to join his father and brother in Red Cloud, Nebraska. It was as if she'd been dropped into an ocean of rough, shaggy red grass from a space capsule, and quite frankly, she never got over the shock of it. As far as her eyes could see, there wasn't a tree, bough, leaf, or a blade of green grass. She would later describe her prairie surroundings as having erased her personality, while it forged her character. She came to see the relinquishment of Old West country ways by the second generation of immigrants as spiritually threatening. "The generation now in the driver's seat hates to make anything, wants to live and die in an automobile, scudding past those acres where the old men used to follow the long cornrows up and down," she wrote in 1923. "They want to buy everything ready-made: clothes, food, education, music, pleasure."

What makes this tart opinion so fascinating, bewildering, really, is that Willa Cather had already been in Greenwich Village since 1906, and she would live in New York City until her death in 1947. Her prairie years were few, between the ages of nine and fifteen, including a stint as a mail pony girl, delivering the post to her few and far-between neighbors. But these early years informed her art all her adult life, particularly because she had found spiritual refuge—her sense of belonging—by spending her mornings with neighbor immigrant women baking or butter-making. "My mind and my stomach are one," she told an audience in 1925: "I think and work whatever it is that digests. I think the preparation of foods the most important thing in life. And America is too young a nation to realize it. It makes musical discords in the cooking."

Is it any wonder that Ántonia in *My Ántonia* doesn't want "to die and stop cooking."

This is a lovely thought for those of us who will be doing a lot of cooking in the next couple of weeks. "I have never had any intellectual excitement more intense than spending a morning with a pioneer woman at butter-making and hearing her talk," Willa Cather confessed. Still, while she wrote of food, she was more often writing than she was cooking. Although she would go on to win the Pulitzer Prize in 1922 for her novel *One of Ours,* set during the first World War, many believed it was because she did not win one for *My Ántonia.*

As you create the rich autumn hues of gracious plenty on your Thanksgiving table this year, may you know much contentment and a sense of peace. "The farmer's wife who raises a large family and cooks for them" expresses "the real creative joy...which marks the great artist." Always remember, women are Artists of the Everyday. *You* are an Artist of the Everyday.

I always loved Willa Cather's wisdom in pointing out that "One cannot divine nor forecast the conditions that will make happiness; one only stumbles upon them by chance, in a lucky hour, at the world's end somewhere, and holds fast to the days, as to fortune or fame."

Hold fast to that moment, hold fast to the benediction, bend your knees and acknowledge that blessed are you among women to know that moment and give thanks. Cherish it. "Some memories are realities and are better than anything that can ever happen to one again," Willa Cather confessed to console. For the writing that breaks the heart holding the pen only soothes the soul of her who turns the page, when writers find the strength to write not about what they love, but what they have lost.

Pilgrim's Progress

Beauty and grace are performed whether or not we will or sense
them. The least we can do is try to be there.
—Annie Dillard
American Pulitzer Prize–winning author

In November 1929, just one month after the famous stock market crash that set in motion the Great Depression, an editorial in *The Household Magazine* encouraged their readers to take heart and have courage as they faced the unknown:

"Thanksgiving Day was meant to be something more than a mere period of time between Wednesday and Friday of the last week in November. It may be something more than a holiday, or it may have none of the characteristics of one.

"What it is depends on the state of mind."

By the third Thanksgiving of the Great Depression in November 1932, American homemakers and the women's magazines they read had passed through the same desperate psychological stages a person experiencing profound loss endures—shock, denial, anger, bargaining, and great grief—before settling in for what is often the longest stage of any traumatic change: depression. A new Democratic president-elect, Franklin Delano Roosevelt, was getting ready to take over the White House, but it would be another few months before FDR's rousing inaugural address, which reminded Americans that "all they have to fear is fear itself."

There would be seven more lean Thanksgivings of economic uncertainty followed by five years of world war. How did our grandmothers and great-grandmothers drag themselves out of bed to make biscuits for breakfast? An image of my Kentucky granny rolling out dough in her salmon-pink chenille bathrobe and slippers has come to represent grace under pressure in the archives of my heart.

You might be approaching this Thanksgiving with dread for the future and sorrow for what is happening now. When deep discouragement comes, I comfort myself by thinking of the long line of heroic women who came before me—not only those in my family, but every woman settler, explorer, adventurer, native American mother, and prairie homemaker, who tamed wild lands and wild times to make homes for those they loved. I particularly love to meditate on the first band of Pilgrim women.

There were eighteen women on the *Mayflower*, and although none of them died during the crossing from England to Massachusetts, by the time of the first "Thanks Giving" meal, a year later in 1621, there were only four women who had survived the brutal winter, spring sowing, and autumn harvest. Four very tired women who needed to take care of fifty men and children daily.

With the men almost entirely focused on building houses and the village, the women had so many chores, they performed in shifts. For aside from cleaning and cooking, there were plowing and planting, preserving and putting away, caring for livestock, making soap and candles from tallow (animal fat), tending the sick, and creating herbal medicines. There was so much work that they lived on one portion's grace, and if they didn't drop down dead with their hand to the plow or wither away in a nighttime sweat from a succession of diseases contracted on the voyage, they took it as a sign that God meant for them to go on. And, you know, they were right.

I love the bare bones simplicity of this truth. Sometimes in life, all we can do is put one foot out of the bed and then in front of the other, literally. I figure if you wake up in the morning, you're meant to go on—continue at what you're doing and ask Heaven to show you what you're doing wrong, if you are. Since God knows we're not meant to manage alone, Providence will be there to help if we ask for it.

These are the same gifts all women are endowed with. We are born with a blessed DNA—the genetic code of resilience, strength, ingenuity, creativity, perseverance, and determination. Our Destiny, Nature, and Aspirations are Heaven endowed, so why wouldn't we be given the wherewithal to fulfill them?

While our historical attention is drawn to the Pilgrims and early settlers of this wild and beautiful land, we should not overlook the women who were here before the Pilgrims arrived. Author Dina Gilio-Whitaker, an Indigenous researcher and activist, broadens our horizons on the heroism and humanity of Native American women. Dina shares the authentic stories of Native American women we should know more about. Nanye-hi (Nancy Ward) is a Cherokee leader granted the designation of *Ghigau*, which Dina explains means "most beloved woman" and also "war woman." While her exploits are grand, it is her wisdom we hope resonates forever. Dina writes that while negotiating the Treaty of Holston in 1781, Nanye-hi reminded the U.S. treaty commissioners, "We are your mothers... you are our sons."

So this Thanksgiving week as you go about cooking and laying the table, as you make preparations for gathering together with friends and loved ones, whenever anything happens that triggers the feeling of angst or distress, take a deep breath and silently ask yourself a few questions as I do when I'm in the midst of trying to do everything:

Is my family safe today?

Is there a roof over our heads today?

Do I have to chop wood to keep warm, today?

Today, do I have to carry water from a creek two miles away?

Did I have to shoot the turkey for our meal today?

One of my favorite quotations is from the *Ladies Home Journal* in October 1932. "When money is plenty this is a man's world. When money is scarce it is a woman's world. When all else fails the woman's instinct comes in. She gets the job. That is the reason why in spite of all that happens, we continue to have a world."
Thank Heavens, some things never change.

NOVEMBER 27

The Prosperity of Living

Woman must be the pioneer in this turning inward for strength. In a sense, she has always been the pioneer.
—Anne Morrow Lindbergh (1906–2001)
American pioneering aviatrix and author

These are challenging times in which to live. But we are not the only generation of women to have known difficult days. It is comforting to realize that others before us have persevered and prospered. During the dark days of the Depression an editorial in the October 1932 issue of *Ladies' Home Journal* encouraged readers to remember that "The return of good times is not wholly a matter of money. There is a prosperity of living which is quite as important as prosperity of the pocketbook." But the magazine stressed, "It is not enough to be willing to make the best of things as they are. Resignation will get us nowhere. We must build what amounts to a new country. We must revive the ideals of the founders. We must learn the new values of money. It is a time for pioneering—to create a new security for the home and the family..."
I found the above paragraph more than twenty-five years ago, at a time in my life when I was completely in the dark and struggling to know what my Divine calling and purpose was. I realize now, with the wry wisdom of the backward glance, that I wrote those words in an effort to console myself because I didn't know if they would ever be read by another pair of eyes. I was very discouraged; I felt like such a complete failure at forty-four and as if I'd achieved nothing. By then, I'd spent more than two years writing a book that no publisher in America

wanted to publish. I needed a lot of comfort, consoling, and encouragement, and with no one to talk to except Heaven, which didn't seem to be holding up its end of the conversation, I returned daily to my treasure chest of women's periodicals from the late Victorian era through the 1950s, which I called "The Mother Lode," a personal vein of gold which I worked every day. The way I wrote was to find a quote to start and then see where the crumbs led me. That day, I was back on the pioneer trail.

I was always deeply moved by how "the woman's view" in periodicals changed every decade, especially from the Great Depression with its emphasis on homemaking to abruptly taking the apron off for the factory floor during the years of World War II. But always, the goal was to spoon-feed readers doses of optimism, hope, comfort, or ways to find contentment, so they could continue on meeting the challenges of their daily rounds with courage and good cheer.

I particularly loved the home-centered rituals they inspired: drawing the curtains, turning on the soft golden lights, turning down the bed, and slipping in a flannel-covered hot water bottle to warm the sheets. If I could create and keep a safe place on the page like my illustrious, often anonymous mentors did for me, then perhaps I could create a refuge from all the hullabaloo of the outside world for other women.

We read for pleasure or we read to quiet the pain from a deafening roar to a dull throb. We read to forget who we are or discover it; we read to understand or be understood. That is why I write as well.

What's fallen through the cracks of social and domestic history during the last seventy years is the very sacred need to keep up women's morale on the home front through whatever social, political, or economic turmoil or upheaval we are going through. Women have always cared for the world, one way or another, but we still don't know how to take care of ourselves. If we can't do one, then we can't do the other. I just love to share what I have sought: Divine connection and the courage to go on, wherever the pioneer trails lead us. We will not, cannot forget the legacy of love passed down to us, our daughters, and granddaughters, from generations of beautiful, brave, and heroic women over the last centuries, who reach through the portcullis of the past watching over us and encouraging us to go on, further than they could even imagine.

So this Thanksgiving, I will celebrate and consecrate that indomitable spirit with every word in my dictionaries. To be called to be a *caretaker* is the most beautiful compliment and description of my work in the world that I can imagine.

NOVEMBER 28

True Thanksgiving

An open home, an open heart, here grows a bountiful harvest.
—Judy Hand (1943–2007)
American artist

The turkey is in the oven, filling the air with the fragrance of anticipation, and my heart is glad. The pies are cooling on the rack, overflowing with the fruits of the earth, and my heart is full. Conversation, companionship, and conviviality transform the rooms of this beloved home, and my heart is at peace.

Soon dear ones—family and cherished friends—will gather at the table to rejoice in our bounty of blessings, and with us lift up their hearts in thanksgiving. As the table is set, my heart gratefully remembers the legacy of love and tradition represented in the talismans of freshly laundered linens, sparkling crystal, and gleaming china. The silver shines, the candles glow, the flowers delight us with their beauty.

This is good. This is very good. Let us hold fast to this authentic moment of *Simple Abundance*. Let us cherish this feeling of complete contentment. Let us rejoice and praise the Giver of all good. The English novelist Thomas Hardy believed that the days of declining autumn created an inner season in which we could live "in spiritual altitudes more nearly approaching ecstasy" than at any other time of the year. Let us exult in our souls' ecstatic accord.

Come, my thankful sisters, come. Offer grace for the bounty of goodness. Raise the song of harvest home, the glass of good cheer, the heart overflowing with joy. We have so much for which to be thankful. So much about which to smile, so much to share. So much, that in this season of plenty, we can embrace the season of relinquishment. All we have is all we need.

O beloved Spirit, truly you have given us so much, an extravagance of riches. Give us, we pray, one thing more: the gift of grateful hearts. Hearts that will not forget what You have done.

NOVEMBER 29

The Blessing of Health

The first wealth is health.

—Ralph Waldo Emerson (1803–1882)
American philosopher and poet

No sooner than we get up from the table, our conscious attention often turns to what we don't have rather than what we do—and for a very good reason. Black Friday arrives dressed as the walking dead, only to be followed by Cyber Monday. Ah, yes, the season of nonstop shopping has arrived. With the advent of four frenetic weeks of looking, finding, ordering, and buying, suddenly we feel overwhelmed by a season of lack.

So before we head to the mall, it would do our souls good to have a reality check, in the form not only of counting our blessings but of focusing on them. Money is going to have to buy a lot in the next few weeks, but it can't buy the gifts that count most: good health, a loving and supportive marriage, healthy children, the fulfillment of creative expression, and inner peace. We forget this, not because we're ungrateful louts, but because we get distracted with the razzmatazz of real life. Now is the time to remember.

What if I gave you a choice? You're guaranteed all the above joys but not a BMW in the driveway. Or you are guaranteed a BMW in the driveway, with the cash to pay comfortably for the luxury home adjacent to it, but you'll have to throw the dice for the real-life blessings. Which would you choose?

The blessing we'll meditate on today is health. We can't buy good health, no matter how much money we have. We can purchase the best medical treatment available in the world, but good health is not for sale. Health is a priceless gift from Spirit that most of us take for granted until we become sick. "One of the most sublime experiences we can ever have is to wake up feeling healthy after we have been sick," Rabbi Harold Kushner reminds us in *Who Needs God.* "Even if it is only relief from a headache or toothache, the health we take for granted most of the time is suddenly seen to be an incredible blessing." Today, realize if you have nothing else but your health, you are a wealthy woman. If you have a healthy mind, a healthy heart, and reserves of stamina and creative energy to draw upon, the world is literally lying at your feet. With your health you have *everything.*

But health is not just the absence of sickness. Good health is vitality, vigor, high energy, emotional equilibrium, mental clarity, and physical endurance. *These* are the gifts to pray for, not just that your credit card purchases will be approved and you won't have to slink away in disgrace.

Take your vitamins. Thank Spirit for the health you enjoy, and ask for more. If there is only one spiritual lesson I can inscribe on your consciousness, it's to ask. Ask and you shall receive. Ask and if you don't get it, at least you tried. Ask and be *specific*. Today, why not ask for the creative and physical energy you'll need, not just to survive the holiday season, but to enjoy it?

NOVEMBER 30

Do Try This at Home: Let There Be Light

In the full light of day,
I don't want to think about the sunset.
　　　　　—Shakira
　　　　　Latin music star, humanitarian, and UNICEF
　　　　　Goodwill Ambassador

Light is one of those amazing miracles that we don't really think about when it's present. But let the night creep in on the tail of a thunderstorm and we quickly remember how important it is to life and safety. So, as we settle in for winter nights, let's double check on extra light sources in our Caution Closet. In fact, let's double down on backups.

Candles may set the tone for relaxation and romance, but during times of no power and raging storms, they aren't going to be our primary go-to item. When choosing our light sources—the brighter the better. Without electricity we'll do well with portable lights and Goal Zero's crush lights in the home, Caution Closet, and backpack. These solar collapsible lanterns store flat and can be charged by the sun or a mini USB cable (included). They are lightweight and affordable and provide three hours of strong light on high or thirty-five hours of steady light on low. These are not your reading lights but will light your way.

　　✐ The Caution Closet's portable light sources can be found at the website www.goalzero.com and, for flashlights, *Popular Mechanics* (www.popularmechanics.com/technology/gadgets/g3035/best -flashlight/) gives a great tutorial. My interest in all things tactical was piqued by a well-known brand: MagLite's ML300LX with 625 lumens of light and different settings to brighten any situation. It will last for years!

　　✐ Practical, but less portable, are battery-operated lanterns. While there are many on the market in different price ranges, I personally have a few four-sided panel lanterns. They light up all sides, and I have used them during power outages to light my front step and the sidewalk. Look for a brand you know, like those made by Coleman for camping (www.coleman.com) and don't forget to stock the eight D batteries you'll need to keep them going.

ᴥ No matter what your preference, it is important to remember that all of these devices will need a power source. Keeping a variety of battery sizes, from AAA to D, on your closet shelves will be helpful in any situation. If your family uses electronic devices—and let's face it, we all do—it is wise to invest in a portable power bank. These small devices can charge a mobile phone or a tablet. Wirecutter (thewirecutter.com/reviews/best-usb-c-battery-packs-and-power-banks/), a *New York Times* company, has done a great review on power banks that can even charge your laptop. Of course, you will want to double check that your power bank is compatible with your current brands and models of products.

Don't forget to recharge your internal battery as well, for as cinematographer Aaron Rose reminds us, "In the right light, at the right time, everything is extraordinary." This is the time to pack a spiritual talisman, whatever that might be. If you ever need to unpack it, may it symbolize that you're never alone, especially during those crisis moments when we're convinced otherwise.

Joyful Simplicities for November

Some of the days in November carry the whole memory of summer as a fire opal carries the color of moonrise.
—Gladys Taber (1899–1980)
American columnist and author

ᴥ Native American legend reminds us that both good and bad dreams hover over us while we sleep, waiting to capture our minds for the night. In order to ensure a peaceful night's sleep, "dream catchers" were prepared: webs of colored string with a hole in the middle to let happy dreams pass through to the subconscious mind. Bad dreams are caught in the dream catcher's net, where they disappear with the first light of a new day. Dream catchers made by Native Americans (as well as kits for making them) are available from large craft stores, gift shops, and catalogs. You can also make one yourself by taking a small embroidery hoop and stringing it with a net made of colored embroidery thread. (Be sure to leave a hole in the middle.) Add festive colored beads (green is the color of abundance; rose or red is the color of love;

blue is the color of healing and protection; purple is the color of inner power) and feathers. Hang it over your bed.

- Write your own personal grace and offer it for the first time on Thanksgiving. This is a wonderful restorative, because you must carefully consider those things for which you are truly grateful. To inspire you, peruse *One Hundred Graces*, edited by Marcia and Jack Kelly.

- Fill a basket of food and take it to a shelter the day before Thanksgiving. Re-create your family dinner as much as possible, if you can, starting with the turkey. But any contribution you make will be welcome. If you have children, let them help you shop, load the basket, and deliver it with you. This is a very real reminder of how much we have for which to give thanks.

- Watch the Macy's Thanksgiving Day parade.

- Have fun choosing your own Advent calendar, if this is part of your tradition.

- If you plan to send holiday cards, this is the week to pick them out or create a plan with the family to make cards together. What I do is send New Year's cards, because no one expects them, and that also allows me a little extra time to add a note.

- "You say grace before meals. All right. But I say grace before the play. And the opera. And grace before the concert and pantomime. A grace before I open a book. And grace before sketching, painting, swimming, fencing, walking, playing, dancing. And grace before I dip the pen in the ink," G. K. Chesterton, the English writer and poet, admitted. It's a great idea to change up the Gratitude Journal. See how many times during the day you start different activities and offer a nod of the head to the very fact that all these opportunities are available to you.

- Don't rush out the day after Thanksgiving to do holiday shopping with the rest of the world. Instead, make a pot of homemade turkey vegetable soup, write out a shopping list for your festive desserts such as Christmas plum pudding and rum or Guinness cake ingredients. Create an Advent wreath, prepare the menorah, and start listening to holiday music.

DECEMBER

December, the diamond-frosted clasp
linking twelve jeweled months to yet another year.
                                        —Phyllis Nicholson
                                        English country memoirist

December's gifts—custom, ceremony, celebration, consecration—
come to us wrapped up not in tissue and ribbons but in cherished
memories. This is the month of miracles. The oil that burns for
eight days, the royal son born in a stable, the inexplicable return
of Light on the longest, darkest night of the year. Where there is
Love, there are always miracles. And where there are miracles,
there is great joy. Gratefully we weave the golden thread of the
sixth Grace of Simple Abundance—Joy—into our tapestry of contentment. At last we embrace the miracle of authenticity, changing
forever how we view ourselves. Our daily round. Our dreams.
Our destinies. Days we once called common, we now call holy.

DECEMBER 1

Charmed Lives

There is entirely too much charm around, and something must be done to stop it.

—Dorothy Parker (1893–1967)
Founding member of the Algonquin Round
Table

Charmed lives. Crammed down our throats in the glossy pages of lifestyle magazines, blogs, and Instagram feeds. Paid for with a portion of our life energy. You know who was celebrated for having a charmed life? Macbeth. Now there's a thought worth meditating on. Did Lady Macbeth share this opinion?

We all have charmed lives. We just don't have a conscious awareness of it, especially after reading about the airbrushed lives of other women. It takes the story of a modern Everywoman to help us see.

This had been one hell of a year for Everywoman. Just about everything that could go wrong had gone wrong. Or so it seemed. Money was tight because Everywoman's pay was based on commission and the size of her social media posse. It didn't seem to matter how hard she worked, the paychecks were irregular.

Because finances were tight, there was tension in her marriage, which increased when the government shut down and her husband missed two pay periods. He took a temporary shift job at the superstore to help. Now he was working two jobs at all hours but only being paid for one. Many of their conversations (when they were speaking) were about her finding a more reliable form of employment. Everywoman enjoyed her work and was good at it; she just needed a little more time to make it pay off. But time seemed to be running out.

That year, her various aches and pains had turned out to be due to a chronic condition. Her doctor told her she needed to make a lifestyle adjustment: eliminate the stress and fatigue that triggered flare-ups. When was that going to happen? One of her children had required special attention to get him through a rough emotional patch, which only made the other children resentful. Last spring her dad had died suddenly. Soon afterward, her mother had a debilitating stroke. Unable to care for herself, she had to be put into a nursing home. Her widowed mother-in-law fared better: She came to stay "temporarily" during the summer and hadn't left yet. Her teenage daughter frequently complained about having to give up her bedroom for Grandma. Seeing her mother-in-law at the dinner table made Everywoman feel guilty and resentful that she couldn't do the same for her own mom. Everywoman felt worn to a raveling. Today she begged Anyone Who Might Be Listening to give her a break.

"You're right. It's been tough," the kindly voice of her guardian angel agreed. "Take heart. Every life comes with its hard times. The Boss says there's a holiday special going on right now. Come up and choose another life or choose the Strength-Wisdom-Grace package. Strength to meet your challenges, Wisdom to embrace real life, and the Grace to be grateful not only for what you have but what you've escaped."

"I want a charmed life," Everywoman said.

"A charmed life, is it? Well, let's see what's available."

The next thing Everywoman knew she was sitting in front of a celestial computer, as the charmed lives of women all around the world came online. The faces were familiar but not so glamorous in private as they seemed in public. She was told she could exchange her life for the life of any other woman. A woman's life appeared. "How about her?" an angelic life-exchange counselor asked. "Comfortable—there's a live-in housekeeper—but rather hectic. Had to put aside her career as a famous trial attorney because of her twin daughters' cystic fibrosis."

Everywoman asked to be shown other lives...

There was the beautiful woman beaten by her superstar husband... The woman whose child was hit by a drunk driver and is now in a coma... The infertile woman who finally became pregnant only to discover she had breast cancer... The famous woman whose very public husband had a reputation for being a philanderer... The wealthy woman whose husband is about to go to prison for insider financial manipulation.

Everywoman was shaken. "I asked for women with charmed lives," she moaned. "You've only shown me women with great sorrow, humiliation, pain, and despair in designer clothes."

"Each of these women has been celebrated for her charmed life in those magazines and blogs you're so fond of. Still believe everything you see?

"So, which one will it be?"

"Is it too late to choose Strength, Grace, and Wisdom?" Everywoman asked hesitantly.

"Good choice. Has anyone told you lately that you lead a charmed life?"

What Women Want

The great question…which I have not been able to answer, despite my thirty years of research into the feminine soul, is "What does a woman want?"

—Sigmund Freud (1856–1939)
Austrian neurologist and founder of
psychoanalysis

A nap, Dr. Freud. A nap.

Now. Today. All right, if not today, at least on Sunday afternoon. This is the campaign platform I'll run on: eight hours of work, eight hours of rest, eight hours to do whatever we please. Should one of those pleasant hours be spent napping on your bed under a cozy comforter, door closed, curtains drawn, I would pronounce you a woman of great discernment.

A nap is not to be confused with sleeping. We sleep to recharge our bodies. We nap to care for our souls. When we nap, we are resting our eyes while our imaginations soar. Getting ready for the next round. Sorting, sifting, separating the profound from the profane, the possible from the improbable. Rehearsing our acceptance speech for the Nobel Prize, our surprise on receiving the MacArthur genius award. This requires a prone position. If we're lucky, we might drift off, but we won't drift far. Just far enough to ransom our creativity from chaos.

Where to have a proper nap? Your own bedroom. On your living room couch if you're single, or your parents' couch when you visit because they've taken charge of the grandchildren, who've been told to leave their poor mother alone and go outside to play (just the way you were told when you were little and *your* poor mother wanted to be alone). Or in a hammock. On a chaise longue. Under an umbrella on the beach. In a wingback chair in front of a fire.

How long do we nap? Personally, I book the one-hour slot, but you might like to introduce naps gradually, such as a half hour at a time, so you don't completely drop off the end of the world. Power nappers rave about twenty-minute revivers.

How do we do this if we have small children at home? We nap when they nap. But they *don't* nap, you say. They do now.

How do you nap at the office? Unfortunately, you don't, unless you shut the door and put your head on the desk for a quickie. Usually this is reserved for when our eyes need toothpicks to hold up our lids. This makes the tradition of the Sunday nap all the more essential. If you want to be happy for the rest of your life, napping is not optional.

How do you begin this tradition? Sunday at three o'clock, after the potatoes are peeled and the roast is in the oven, you disappear up the stairs or down the hall. Reassure them you will be back. Tell anyone who might be interested in your whereabouts that you need to sort something out. Alone. If you must look like you're about to do something productive, bring the newspapers, your iPad, or a book with you as if you're going to read. What they don't know can only help you. Now crawl under the covers. Good. You've done it.

"No day is so bad it can't be fixed with a nap," the American stand-up comedian Carrie Snow insists. Or no day so good that it can't be made better with a terrific time-out.

DECEMBER 3

When You're Sick

Illness is the doctor to whom we pay most heed; to kindness, to knowledge, we make promises only; pain we obey.
—Marcel Proust (1871–1922)
French novelist best known for *A Remembrance of Things Past*

You feel like you're dying, you look like you're dying, and you sound like you're dying," my doctor said while studying my lab slips and X ray. "Thankfully, you're not. You've got a relapse of the flu, infected sinuses, and now pleurisy. I want you to take an antibiotic and go back to bed where you belong until you're well enough to be up, which could be another week to ten days." When I feebly protested that I'd already been sick with the flu for three weeks and that I was far behind in my work, my doctor nodded sympathetically. "Well, go home then, take your medicine, put on your pajamas," she advised, "and write a meditation about how important it is to take care of yourself when you're sick. But I will be very angry if the next time we meet it's in the hospital."

I did as I was told. Sort of. I send this dispatch from underneath the covers.

Most women don't go to bed when they're sick because they can't. The children still need to be taken care of, the work still must get done, the meals still must be made, life marches on. So you stagger around like Typhoid Mary until you drop. One morning you just can't move, and with good reason. You're sick. For a day or two—at the most—you allow yourself a reprieve. Your mate and/or the children of the household solicitously inquire if there's anything you need, then quietly close the bedroom door so you can rest. Frequently, they'll poke their heads in to check on you because the sight of a woman prone on the bed for more than two hours registers a 7.5 on their personal Richter scales.

"Feeling better yet?" you're asked cheerfully. Eventually, after this question has been posed enough times, you say you do, even if you don't. You get out of bed, get dressed, and get ready once again to swallow swords while juggling flaming torches. The show must go on.

But sometimes we can't get up. Sometimes we're so run-down that we can't shake the flu standing up, or our bad cold becomes bronchitis, or we break a bone, slip a disc. Sometimes the unthinkable confronts us: a lump in the breast, a high white blood cell count, a whack on the head, chest pains that stun us into submission. We're not asked politely if we'd like to pause on the path for a refreshing respite. We're abruptly ordered to a halt.

The deeply spiritual Southern writer Flannery O'Connor came to believe, "In a sense sickness is a place more instructive than a long trip to Europe, and it's always a place where there's no company, where nobody can follow." The next time you're sick, stop feeling guilty about it. And quit operating under the deranged and dangerous delusion that *it's all under your control.* Instead of setting yourself up for a fall, give yourself permission to drop out for as long as you really need to in order to (1) get well and (2) gently explore this strange but temporary detour. Be as open to new insights as an inquisitive tourist would be.

If I'd never sustained a head injury years ago, I don't think I would have started my own business, written a syndicated newspaper column, or eventually published fourteen books. Having been forced into nearly two years' arbitrary sabbatical gave me the opportunity to strike out on a new path after I recovered. Every illness, from a cold to cancer, has a life-affirming lesson for us if we're willing to be taught. It can be simple or profound. Learning to take better care of ourselves in the future in order to stay healthy. Bringing more harmony into our daily affairs. Balancing our need for rest and recreation with the demands of responsibility. Appreciating the subtle nuances of the dark days as well as the light-filled ones. Seeking Wholeness as well as healing. Searching not just for a possible cure, but for the probable cause.

Flannery O'Connor searched for the positive aspects of her illness until she viewed her tutorial with lupus as "one of God's mercies." We may never become that enlightened. But the next time you're not feeling well, *please* cradle yourself gently with kindness and compassion. You'll be better for it.

DECEMBER 4

Romancing the Cold

The happiest people in this world are the convalescents.
—Mary Webb (1881–1927)
Victorian English Romantic novelist

Influenza and snowdrops come with linked hands. At winter's end, as in the hours between midnight and dawning, vitality is at its lowest," one of my favorite English country muses, Phyllis Nicholson, wrote in 1941.

"But here, we have compensations. We can, at least, be ill in comfort, and maintain complete independence. The worst condition on earth is to be stretched out on a bed of sickness under somebody's thumb. How we bless our warm, comfortable room with its ample radiator, its electric fire, the telephone within an arm's reach, and a private bathroom. We can make our own hot drinks, renew hot-water bottles, ring up the grocer; and still remain segregated from the outside world."

The last thing a woman wants to think about when she's about to drop like a stone—eyes sizzling out of their sockets, red and runny nose, raspy throat, hacking cough—is how fetching she looks. In that case, we might aspire to appear ravishing when we're caught up in a romantic fever, especially if it precedes flirtation. But when we're really ill, we battle the desire just to be left alone against the ache for extra pampering and a loving touch.

Happily, many soothing solutions are right at hand. No need to struggle out to shop, no need to call for reinforcements. If you open your closet, you'll find a nice large square Rx basket filled with necessities in anticipation that this day might come upon you. Just pull it out and let the recuperation begin.

Let's start with your sleeping arrangements. Slip into something light and loose. Like most simple pleasures and home comforts in my life, what to wear when I'm succumbing to the annual cold is not just the first old, odd, clean thing I can find.

Instead, I search the basket for my "comfy" jersey pajamas, folded and wrapped in lavender scented tissue paper. I've had them for over a decade, but time only brings out their beauty and sheen. Don't trap achy limbs within garments that bind or stick. The same goes for your bedding: lightweight, layered covers that can be drawn up over your shoulders or kicked off is what the lie-abed lady needs. Have a couple of extra-comfy pillows close by, so that you can hug one when you thrash to the left or heave to the right. Raise your head with an extra pillow. And keep some extra bedding (sheets, blankets) and nightclothes nearby, so if you become at all uncomfortable, hot, sweaty, or stinky, you can remake your bed and change into a fresh set. And yes, it is worth the effort. But the real worthy effort is planning for sick days when we're well. You might think these preparations are unnecessary, but then you'll have a bad bout and realize in your feverish state how much easier it would have been if you'd listened to me.

Ah, now what do my eyes land upon? A hot-water bottle. For those of you who live on the U.S. side of the Atlantic and always wonder what in the world is being placed at the foot of the bed in those classic black-and-white British films—it's a hot-water bottle. Get one that has a removable flannel cover. If this is a splurge gift, it could be a cashmere cover. The comfort and joy it brings are more than words can convey. You'll be telling everyone how it's the best purchase of your life.

Staying fresh and clean when you're sick seems impossible, but it makes you feel so good. When I was little, my mother would wash my arms, face, and neck with a moist cloth, wiping the "sick" away as she called it, and I always believed her, as did my daughter when I performed that loving ritual with her. But if you can muster the energy, a long, warm shower or leisurely eucalyptus-scented bath gel and shampoo will do wonders for respiratory ailments. And I love having the mist of a humidifier moisten the bedroom air. You can sweeten the air by simmering a few drops of lavender, eucalyptus, peppermint oil, dried rosemary, lavender, or ground cinnamon in a pot of water. If you're lucky enough to live in building with old-fashioned radiators, put your pot on top. It's something a Victorian nanny would do for her little charges.

Your nose is *so* sore, poor thing. Are you using the softest tissues? Keep a pot of lip balm and scented skin lotion on your nightstand in a pretty little basket. Pure almond oil is soothing, as is argan oil lip balm. Keep these together, along with rose-scented pastilles, your favorite cough drops, zinc tablets, a small bottle of reviving smelling salts, a nail file, tweezers, hand crème, and hand sanitizer. Prepare yourself for surrendering without feeling like a prisoner.

Drink through a straw if you have cold sores; have a small jar of flavored honey to dip a little spoon into and every so often suck on it.

Remember to wash your hands frequently (all winter long); a lovely lavender-scented liquid soap in a pump bottle at the sink is a good reminder, even if you're too stuffed to smell its fragrance. But don't give up the hand sanitizer. Keep small bottles in different places. And remember to wash your glasses and cups and change your hand towels frequently. When you're in the initial throes of it and if you live alone, have a plastic washbasin that can hold your dirty cups; they can be washed later. Don't worry about doing anything except rest and recuperation. However, you don't want to pass your own germs back to yourself! So fresh glasses and cups every day.

There are stages in the progress of every cold or flu. To fill the hours when you are too bleary-eyed or feverish to read, listen to soothing music that lets you drift in and out of pleasant hallucinations. During one nasty bout, Johnny Mathis kept me company, just as he did during my high school years. It was great. Chances are that old favorites you haven't heard in a while can induce pleasant reveries for you, too. I also keep a "Wonder Years" box—for me it's filled with Nancy Drew novels (the originals), Archie and Veronica comic books, and a couple of old issues of *Seventeen* that I found at a flea market. They're so amusing to flip through when I'm feeling poorly (I can't get over how mature the teenage models look). The whole point, when you're sick, is to entertain yourself as much as you can.

"The sad truth is that there is no point to getting sick when you're a grown-up. You know why. It's because being sick is about you and your mother," Adair Lara reminisces in her memoir, *Welcome to Earth, Mom* (1992). "Without that solicitous hand on your forehead, there is no one to confirm that you are really sick."

Ah, but we know better, dearest Reader. Take care of yourself.

P.S. Preparing a "Romancing the Cold" box for holiday gifts is absolutely genius on your part, and your lucky recipients will be grateful and astonished at your cleverness. You can find boxes to fill up under wedding supplies on Etsy.com.

DECEMBER 5

Passionate Kisses

A kiss can be a comma, a question mark or an exclamation point.
—Mistinguett (1875–1956)
French actress

Every woman knows the subtle nuances of puckering up: fly kisses, bye kisses, real kisses. *Lock-the-door* kisses.

Ah, lock-the-door kisses... vaguely, wistfully recalled. It's been a while since we had some of those. This is the season that grips most of us in a relentless cycle of contagion—strep throat, flu, bronchitis—unvanquished despite megadoses of every antibiotic known to modern medicine. At this moment I don't want to be kissed by anyone on this ward, and they certainly don't want to be kissed by me.

The good news is that the same precious natural resources not being pleasurably expended in regular lovemaking can be channeled into your creativity. Waste not, want not. Passion ignites sexual energy or creative energy. Your choice. Every artist, if they're telling the truth, will confess that when they're working at full throttle—writing a book, making a movie, directing a play, preparing for an exhibition, rehearsing for a concert, choreographing a new pas de deux—the sex drive diminishes. Frankly, my dear, we don't give a damn. That's because we can make wild, passionate love or make wild, passionate art. Rarely both at the same time.

This natural sublimation process works just as well in reverse. Found yourself in a solitary space as far as an intimate relationship is concerned? Don't waste time sulking. Try not to get caught up in what's missing but what's presenting itself to you. Dame Fortune is knocking. Invite her in. This is the perfect time to get serious and volunteer at the local food co-op, sign up and *show up* for the photography class, finish your degree, check in to Shepheard's Hotel, fall in love with your Authentic Self. *There is nothing sexier than the woman emitting the pheromone of personal fulfillment.* You'll not be alone for long, unless you want to be.

I can think of only one reason on earth why we shouldn't be able to have all the good stuff as well as passionate kisses: real life. Every woman knows times when she's alone: by choice, by chance, by circumstance. Cheer up. Sometimes you haven't found the lips you want to kiss. Sometimes the lips you want to kiss aren't available. Sometimes the one you'd like to kiss is sweaty and chilled, hacking and moaning in the bedroom just down the hall.

DECEMBER 6

Rx for Harried Hearts and Frazzled Minds

There is hope for all of us. Well, anyway, if you don't die you live through it, day in, day out.

—Mary Beckett (1926–2013)
Irish author

Some nights waves of weariness beat against our brains, crash against our hearts, wash over our bodies, threatening to erode our best defenses like sand dunes upon the shore. The water is cold, dark, and deep. Diversions that have worked in the past—drink, drugs, food, sex, shopping, work—now obscure a dangerous undertow. Nothing seems to hold back the tide. We need someone to throw us a line, to rescue us from drowning in disappointment.

When these nights come and I find I'm stranded alone on the beach of faltering belief, I have found refuge in a very centering and comforting prayer by Dame Julian of Norwich, a thirteenth-century English mystic:

All shall be well,
And all shall be well,
And all manner of things shall be well.

This simple affirmation of faith is especially comforting because it seems to console the dark, submerged sadness of the inexplicable, the unexpressed, the unresolved, the unfair, and the undeniable that stalk my soul after I close my eyes. I'll say the prayer over and over again softly, under my breath like a mantra, not trying to understand the meaning of the words, because I can't. Some mysteries are beyond our comprehension. Some mysteries we will never solve. Never know.

So instead of trying to make sense of it all, I'll simply let the Spirit of the words soothe my frazzled mind and harried heart until sleep comes. Sometimes we can't make sense of it. Sometimes *none of it makes sense.* Sometimes it just is. But if we can hold on long enough for this night to give way to another day, all shall be well, even if it's different from what we had expected. Even if it's different from what we had hoped for and believed with all our hearts would happen.

All shall be well,
And all shall be well,
And all manner of things shall be well.

DECEMBER 7

The Refinement of Everyday Thinking

The whole of science is nothing more than a refinement of everyday thinking.

—Albert Einstein
German Nobel Prize–winning theoretical physicist

There is a significant difference between thinking you know and actually *knowing.* Just as there's a significant difference between superficial change and change on a cellular level. It's one thing to move the furniture around for a fresh new look; it's quite another to rearrange your "DNA"—your destiny, nature, and aspirations—which is exactly what you're doing when you search for your authenticity. Start to do that and you get a fresh new life.

When I started writing this book, I knew that if I integrated Gratitude, Simplicity, Order, Harmony, Beauty, and Joy into my daily round, a sense of lack would diminish as a sense of abundance increased. That seemed to be quite enough. What I didn't know or couldn't possibly anticipate was the potency of the *Simple Abundance* process when combined with passionate and persistent reflection over a year. It is virtually impossible to write a book on authenticity as a spiritual and creative path and not be profoundly challenged and changed by it.

On paper, Einstein's mathematical equation $E = mc^2$ appears rather benign, doesn't it? But it led to the development of the atomic bomb.

On paper, Gratitude/Simplicity/Order/Harmony/Beauty/Joy = Authenticity appears equally harmless, even lackluster. But I've discovered that this equation leads to complete personal and spiritual transformation—a mystical metamorphosis of our particular "DNA" that's so deep our egos don't know whether they're coming or going. One minute we're sure of ourselves; the next, we're second-guessing. This can be very disconcerting to our conscious selves.

Of all the definitions of the *ego* I've ever discovered, my favorite is Joseph Campbell's: "What you think you want, what you will to believe, what you think you can afford, what you decide to love, what you regard yourself as bound to." Your ego has everything to lose with your authenticity, and she's got a stranglehold on your destiny, nature, and aspirations that's so strong it will take nothing less than a Divine detonation before she lets go.

Don't worry. About this time, you're poised for critical mass—that point when a self-sustaining chain reaction occurs.

In physics, nuclear fusion occurs when two separate elements, like hydrogen and helium, are forced together. Through the exertion of extreme pressure and temperature, a surge of energy as powerful as the sun is suddenly released until the hydrogen and helium are completely transformed, producing an entirely new force in the universe. This is how new stars are created.

In your search for authenticity, a similar process occurs. You fuse the six *Simple Abundance* Graces—Gratitude, Simplicity, Order, Harmony, Beauty, and Joy—with your own inner work, or what Einstein called "the refinement of everyday thinking." Now exert real life's pressures and the heat of your own passions on the six Graces and ponder for at least one to two years. The result? One day the transformative process builds to a point at which it can no longer be contained within. A huge surge of creative energy is suddenly released, bringing forth a completely new entity: your Authentic Self, the visible manifestation of your soul.

When this happens, "what you think you want, what you will to believe, what you think you can afford, what you decide to love, and what you regard yourself as bound to" will seem as if they belonged to another woman. They did.

After passionately and persistently exploring the origins of the universe, Albert Einstein came to know that "Something deeply hidden had to be behind things." When you passionately and persistently search for Wholeness, *you'll* know as well.

DECEMBER 8

Daydreams

Reverie is not a mind vacuum. It is rather the gift of an hour which knows the plentitude of the soul.

—Gaston Bachelard (1884–1962)
French philosopher

Were you admonished in no uncertain terms during your wonder years to get your head out of the clouds? Quit daydreaming? Unfortunately, so was I. It's taken me five decades to unlearn the impulse to be practical. Just imagine what you might have accomplished if only you'd been encouraged to honor your creative reveries as spiritual gifts.

Daydreams are the fertile soil in which our imaginations flourish and reach for the Light. Daydreams incubate creativity and make possible reveries, visualization, and maybe even visions. A lot of people think that daydreams are fantasies, but fantasies possess a sense of improbability and often danger. Fantasies are perfectly healthy—we all have them, especially sexual ones—and they're very therapeutic. Fantasies allow our shadows to act out our unacceptable tendencies in the safety of a protective inner hologram. Mrs. Billy Graham was once asked if she ever thought of divorcing her famous evangelist husband to whom she had been married for half a century. No, she confessed, but she'd often thought of murder.

We must enter a daydream—willingly suspend conscious thought of reality with our eyes open—before we can experience the joy of reverie. Poets, artists, writers, musicians, and scientists know that the Muse visits in reverie, even if the subject of the reverie has absolutely nothing to do with the creative project at hand. Reveries seem to be experienced through a veil, just beyond the other side of consciousness. Reveries are always pleasurable but take time. I need at least fifteen minutes of active daydreaming before I can enter the reverie zone. You'll know you've experienced one if you feel as if you've been pulled back into your body when you're snapped out of it.

Visualizations are daydreaming's virtual reality: a deliberate, positive scene-setting of what you'd like to see happen in your future. When we visualize, we make the interior scene as realistic and detailed as possible, coloring the scene with the senses until what we are viewing is so realistic it triggers an emotional response: happiness, ecstasy, joy, relief, thanksgiving.

Since the subconscious mind cannot distinguish between reality and virtual reality, deliberate visualization over a period of time usually results in the desired end. The subconscious mind is the soul's servant; it willingly sets in motion whatever behavior and circumstances are necessary to manifest physically the desired program. The pulse of the subconscious is belief. If you *truly* believe it, you'll eventually see it in your life.

Visions are Divine revelations through supernatural images. Visions are usually the province of saints, mystics, and shamans because these special people are spiritually strong enough to handle them. We can't really induce a vision, although we can invoke one through daydreams. But if you're not successful at visions, think of this as a blessing. Visions utterly, dramatically, vividly, often violently change the course of lives. You don't go back or stay in one place after you've encountered a vision. You're propelled forward in a quantum leap. Those who are able to call forth visions usually prepare themselves for the experience with days of isolation. Native Americans and indigenous people embark upon "vision quests" as ceremonial rites of passage, and while this is an ancient tradition, it's not one that readily translates into a contemporary woman's real life. There are many marvelous books available offering the wisdom of different spiritual paths, but most of them seem to have been written by people who do not have children; people who are free to travel to ashrams, convents, monasteries, power points, and sacred places where Heaven and earth meet.

But I believe with all my heart that today's woman can and must find this sacred intersection in her daily round. We've been given the spiritual tools of prayer, meditation, solitude, Gratitude, Simplicity, Order, Harmony, Beauty, Joy, and daydreams. "A dream is a scripture," the Italian novelist Umberto Eco tells us in *The Name of the Rose*. If we seek divine revelation, we'll find it, even if it occurs during a subway ride or while folding laundry.

DECEMBER 9

Nightscapes

Dreams are illustrations...from the book your soul is writing about you.
—Marsha Norman
American Pulitzer Prize–winning playwright,
screenwriter, and novelist

Last night I dreamed I was at a flea market searching for the Holy Grail, supposedly hidden in a bushel of gold, silver, and copper sugar bowls. I had just spied it when a pink porcelain vase I didn't even know I was holding shattered onto the concrete floor and I had to rush out into a thunderstorm to get the children off a beach. I'm sure there's a message encrypted in there, though I haven't had time today to figure it out. But at least I've written the dream down, so that I can seek divination when an opportunity for reflection presents itself.

While I've been on the path toward authenticity, I've experienced more Technicolor nightscapes than I'd ever previously known. We have dreams every night, though we don't always remember them. As you seek your authenticity don't be surprised if you start remembering more dreams. This is not a coincidence. We communicate our willingness for Divine revelation with daydreams, and our Authentic Self responds with a nightscape.

Our dreams are Divine stories that reveal where we've been and why, where we're headed, and the easiest way to get there. Dreams are our authentic Rosetta stones. Each night new hieroglyphics are inscribed, but instead of Egyptian, our Divine inscriptions are familiar faces, settings, objects, pursuits, dilemmas. We just need to make time to translate them. Dreams are also problem solvers. When we are perplexed about a course of action or need creative direction, we can seek Divine assistance through our dreams. Scientists, inventors, writers, and composers creatively brainstorm with their Authentic Selves in nightscapes. Beethoven and Brahms would jump out of bed in the middle of the night to write down scores. Thoreau kept a pencil and piece of paper under his pillow. Samuel Taylor Coleridge received the entire text of the poem "Kubla Khan" in a dream, and Robert Louis Stevenson worked out plot developments in *The Strange Case of Dr. Jekyll and Mr. Hyde* while dreaming.

The most informative dreams usually occur when we've gotten a good night's sleep and didn't go to bed exhausted or intoxicated. If you can't pick up a pen the moment you get out of bed because you have children, lie quietly before getting up and run the dream consciously through your mind several times so that you can remember the gist of it. If you do find time to write it down sometime during the morning, you'll be surprised that your pen will reveal details you didn't even remember. After a few hours of consciousness, however, even vivid nightscapes tend to fade back into the deep.

Carl Jung believed that all the participants in our dreams are aspects of ourselves. If that's the case, then my dream last night was a clear signal from Spirit that *Simple Abundance*—the search for my Authentic Self—is the path I need to continue following in order to become the woman I really am. But I don't think the message was meant only for me.

The Holy Grail is our authenticity. It's glimpsed hidden among what is familiar to us—home, family, work, pleasures. But what appears on the surface to be ordinary—sugar bowls—is really a treasure, because the sugar bowls are all made of precious metals. The vase that slips to the floor and shatters is who we were before we awakened to our Divinity. Our authenticity begins to emerge in our daily round, but as it does, sudden storms develop as the ego tries to frighten us back into denial. We are the little children huddling on the beach afraid to move forward. We feel alone and helpless. Then, when we look up, we see our Authentic Self rushing toward us—strong, beautiful, and brave. Gently she scoops us into her arms and reassures us there is nothing to fear. She has come to carry us to safety. To return us to Wholeness. To bring us Home.

DECEMBER 10

The Loss of Control

We are most deeply asleep at the switch when we fancy we control any switches at all.

—Annie Dillard
American Pulitzer Prize–winning author

Life is an illusion," the notorious World War I double agent Mata Hari confessed in 1917, as her eyes met a French firing squad. You know what they say about confessions on the way out: It's the truth, whether you believe it or not. Certainly, Mata Hari lived the ultimate illusion. She was all things to all men, at least until she gave herself away by assuming she had it all under control. First, she seduced French officers into divulging military secrets that she passed along to the Germans. Then she cajoled the Germans into giving her information coveted by the French. But the trouble with illusion, as the famous femme fatale discovered to her regret, is that you can't keep it up forever. Eventually it all goes up in a puff of smoke, and you might not be left standing when the smoke clears.

Illusions are the conscious mind's double agents. The ego doesn't like to think that anybody—especially the Authentic Self—can do anything better than she can. So she seduces the rational mind into believing those things that help us make it through the day—that this time he'll stop drinking, that the kid's just going through a phase, that the arguments are over money and not power, that the unworkable will work, *if you just try a little harder*. Now, maybe all of this is true. But if it's not, you're setting yourself up for the double-cross. When that subterfuge succeeds, the master illusion—the mind's Mata Hari—moves in for the kill, convincing you that life can be manipulated.

Life can't. But we can. A few weeks go smoothly, at home and work, and suddenly we secretly succumb to the lure of thinking we can control relationships or the course of events. We line everything up in perfect order so that, through sheer force of will, we'll be at the right place at the right time. But when we become addicted to thinking we can control another person's behavior or a particular outcome, we're as vulnerable as riding out a hurricane on a beach underneath an umbrella. High on determination, we assume we can handle the day, the deal, the deadline, the divorce, or the disease, if we can just keep everything under control. When we can't, we spin dangerously *out of control* and into a nosedive. As Melanie Beattie reminds us in *The Language of Letting Go*: "Whatever we try to control does have control over us and our life."

And while we might walk away from the wreck, we're often more upset by the loss of the illusion than by the reality of the rubble. The good news is that we can pick up the pieces and salvage the best of a bad situation, but only after we become aware that we have unconsciously betrayed ourselves.

You can never lose something if you never had it to begin with. You were never in control and never will be. Let go of that illusion so that you can cut your losses and move on. Acceptance of the inevitable—as difficult and painful it might be today—is the first step toward an authentic trade-off. "We trade a life that we have tried to control," Melanie Beattie reassures us, "and we receive in return something better—a life that is manageable."

DECEMBER 11

Sigh Some More, My Ladies, Sigh Some More

Most of the sighs we hear have been edited.
—Stanislaw Jerzy Lec (1909–1966)
Polish poet

I have a habit that used to drive my former husband crazy. But it keeps me sane.

I sigh.

Obviously, I sigh more than I am consciously aware of. Yet I began noticing that whenever my sighing was brought to my attention—*"Please don't do that"*—I'm taking deep breaths for a very good reason.

Women sigh so that we won't scream. There are several occasions in the course of any woman's day when, without question, screaming is the appropriate response. However, on this side of an electrified fence, screaming is not considered good form.

So we sigh.

First, we breathe in, quickly and sharply, inhaling reality, acknowledging the present situation—the current hassle or disappointment, confrontation or challenge, long wait or lack of cooperation.

We hold our breath for a heartbeat.

Then we breathe out, slowly and deeply, exhaling and letting go of our initial response—our dismay, impatience, frustration, annoyance, disappointment, regret. Letting it out. Letting it go.

The act of sighing is a quiet nod of acknowledgment—of "getting over it," so as to move on.

Women with significant others and/or children sigh more than their solitary sisters because there are more preferences, needs, wants, wills, and demands to be dealt with, especially if there is to be a state of detente in the daily round. More bending in order not to break.

So should you feel the need to sigh today, by all means breathe slowly and deeply. Breathe expressively. Think of sighing as the hot air that makes rising to the occasion possible. Hot air that's pent up will eventually explode, and steam can burn. But steam that's deliberately allowed to escape through a safety valve can be converted into creative energy. Sigh without hesitation. Sigh without guilt. Sigh without embarrassment. Sigh with pleasure.

Sigh some more, my ladies, sigh some more.

DECEMBER 12

Are Women Human?

We are not human beings trying to be spiritual.
We are spiritual beings trying to be human.

—Jacquelyn Small
British psychologist and author

Whether women were human fascinated the English writer D. H. Lawrence, who often explored this conundrum in his work. "Man is willing to accept woman as an equal, as a man in skirts, as an angel, a devil, a baby-face, a machine, an instrument, a bosom, a womb, a pair of legs, a servant, an encyclopedia, an ideal or an obscenity; the one thing he won't accept her as is a human being, a real human being of the feminine sex."

Perhaps the reason men find it so difficult to accept women as human beings is because we're not, and deep down everyone knows it. But often women forget their Divinity as they go about their daily round. How often do we excuse ourselves with the expression, "Well, I'm only human."

No, you're not, I must remind myself this morning, even as a website asks for me to confirm my humanity by identifying all the crosswalks in a group of photographs. I've not got the emotional bandwidth for this nonsense today.

I certainly forgot I was a spiritual being the morning my daughter stayed home from school because she was sick. *Again.* I knew that, in a little while, I'd have to take her to the doctor for a strep test and my entire work day would be upended. I was frustrated and annoyed; not at my girl—at real life, at deadlines, at too little help and too much to do. But did she realize that, when I rolled my eyes at the thought of another day gone awry? I don't think so.

Spiritual beings know that most of what drives humans crazy in real life *is* small stuff, irritations and inconvenience rather than calamities.

A spiritual being knows that the work will be waiting for her when she gets back from the doctor's office. A spiritual being knows that there is no such thing as a deadline. Deadlines are *chronos*, the world's time; Divinity knows only *kairos*, eternity. The deadline will be met if I remember to ask for grace. A spiritual being knows that the only thing that's not small stuff is caring for and comforting a sick child.

This spiritual being might have also known that the morning her daughter was ill, if she'd taken five minutes to center herself.

The Old Testament tells us that men were created a little above the angels. But don't ever forget that women were the climax of the Spirit's creativity cycle. After woman was created, Wisdom realized there was no need to proceed further: this superior being would save the world.

Big things are expected of us.

We better be about it. We need to take care of ourselves so we have the strength and the patience to care for who and what we love.

As for me, there was a lost heart that needed to be comforted by an aspiring spiritual being who answers to "Mom." So if you're asked today to confirm your humanity, why not claim your Divinity?

DECEMBER 13

The Time of Your Life

Yours is the year that
Counts no season
I can never be sure
What age you are.

—Vita Sackville-West, Lady Nicholson (1892–1962)
English novelist, poet, and garden designer

Writers are always nervous when a potential new reader picks up their book for the first time, in front of you, especially at a book event.

When *Simple Abundance* was first published, I noticed this happening, quite often, at my signings. Women flipping pages, reading and breaking into grins. Then a nod to another women, all very conspiratorial using that code of facial expressions that girlfriends have used with each other since time began. Since *SA* was new, it was all a great mystery to me. What passage could possibly spark the same reaction from each reader? Finally, my curiosity got the better of me. I asked a few women what reflection they were discussing: "Oh, my birthday. And you know what? It's just perfect. That's where I am, or who I am…Or where I want to be…How did you know?"

I guess I knew because I'm you and you're me. Feminine eternal twins separated at birth. And I'm so happy and grateful we found each other at last, even if it's just on the page.

Most birthdays are fun, at least when you're little or have littles of your own to plan for. I mean, you wake up and everybody makes a fuss over you and gives you presents and cake. Then, abruptly your mother announces that you're too old to have a birthday party (I think that was at thirteen)—until the marker ones start coming along: sixteen, eighteen, twenty-one, twenty-five, thirty, thirty-five, forty, fifty, sixty, sixty-five, seventy, seventy-five, eighty, eighty-five, ninety, ninety-five, and one hundred. After the century mark, birthday parties once again become annual events. Well, I'm aiming for that century milestone. It will probably take me that long to figure out what the blazes I'm supposed to be doing with my life.

My mother gave amazing birthday parties for her four children, and my sister and I certainly tried to live up to her in that regard. When my daughter was little, the planning for hers began months in advance. This was during the 1980s, when "theme" or destination birthday parties were all the rage: dance studio, decorate your own pottery, tea at the Dollhouse Museum, pony rides, swimming, bowling, ice-skating, and weekend-long sleep-overs. And the goody bags!

Are we having fun yet?

We could tell when the party was over because the birthday girl would eventually dissolve into tears brought on by excitement, exhaustion, too much sugar, and expectations exceeding what's humanly possible. Then her mother would gratefully sigh, "Done, for another year!"

Well, this year I have officially become *la femme d'un certain age.* For women of a certain age, birthdays need to become like sacraments, and I mean this sincerely.

But here's the catch. You are the only person on earth capable of giving yourself the birthday ritual you deserve—one that is nurturing with genuine indulgences, well-spent moments, joyful simplicities, contemplation, closure, beauty, and celebration. Many people who love you will try, but no one can celebrate your birthday exactly the way you need for it to be observed.

That's because no one else truly knows the year you've just completed; no one else has lived through every day of it. But you have. You know what you have endured in silence. You know the desperate prayers. You know the inexpressible gratitude your soul feels after surviving a crisis. What's more, each year in our life is different. Your thirty-second, forty-eighth, fifty-ninth, sixty-fourth, and sixty-ninth birthdays won't begin to even resemble the previous ones.

Your spouse, partner, lover, children, friends, and coworkers can be aware of recent events that have unfolded in your life, but only Heaven and your soul know how deeply these events reverberated in, around, and through you. Perhaps a loved one has died, or a relationship has become estranged; perhaps a child has moved, or a cherished job was eliminated. Perhaps you're still reeling from a diagnosis for either yourself or a loved one, and your days are filled with uncertainty and nights with dread; perhaps the financial crisis never ended for you and you don't know how to replace the future you were planning and counting on. The shock of your own peculiar and particular losses, the navigation of the terra nova you find yourself in must be acknowledged before it can be accepted, traversed, and explored.

Maybe you need, not a boisterous family party, but a few private hours or days to remember and to honor the sacredness of change and transitions. Birthdays are not only new beginnings, they are also moments of personal closure, which are crucial if we are to grow positively into our authenticity.

Every birthday, not just the public "markers," is a significant milestone. Every age brings with it the hope of three hundred sixty-five Real Life lessons in loving, risking, surviving, overcoming, hope, and joy. "We turn, not older with years, but newer every day," Emily Dickinson reassures the birthday girl in all of us. And that is certainly something worth celebrating and giving thanks for. So if your birthday is today, tomorrow, or later this year, happy birthday! Happy birthday to you!

I've got a good feeling about this coming year—and I think it's going to be our best yet. Heaven knows, we certainly deserve a birthday for the books!

DECEMBER 14

Gold-Star Days

*Maybe one of these days I'll be able to give myself a gold star for
being ordinary, and maybe one of these days I'll give myself a gold
star for being extraordinary—for persisting. And maybe one day I
won't need to have a star at all.*

—Sue Bender
American author, ceramic artist, and lecturer

I haven't yet gotten to the point where I don't need gold stars: gleaming, golden, five-pointed proof that I've accomplished something that was a bit of a stretch, especially if it was remembering to treat myself with the loving-kindness that seems so much easier to give to others.

Back in the days of blackboards and chalk, gold stars came in a small cardboard box. You'd take the lid off to find five hundred gold, paper-foil stars, stiff with dry glue backs. Running your fingers through the small pile of possibilities, you'd hear the rustling of self-worth. Nowadays gold stars get pulled off self-sticking sheets. You don't even get the taste of success on your tongue, but I love them just the same.

A good friend of mine has a different memory of gold-star days. Her mother kept star charts for each of her eight children. Every Sunday night after dinner, the past week's reckoning would occur in the dining room as the gridded charts revealed who had excelled at homework, chores, personal hygiene, and behavior—and who hadn't. The striving for gold stars was supposed to be a motivational game. However, accumulating gold stars under duress wasn't fun for Anne, despite the fact that she excelled at everything and was a model "good girl." For her, the pressure of constant evaluation was excruciating. Opening the cardboard box was a psychological and emotional stretching on the rack of self-respect.

But gold-star days are *very* different when we give them to ourselves. When you give yourself a gold star, sticking it to an empty calendar block, the star twinkles, winks, and whispers, "Good for you, girl!" I particularly like to give myself gold stars when I'm embarking on a new self-nurturing pastime or reviving one that has fallen by the wayside: walking, creative movement, healthy eating, playing hooky, taking a nap, meditation, slowing down, balancing work and play. The spirit may be willing, but all too often the flesh gets sidetracked.

The extraordinary days in our lives don't need gold stars. But ordinary days sure can be brighter with a shiny, five-pointed pat on the back.

Joy to the Girl

Gloom we have always with us, a rank and sturdy weed, but joy requires tending.

—Barbara Holland (1933–2010)
American author

And we're off, as a sprinter to a starter pistol, for the holiday season. This is the week that women's shoulders begin to droop as their list of festive should-dos becomes as long and heavy as Jacob Marley's chains. There's card writing, card mailing, gift buying, gift wrapping, gift sending, tree buying, tree trimming, cookie baking, party giving, turkey roasting. By next week, unless a Power greater than ourselves restores us to sanity, women will be dropping in their tracks. Not surprisingly, the holidays are the height of the flu season. It makes any sane person want to take a pass, but let's get serious, could that ever really be an option? Didn't think so. In anticipation, perhaps you try to jolly yourself by buying all your favorite magazines, which display picture-perfect Christmas spreads that simultaneously excite and then diminish your Spirit before you even turn the page.

No one used to love curling up with a fresh pile of monthly magazines and a glass of cheer better than I, but I have given them up, especially the "Best Christmas Ever" editions, in an annual pursuit of sacred self-nurturance. Why? Because I know, from personal experience, that they are not true. And that is why I feel I must bring a little full disclosure and "Joy to the Girl," and that girl is you.

"Christmas comes but once a year. Don't ever say that to a cookery journalist," the renowned English food writer Elizabeth David (1913–1992) begins her classic holiday essay collection *Elizabeth David's Christmas*.

"Cookery journalists know different. For them, three times a year would be nearer the mark. First, around mid-August, when they must work on the recipes, at any rate if they contribute to a glossy monthly. There'll probably be color photographs to cook for and supervise as well. The next round comes about the end of September when the articles have to be written and something original—well, anyway, different from last year—dredged up in the way of advice about when it's all cooked for real, although not without notes being made for next year's stint. In between the delivery of the monthly article there will almost certainly be another couple of Christmas pieces to write, for a weekly, a wine merchant's newsletter, a Sunday, a daily."

I must confess that annually rereading Elizabeth's depiction of

Christmas through the New Year is one of my favorite holiday rituals, because her ironic and truthful insights always trigger a smile and nod in agreement to this ultimate confession:

"If here and there in my account of a cookery journalist's Christmas a note of desperation is clearly audible, I don't make apologies. Christmas, at any rate, the way we are supposed to celebrate it nowadays, does tend to unbalance people, particularly those people responsible for the catering, the cooking, the presents, the tree, the decorations... the frantic shoppers in the stores,... the season of the Great Too Much... [which has] also become the Great Too Long. A ten-day shutdown, no less, is now normal at Christmas."

There we have it in a gilded nutshell game: the season of the Great Too Much for Great Too Long. Not to worry. Doesn't it feel good just to acknowledge the truth?

Back to those glossy magazines: Is there a woman with soul so dead that never to herself hath said, "I wish my life could look like it was out of a magazine." Well, it can, darling, if you have a home décor stylist, a wardrobe and prop stylist, a hair and makeup artist, a photographer, and a slew of assistants, for a two-day shoot that will appear as a spontaneous Christmas article next year. I've been very flattered to have been featured in two glossy Christmas magazine spreads, and while it is fun to gaze back in astonished amusement, I've always felt that, rather like the signs on rearview mirrors that read "objects may appear larger than they really are," those glossy magazines should come with the warning, "No perfect lifestyle pictured in this month's issue is real."

The celebration of Christmas as we know it today, with its whirl of festivity, decorations, lavish gifts, parties, and family-centered traditions, was a creation of middle-class Victorians in both England and the United States in the mid-nineteenth century. Victorian women, who were full-time homebodies, began "doing" Christmas in July. However, since the final two decades of the twentieth century, women have been doing lots of other things while we're doing Christmas. Which is why we end up doing ourselves in every December. For many women, this is the season of misery and angst: tears, tantrums, screaming, yelling, hustle, bustle, cash conflicts, royal pain relations, and holiday humbug.

Wouldn't the real Christmas miracle be if we slowed down long enough to remember the reason for the season, so that our holiday celebrations became authentic and meaningful?

So be of good cheer. Be not frazzled, frustrated, nor frantic, for I bring you tidings of comfort and joy. If *you* do Christmas at your house, you can choose to do it your way. Whatever that way might be. You *can* consciously decide to be happy, loving, fulfilled, generous, peaceful, contented, spiritual, joyous, calm, festive, and emotionally connected to the important people in your life for the holidays this year.

Or you can, unconsciously, choose to be a wreck.

Today, *realize* that you can't do everything. Not all at once. Not in the next ten days. Not at all. Period.

Now, *recognize* that one of the reasons Christmases past probably didn't live up to your expectations is that you've tried to do too much, too perfectly.

Look at that list.

Choose to let only what you love best about the holidays remain. Cross out two more "musts." Now there's time for gazing out the window at gently falling snow, delighting in the sounds of bells and joyful music, savoring the sweet aromas of hot cider, roast turkey, and gingerbread, sipping hot chocolate and homemade eggnog, reading a holiday story each night at dusk, basking in a fire crackling on the hearth, and re-creating cherished customs that care for your soul as well as the souls of those you love.

"I do hope your Christmas has...a little touch of Eternity in among the rush and pitter patter and all," the English mystic Evelyn Underhill recommends. "It always seems such a mixing of this world and the next—but that, after all, is the idea!"

DECEMBER 16

Gifts of the Magi

Christmas won't be Christmas without any presents.
—Jo March in *Little Women* by Louisa May Alcott

Jo's right. Remember when she grumbled about not having any money for presents in *Little Women*?

Christmas is about gifts.

Always has been. But we feel uncomfortable with this emphasis on gimme, gimme, gimme. Buy, buy, buy. Charge, charge, charge. We admonish our children to remember the reason for the season, even though we have difficulty remembering it ourselves when we're caught up in the chaos and commotion of the holidays.

Today let's ruminate on the real role of gifts in the Christmas story. Those gifts were wrapped in miracles, which is probably why we can't find them online or in gigantic box stores.

The first gift was of Spirit: unconditional Love. The next gift came from a Jewish teenager named Miriam, who was known to her family and friends as Mary. Her Christmas present was selflessness, the complete surrender of ego and will needed to bring Heaven down to earth. The gifts of her fiancé, Joseph, were trust and faith. He trusted that Mary wasn't pregnant with another man's child; he believed there really was a Divine Plan to get them through this mess. The Child brought forgiveness. Wholeness. Second chances. Third chances. As many chances as you need.

The angels' gifts were tidings of comfort, joy, and peace, the reassurance that there was nothing to fear, so rejoice. The shepherd boy's gift was generosity: his favorite lamb for the baby's birthday present. The innkeeper's wife's gifts were compassion and charity: a warm, dry, safe place for the homeless family to stay, her best coverlet to wrap the new mother and little one, a meal for Joseph, the donkey's fresh hay.

Three kings from the east traveled many hot, dusty miles following a bright star in search of a royal birth. The sages' divination foretold the coming of the "King of Kings"; on their camels' backs were treasures with which to honor his arrival. But when they arrived in Bethlehem, they found the newborn prince in a cow stall instead of a palace. The shocked Wise Men unwrapped gold, frankincense, and myrrh, but their Real gifts were wonder, acceptance, and courage. They offered wonder by surrendering logic, reason, and common sense. Accepting the impossible, they suspended skepticism long enough to double-cross the insane King Herod, frantically searching for the child who would change the world. With courage—at the risk of their own lives—the Wise Men helped the young family escape to a safe haven in Egypt.

Oh, yes. Christmas *is* all about gifts. Nothing but gifts. But such gifts! Gifts tied with heartstrings. Gifts that surprise and delight. Gifts that transform the mundane into the miraculous. Gifts that nurture the souls of both the giver and the given. Perfect gifts. Authentic gifts. The gifts of Spirit, a frightened teenage girl, her bewildered sweetheart, the Child, the angels, the shepherd boy, the innkeeper's wife. The gifts of the magi.

Unconditional Love. Selflessness. Trust. Faith.
Forgiveness. Wholeness. Second Chances. Comfort. Joy.
Peace. Reassurance. Rejoicing. Generosity. Compassion.
Charity. Wonder. Acceptance. Courage.

To give such gifts. To truly open our hearts to receive such gifts gratefully.

Christmas just won't be Christmas without any presents.

A Partridge in a Pear Tree

While we are all so wrapped up in the presents we are giving to gladden hearts at Christmastime, we might pause to think of that other side of giving that means much more in every home—the giving of ourselves. The Christmas Present, after all, is only a token of our feelings, and more important are the daily contributions we each make to the happiness of those near us.
—House and Garden, *December 1938*

I don't think many of our true loves are waiting with bated breath for a partridge in a pear tree this year. But I do know a one-size-fits-all gift that would be absolutely thrilling for everyone on your list: the gift of yourself. Unfortunately, this most personal gift is very expensive, for it requires large expenditures of our precious, but dwindling, natural resources. Time. Creative Energy. Emotion. It would be far easier to give everyone two turtle doves and be done with it.

This doesn't mean that we don't want to give of ourselves during the holidays. That's what we're desperately trying to do. Obviously, we're not doing it very well. Which is why many of us end up feeling depressed and discouraged as we pack away the ornaments. How did Christmas slip out of our grasp *again*?

Because we were holding too many things at once: obligations, promises, should-dos, conflicting commitments. "Oh, sure, no problem" is the first symptom of the discombobulated mind.

First thing: Excuse yourself from every evening meeting for the rest of the month. Only accept social events that you *really* want to attend. Your absence might be noticed any other time of the year, but not during the holidays. Everybody's focus is as scattered as yours. You'll not be missed.

Now about those gifts. All those bright, pretty baubles blowing your budget are only symbols of the gifts you really long to give. So this year why don't you try to give them the right stuff?

On the first day of Christmas, I gave to my true loves:
The gift of my Undivided Attention

On the second day of Christmas, I gave to my true loves:
The gift of Enthusiasm

On the third day of Christmas, I gave to my true loves:
The gift of Creative Energy

On the fourth day of Christmas, I gave to my true loves:
The gift of Simple Seasonal Pleasures

On the fifth day of Christmas, I gave to my true loves:
The gift of Tenderness

On the sixth day of Christmas, I gave to my true loves:
The gift of Good Cheer

On the seventh day of Christmas, I gave to my true loves:
The gift of Beauty

On the eighth day of Christmas, I gave to my true loves:
The gift of Communication

On the ninth day of Christmas, I gave to my true loves:
The gift of Surprise

On the tenth day of Christmas, I gave to my true loves:
The gift of Wonder

On the eleventh day of Christmas, I gave to my true loves:
The gift of Peaceful Surroundings

On the twelfth day of Christmas, I gave to my true loves:
The gift of Joy

"Be ready at all times for the gifts of God, and always for new ones," the thirteenth-century German mystic Meister Eckhart urges us in this season of giving. Be ready at all times to give those you love the simply abundant gifts of Spirit. If you do, they'll give you Christmas gifts you'll never forget: happy smiles and contented hearts. And you won't want to exchange them.

DECEMBER 18

The Spirit of Mother Christmas

Twenty-five years ago, Christmas was not the burden that it is now; there was less haggling and weighing, less quid pro quo, less fatigue of body, less weariness of soul; and, most of all, there was less loading up with trash.
—Margaret Deland (1857–1945)
American novelist, short story writer, and poet

Pause for a moment and take in with a big breath, laugh, or both, Margaret Deland's staggering observation of the Victorian Christmas. This was written in *1904*, over a century ago, and she was throwing up her hands while grabbing her pen.

What was Christmas to Margaret and her generation of women? A burden? Haggling? Fatigue? Weariness of soul? Loading up with trash? God bless Margaret. If she were to arrive with the Spirit of Christmas Past to visit our Christmas Yet to Come, she'd think she was waking up to the Nightmare Before Christmas.

I think women veer between two extremes during the holiday season: blessed Hildegard of Bingen and Auntie Mame. One minute we're performing saintly acts of will as we plow through that formidable to-do list by the power of Grace, and the next we're trying to fit into that red sequined dress to deck the halls and be merry about it if it kills us.

I'm not quite sure how it happened, but I've misplaced at least a week. Somehow, I've run out of everything—time, creative energy, emotional bandwidth, and budget. However, hasn't this become your typical approach to Christmas—so exhausted and drained that all that can save you is a miracle? A miracle so gigantic you can't even conceive of it. That's what I'm believing in.

Let's return again to the subject of my favorite holiday meditation. The first Christmas unfolded the way it did because, one ancient night, a tired and harried innkeeper's wife stopped long enough to be moved by the power of Love. She improvised so that a frightened, unmarried teenage girl about to give birth to her first child could be comforted. And in so doing she midwifed a miracle that would change the world forever. Forgive me, if you must, but may I gently point out that on the first Christmas Eve, God the Father was in Heaven. God the Great Mother was on earth. In my heart, I see the older woman leaving the crowded, rowdy dining room and rushing up the stairs to her bedroom, opening up a trunk, and bringing forth her best, making sure that all she had would be all the mother and baby would need. She gathers in her arms linen and silk, the blankets from her own bed, her favorite shawl.

In my imagination, I can also see the young woman's thankful smile, hear her sigh of relief, taste the salt in her tears. I smell not only the barn, but the aroma of the broth the older woman helped the younger sip to keep up her strength. As I hug my own daughter, I can feel the reassurance both women felt in each other's presence. I know that the older woman's sacred gift of generosity and the younger woman's gratitude are not insignificant footnotes to what has been called the Greatest Story Ever Told. It's how the Wonder unfolded.

Sometimes women need a gentle reminder when to take a break and a breather, so I thought I'd send a little prayer for both of us.

Blessed Mother Courage, Weaver of Dreams, Spirit of Christmas, hush the harried heart of your Beloved, and hear her sighs this eventide. Please gift this sweet woman with a respite from all her crises—both the big challenges that overwhelm her and the little things that gnaw at her strength. As the shadows lengthen, let her sorrows disappear and fears fade. Gentle Shepherdess who watches over all her lambs, no matter where they may have wandered, let her not be restless, wakeful, in danger or despair. Soothe her frazzled mind and brush from her brow the cares she has courageously carried for others for so long.

Ransom, retrieve, and return to her the strayed or shattered and scattered parts of her soul. Restore in this night's reveries her grace, repose, and good humor. Replenish her energy consumed by overwork and good intentions. Stretch her purse even as you expand her Spirit with the true meaning and wealth of this blessed season. Infuse her with endless patience and boundless enthusiasm for all the tasks she must complete to ensure that those in her care are well provided for this Christmas, Hanukkah, and Kwanzaa.

As she snuggles down in the Simple Abundance *you have set apart for her, wrap her in comfort and tuck her in safety. Bless, protect, and preserve all she loves, especially those darlings whose safety she worries about, and keep watch over her until the darkness dissipates. And when the miracle of morning arrives, awaken her at first Light, with the deep knowledge that all will be well, even if it is different than she expected.*

May this blessed woman know that all her efforts are not, nor ever have been, in vain. To this we offer Heaven the deepest gratitude our hearts can express.

Amen. And so it is.

May you find an unexpected blessing in today's gifts of Divine Strength, Wisdom, and Grace, wrapped most assuredly in brown paper and string.

DECEMBER 19

Becoming Real

Once you are Real you can't become unreal again. It lasts for always.

—Margery Williams (1881–1944)
English-American Newbery Medal–winning
author

On Christmas morning the bunny sitting in the top of the boy's stocking with a sprig of holly between his paws looked quite splendid. He was fat and bunchy in all the right places, with a soft, spotted white-and-brown coat, thread whiskers, and ears lined in pink sateen. The boy was enchanted and played with the rabbit for two whole hours until the family directed his attention to all the other wonderful parcels lying under the tree "and in the excitement of looking at all the new presents the Velveteen Rabbit [was] forgotten."

For a long time, the bunny remained just another plaything in the nursery. But he didn't mind because he was able to carry on long, philosophical discussions with the old Skin Horse who was very old, wise, and experienced in the strange ways of nursery magic. One of the rabbit's favorite topics of conversation was on becoming "Real." Here is the heart of Margery Williams's mystical tale of the transformative power of love, *The Velveteen Rabbit*, written in 1927.

The Skin Horse patiently explained to the bunny, "Real isn't how you are made. It's a thing that happens to you. When a child loves you for a long, long time, not just to play with, but REALLY loves you, then you become Real."

Becoming Real doesn't happen overnight to toys or people. "Generally, by the time you are Real, most of your hair has been loved off, and your eyes drop out and you get loose in the joints and very shabby. But these things don't matter at all, because once you are Real, you can't be ugly, except to people who don't understand."

In order for toys to become Real, they must be loved by a child. In order for us to become Real, we must become lovers of real life in all its complexity and uncertainty. Like the Velveteen Rabbit, we long to become Real, to know what authenticity feels like. Sometimes this hurts. The thought of losing our whiskers and having our tail come unsewn is frightening. In a world that judges by appearances, it's embarrassing having all the pink rubbed off your nose. The Velveteen Rabbit isn't alone in wishing to become Real without any uncomfortable or unpleasant things happening.

One of the ways that we become Real without too much discomfort is by growing gradually into our authenticity. As you learn to acknowledge, accept, and appreciate what it is that makes you different from all the other toys in the cupboard, the process begins. As you learn to trust the wisdom of your heart and make creative choices based on what you know is right for you, process becomes progress. As you learn to endow even the smallest moment of each day with Love, progress becomes reality perfected. Your black-button eyes might have lost their polish, but now these windows to the soul see only beauty. You become not only Real to those who know and love you, but Real to everyone. You become authentic.

The Winter Solstice

*The Winter Solstice is the time of ending and beginning, a power-
ful time—a time to contemplate your immortality. A time to forgive, to be forgiven, and to make a fresh start. A time to awaken.*
—Frederick Lenz (1950–1998)
American Buddhist teacher

In ancient times, as the days grew shorter and darker, people became increasingly anxious and depressed, fearing that the sun was dying. Without the sun, whom they worshipped as a god, people knew they would perish. In order to coax back the source of their warmth, light, and abundance they created midwinter rituals, culminating in a great festival at the Winter Solstice, on or about December 21–22, the longest night of the year. The women would gather greenery to decorate dwellings and prepare elaborate communal feasts. The men would light huge bonfires; in the bright glow of the flames representing the energy of the sun, they would hold revels with music and dance.

Today, celebrating the Winter Solstice is becoming very popular. For people who don't feel comfortable with organized religion or even with exploring an individual spiritual path, honoring the festivals of the natural world fulfills a deep, primordial need to connect with a Power greater than humanity, no matter what that Power is called. Women reviving the ancient feminine traditions celebrate the Solstice as the birthday of the Great Mother. Ecology-minded people, such as many Native Americans, honor the sacredness of their connection with the earth. Women who have interfaith marriages and can't make a choice between celebrating Hanukkah and Christmas often view the Winter Solstice as a neutral holiday the whole family can celebrate.

One meaningful way to celebrate the Solstice is to consider it a sacred time of reflection, release, restoration, and renewal. "Winter is the time for comfort, for good food and warmth," the English writer Dame Edith Sitwell reminds us, "for the touch of a friendly hand and for a talk beside the first. It is the time for home." The Winter Solstice is also the time to send reconciliation notes to heal a breach, a longtime family dispute that no one can remember how or why it started, and to send that apology you've been writing in your heart for so long. Or a card that simply tells someone how much they are missed. It's the season. For a reason.

DECEMBER 21

Seasonal Soul-Craft

Live in each season as it passes; breathe air, drink the drink, taste the fruit, and resign yourself to the influences of each.
Let them be your only diet drink and botanical medicines.
—Henry David Thoreau (1817–1862)
American philosopher and author

The winter air outside is thin and bracing: sharp, frigid, icy, stinging. We do not saunter; the pace of our steps is quick, mirroring on the outside the accelerated forward motion within as holiday preparations take center stage. Once we close the door, the winter air is warm, heavy, and aromatic: wood burning, fresh evergreens, spicy cinnamon and ginger. Breathe in deeply the fragrance of contentment.

In winter we live in anticipation. Friends come in from the cold to be embraced by the convivial chaos of our family's annual holiday open house. "All year long I dream about your homemade eggnog," a guest confides as soulful gifts are exchanged: heartfelt compliments and a cup of cheer. In the kitchen, frothy hot wassail—spiced cider and dark English ale— is ladled into cups, ransoming hands and hearts from winter's chill. The dining room table groans good-naturedly from the bounty of abundance: roast turkey, baked ham, cheeses, fresh breads. Children of all ages crowd around seasonal sweets and winter's fruits: candy canes and sugarplums; pumpkin, mince, and apple pies.

Souls, sip and savor. Take thine ease. Eat, drink, and be merry in this season of joy.

"The most ancient spiritual wisdom was centered around the predictable shifts in seasonal energies. Rituals revolved around sowing, reaping and the cycles of light and darkness," Joan Borysenko, the respected scientist, gifted therapist, and unabashed mystic, reminds us in her tiny contemplative jewel, *Pocketful of Miracles: Prayers, Meditations, and Affirmations to Nurture Your Spirit Every Day of the Year.* "The seasonal rhythms correlate with our bodily rhythms...Our dream life and inner life grow more insistent in the winter darkness... The old year is put to bed, one's business is finished, and the harvest of spiritual maturity is reaped as wisdom and forgiveness."

For centuries, Eastern healers—particularly practitioners of Chinese medicine—have taken into consideration the impact the seasons have on our bodies, minds, and souls. But the symbiotic relationship between human beings and nature has virtually been ignored by Western medicine until recently. Now physicians acknowledge that some people suffer from a deep depression in the winter because they're extremely sensitive to darkness. Light therapy restores their subtle energies to a healthy balance.

Learning the soul-craft of seasonal healing can bring new depth to our journey toward Wholeness. In the natural world, winter is the season of rest, restoration, and reflection. There's not much of that going on this week, but after the holidays are behind us, consider how you spend whatever time you have at your personal disposal. And if you have as little as I think you do, reflect on how you can change that next year.

The twelfth-century German mystic Hildegard of Bingen suggests a simple way for us to begin exploring the richness of seasonal soul-craft:

> *Glance at the sun.*
> *See the moon and the stars.*
> *Gaze at the beauty of earth's greenings.*
> *Now, think.*

DECEMBER 22

The Festival of Lights

They carried their land upon their shoulders
And their sanctuary in their hearts.

—Jessie Sampter (1883–1938)
Jewish educator and poet

In the dark days of December comes the wonderful holiday of Hanukkah, celebrated in Jewish homes. Originally known as the "Festival of Lights," Hanukkah commemorates a miracle that occurred in 165 B.C., after Judas Maccabeus and his followers reclaimed Jerusalem from a Greek emperor who considered Israel a Greek province.

In an attempt to assimilate conquered nations into a cohesive and controllable society, the Greek empire prohibited any other religion; Jews were forced to abandon their faith and ordered to worship Greek gods. By decree, the Temple of Jerusalem was turned into a Greek shrine, and Jews were forbidden to study the Torah, celebrate their holidays, or practice Jewish customs. Many Jews, disobeying the edict, died for their beliefs. After a three-year guerrilla campaign, the Maccabees were victorious, and the temple was restored to Jewish worship. As part of their rededication ceremony (the word "Hanukkah" means dedication) the Maccabees began an eight-day purification rite, only to discover there was barely enough sacred oil to keep the temple *menorah*—a candelabrum with eight branches—lit for one day. Miraculously, the temple lamp burned continuously for eight days. Ever since that time the Jewish people have observed Hanukkah in remembrance of their struggle for religious freedom and the miracle of restoration, symbolized by the abundance of oil.

Many who celebrate Christmas believe that Hanukkah is a festival reserved solely for those who practice Judaism. But as Rabbi Harold Kushner points out in his enlightening and engaging meditation *To Life: A Celebration of Jewish Being and Thinking*, if it weren't for Hanukkah, we wouldn't be celebrating Christmas. Had the Maccabees not rebelled against the Greeks, the Jewish faith would have faded into Greek culture, never to be heard of again. "There would have been no Jewish community for Jesus to be born into a century and a half later. No one would have remembered the messianic promises he claimed to fulfill. Without Hanukkah, there would have been no Christmas."

When one follows any family tree back far enough, there are bound to be surprises. And those who follow the Christian path will discover, if they truly search for their roots, that by faith we belong to the House of David. Jesus lived his entire life as an observant Jew. He celebrated Hanukkah as a child; the Last Supper was a Passover Seder. All the apostles and most of those who became his early followers were Jewish. The crowds who came to hear Jesus preach called him "Rabbi," the Hebrew word for teacher. Perhaps our similarities and heritage are greater than our differences after all.

Personally, I've come to think of Hanukkah as a celebration of authenticity. The Maccabees refused to surrender what made them authentic—their faith—even if it cost them their lives. Not to be able to live as observant Jews was not to live at all. I also consider the Hanukkah miracle the earliest recorded demonstration of *Simple Abundance*. Two thousand years ago there was only enough sacred oil for one night. But all that these faithful, courageous, and grateful people had *was all that they needed*.

Sacred oil in a temple. Loaves and fishes on a mountainside. Miracles are of Spirit, not any one faith. Miracles are for anyone who believes. That is the heart of Hanukkah and the soul of Christmas. The more we allow ourselves to recognize the wisdom and truth in other spiritual paths, the closer to Wholeness we become.

It's a Wonderful Life

*Instead of the usual "Why can't we make movies more like real
life?" I think a more pertinent question is "Why can't real life be
more like the movies?"*

> —Ernie Pyle (1900–1945)
> American Pulitzer Prize–winning war
> correspondent

Some holiday traditions are sacred. In our house one such tradition is
the annual Christmas classic cinema celebration. Over the course of a
week, as we hang stockings, wrap packages, and munch more popcorn
than we string, we watch *White Christmas, Holiday Inn, Christmas
in Connecticut, The Bishop's Wife, Miracle on 34th Street, National
Lampoon's Christmas Vacation, A Christmas Story, A Muppet Christmas Carol,* and, of course, *It's a Wonderful Life,* the fabulous three-
hanky film fable starring James Stewart and Donna Reed. After nearly
fifty holiday seasons, its potent alchemy of idealism and irony still con-
jures up movie magic.

In 1946, Frank Capra had no idea his sentimental small-town fantasy would become a seasonal favorite for the ages. "In its own icky
bittersweet way, it's terribly effective," *The New Yorker* begrudgingly
conceded. It's Christmas Eve, the night of miracles, and George Bailey
certainly needs one. After a lifetime of saving the lives of others, he's
giving up on his. He's broke, disgraced, facing prison, and in despair
over a savings and loan shortage that is truly not his fault. After angrily
wishing he'd never been born, he's about to jump off a bridge, when
he's rescued by his guardian angel, Clarence Oddbody, who temporarily grants his wish by showing him what the world would have been like
without his authentic contribution.

George believes he's never had a lucky break. But when he steps back
to reconsider his choices, he realizes they were the right ones. He's also
a rich man: He has a loving and supportive wife, healthy children, work
that makes a difference, and more friends than his house can even hold
at one time. Quite frankly, it's a wonderful life he was about to throw
away.

We can discover just how wonderful our lives are—exactly as they
are right at this moment—by doing what George did (without the
bridge scene!). We can step back and take another look at our lives and
the lives we've touched. One of the unexpected blessings of writing
this book is that I've gone back over the ordinary moments of my life,
mining them for meaning. Writing a meditation around an encounter,

mistake, regret, or conversation is very revealing and intimate—even more so than is keeping a journal. Every day in the five years it has taken me to write *Simple Abundance*, I've had a topic to muse upon, usually a title, often a quote, but always a blank page. Most of the time I've found out what I was writing about only after I was well into it. And what I've discovered—as you can—is that I've enjoyed a wonderful life. That knowledge has resonated deep within me, and I'm truly grateful. Obviously, there are many things I wish I hadn't done or crises I brought upon myself, but now I see that every experience is a loving teacher.

Next year I want you to seriously consider writing your own authentic meditations. Start slowly. Only write one every week or every month. Search for the Sacred in the ordinary and you'll find it. Nothing in your life is too insignificant to be a source of inspiration. As you begin to write your own meditations regularly, you'll be amazed at how much you start remembering or recognizing. The English poet Cecil Day-Lewis confided: "We do not write in order to be understood; we write in order to understand." If you start writing your own authentic meditations, what you'll remember, recognize, and understand is that yours is a wonderful life.

DECEMBER 24

Here Is All I've Counted Splendid

Write it down, when I have perished:
Here is everything I've cherished;
That these walls should glow with beauty
Spurred my lagging soul to duty;
That there should be gladness here
Kept me toiling, year by year...
Every thought and every act.

Edgar A. Guest (1881–1959)
English-born American poet known as
"The People's Poet"

Tonight is my favorite night of the year. In this quiet moment, *Simple Abundance* is not a philosophy but reality perfected. My heart is full of Gratitude; striving for Simplicity in our holiday obligations has preserved my sanity; Order has kept all the moving parts moving; a sense of Harmony has emerged because I finally stopped long enough to balance work and family at least for the holidays; Beauty surrounds me in the festive decorations throughout the house, now illuminated and intensified with the glow of candles and a cozy fire; and Joy, the child of laughter and contentment has arrived, the guest of honor at our festive family feast.

After dinner, after we have each opened just one gift and other members of the household are snug in their beds, it's time for my own private Christmas ritual: the preparation of a Nativity tray, an English medieval custom that never fails to bring the true meaning of this special night into sharp focus.

Legend has it that on the night of the Nativity, whosoever ventures out into great snows bearing a succulent bone for a lost and lamenting hound, a wisp of hay for a shivering horse, a warm cloak for a stranded wayfarer, a garland of bright berries for one who has worn chains, a dish of crumbs for all huddled birds who thought their song was dead, and sweetmeats for little children who peer from lonely windows—whosoever prepares this simply abundant tray "shall be proffered and returned gifts of such an astonishment as will rival the hues of the peacock and the harmonies of heaven."

So I quietly take down from the top of the cupboard a huge willow tray, line it with cloth, and place on it a juicy bone from our standing rib roast dinner; a bowl of cat food; hay from the bale I used for autumn decorations; a warm coat someone has outgrown or grown tired of; a string of cranberries; a dish of fresh bread crumbs and sunflower seeds; and a plate of sugarplums.

Quietly, I sneak out the door and bring it down to the top of the stone wall in front of our house near the street. Sometimes there's snow, sometimes there's not, but it's always cold. I look up to find a bright star; is it *the* Star? It is to my eyes. I'm freezing. Now it's impossible on this holy night not to think of the homeless as I settle the tray into a drift or dirt. Two thousand years ago another homeless family depended on the charity of strangers. Mine now tugs with guilt; that a basket and presents were dropped off earlier this afternoon to a shelter salves the sting a bit, but I'm disappointed and saddened that I didn't, don't, do more. I will next year, I promise. Sometimes I keep those well-intentioned promises, sometimes real life distracts me from Real Life. I don't do enough, and both Spirit and I know it. Next year I can try.

Many years ago I started preparing the Nativity tray because an almost palpable mysticism seemed to surround the legend. I was also very interested in the promise of astonishing gifts to rival the harmonies of heaven. Every year when I go out onto my suburban front yard on Christmas morning to collect the tray, many of the offerings are gone. One year, even the coat. For all I know, I'm the squirrels' Santa Claus. But it does give me happy pause, wondering whose Christmas dreams came true.

And the astonishing gifts to rival heaven? Everywhere I look. But the best one is that now I can truly see them.

Christmas

If, as Herod, we fill our lives with things, and again with things; if we consider ourselves so unimportant that we must fill every moment of our lives with action, when will we have the time to make the long, slow journey across the desert as did the Magi? Or sit and watch the stars as did the shepherds? Or brood over the coming of the child as did Mary? For each one of us, there is a desert to travel. A star to discover. And a being within ourselves to bring to life.

—Anonymous

I first discovered this profound expression of the essence of *Simple Abundance* as I began writing this book. While browsing in a gallery in Vermont, I was drawn across the room to a display of work by the gifted calligraphy and graphic artist Michael Podesta. There it was—an elegant script rendering of exquisite grace. "That's it," my Authentic Self whispered. "That's *Simple Abundance*." Of course it was, and I had to have it. But when I spotted the price tag, I knew it wouldn't be at that moment. That's okay, I reassured Herod's daughter, writing the quote down. Just accept the gift of the quote right now; the print will come when it's supposed to. I picked up the artist's mail-order catalog and continued to enjoy a wonderful day with Katie, her cousins, and my sister. Back at my mother's, I mentioned the print and how this quote was the very first one I had for the book. "It's perfect for the Christmas quotation," I told her. "It sums up the book in one amazing paragraph."

When I arrived home, Michael Podesta's print was waiting for me, a good luck gift from my mother. After I had cried and laughed and called to thank her, I hung it over my meditation table. It has traveled with me on both sides of the Atlantic for the last twenty-five years. Its beauty acts as an anchor to my bedroom, the place where I sit, work, dream, sleep, love, and pray; its timeless message a deep harbor for my restless heart, a soulful safe haven. When I called Michael to ask where the quote came from, he told me that he didn't know; someone had sent it to him anonymously in the mail without attribution. But it spoke to his heart, and he knew he needed to make a print using it.

To the unknown poet, giver of wisdom and truth, thank you for this very special gift that has inspired so many of us.

"Oh, would that Christmas last the whole year through, as it ought," Charles Dickens lamented. "Would that the spirit of Christmas could live within our hearts every day of the year."

But what is the Christmas spirit? Perhaps the Christmas spirit, like the nature of the Beloved, is meant to be a Holy Mystery. Perhaps the Christmas spirit is our souls' knowledge that things, no matter how beautiful, are only things; that we were created, not always to do, but sometimes simply to be. Perhaps the Christmas spirit is a loving reminder that we must *make* time for the long, slow journey across the desert; we must *take* time to discover our star; we must *honor the time necessary* to brood over the coming of the authentic women we were created by Love to become. It has been said many times that our lives are gifts from God—that what we do with them is our gift in return. Today is the perfect day to remember this.

So this is my Christmas wish for both of us: that behind the toys, tinsel, carols, cards, and convivial chaos, there will come a moment of quiet reflection and peace. That it may be truly said of each of us that we know how to keep Christmas well, if any woman does.

Merry Christmas! And God bless us, God bless us everyone!

DECEMBER 26

The Courage to Create the World You Want

Your story is what you have, what you will always have.
It is something to own.

—Michelle Obama
American lawyer, writer, and former first
lady of the United States

The first time you think you'd like to do something a little differently from the way you've always done it—maybe bring Creole shrimp stew to the potluck supper instead of your delicious-but-predictable potato-and-peas casserole—you pick up a pebble. The first time you actually do it differently—whether you're delighted or disappointed in the results—you throw the pebble into the pond. The pebble sends out tiny, barely visible ripples of movement toward the center. No one else notices. But the woman who threw the pebble or spent two hours in the kitchen cooking a simple pleasure does if she's paying attention.

It's the same with courageous acts in your daily round. They may be so small that only you realize something's going on. But one day, all those small but indelible moments of private courage will burst through. And both you and your world will have changed in an authentic moment.

We become authentic the same way we become courageous. By doing it. Not by thinking about it. Rosa Parks didn't think about becoming the symbol of the civil rights movement when she refused to give up her seat and go to the back of the bus.

She was tired. She just wanted to get home. But her authentic and exuberant commitment to equality pushed through her reserve, joining with the energy that created the world. *Exuberant* means not only "joyously unrestrained" but "displaying something in abundance." Rosa Parks displayed an abundance of authentic courage. And at that defining moment, can we doubt that her soul was "joyously unrestrained," even if her heart was trembling?

This week many African-American women begin celebrating a festival honoring faith, unity, heritage, and values. *Kwanzaa*, which means "first fruits of the harvest" in Swahili, was started in 1966 by civil rights activist Maulana Karenga. Over the last five decades the holiday has become widely celebrated by black women who cherish their authenticity. The seven-day celebration, which starts today, is observed by lighting a candle each night to honor a specific value. They are, in order: unity, self-determination, cooperative work and responsibility, cooperative economics, purpose, creativity, and faith. There is no prescribed way to celebrate Kwanzaa except with great festivity.

Not all of us celebrate Kwanzaa, but the courage to embrace authenticity with joyous unrestraint is certainly something to celebrate by lighting a candle, raising a glass, and doing something completely unexpected that lifts our spirits. "We need to feel the cheer and inspiration of meeting each other," Josephine St. Pierre Ruffin believed. "We need to gain the courage and fresh life that comes from the mingling of congenial souls, of those working for the same ends."

DECEMBER 27

A Woman of Substance

First, we have to believe, and then we believe.
—G. C. Lichtenberg (1742–1799)
German physicist and Anglophile

As the season of believing seems to wind down for the rest of the world, please let me gently make something very clear. Many dreams still wait in the wings. Many aspirations are just within our grasp if we keep stretching. Many hungers need nourishment. Many yearnings must be acknowledged, so that they can be fulfilled. Many authentic sparks must be fanned before Passion performs her perfect work in you. Throw another log on the fire.

This is not the day you quit.

This is not the day you cry.

This is the day you stare down every naysayer in your life who doesn't get it yet. Because *you* do. Finally. And now you *know* that *faith is the substance of things hoped for, the evidence of things not seen.*

This is the day you shout, "I believe!" Keep on shouting it until you're hoarse. No more muttering under your breath.

Do you know what happens every time a child says, "I don't believe in fairies!" A fairy falls down dead.

Do you know what happens every time a woman says, "I don't believe. It's taking too long!"? The woman dies a little bit inside. But it just might take another forty years before they get around to burying you. And do you know what they'll say as your ashes are scattered? "I don't think I can ever remember a time when she was truly happy." And they'll be right.

This is *not* the time you stop believing. You simply can't afford the luxury of skepticism. And what must you believe with every breath, until you do *believe*? How about the mystical alchemy of style and Spirit? In the past a woman's spirituality has been separated from her lifestyle. But now you know this doesn't make any sense. Never did. Never will.

Now you know that the union of authentic style and Spirit creates a woman of substance.

You.

So keep on believing that you have the passion, intelligence, brilliance, creativity, wisdom, clarity, depth, and savvy to find that quiet center of solace, serenity, and strength necessary to create and sustain an authentic life. Every day is the prayer. An authentic life is the most personal form of worship. When you start believing, you'll discover that all things are really possible.

Clap.

Clap once again.

But let's really hear it this time!

Wow! That's better! Why, it's so loud, it'll wake up the dead.

Good for you.

A Success Unexpected in Common Hours

I learned this, at least, by my experiment: that if one advances confidently in the direction of [her] dreams, and endeavors to live the life which [she] has imagined, [she] will meet with a success unexpected in common hours.

—Henry David Thoreau (1817–1862)
American philosopher and author

Some days—and today is one of them—I think of *Simple Abundance* as a distinctly female *Walden*. But Thoreau went off alone to a hut in the woods, whereas we're surrounded by our offspring on vacation, many of them mopey and miserable because "there's nothing to do." When we point out that there's plenty to do, it's not exactly what they had in mind.

Henry, can we trade?

Today is the day the post-holiday blues usually drop in for their annual visit. After any strenuous exertion, especially one that's lasted several weeks, there's a natural letdown in energy and enthusiasm. "The life in us is like the water in a river," Thoreau tells us. It rises, even floods, but then it recedes until it finds its true level.

The year is ending; and whether we're aware of it or not, we're balancing our personal books, tallying up the profits and losses. If we're in the red as far as achieving goals, surrendering expectations, reaching for aspirations, coming to terms with situations we can't change, or acknowledging that we could have made changes but chose not to, we're going to end up feeling blue. If we've blown our budget, it's likely our purses will be leaner for a couple of months. Not fun.

To make matters even worse, you're probably not feeling very well. Don't be surprised by nasty colds or lingering chest congestion. Practitioners of Eastern medicine expect these ailments in the winter; metaphysically the lung is the organ that processes grief. If we've experienced a loss—and all of us have in one way or another this year—we might still be grieving, unable to accept and release it. Old pain is very difficult to give up; by now it's a familiar friend, just not a very nurturing one.

When this happens we need to remember to treat ourselves kindly. This is the time to trust, not make judgments. Soon the children will go back to school. The company will leave. The work will get completed. The bills will be paid. The quiet moment will come. You'll be able to catch your breath, and then you'll notice that it doesn't hurt anymore. Your creative energy and enthusiasm will return. Once again, you'll start to advance confidently in the direction of your dreams.

Most days this is what I truly love about the human experience: that we all share it. The rest of the time I'm trying to cope. Still, nothing we're doing or facing or fearing or worrying about is original. Somewhere, at some time, some woman has pondered in her heart whatever troubles us. When I can stop the centrifugal motion that has me swirling in anxiety long enough to put the kettle on, I can take a deep breath and ask Mother Plenty first for grace and second for joy. This girl's season is not over yet!

Learning to live in the present moment is part of the path of joy. When I was writing *Simple Abundance*, every single day for five years I existed in the compartmentalized space it took for me to write every meditation. I was so focused on the good and so *committed to it being a happy book* for both of us, even though that period of my life was difficult and fraught, there isn't a sour or distressed note in it. That's the miracle of *Simple Abundance*. Blessed be the Great Creator.

Looking back, I understand now that the Book knew so much more than I did (creative projects always do); I just had to get out of the way of Spirit and show up for work. And because I had only so many hours in the day to write, I couldn't allow myself the luxury of a bad thought during that time. Let me write that sentence again, so we both understand what I'm trying to say: *I could not allow myself the luxury of a bad thought.* If I was feeling sick or depressed or frightened, I'd say: "You can think about that tonight. Not now." And of course, after spending a day focused on Gratitude, Simplicity, Order, Harmony, Beauty, and Joy, all I wanted to do at the end of the day was give thanks for my curated contentment.

So let's forget the reality of the rest of the world for a moment, which is fraught with doom and gloom. Many of us unconsciously create dramas in our minds—in part because we're copying or reinforcing the constant dramas playing out in the 24/7 "Breaking News" culture we exist in.

When we create dramas in our minds—about our finances, our health, our children, our grandchildren, our relationships, our work; when we set ourselves up to expect the worst from every situation, our brilliant subconscious never lets us down. Trust me, few of us have the ability to go from zero to a hundred in the calibration of ecstasy. But imagine a tragedy (or see someone else's nightmare playing out before our eyes in real time or on television) and we're already there, ready for our personal close-up. We know that when we expect the worst from a situation it becomes a self-fulfilling prophecy. Inadvertently, we become authors of our misfortune.

This holiday season I would love for us both to learn how to stop the cycles of drama and experiment in trusting the flow of life and the goodness of Spirit.

This is how I'm starting: Each morning I'm praying for one day's portion of Grace and a respite from crises into our New Year. Let's suspend our disbelief and take that leap of faith. Begin today by recording in your Gratitude Journal not just what you're grateful for today but all the wishes and prayers you yearn to come true tomorrow. First the gesture, then the Grace.

"However mean your life is, meet it and live it; do not shun it and call it hard names. It is not bad," Thoreau tells us. "It looks poorest when you are richest. The fault-finder will find faults even in paradise. Love your life, poor as it is. You may perhaps have some pleasant, thrilling, glorious hours, even in a poor-house," Henry reassures us. "The sun is reflected from the windows of the almshouse as brightly as from the rich man's abode; the snow melts before its door as early in the spring."

DECEMBER 29

Do Try This at Home: Some Thoughts to Take into the New Year

One day my life will end; and lest
Some whim should prompt you to review it,
Let her who knows the subject best
Tell you the shortest way to do it:
Thus say, "Here lies one doubly blest."
Say, "She was happy." Say, "She knew it."
— Jan Struther (1901–1953)
Pen name of Jan Maxtone Graham
English author, poet, hymn writer

While we have explored becoming Mrs. Miniver, we have embodied the spirit of a woman who faced life's circumstances with courage and calm but also good cheer. Mrs. Miniver loved her comforts and little treats.

Now that the *Simple Abundance* Caution Closet is full and our backpacks and car trunks are laden with sustenance for life's rainy days, there is only one last item that is essential: comfort.

Let's go on a treasure hunt of comforts for you and your family. Is there a favorite, long ago discontinued stuffed animal for which you can find a duplicate on eBay? Perhaps an empty diary and pen for your journaling daughter, a favorite sweater or socks, or a Nintendo Switch with a backup battery pack. If you have a partner or a spouse, is there a special hobby they enjoy? Let's say you live with a fly-fishing enthusiast. Wouldn't their eyes light up with a couple of old books on the subject or a few magazines?

What about yourself? Do you have a playlist of favorite music? Do you have a few favorites from your Comfort Drawer? There is plenty of room for your go-to moisturizer, hand crème, and lip balm. How about a fresh Gratitude Journal? And don't you forget to pack a good book! What about a mystery anthology if you are a detective fan? If you love novels, have you ever enjoyed short stories? Or a new craft project kit? Only you would know what your treats are, so pack them.

Where would we be without our favorite teas or instant coffee in a pinch? A family size bag of chocolate kisses with long expiration dates of course will have to be refreshed from time to time. Such a sweet problem to have.

There is plenty of room for a crossword puzzle or sudoku book. How about a graphic novel for your teenage fan? When you start to ponder the biggest comforts for the smallest space, think about adding a note of acknowledgment on the strengths and emotional gifts your family brings to you. In the fervor of the moment, these treasures are well packed beforehand to be discovered later.

Out of all the books on disaster preparation out there, these are the two I have on my shelves that cover all the basics in more depth but without the scare tactics. I highly recommend them.

Just in Case: How to Be Self-Sufficient When the Unexpected Happens by Kathy Harrison (Storey Publishing)

Mind of a Survivor: What the Wild Has Taught Me About Survival and Success by Megan Hine (Coronet Publishing)

Well, you've done it, and I'm proud of you. If your procrastinator has been in charge, a new year is right around the corner for you to begin again. As the Irish painter Maria Dorothea Robinson was fond of saying, "Nobody can go back and start a new beginning, but anyone can start today and make a new ending."

God bless.

Ithaka

As you set out in search of Ithaka
Pray that your journey be long,
full of adventures, full of awakenings.
Do not fear the monsters of old...
You will not meet them in your travels
if your thoughts are exalted and remain high,
if authentic passions stir your mind, body and spirit.
You will not encounter fearful monsters
if you do not carry them within your soul,
if your soul does not set them up in front of you.

> —Constantine Peter Cavafy (1863–1933)
> Most distinguished Greek poet of the
> twentieth century

At the funeral of Jacqueline Kennedy Onassis, many of us heard for the first time the poem "Ithaka," written in 1911 by the Greek poet C. P. Cavafy. This exquisite song of encouragement to travelers setting out on a voyage of self-discovery is often read as an elegy. But I believe "Ithaka" is even more powerful when it becomes a personal affirmation of our real-life journey.

Ithaka was the beloved island home of the legendary Greek hero Odysseus. After playing a leading role in the Trojan War, Odysseus roamed the world for ten years, having adventures, meeting challenges, and learning lessons that profoundly changed him. Today an *odyssey* means a long, often exhausting, exhilarating and/or excruciating transformative journey.

The search for authenticity is our personal odyssey. As we move through our daily rounds on the *Simple Abundance* path as daughters, friends, lovers, wives, mothers, and Artists of the Everyday—what we are really seeking is the Ultimate Reality. We are seeking Ithaka.

Over the last fifty years, there have been several fine translations of Cavafy's poem, but for me, they've always seemed as if they had been written for men. This is not too surprising, as they were all translated by men. However, since "Ithaka" has become an emotional touchstone for me, a poem I find myself meditating on a great deal, I was inspired to create a personal translation/adaptation of Cavafy's classic for women:

Pray that your journey be long,
full of many summer mornings
when with much pleasure and much joy

you anchor in harbors never seen before;
Browse through Phoenician markets,
to purchase exquisite treasures—
mother-of-pearl and coral, ebony and amber
and sensual perfumes of all kinds—
as much as you desire.
Visit many Egyptian cities, content
to sit at the feet of sages, eager
and open to receive learning.
Keep Ithaka always in your mind.
Your arrival there is your destiny.
But do not hurry the journey at all; be patient.
Better that it lasts for many years—
longer than you can even imagine.
So that finally, when you reach this
sacred isle, you will be a wise woman,
abundantly fulfilled by all you have gained along the way;
no longer expecting Ithaka to make you wealthy,
no longer needing Ithaka to make you rich.
Ithaka offered you the profound journey,
the chance to discover the woman you have always been.
Without Ithaka as your inspiration, you
never would have set out in search of Wholeness.
And should you find her poor, Ithaka did not deceive you.
Authentic as you have become, full of wisdom, beauty, and grace
enriched and enlightened by all you have experienced
You will finally understand what all of life's Ithakas truly mean.

DECEMBER 31

Pray the Journey Is Long

The world is round and the place which may seem like the end may
also be only the beginning.

—Ivy Baker Priest (1905–1975)
Thirtieth Treasurer of the United States
of America

Life as a journey. Life as safari. Life as a pilgrimage. Life as a garden.
Life as the highest art.

Pathfinders. Prospectors. Pioneers. Detectives. Explorers. Archaeologists. Pilgrims. Poets. Sojourners. Gardeners. Artists of the Everyday.

Women of Spirit. Women of substance. Women with style. Women who have lived the questions. Women ready to embrace the answers. Women who look great in hats. That's why we wear so many different ones.

Seekers of the Sacred in the ordinary. Real Life. The Mystical in the madness. The Holy Mysteries of the mundane.

Seekers of Love. Passion. Wholeness.

Authenticity.

Where are we headed?

We're headed Home.

Ithaka.

But before we arrive, there are vast worlds awaiting exploration. Worlds within. Worlds without. Earth. Heaven.

Heaven on earth.

Sometimes the terrain is rocky and the slopes steep. Sometimes the jungle is thick and its interior very dark. Sometimes the water is deep and the waves extremely rough.

Do you see now why we need some variety in our approaches?

How will we know when we get there?

You'll know.

It's that simple. Real things are.

Are we there yet?

Not quite.

But it's taking too long.

Often it seems that way. Chronologically we're at the end of the year but the beginning of the journey. Not to worry. We'll have all the time we need in *kairos* to find ourselves.

Here's where we must part company. At least for a little while. I've got some discoveries I need to make on my own. And so do you.

But you won't be alone. Someone who loves you unconditionally is at the helm. Divine Love sustains you, surrounds you, enfolds you, protects you. Go in peace. You're as ready as you ever will be, well equipped for the adventures awaiting. Divine Substance—which is your only Reality—provides abundantly. But you must ask. Ask for help, supply, guidance, Grace. Ask for the Power to be switched on. Ask to catch the flow. Ask to soar.

Ask. Ask. Ask.

Ask for a respite from all your crises. Surrender suffering, sorrow, pain. Surrender expectations. Ask to be surprised by joy.

Give thanks. Wait. Watch what happens. Get excited. Open your arms as wide as you can to receive all the miracles with your name on them.

Never forget that all you have is all you need.

Simple Abundance is a creative and practical path, full of Joyful

Simplicities waiting to be revealed in the small moments. But don't forget, the path is a spiral. If you get stuck, look out at the wider vista and see how far you've traveled. For the parts of the journey when only the far horizon is in sight, *Simple Abundance* becomes a caravel of contentment—a small but sturdy vessel, strong enough to withstand storms. Her triangular sails have been spiritually designed to take advantage of winds blowing from either side of real life—the shadows and the Light.

Let's see. Do you have everything? Get out your Gratitude Journal. Think of your *Illustrated Discovery Journal* as your ship's logbook. Your wise and loving heart is your compass to determine the latitude and longitude of longing. Check it every day. Trust it to keep you steady and on the mark. Love will not fail you.

Believe. Believe in yourself. Believe in the One who believes in You. All things are possible to She who believes.

Navigate by the stars. Search the Heavens for yours. Follow it. Keep on the lookout for soulful markers. They surround you. The Soul's awakening is gratitude. The Soul's essence is simplicity. The Soul's serenity is order. The Soul's repose is harmony. The Soul's passion is beauty. The Soul's purpose is joy.

Pray your journey be a long one. Savor the stops along the way. They make the search marvelous. Meaningful. Memorable. Find and honor your own pace. There are still so many harbors to be seen for the first time. You're headed for someplace you've never been before. Keep your thoughts held high. Let personal passions stir your mind, body, and spirit.

Set your course for Authentica. Legend has it that once you reach her shores, you'll not leave the same woman. For if you find this sacred isle, you will remember what you have always known. You will discover the woman you have always been. No longer will you see things as they are. You will see things as you are. Through the parting of the mists where doubt and faith meet, you will see *the Authentic Self is the soul made visible.*

Blessings on your courage, my darling girl, my dearest friend. Godspeed.

Joyful Simplicities for December

There are times when Life surprises one, and anything may happen, even what one had hoped for.
—Ellen Glasgow (1873–1945)
American Pulitzer Prize–winning novelist

❧ One of the loveliest gifts of the *Simple Abundance* philosophy is that you get to start your life over at any point—and if ever Christmas felt like a chance to start over, it's this year. This is when we get to rethink certain holiday rituals we've taken for granted to see if they're still bringing us comfort and joy. The heart of *Simple Abundance*, as I've discovered through the years and different configurations of the family, is its adaptability.

✍ Really deck the halls. Spread holiday cheer throughout your entire home with seasonal decorations, no matter what holiday you celebrate. Evergreens, beautiful flowering plants, candles, tiny lights, and natural decorations don't have to be associated with any one holiday unless you make them so. When you make a special effort to create beauty in your home, you set the stage for festivity, an authentic quality of Hanukkah, Winter Solstice, Christmas, and Kwanzaa.

✍ If you're one singular sensation this year and want a low-key but festive observance, treat yourself to a beautiful amaryllis or two (the pink is gorgeous) and a small tree-shaped rosemary plant, and you'll be so pleased every time you come home to yourself. Add a scented candle and a new throw. Now for something to read: *Elizabeth David's Christmas* (edited by Jill Norman; Michael Joseph Publishing), where David celebrates by going solo in bed with salmon and champagne. And begin a holiday mystery marathon as I do with these two anthologies: *The Big Book of Christmas Mysteries* (edited by Otto Penzler; Vintage Crime/Black Lizard) and *The Big Book of Female Detectives* (edited by Otto Penzler; Vintage Crime/Black Lizard). You'll have such fun.

✍ Christmas stockings, plump with promise, lend enchantment to children of all ages who have a deep, primordial need to believe in a Great Gift bringer who rewards the good (and that includes all of us!). What a thrill it is to reach out for the stocking in the darkness, pull it under the covers, clasp the contents with the imagination running wild, until by dawn's early light it can be emptied out onto the bed and the wrappings furiously pulled off with glee. If you have a blended family that requires a Christmas celebration at both Mom's and Dad's and gifts for stepchildren, a tree at one house and stockings at the other gracefully fills the bill without anyone feeling left out. The Victorian Christmas stocking recipe is: something to eat, something to read, something to play with, something they need. And this recipe never fails—for children of all ages. The "recipe" also works wonders for Easter baskets.

✍ Delicious food is each winter holiday's gift. Enjoy potato latkes, Christmas pudding, sugarplums, eggnog, wassail, spicy Creole shrimp. You don't have to bake to enjoy Christmas cookies. Start thinking about calories on January 2. Forget about fruitcake. Think about Black Cake. "There is fruitcake, and there is Black Cake, which is to fruitcake what the Brahms piano quartets are to

Muzak," Laurie Colwin tells us. She'll tell you how to make one in *Home Cooking: A Writer in the Kitchen*.

- Hold a holiday classic-film fest. Besides familiar favorites, there are many more marvelous movies you probably aren't familiar with that celebrate Christmas as the star or the subplot. You'll find a list of them in *The Great American Christmas Almanac* by Irena Chalmers and friends. Most of them are easy to find on streaming services.

- Fulfill the holiday dreams of a child who isn't yours.

- Share your blessings with a shelter for women or the homeless.

- Prepare a Nativity Tray.

- Find your star. Follow its Light. If you really want a star you can call your own, you can have one. Each day new stars are discovered in the heavens. The International Star Registry will name one after you, a dream, or a loved one as a memorial. Contact them online at www.intlstarregistry.com.

- Michael Podesta's inspirational calligraphy art is exquisite. Visit his lovely website: www.michaelpodesta.com.

- Look back on the aspirations you wrote on January 1. Don't be discouraged if you haven't achieved them. It's the reaching for them that's important. Make a new list. Carry whatever's still meaningful to you over to the New Year's list. Now confide your new dreams to a close friend, who will act as your witness.

- Before we can welcome in the New Year, we need to put the Old Year's unfinished business—mistakes, regrets, shortcomings, and disappointments—behind us. Here's how: Write down on small slips of paper whatever you'd like to forget, then place the slips of paper in a small cardboard box. Next, with ceremony, wrap the box in black or very dark paper, sealing in the sorrow and hard luck. Say, "Good riddance," and toss the box into the fireplace to burn away the past. If you don't have a fireplace, toss the bad memories from the past into the trash where they belong. Keep only the good.

- Chill something bubbly. Honor the Old Year with a farewell toast, welcome the New Year within. Offer thanks. Celebrate how far you've come, how much you've learned, and the glorious woman you really are.

- Happy New Year!

With Thanks and Appreciation

If the only prayer you ever say in your entire life is "Thank you," it will be enough.

—Meister Eckhart
13th century German mystic

Books. Darned if I know how they come alive other than through miraculous inception. I've got to confess, the hardest part of writing any book isn't the beginning or the ending, but the appreciations. For in between "It was a dark and stormy night" and "The End," the Book is a collaborative art. Your name might be on the cover, but you know the talents of many others contributed—like a thousand angels on a pinhead—just when you, or the Book, needed them.

During the long time it took to realize the dream of this book, a close circle of family, friends, creative colleagues, and "unseen hands" assisted me and nurtured *Simple Abundance* as if it were their own. I want to acknowledge the love, support, time, creative energy, emotion, guidance, inspiration, and faith so generously bestowed on me as I followed my bliss.

With all my heart I thank God for entrusting me with *Simple Abundance*, both the original, published in 1995, and now the revised twenty-fifth edition of *SA*. Among my many blessings was being led to Liv Blumer at Warner Books. Her generosity, thoughtfulness, passion, intelligence, wit, and respect for my work moved me deeply. A special note of heartfelt affection and respect goes to Caryn Karmatz Rudy, who also superbly edited portions of the original *SA* and then became my editor on four succeeding books. Caryn always responded to my requests and concerns with cheerful élan and much-appreciated kindness. From the very beginning it was apparent to me that Liv and Caryn really loved *Simple Abundance*, confirming what Victorian philosopher John Ruskin said about the harmony that results "when love and skill work together."

Warner Books became Grand Central Publishing in 2006. My thanks to all who worked behind the scenes at Grand Central for *Simple Abundance: 365 Days to a Balanced and Joyful Life*, shepherding my work through the labyrinth of time, space, budget meetings, and production schedules with care and consideration. Let me start with Karen Kosztolnyik, Grand Central's editor in chief, whose keen enthusiasm for the new *SA* is so appreciated. Karen's elegant grace is evident on every page.

I don't know how Elizabeth Kulhanek juggles those flaming torches so deftly, but she was amazing assuaging the editor, production, and author at the same time with her sleight-of-hand skills. Thanks so much.

Thank you, Rebecca Maines, for affectionately hovering over these pages with such savvy dedication and sleuthing skills, continuing to perpetuate the illusion that I have command over the English language.

Much appreciation for Luria Rittenberg, the production editor, and the senior production associate, Laura Eisenhard, on the manufacturing side; and the digital production coordinator, Melissa Mathlin.

To Ben Sevier, my print publisher, and digital publisher Beth de Guzman, thank you.

No matter how wonderful your book might be, you need the talented people in marketing and publicity to get the word out. Thank you, Amanda Pritzker and Alana Spendley; associate publisher/marketing director Brian McLendon. In publicity, my gratitude to Kamrun Nesa.

In sales, how happy I am to have Karen Torres still watching over the new twenty-fifth anniversary *SA*, along with Ali Cutrone, Alison Lazarus, and Chris Murphy.

For the audio version, thank you to Anthony Goff and my producer, Christine Farrell.

Readers attempting to find a new favorite do judge books by their covers. I have no worries there. Thank you so much, creative director Albert Tang and cover designer Jim Tierney for a fresh look for *SA* while keeping her in the family of my other Grand Central books.

Blessings to my dear friends Dawne Winter, Dona Cooper, and MJ Brant for their abiding prayers, incredible hospitality, genuine comfort, and jubilant celebrating on this journey. My sister, Maureen O'Crean, has been the connective tissue between my *SA* readers and me from the beginning. I could not do the webinars without her enthusiasm, empathy, and encouragement, especially when I'm overwhelmed by other commitments.

My brother, Pat Crean, supported me in countless ways during the writing of the twenty-fifth anniversary edition of *SA*, checking in with me a couple of times a week to make sure I wasn't losing my mind as I was making my deadline. When in doubt, a subscription for cat food started to arrive, so that my most pressing "adulting" duty could be checked off. His sage advice for any bump in the road, "It's too late to go home early" and "Keep calm and type on," always seemed to work.

To Oprah Winfrey, who became *Simple Abundance*'s godmother, unbounded thanks for your enormous generosity of spirit in supporting my work these last twenty-five years. My gratitude begins with "thank you" and does not end, because the depth of my thankfulness is simply more than words can say.

To my creative and intuitive son-in-law, Jeff Lichtfuss, thank you for pointing out (in fact, several times) that I was receiving a growing number of requests from millennial fans who wondered on social media if I could update *Simple Abundance* for a new generation. I hope you like the results, and any new idea for the future is most welcome.

This book—both versions—could not have been written without my agent and close friend, Chris Tomasino. Her unconditional faith in me and her deep and fervent belief that women needed to read what I needed to write made *Simple Abundance* possible. She was the first to read my drafts in monthly installments (cutting the manuscript down from over 1,200 pages!), and her vision of what this book could be stretched and sustained me during our long, difficult journey to publication. Her steadfast support gave me the courage to take the creative risks necessary to hear my authentic voice after two decades of journalism. I learned to soar on these pages because I knew Chris was holding the net.

My darling daughter, Kate, was eight when the *Simple Abundance* dream began. For over half her life she has graciously accepted the overwhelming presence of "The Book" in her daily round, one way or another, with great humor, patience, and consideration. She's always kept the faith, especially when mine faltered, and it is a privilege to reverse roles as she now follows her exciting, authentic path as a film producer. It is my dearest wish that we will work on new projects in the future, because she's simply the best.

How blessed I am to have both Kate and Chris with me on this new creative chapter in my work and life. And I know it.

May I end this note of thanksgiving wishing that everyone connected with *Simple Abundance*, especially you, dear Reader, reap the rich harvest sown by my love. As Meister Eckhart tells us, and *Simple Abundance* proves, we should "Be always ready for the gifts of God, and always for new ones" because "God is a thousand times more ready to give than you are to receive."

Your names are forever engraved in the Gratitude Journal of my heart.

Soli Deo gloria.

Sarah Ban Breathnach
July 2, 2019

About the Author

A writer of remarkable wisdom, warmth, and compassion, **Sarah Ban Breathnach** (pronounced "Bon Brannock") has become a trusted voice to women around the world. Sarah is the author of fourteen books, including the number one *New York Times* best-sellers *Simple Abundance: A Daybook of Comfort and Joy* and *Something More: Excavating Your Authentic Self*, and she is the creator of *The Simple Abundance Journal of Gratitude*. Sarah's work celebrates quiet joys, simple pleasures, and well-spent moments. By reminding us to search for the small and the sweet in our daily round with appreciation and awe, we find the beauty in the everyday. *Simple Abundance* was named one of the top ten best-selling books in the United States during the nineties according to *USA Today*.

Sarah Ban Breathnach is also the president and CEO of Simple Abundance®, Inc., a consultancy firm specializing in publishing and multimedia projects that give creative expression to the Simple Abundance® philosophy and the concept of personal authenticity.

Sarah's other titles include: *The Best Part of the Day* (her first children's book), *Peace and Plenty: Finding Your Path to Financial Serenity*, *The Peace and Plenty Journal of Well-Spent Moments*, *Romancing the Ordinary*, *The Simple Abundance Companion*, *The Illustrated Discovery Journal*, *A Man's Journey to Simple Abundance*, *Moving On*, *The Victorian Nursery Companion*, and *Mrs. Sharp's Traditions*.

Oprah Winfrey has called Sarah's work "life-changing," and Sarah has been a frequent guest on *The Oprah Winfrey Show* and OWN's *Super Soul Sunday*. Additionally, Sarah was named as one of the fifty women redefining what it means to be fifty today by *MORE* magazine.

In 1995, Ban Breathnach founded the Simple Abundance Charitable Fund, which has aided more than 100 nonprofit organizations by awarding over one million dollars in financial support.

Time magazine has called Sarah "the Martha Stewart of the soul," and Deepak Chopra has said, "Sarah Ban Breathnach is a one-woman women's movement, an awakener of awareness whose simple message has timeless roots...She exemplifies a surging social movement much greater than herself. This is just the subversively cosmic voice society needs."

Sarah lives in Southern California near her daughter, Kate, and their beloved animals.

Visit her on the web at:
www.sarahbanbreathnach.com
www.simpleabundance.com

What's in a Name?

Both legally and familiarly, as well as in my books, I now have only one name, which is my own.

—Colette
La Naissance du Jour (1928)

Like the French writer, Colette, I also have a name, both familiar and legal, which is found in my books and which I own: *Simple Abundance®*. Please do not use it for your garden center, B&B, cooking courses, workshops, or magazine features (unless, of course, you're writing about my work). If you're thinking about naming a rose or a health food supplement after *Simple Abundance*, I'm flattered, but you still must write for permission.

Intellectual property pilfering is spiritually distressing and now, thank goodness, it's also internationally prohibited by law.

Sarah Ban Breathnach

Bibliography

I am a part of all I have read.

—John Kieran (1892–1981)
American author and editor

My sources for the quotes have been many and varied. Collecting the pithy and the profound has been an absorbing pastime for more than forty years, and I gather them from many sources: books, magazine articles, reviews, newspaper features, radio interviews, television broadcasts, plays, and films. My favorite collections of quotations are: *The New Beacon Book of Quotations by Women*, compiled by Rosalie Maggio (Boston: Beacon Press, 1998); *Bartlett's Familiar Quotations*, Sixteenth Edition, edited by Justin Kaplan (Boston: Little, Brown and Company, 1992); and *The Columbia Dictionary of Quotations*, compiled by Robert Andrews (New York: Columbia University Press, 1993). The vintage source materials have come from my personal collection of women's magazines circa World I, the Great Depression, and the home front years of World War II.

Ackerman, Diane. *A Natural History of the Senses*. New York: Random House, 1990.

Anthony, Evelyn. *The Avenue of the Dead*. New York: Coward, McCann & Geoghegan, 1982.

Antin, Mary. *The Promised Land*. Boston: Houghton Mifflin, 1969.

Armstrong, Karen. *A History of God: The 4,000-Year Quest of Judaism, Christianity and Islam*. New York: Alfred A. Knopf, 1993.

Austen, Jane. *Mansfield Park*. New York: Oxford University Press, 1990.

Baldwin, Christina. *Life's Companion: Journal Writing as a Spiritual Quest*. New York: Bantam, 1990.

Beattie, Melody. *The Language of Letting Go*. New York: Hazelden/Harper-Collins, 1990.

_____. *Gratitude: Affirming the Good Things in Life*. New York: Hazelden/Ballantine Books, 1992.

Beck, Martha. *Finding Your Own North Star: Claiming the Life You Were Meant to Live*. New York: Three Rivers Press, 2001.

_____. "Lies About Love." *Real Simple*, February 2001.

Beeton, Isabella. *The Book of Household Management*. London: 1861.

Bender, Sue. *Plain and Simple: A Woman's Journey to the Amish.* New York: HarperOne, 1989.

Bennett, Arnold. *How to Live on Twenty-Four Hours a Day.* London: 1910; Plainview, New York: Books for Libraries Press, 1975.

Berenbaum, Rose Levy. *The Cake Bible.* New York: William Morrow and Company, Inc., 1988.

Bogan, Louise. *Journey Around My Room: The Autobiography of Louise Bogan.* New York: Penguin Publishing Group, 1981.

Bolen, Jean Shinoda. *Goddesses in Everywoman.* New York: Harper & Row, 1984.

Borysenko, Joan. *Minding the Body, Mending the Mind.* New York: Addison-Wesley, 1987.

_____. *Guilt Is the Teacher, Love Is the Lesson.* New York: Warner Books, 1990.

_____. *Fire in the Soul: A New Psychology of Spiritual Optimism.* New York: Warner Books, 1993.

_____. *Pocketful of Miracles: Prayers, Meditations, and Affirmations to Nurture Your Spirit Every Day of the Year.* New York: Warner Books, 1994.

Brant, Mary Jane Hurley. *When Every Day Matters: A Mother's Memoir on Love, Loss and Life.* New York: Simple Abundance Press, 2008.

Breathnach, Sarah Ban. *Mrs. Sharp's Traditions: Reviving Victorian Family Celebrations of Comfort & Joy.* New York: Simple Abundance Press, 1990, 2001.

_____. *The Victorian Nursery Companion.* New York: Simon & Schuster, 1992.

_____. *The Simple Abundance Journal of Gratitude.* New York: Warner Books, 1997.

_____. *Something More: Excavating Your Authentic Self.* New York: Warner Books, 1998.

_____. *The Simple Abundance Illustrated Discovery Journal: Creating a Visual Autobiography of Your Authentic Self.* New York: Warner Books, 1999.

Brontë, Emily. *Wuthering Heights: Complete Authoritative Text with Biographical and Historical Contexts.* Boston: Bedford Books, 1992.

Browning, Dominique. *Around the House and Through the Garden: A Memoir of Heartbreak, Healing and Home Improvement.* New York: Scribner, 2002.

Brussat, Frederic, and Mary Ann Brussat, editors. *100 Ways to Keep Your Soul Alive.* New York: HarperOne, 1994.

Büchmann, Christina, and Celina Spiegel, editors. *Out of the Garden: Women Writers on the Bible.* New York: Fawcett Columbine, 1994.

Budapest, Zsuzsanna E. *The Grandmother of Time: A Woman's Book of Celebrations, Spells and Sacred Objects for Every Month of the Year.* New York: Harper & Row, 1989.

Burnett, Frances Hodgson. *The Secret Garden.* New York: Frederick A. Stokes, 1911.

Burnham, Sophy. *A Book of Angels.* New York: Ballantine, 1990.

Caddy, Eileen. *Opening Doors Within.* Forres, Scotland: The Findhorn Press, 1987.

Cameron, Julia. *The Artist's Way: A Spiritual Path to Higher Creativity.* New York: Jeremy P. Tarcher/Perigee Books/Putnam Publishing Group, 1992.

Cantwell, Mary. "The Mauv-ing of America." *New York Times Magazine,* March 17, 1991.

Carter, Mary Randolph. *American Junk.* New York: Viking Studio Books, 1994.

Chisholm, Anne. *Rumer Godden: A Storyteller's Life.* London: Macmillan, 1999.

Clampitt, Amy. *The Kingfisher.* New York: Alfred A. Knopf, 1983.

Clurman, Carol. "Family vs. Career: A Woman on the Road to Power Takes a U-Turn." *USA Weekend,* December 2–4, 1994.

Colwin, Laurie. *Home Cooking: A Writer in the Kitchen.* New York: Alfred A. Knopf, 1988.

_____. *More Home Cooking: A Writer Returns to the Kitchen.* New York: HarperCollins, 1993.

Conwell, Russell H. *Acres of Diamonds.* New York and London: Harper & Brothers, 1915.

Cooper, Dona. *Writing Great Screenplays for Film and TV.* New York: Prentice Hall, 1994.

Coupland, Ken. "Is There a Doctor for the House?" *New Age Journal,* November/December 1991.

Csikszentmihalyi, Mihaly. *Flow: The Psychology of Optimal Experience.* New York: Harper & Row, 1990.

Damrosch, Barbara. *The Garden Primer.* New York: Workman Publishing, 1988.

David, Elizabeth. *Elizabeth David's Christmas,* edited by Jill Norman. London: Michael Joseph, 2003.

Davidson, Diane Mott. *Dying for Chocolate.* New York: Bantam, 1992.

_____. *Cereal Murders.* New York: Bantam, 1993.

_____. *Catering to Nobody.* New York: Bantam, 2002.

Davis, Bette. *The Lonely Life.* New York: Putnam, 1962.

Deval, Jacqueline. *Reckless Appetites: A Culinary Romance.* Hopewell, New Jersey: Ecco Books, 1993.

de Wolfe, Elsie. *The House in Good Taste.* New York: The Century Company, 1913.

Dickinson, Emily. *Emily Dickinson: Selected Letters,* edited by Thomas H. Johnson. Cambridge, Massachusetts: The Belknap Press of Harvard University Press, 1985.

Didion, Joan. *Slouching Towards Bethlehem.* New York: Farrar, Straus and Giroux, 1998.

Dillard, Annie. *Pilgrim at Tinker Creek.* New York: Harper & Row, 1974.

_____. *The Writing Life.* New York: Harper & Row, 1989.

Dolmar, Alice D. and Henry Dreher. *Self-Nurture: Learning to Care for Yourself as Effectively As You Care for Everyone Else.* New York: Penguin Books, 2001.

Dolnick, Barrie. *Instructions for Your Discontent: How Bad Times Can Make Life Better.* New York: Simple Abundance Press, 2003.

du Maurier, Daphne. *Rebecca.* New York: Doubleday, Doran and Company, 1938.

Eliot, George. *The Mill on the Floss.* New York and Chicago: Scott Foresman & Company, 1920.

Eliot, T. S. *Collected Poems 1909–1962.* New York: Harcourt Brace Jovanovich, 1963.

Emerson, Ralph Waldo. *The Best of Ralph Waldo Emerson.* New York: Walter J. Black, Inc., 1941.

_____. *Self-Reliance: The Wisdom of Ralph Waldo Emerson as Inspiration for Daily Living* (selected and with an introduction by Richard Whelan). New York: Bell Tower, 1991.

Engelbreit, Mary. *Mary Engelbreit's Home Companion: The Mary Engelbreit Look and How to Get It*. Kansas City: Andrews and McMeel, 1994.

Erlanger, Micaela. *How to Accessorize: A Perfect Finish to Every Outfit*. New York: Clarkson Potter, 2018.

Esquivel, Laura. *Like Water for Chocolate*. New York: Doubleday, 1992.

Estés, Clarissa Pinkola. *Women Who Run with the Wolves*. New York: Ballantine Books, 1992.

Ferguson, Sheila. *Soul Food: Classic Cuisine from the Deep South*. London and New York: Weidenfeld & Nicolson, 1989.

Fernea, Elizabeth Warnock, editor. *Women and Family in the Middle East: New Voices of Change*. Austin, Tex.: University of Texas Press, 1985.

Ferrucci, Piero. *Inevitable Grace*. New York: Jeremy P. Tarcher/Putnam Books, 1990.

Field, Joanna (pen name of Marion Milner). *A Life of One's Own*. London: Chatto & Windus, 1936; Los Angeles: Jeremy P. Tarcher, 1981.

Fields, Rick, with Peggy Taylor, Rex Weyler, and Rich Ingrasci. *Chop Wood, Carry Water: A Guide to Finding Spiritual Fulfillment in Everyday Life*. New York: Jeremy P. Tarcher/Perigee/Putnam, 1984.

Fisher, M. F. K. *How to Cook a Wolf*. New York: Duell, Sloan and Pearce, 1942.

Fitzgerald, Sally, editor. *The Habit of Being: Letters of Flannery O'Connor*. New York: Farrar, Straus, and Giroux, 1979.

Foster, Patricia, editor. *Minding the Body: Women Writers on Body and Soul*. New York: Doubleday, 1994.

Fox, Emmet. *Power Through Constructive Thinking*. New York: HarperCollins, 1989.

Fox, Matthew. *The Reinvention of Work: A New Vision of Livelihood for Our Time*. New York: HarperCollins, 1994.

Fraser, Kennedy. *The Fashionable Mind*. Boston: David R. Godine, 1985.

Freeman, Eileen Elias. *Touched by Angels*. New York: Warner Books, 1993.

_____. *Angelic Healing: Working with Your Angels to Heal Your Life*. New York: Warner Books, 1994.

Gibson, Cynthia. *A Botanical Touch*. New York: Viking Studio Books, 1993.

Glasgow, Ellen. *Barren Ground*. New York: Doubleday Page & Co, 1925.

Glaspell, Susan. *The Visioning*. New York: Frederick A. Stokes, 1911.

Godden, Rumer. *A House with Four Rooms*. New York: William Morrow and Company, Inc., 1989.

Goldberg, Natalie. *Writing Down the Bones: Freeing the Writer Within*. Boston: Shambhala, 1986.

_____. *Wild Mind: Living the Writer's Life*. New York: Bantam, 1990.

Graham, Abbie. *Ceremonials of Common Days*. New York: Womans Press, 1923.

Graham, Ysenda Maxtone. *The Real Mrs. Miniver: Jan Struther's Story*. London: John Murray, 2001.

Guest, Edgar A. *Collected Verse of Edgar A. Guest*. Chicago: Reilly & Lee Co., 1934.

Hampton, Mark. *Mark Hampton on Decorating.* New York: Condé Nast Books/Random House, 1989.

Hancock, Emily. *The Girl Within.* New York: Fawcett Columbine, 1989.

_____. "Growing Up Female." *New Woman,* May 1993.

Hanh, Thich Nhat. *The Miracle of Mindfulness: A Manual on Meditation.* Boston: Beacon Press, 1987.

Harrison, Kathy, and Alison Kolesar. *Just in Case: How to Be Self-Sufficient When the Unexpected Happens.* North Adams, Mass.: Storey Publishing, 2008.

Hepner, Harry. *The Best Things in Life.* New York: B. C. Forbes & Sons, 1953.

Hersey, Jean. *The Shape of the Year.* New York: Charles Scribner's Sons, 1967.

Hine, Megan. *Mind of a Survivor: What the Wild Has Taught Me About Survival and Success.* London: Coronet Publishing, 2017.

Holland, Barbara. *Endangered Pleasures.* Boston: Little, Brown and Company, 1995.

Holmes, Marjorie. *I've Got to Talk to Somebody, God.* New York: Doubleday, 1968.

Holt, Geraldene. *The Gourmet Garden.* Boston: Bullfinch Press Books/Little, Brown, 1990.

Huxley, Judith. *Table for Eight.* New York: William Morrow and Company, 1984.

Hyatt, Carole, and Linda Gottlieb. *When Smart People Fail: Rebuilding Yourself for Success.* New York: Penguin Books, 1988.

Irion, Mary Jean. *Yes, World: A Mosaic of Meditation.* New York: R. W. Baron, 1970.

James, William. *The Principles of Psychology.* New York: Henry Holt & Co., 1890; Cambridge, Mass.: Harvard University Press, 1983.

Johnson, Samuel. *Samuel Johnson/Oxford Authors.* Oxford/New York: Oxford University Press, 1984.

Johnston, Mireille. *The French Family Feast.* New York: Simon & Schuster, 1988.

Keane, Molly. *Molly Keane's Nursery Cooking.* London: Macdonald, 1985.

Kelly, Marcia, and Jack Kelly. *One Hundred Graces.* New York: Bell Tower, 1992.

Kondo, Marie. *The Life-Changing Magic of Tidying Up.* New York: Ten Speed Press, 2014.

Kornfield, Jack. *A Path with Heart: A Guide Through the Perils and Promises of Spiritual Life.* New York: Bantam, 1993.

Kosinski, Jerzy. *Being There.* New York: Harcourt Brace Jovanovich, 1971.

Kripke, Pamela. "Create Your Own Decorator's Notebook." *Mary Emmerling's Country,* August 1993.

Kron, Joan. *Home-Psych: The Social Psychology of Home and Decoration.* New York: Clarkson Potter, 1983.

Kushner, Harold. *Who Needs God?* New York: Summit Books, 1989.

_____. *To Life! A Celebration of Jewish Being and Thinking.* New York: Warner Books, 1993.

Lamott, Anne. *Bird by Bird: Some Instructions on Writing and Life.* New York and San Francisco: Pantheon Books, 1994.

Lange, Dorothea. "The Assignment I'll Never Forget: Migrant Mother." *Popular Photography,* February, 1960.

Lawlor, Anthony. *A Home for the Soul: A Guide for Dwelling with Spirit and Imagination*. New York: Clarkson Potter, 1997.

Lawrence, Brother. *Practicing the Presence of God*. Wheaton, Ill.: Harold Shaw, 1991.

L'Engle, Madeleine. *A Circle of Quiet*. New York: Farrar, Straus and Giroux, 1972.

_____. *The Irrational Season*. New York: The Seabury Press, 1979.

_____. *Walking on Water: Reflections on Faith and Art*. Wheaton, Ill.: Harold Shaw, 1980.

Lewis, C. S. *Miracles*. New York: Macmillan, 1947.

Lindbergh, Anne Morrow. *Gift from the Sea*. New York: Pantheon Books, 1955.

Markham, Beryl. *West with the Night*. Boston: Houghton Mifflin Company, 1942.

Martin, Tovah. *The Essence of Paradise: Fragrant Plants for Indoor Gardens*. Boston: Little, Brown, 1991.

Matthews, Caitlin. *Celtic Devotional: Daily Prayers and Blessings*. New York: Harmony Books, 1996.

May, Rollo. *The Courage to Create*. New York: W. W. Norton, 1975.

McCall, Anne Bryan. *The Larger Vision*. New York: Dodd, Mead & Company, 1919.

McDonald, Carla, and Kristen O'Brien on Madame Sophie Swetchine. www.salonniere.com.

McGinley, Phyllis. *Sixpence in Her Shoe*. New York. Dell Publishing, 1964.

_____. *Saint-Watching*. New York: Viking, 1969.

McManus, Erwin Raphael. *The Artisan Soul: Crafting Your Life into a Work of Art*. New York: HarperOne, 2014.

Mendelson, Cheryl. *Home Comforts: The Art and Science of Keeping Home*. New York: Scribner, 1999.

Merker, Hannah. *Listening*. New York: HarperCollins, 1994.

Miller, Ronald S., and the Editors of *New Age Journal*. *As Above, So Below: Paths to Spiritual Renewal in Daily Life*. Los Angeles: Jeremy P. Tarcher, 1992.

Mitchell, Stephen. *Tao Te Ching, A New English Version*. New York: Harper & Row, 1988.

Moore, Thomas. *Care of the Soul: A Guide for Cultivating Depth and Sacredness in Everyday Life*. New York: HarperCollins, 1992.

_____. *Soul Mates: Honoring the Mysteries of Love and Relationship*. New York: HarperCollins, 1994.

Morris, Mary. "Hello, This Is Your Destiny." *New Woman*, February 1993.

Moss, Charlotte. *A Passion for Detail*. New York: Doubleday, 1991.

Murphy, Joseph. *The Power of Your Subconscious Mind*. New York: Bantam Books, 1982.

Nicholson, Phyllis. *Norney Rough*. London: John Murray, 1941.

_____. *Country Matters*. London: John Murray, 1947.

Norris, Gunilla. *Being Home*. New York: Bell Tower, 1991.

Nouwen, Henri J. M. *Life of the Beloved: Spirituality Lessons in a Secular World*. Anniversary edition. New York: New York: Crossroad Publishing. 2002.

O'Connor, Elizabeth. *Eighth Day of Creation: Gifts and Creativity*. Waco, Tex.: Word Books, 1971.

O'Donohue, John. *Anam Cara: A Book of Celtic Wisdom*. New York: HarperCollins, 1998.

_____. *To Bless the Space Between Us: A Book of Blessings*. New York: Doubleday, 2008.

Ohrbach, Barbara Milo. *The Scented Room*. New York: Clarkson Potter, 1986.

Olsen, Tillie. *Silences*. New York: Seymour Lawrence/Delacorte Press, 1978.

_____. *Tell Me a Riddle*. New York: Seymour Lawrence/Delacorte Press, 1979.

Palmer, Derek. *The Dream of Perpetual Motion*. New York: St. Martin's Press, 2011.

Pascale, Richard Tanner. "Zen and the Art of Management." *Harvard Business Review*, March/April 1978.

Peck, M. Scott. *The Road Less Traveled*. New York: Simon & Schuster, 1978.

_____. *Further Along the Road Less Traveled*. New York: Simon & Schuster, 1993.

Perenyi, Eleanor. *Green Thoughts: A Writer in the Garden*. New York: Vintage Books, 1983.

Phipps, Diana. *Affordable Splendor*. New York: Random House, 1981.

Ponder, Catherine. *The Prosperity Secrets of the Ages*. Marina del Rey, Calif.: DeVorss & Company, 1954.

_____. *Open Your Mind to Prosperity*. Marina del Rey, Calif.: DeVorss & Company, 1971.

Porter, Eleanor Hodgman. *Pollyanna*. Boston: The Page Company, 1913.

Post, Emily. *The Personality of a House*. New York and London: Funk & Wagnalls, 1948.

Priestly, J. B. *Delight*. London: Heinemann, 1949.

Radner, Gilda. *It's Always Something*. New York: Simon & Schuster, 1989.

Raynolds, Robert. *In Praise of Gratitude: An Invitation to Trust Life*. New York: Harper & Brothers, 1961.

Redfield, James. *The Celestine Prophecy*. New York: Warner Books, 1993.

Rilke, Rainer Maria. *Letters to a Young Poet*. New York: W. W. Norton, 1934.

Ripperger, Henrietta. *A Home of Your Own and How to Run It*. New York: Simon & Schuster, 1940.

Robbins, John, and Ann Mortifee. *In Search of Balance*. Tiburn, Calif.: H. J. Kramer, Inc., 1991.

Robyn, Kathyrn L. *Spiritual Housekeeping: Healing the Space Within by Beautifying the Space Around You*. Oakland, Calif.: New Harbinger Publications, 2001.

Roesch, Diana K. "Body Language." *Lear's*, February, 1994.

Sacks, Oliver. *Awakenings*. New York: Summit Books, 1987.

Sangster, Margaret E. *Ideal Home Life*. New York: The University Society, Inc., 1910.

Sarton, May. *Plant Dreaming Deep*. New York: W. W. Norton, 1968.

_____. *Journal of a Solitude*. New York: W. W. Norton, 1973.

Schaef, Anne Wilson. *Meditations for Women Who Do Too Much*. San Francisco: HarperCollins, 1990.

_____. *Meditations for Living in Balance*. San Francisco: HarperCollins, 2000.

Seal, Mark. "Laura Esquivel's Healing Journey." *New Age Journal*, May/June 1994.

Seuss, Dr. *Oh, the Places You'll Go!* New York: Random House, 1990.

Shain, Merle. *Hearts That We Broke Long Ago*. New York: Bantam, 1983.

_____. *Courage My Love: A Book to Light an Honest Path*. New York: Bantam, 1989.

Sheehy, Gail. *Pathfinders*. New York: William Morrow, 1981.

_____. "The Flaming Fifties." *Vanity Fair*, October 1993.

_____. *New Passages: Mapping Your Life Across Time*. New York: Random House, 1995.

Shi, David E. *In Search of the Simple Life*. Layton, Utah: Peregrine Smith/ Gibbs M. Smith, Inc., 1986.

Shinn, Florence Scovel. *The Wisdom of Florence Scovel Shinn*. (Includes four complete books: *The Game of Life and How to Play It*; *The Power of the Spoken Word*; *Your Word Is Your Wand*; *The Secret of Success*.) New York: Fireside/Simon & Schuster, 1989.

Siegel, Alan B. *Dreams That Can Change Your Life*. Los Angeles: Jeremy P. Tarcher, 1990.

Sinetar, Marsha. *Do What You Love and the Money Will Follow*. New York/ Mahwah: Paulist Press, 1987.

_____. *Reel Time: Spiritual Growth Through Film*. Ligouri, Missouri: Triumph Books, 1993.

Starhawk. *The Spiral Dance*. New York: Harper & Row, 1979.

Steindl-Rast, Brother David. *Gratefulness, the Heart of Prayer: An Approach to Life in Fullness*. New York/Ramsey, New Jersey: Paulist Press, 1984.

Steinem, Gloria. *Revolution from Within: A Book of Self-Esteem*. Boston: Little, Brown and Company, 1992.

Stern, Jane and Michael. *Square Meals*. New York: Alfred A. Knopf, Inc., 1984.

Stern, Janet, editor. *The Writer on Her Work*. New York: W. W. Norton, 1980.

Stevens, Wallace. *The Collected Poems of Wallace Stevens*. New York: Alfred A. Knopf, 1954, 1982.

Stoddard, Alexandra. *Daring to Be Yourself*. New York: Doubleday, 1990.

_____. *Creating a Beautiful Home*. New York: William Morrow, 1992.

Struther, Jan. *Try Anything Twice*. New York: Harcourt, Brace and Company, 1938.

_____. *Mrs. Miniver*. New York: Harcourt, Brace and Company. 1940.

Sullivan, Rosemary. *Labyrinth of Desire: Women, Passion and Romantic Obsession*. Washington, D.C.: Counterpoint, 2001.

Taylor, Terry Lynn. *Messengers of Light: The Angels' Guide to Spiritual Growth*. Tiburon, Calif.: H. J. Kramer, Inc., 1990.

_____. *Guardians of Hope: The Angels' Guide to Personal Growth*. Tiburon, Calif.: H. J. Kramer, Inc., 1992.

_____. *Creating with the Angels*. Tiburon, Calif.: H. J. Kramer. Inc., 1993.

Terkel, Studs. *Working: People Talk about What They Do All Day and How They Feel about What They Do*. New York: Pantheon Books, 1974.

Thoreau, Henry David. *Walden and Other Writings of Henry David Thoreau*. New York: Modern Library, 1992.

Thurman, Judith. *Isak Dinesen: The Life of a Storyteller*. New York: St. Martin's Press, 1982.

_____. "A Boudoir of One's Own." *Victoria*, August 1992.

Tisserand, Robert B. *The Art of Aromatherapy*. New York: Inner Traditions International, 1977.

Uchida, Yoshiko. *A Jar of Dreams*. New York: Atheneum, 1981.

Underhill, Evelyn. *Mysticism*. New York: World Publishing, 1955.

Wasserstein, Wendy. *Uncommon Women and Others*. New York: Dramatists' Play Service, 1987.

_____. "The Me I'd Like to Be." *New Woman*, December 1994.

Watts, Alan W. *The Way of Zen*. New York: Random House, 1965.

White, Katharine S. *Onward and Upward in the Garden*. Edited by E. B. White. New York: Farrar, Straus and Giroux, 1979.

Wickham, Cynthia. *House Plants through the Year*. London: William Collins Sons & Co. Ltd., 1985.

Williams, Margery. *The Velveteen Rabbit, or How Toys Become Real*. Garden City, New York: Doubleday, 1960.

Williamson, Marianne. *A Return to Love: Reflections on the Principles of a Course in Miracles*. New York: HarperCollins, 1992.

_____. *A Woman's Worth*. New York: Random House, 1993.

Winfrey, Oprah. *The Wisdom of Sundays: Life Changing Insights from Super Soul Conversations*. New York: Flatiron Books, 2017.

_____. *The Path Made Clear: Discovering Your Life's Direction and Purpose*. New York: Flatiron Books, 2019.

Witty, Helen. *Fancy Pantry*. New York: Workman Publishing, 1986.

Wolfe, Thomas. *Look Homeward, Angel*. New York: Charles Scribner, 1957.

Wolfman, Peri, and Charles Gold. *The Perfect Setting*. New York: Harry N. Abrams, Inc., 1985.

Woolf, Virginia. *A Room of One's Own*. New York: Harcourt Brace Jovanovich, 1929.

Yancey, Phillip. "Reading Wars," www.philipyancey.com, July 20, 2017.